Advances in Medicine and Health Science

Advances in Medicine and Health Science

Edited by Anna Garner

hayle
medical

New York

Hayle Medical,
750 Third Avenue, 9th Floor,
New York, NY 10017, USA

Visit us on the World Wide Web at:
www.haylemedical.com

ISBN: 978-1-63241-797-8

Cataloging-in-Publication Data

Advances in medicine and health science / edited by Anna Garner.
    p. cm.
Includes bibliographical references and index.
ISBN 978-1-63241-797-8
1. Medicine. 2. Medical sciences. 3. Health. 4. Diseases. 5. Physiology.
6. Medical innovations. I. Garner, Anna.
R130 .A38 2019
610--dc23

Table of Contents

Permissions

List of Contributors

Index

Preface

Medicine is a broad field comprising of the science and practice of the study, diagnosis, treatment and prevention of disease. Modern medicine encompasses the application of genetics, biomedical sciences and technology, therapies, biologics, medical devices, etc. In current clinical practice, the first step is an examination of the patient's medical history, medical interview and physical examination. This is followed by medical diagnostic tests. Various medical imaging technologies such as PET scan, MRI, CT scan, ultrasound, microscopy, etc. are part of medical diagnostics. The medical decision-making process is characterized by an analysis of all pertinent information for obtaining a differential diagnosis and designing a strategy for the management of the condition. Medical specialties can be categorized as diagnostic or therapeutic, surgical or internal medicine, organ-based or technique-based, etc. Some of the common medical specialties are allergy and immunology, pathology, cardiology, dermatology, emergency medicine, gastroenterology, geriatrics, nephrology, etc. The aim of this book is to present researches that have transformed the field of health care and aided its advancement. Different approaches, evaluations, methodologies and advanced studies on medicine and health science have been included in this book. It includes contributions of experts and scientists, which will provide innovative insights into this field.

The researches compiled throughout the book are authentic and of high quality, combining several disciplines and from very diverse regions from around the world. Drawing on the contributions of many researchers from diverse countries, the book's objective is to provide the readers with the latest achievements in the area of research. This book will surely be a source of knowledge to all interested and researching the field.

In the end, I would like to express my deep sense of gratitude to all the authors for meeting the set deadlines in completing and submitting their research chapters. I would also like to thank the publisher for the support offered to us throughout the course of the book. Finally, I extend my sincere thanks to my family for being a constant source of inspiration and encouragement.

Editor

Healthcare service delivery to refugee children from the Democratic Republic of Congo living in Durban, South Africa: a caregivers' perspective

Anna Meyer-Weitz[1], Kwaku Oppong Asante[1,2]* and Bukenge J. Lukobeka[1]

Abstract

Background: Refugees are generally considered a vulnerable population, with refugee children (newborn and young children) being particularly so. Access to healthcare for this population remains a challenge. The main purpose of this study was to explore refugee caregivers' perceptions of their children's access to quality health service delivery to their young children in Durban, South Africa.

Methods: This study used an explanatory mixed methods design, purposively sampling 120 and 10 participants for the quantitative and qualitative phases, respectively. Participants were administered a self-developed questionnaire that assessed demographic information of participants, socioeconomic status and living standard, medical history of children, satisfaction and experiences with healthcare services and refugees' networks and social support. A semi-structured interview schedule was developed to elicit in-depth and more detailed information from the participants on the quantitative areas that were investigated. Frequencies were calculated and a χ^2 test was used to explore the factors associated with refugees' satisfaction of the healthcare provided and thematic analysis was used to analyse the qualitative data.

Results: The majority (89%) of caregivers were women, with over 70% of them aged between 30 and 35 years. Over 74% of caregivers visited public clinics for their children's healthcare needs. The majority of caregivers (95%) were not satisfied with healthcare services delivery to their children due to the long waiting hours and the negative attitudes and discriminatory behaviours of healthcare workers, particularly in public healthcare facilities.

Conclusion: These findings underscore the need to address health professionals' attitudes when providing healthcare for refugees. Attitudinal change may improve the relationship between service providers and caregivers of refugee children in South Africa, which may improve the health-related outcomes in refugee children.

Keywords: Refugee children, Healthcare services, Accessibility, South Africa, Democratic Republic of Congo

Background

Globally, mass movement of people often occurs as a result of political and economic instability, poverty and armed conflict [1]. These critical conditions push people out of their home countries in search of what they believe to be a better place to live [1]. The mass relocation of people can lead to major challenges to public resources during their movement and in the various countries of destination. African countries that agree to receive refugees are faced with challenges to address the needs of their own people as well as those of refugee populations entering their countries [2].

Refugees are generally considered a vulnerable population, with refugee children (newborn and young children) being particularly so [1, 3]. Infants and young children are often the first and most frequent victims of violence, infectious diseases and malnutrition, all of

* Correspondence: kwappong@gmail.com
[1]Discipline of Psychology, University of KwaZulu-Natal, Durban, South Africa
[2]Department of Psychology, University of Ghana, P. O. Box LG 84, Legon, Accra, Ghana

which frequently accompany displaced populations and refugee movements [3, 4]. These children face far greater dangers to their safety and well-being than the average child as a result of the sudden and violent onset of emergencies and related uncertainties [3, 5]. Despite a reduction in early child mortality due to improved child survival interventions such as immunisation, nutrition control and treatment of childhood diseases [5], the improvement in child mortality remains a challenge in developing countries accounting for 41% of under-five deaths [6].

The complex interactions between refugee status and health shows that such a status may have either adverse or positive impacts on health and well-being [5, 6]. A compromised health status and access to adequate healthcare are two major areas of vulnerability that refugees face. Maintaining good health among refugees is a challenge, not only because of the health risks commonly associated with the movement of people, but also because of the economic hardships that refugees face and the undesirable conditions in which many refugees live [7]. It is therefore critical for refugee children to access the host country's local primary healthcare services [7].

Previous studies have highlighted several factors that adversely influence access to healthcare by refugees. Lack of knowledge about refugees' rights, low socioeconomic status, language barriers and poor understanding of a host country's healthcare system are factors found to influence access to healthcare for migrants living in South Africa [8–10]. The attitudes of healthcare workers towards migrants and refugees can be linked to their understanding of refugee status and their accompanied legal rights, including eligibility to free, accessible and quality healthcare services as delivered to South African citizens (referred to above); their own levels of work satisfaction, where greater levels of satisfaction are expected to translate into better healthcare delivery [11]; and personal prejudice in the form of xenophobia, evident in recent expressions of violent attacks on foreign nationals, looting of businesses and homes, as well as verbal abuse, all which received wide media coverage and caused public outrage [12]. Medical xenophobia in South Africa has also been reported [10, 13, 14].

Despite the abovementioned studies, there is a dearth of research regarding refugee children's healthcare access. The main purpose of this study is to understand caregivers' perceptions of the healthcare needs of refugee children (10 years and younger) as well as their perceived access to primary healthcare, including their satisfaction with healthcare services for their children. The study focuses on the caregivers of refugees from the Democratic Republic of Congo (DRC) by using an explanatory mixed methods design. The findings of this study will help to formulate policies to improve service delivery to refugee children as well as to address the key health challenges faced by parents and caregivers of refugee children.

Theoretical frameworks

The health access model and the household resources model were used as conceptual frameworks to explain the factors that affect access to healthcare for refugee children [15, 16]. The health access model by Peters et al. [15] addresses the compromised health service access of people in poor countries and contexts. It is argued that, while a lack of financial resources creates barriers to accessing healthcare, the complexities of environmental aspects in combination with individual and household characteristics denote poverty, which impacts on other factors that may inhibit access. The cycle of poverty is viewed to impact health and well-being, which in turn maintains ill health and access to healthcare. Quality of care is central to healthcare access, which in turn is determined by geographical accessibility, availability of services, financial accessibility and acceptability of services. The policy and macro environment, in combination with individual and household characteristics, determine health status but also impact healthcare access. Due to the relatively low level of socioeconomic status and available household resources [17], the health status and general well-being of migrants and refugees are compromised. In applying this model to the study, it is expected that access to healthcare will not only be influenced by the financial and geographical location but also by users' attitudes, beliefs, expectations and characteristics of the health facilities.

The household resource model [16] explains accessibility to healthcare services in terms of material resources, investment potential and social resources. These authors argue that material resources, investment potential and social resources are important key resources that facilitate access to better healthcare. With inadequate material and investment resources, it is expected that social networks among refugees will play an important role in their access to healthcare. A strong social network may, for example, assist in the decisions to seek refuge in a particular country and obtain information, including healthcare related, social support and even employment in the new host country [18]. In this study, we expect that social networks in the form of interpersonal ties of kinship, friendship and shared community origins, which have been found to connect refugees, former refugees and non-refugees in countries of origin in the new host country [2, 19], will help in the facilitation of better healthcare for refugee children.

Methods

Research design and setting

This study used an explanatory mixed methods design in which the quantitative cross-sectional survey was followed by a small qualitative study. These methods were chosen because it allowed the researchers an opportunity to understand different aspects of the quantitative data in more detail [20]. As the study quantitatively investigated refugee parents' or caregivers' perceptions of their children's health status, the experiences in seeking healthcare as well as accessibility and satisfaction with health service delivery are explored qualitatively. The added value of the qualitative component was to gain a deeper understanding of the caregivers' perceptions and experiences. The study was conducted in Durban, KwaZulu-Natal province of South Africa. The province of KwaZulu-Natal has the second largest populace of the country, with 10.5 million people, approximately 19.8% of the country's population [21], and is known to host a great number of refugees from the DRC [22, 23].

Sampling and participants

A non-probability purposive sampling in combination with snowball sampling was used to recruit participants in this study as it allowed the researchers to select participants able to provide rich information about the phenomenon being studied [24]. This sampling strategy was used to select the research participants who are parents and/or caregivers of refugee children (aged 0 to 10 years), from the DRC, living in Durban, KwaZulu-Natal. Within the community of refugees from the DRC, the different networks that exist were used to gain access to the parents/caregivers before approaching them to seek their participation in the study. Participants were included in the study if they met the inclusion criteria, namely being a DRC refugee living in Durban, aged 18 years and over, had a child or taking care of other children, and willing to take part in the study. Based on the inclusion criteria, 120 parents or caregivers of young children (< 1 to 10 years of age) were recruited for the quantitative phase of the study. Ten of the participants from the quantitative study were purposively selected to provide further information on different aspects explored in the qualitative phase. Principles of data saturation were applied and no additional data was obtained after approximately 10 interviews [25].

Measures

A structured questionnaire was developed by the researchers based on a good understanding of the literature, the theoretical framework, and the aims and objectives of the study. The questionnaire consisted of five main sections, namely demographic information of participants, socioeconomic status and living standard,

medical history of children, satisfaction and experiences with healthcare services, and refugees' networks and social support. The demographic information included age, sex, level of education, religious affiliation, marital status, English language proficiency and number of children had by caregivers. The socioeconomic statuses of participants focused on employment status and living standard of caregivers of refugee children. Some of the questions asked were 'Are you currently employed?', 'How many people are you supporting in your household?', 'How many people are you sharing your accommodation with?' The third section on medical history of children asked questions that assessed the health status of both the caregivers and the children. Some of the questions asked included 'Has your child been immunised?' and 'Where was your child immunised?' The response format for these questions was in the form of 'Yes' or 'No'. Participants were also asked the type of vaccination children received and at what age this was done. Questions on accessibility, experiences and satisfaction with the healthcare services focused on caregivers' general satisfaction with the healthcare services, healthcare consultation process, and their perceptions and experiences with private and public healthcare services. Examples of some of the questions asked included 'On a scale of 0–10, rate your satisfaction with the healthcare service your children received from the private medical doctor, local clinic, a faith healer, local herbalist and the traditional healer', 'Were you able to ask all the questions you wanted to when you last visited a public clinic/hospital?' and 'Did the attending nurse spend enough time with you?' The final section of the questionnaire, which focused on refugee networks and social support, elicited information about the availability of support from other refugees living in Durban. Some of the questions asked were 'Have you received any help from your refugee community?' and 'How often do you meet with your family members?' Questions about sources of information about healthcare, such as friends, family members and other individuals from church, were also asked.

For the qualitative study, a semi-structured interview schedule was developed in English, translated into French and translated back into English, based on the key research areas of the quantitative research instrument. Open-ended questions were developed in this regard to elicit in-depth and more detailed information from the participants on the quantitative areas that were investigated. Some of the questions asked were 'What are the kinds of illnesses that your children suffer from for which you sought medical treatment?', 'How did the healthcare workers make you feel when you visited the clinics?', 'Why did you choose the private doctor?', and 'What were your experiences with the clinic services?' Additional file 1 provides a full description of the questionnaire.

Data collection and procedures

Before data collection commenced, ethical approval to conduct the study was obtained from the Ethics Committee of the University of KwaZulu-Natal, Durban, South Africa (Reference: HSS/0123/013 M). Caregivers were approached to participate by explaining the aims and objectives of the study in a language they understood, in most instances French and Swahili. Those who agreed to participate in the study were given a written informed consent to sign after being informed that their participation was voluntary and that confidentiality and anonymity would be maintained. The anonymity of the participants was guaranteed through the use of pseudonyms, and they were assured of their rights to withdraw from the study at any point in time without any negative consequences to them. Permission was also gained to audio tape the qualitative interviews. An interview was scheduled with the participants at a place and time most convenient to them. The administering of the questionnaire took an average of 35 minutes, while the qualitative interviews took approximately 45 to 60 minutes. Data collection lasted for 3 months. Qualitative data collection lasted for a further 4 weeks.

Data analysis

The Statistics Package for Social Sciences (SPSS) version 23 was used to analyse the quantitative data. The data was first entered into Microsoft Excel before later being imported into SPSS. Frequencies and descriptive statistics were conducted to describe the sample and on all the items guided by the objectives of the study. χ^2 tests were used to explore relationships among categorical variables, namely (1) the relationship between demographic variables (level of education, sex and age), satisfaction of healthcare provided and socioeconomic status of caregivers, (2) the relationship between demographic variables (level of education, sex and age), the different resources adopted in the research framework (i.e. Material Resources, Investment Potential and Social Resources), as well as social networks of refugee caregivers. The Mann–Whitney U test was used to test for differences between two independent groups, i.e. demographic data in relationship with satisfaction with healthcare services at both public and private facilities. It was also used to evaluate differences regarding caregivers' experiences with the healthcare system.

All the qualitative interviews were transcribed verbatim, and thematic analysis was used to analyse the data using the guidelines of Braun and Clark [26]. The first step in analysing the data for this study involved familiarising and immersing oneself in the data to identify the common themes. In the second step, themes that shared the same words, styles and terms used by participants and the ways in which they were connected, were identified. This was followed by coding of the themes and sub-themes linked to the broad objectives of the study. The last step in the process involved the interpretation of the data and cross checking.

Results

Sociodemographic characteristics of participants

The demographic characteristics of the participants are presented in Table 1; 89% of the participants were females and approximately 61% of the respondents were aged 30–35 years. The majority of the participants (80.0%) were married, and 90% were actual caregivers of their own children. Approximately 71% of the respondents in the study had senior secondary education, 90% were Christians and over 70% of the participants had three children. Overall, 46.7% of the participants in the study were not able to communicate in English (i.e. could not speak, understand or write in English), while 27.5% reported than they could understand but cannot speak English, and 25.8% revealed that they could speak and write in English. The majority of the participants (86.7%) were asylum seekers (i.e. not classified as refugees by the United Nations High Commissioner for Refugees (UNHCR)), while 13.3% were officially refugees. Approximately half of the refugee caregivers decided to relocate to Durban as they already had relatives living there. A substantial group (38.5%) indicated that, because they had hentered South Africa through Mozambique, they felt safe and decided to stay in Durban.

Socioeconomic and social support of participants

Information on the socioeconomic conditions, household resources and available social capital is presented in Table 2. With regards to the economic challenges refugees face, the majority of the participants (66.7%) reported that they did not have enough money for basic things like food and clothes, with only 0.8% of the respondents indicating that they had money to afford more expensive items such as a TV, radios, etc., but not enough money to buy any expensive commodities. Participants who reported having enough money for food and clothes were also more likely to report having a post-school qualification ($\chi^2 = 4.406$, $df = 1$; Fisher's exact test $p = 0.42$). Interestingly, further analysis did not reveal any significant difference between those who had money for basic food and clothes and those that had enough only for the basics and their English language proficiency ($\chi^2 = 1.070$, $df = 2$; Fisher's exact test $p = 0.589$). When participants were asked about their source of income, the majority of respondents (96.7%)

Table 1 Sociodemographic information of the participants (N = 120)

Characteristics	Number	%
Sex		
Male	13	10.8
Female	107	89.2
Age groups		
23–29 years	21	17.5
30–35 years	73	60.8
36–40 years	14	11.7
> 40 years	12	10.0
Marital status		
Married	96	80.0
Separated	17	14.2
Divorced	6	5.0
Widower	1	0.8
Relationship with child		
Mothers	108	90.0
Fathers	12	10.0
Number of children		
3 children	85	70.8
4–5 children	28	23.3
6–7 children	7	5.9
Caregivers' level of education		
Primary school (Grade 1–6)	5	4.2
Junior secondary school (Grade 7–9)	22	18.3
Senior certificate (Grade 12)	85	70.8
Tertiary	8	6.7
Religious affiliation		
Christian	108	90.0
Muslim	12	10.0
English language proficiency		
Write and speak English	31	25.8
Understand but cannot speak	33	27.5
Neither speak, understand nor write	56	46.7
Reasons for relocating to Durban		
Had relatives living in Durban	61	50.8
Came through Mozambique and stayed	46	38.4
Job opportunities	7	5.8
Clean city	3	2.5
Feel secure in Durban	3	2.5

Table 2 Frequencies of items regarding household resources and social capital

Items linked to household resources	N	Yes %	No %
Material resource items			
Working full time	120	3.3	96.7
Work part time	120	12.5	87.5
Sell some of my possessions to get money	120	5.8	94.2
Have enough money for basics like food and clothes	120	33.3	66.7
Social Resource items			
Getting financial help from family/friends in South Africa	120	85	15
Getting financial help from church/pastor	120	75.8	24.2
Getting money from family/friends in the Democratic Republic of Congo	120	0	100
Investment potential resources			
Trading	119	88.2	11.8
Have many unused skills	111	100	0.0
Using skills to provide services to refugee community	120	53.3	46.7
Social capital items (bridging)			
Know people who can help	120	97.5	2.5
Know people who are well connected with others	120	100	0.0
Know people who are willing to help when there is a need	119	72.3	27.7
Give assistance to other refugees	120	70.8	29.2
Received assistance from my community	120	64.2	35.8
Social capital items (linking)		N	%
Have contacted UNHCR			
Yes		9	07.5
No		111	92.5
If Yes, reason for the visit (n = 9)			
Social support		3	33.3
Refugee documentation		4	44.4
Information to relocate back home		2	22.2
Ever visited an office of an NGO working with refugees			
Yes		93	77.5
No		27	22.5
Received help from NGOs			
Received no assistance		48	51.6
Paid rent for few months		19	20.4
Received food vouchers when first arrived in South Africa		17	18.3
Paid school fees		9	9.7

reported that they were not fully employed. Most (85%) relied on family members/friends and 75.8% received help from their church (pastors). Additionally, 53.3% of the participants indicated that they relied on their own skills to receive an income by providing services needed by the refugee community.

With regards to household resources, 26%, 42.2% and 58.2% of the respondents had some material resources, social resources and investment potential, respectively. As reported in Table 2, the majority of respondents also relied on social networks for help; 97% of the participants knew someone who could help, 72.2% were aware of people willing to help whenever there is a need, and all participants were aware of people who are well connected with others. Only few ($N = 9$; 7.5%) participants had visited the UNHCR for support. The key issues that they sought help from the UNHCR for included social support ($N = 3$; 33.3%), refugee documentation ($N = 4$; 44.3%) and advice on the relocation back to their country of origin ($N = 2$; 22.2%). The results also showed that refugees received help from non-governmental organisations. However, 51.6% indicated that they never received any assistance, while those who received assistance were supported to pay rent (20.4%) and some indicated that they were given food vouchers when they first arrived in South Africa (18.3%). The remaining 9.7% reported receiving help with regards to the payment of school fees.

The qualitative findings highlighted the inconsistency in support rendered to the refugee community and the limited support they actually receive. Additionally, these refugees feel discriminated against, as shown by a narrative of a female caregiver:

"With regards to the Refugee Social Services, I can say it does not help. This is because the services that they provide to us are based on some kind of partiality, just like the nurses do at the clinics. If you do not have a friend who is working in their offices, you will not get help. However, I have heard from some of my friends that they received help from them, where they paid 2 months' rent for them and also gave them food" (Female, participant 3).

Healthcare seeking for children
The responses of caregivers regarding healthcare seeking for children are shown in Table 3. In general, the majority of the participants (74.2%) indicated that they primarily seek healthcare from the public healthcare clinics (which are generally free of charge), while the very few (2.5%) who use private medical practitioners indicated that they prefer them primarily because of the higher quality of healthcare received from them. The majority (52%) of the participants also indicated that they usually prefer seeking healthcare from private doctors who are Congolese. There were delays in seeking formal healthcare by the caregivers as 57.5% waited longer than 4 days before they sought help. Key reasons attributed to this delay were their inability to communicate in English and IsiZulu (62.3%) and the negative attitudes of healthcare workers towards refugees (30.4%). Over 65.0% used public transport as means of travel to the various healthcare

Table 3 Healthcare seeking behaviours description

Healthcare seeking items	N	%
Healthcare facilities normally visited for ill health ($N = 120$)		
Public clinic	89	74.2
Public hospital	28	23.3
Private doctor	3	2.5
Actions taken after unsuccessful treatment at public facilities ($N = 120$)		
Seek help from private hospital	74	61.7
Go to another clinic	26	21.6
Get medicine from the pharmacy	9	7.5
Prayer	11	9.2
Actions taken recently when child was ill ($N = 120$)		
Went to local clinic	97	80.8
Bought medicine at the pharmacy	10	8.4
Prayed to God	9	7.5
Ask friends/neighbours for advice	4	3.3
Normal waiting time before seeking medical care ($N = 120$)		
No delay – same day	14	11.7
After 1 day	23	19.2
After 2 to 3 days	14	11.7
4 days and longer	69	57.4
Reasons for the delay of 4 days and longer ($N = 69$)		
Unable to speak English or Zulu	43	62.3
Healthcare workers hold negative attitudes towards refugees	21	30.4
Do not have valid documentation to stay in South Africa	2	2.9
Other reasons	3	4.4
Information/advice received about health issues[a]		
Friends	53	44.2
Neighbours	78	65
People at church	47	39.2
Health clinic	120	100
Private doctors	62	51.7

[a]Multiple responses to the variable, therefore total percentage is more than 100

centres. For participants using public transport, the average transport ranges from 10 ZAR to 20 ZAR (US$ 0.73 to US$ 1.47), considered by most as expensive when not having enough money for food.

Satisfaction with healthcare service delivery
The caregivers were asked to rate their level of satisfaction with both public health clinics and private doctors over the last 6 months on a 10-point scale (0 = not satisfied at all, to 10 = highly satisfied). The results on the satisfaction of the healthcare service delivered to their

children showed that most of the caregivers were dissatisfied with the quality of healthcare rendered to their children, particularly when referring to public healthcare services. Very low ratings were noted for the public facilities; a rating of 0 was given by 11.7%, a rating of 1 by 45% and a rating of 2 by 43.3%. However, private doctors received ratings of 5 by 3.3%, a rating of 6 by 21.7%, a rating of 7 by 34.2% and a rating of 8 by 40.8%. It is clear that the response options on the rating scale for caregivers' satisfaction with public clinics were very restrictive and at the lower end of the rating scale, ranging from 0 to 10, showing mainly dissatisfaction with the clinic health services.

Further results showed that caregivers with a higher number of social networks were more satisfied with public healthcare delivery ($p = 0.025$) and the healthcare services by private doctors ($p = 0.003$).

Participants were asked to evaluate their level of satisfaction with the last health service consultation regarding their children at the public healthcare clinic and private doctor (Table 4). The results showed that caregivers generally had a more negative experience from their last visit to a public clinic when compared to service received from a private health facility or private general practitioner. With regards to the public clinic service,

most felt that they were not able to ask the questions they wanted to (93.1%; $n = 81$), that not enough information was provided to them (91.0%; $n = 81$), that the nurses did not spend enough time with their children (100%; $n = 89$), and that their views about the healthcare needs of their children were not respected (100%; $n = 89$).

The qualitative findings support the quantitative results in the sense that dissatisfaction with the public health sector was reiterated. However, greater clarity was given to understand the issues that are problematic. The findings suggested that the participants' dissatisfaction with healthcare services was due to a range of issues, including structural limitations as well as direct and indirect discriminatory tendencies towards refugees. With regard to structural impediments, the participants talked about the long waiting times before being attended to by healthcare workers:

"For my first time I was with my husband, it was terrible. We stood for more than four hours since 6am to 9am. The queue was so long. After 8am they gave us numbers. We were seen by the healthcare workers after being tired, the nurse who received my child was nice, He was so cool and polite, but the one who was taking measurements was different - she was not talking to me. On the appointment day for immunisation, we face hard times at the clinic. Some nurses don't treat foreigners like people who don't have a country. They talk to any way - they insult people and all their healthcare communication to us was done in IsiZulu. If you ask them questions, they don't respond to your questions, but they respond nicely when their people do same." (Female, participant 2)

"I have never been happy at the local clinic as there are many things that can make you angry. You have to be there all day from 6am until the end of the day, and at the end, they will give you just Panadol (a pain killer). Sometimes you spend all your time and you worry about what the family will eat." (Female, participant 4)

Furthermore, the qualitative findings revealed that nurses' negative attitudes in the public hospitals as compared to the good services provided by private medical practitioners compel them to use private hospitals rather than public.

"There is big difference between these two clinics [i.e. public and private]. At the private clinic, patients feel at home and they feel more comfortable, not only because we pay the money but the way healthcare workers treat you even before you receive any

Table 4 Frequencies of healthcare services experiences during the last child healthcare consultation

Experiences during last clinic visit	Yes N (%)	No N (%)
Public clinics ($N = 89$)		
Were you able to ask all the questions you wanted to?	6 (6.9)	81 (93.1)
Did the nurse provide you with enough information?	8 (9.0)	81 (91.0)
Did the nurse spend enough time with your child?	–	89 (100)
Will you recommend the clinic to others?	23 (25.8)	66 (74.2)
Did you have to wait too long before being attended to?	89 (100)	–
Did the nurse respect your views about your child's healthcare needs?	–	89 (100)
Private doctor ($N = 3$)		
Were you able to ask all the questions you wanted to?	2 (66.7)	1 (33.3)
Did the doctor provide you with enough information?	2 (66.7)	1 (33.3)
Did the doctor spend enough time with your child?	3 (100)	–
Will you recommend the doctor to others?	3 (100)	–
Did you have to wait too long before being attended to?	–	3 (100)
Did the doctor respect your views about your child's healthcare needs?	2 (100)	–

medication. *They welcome a patient so nicely and they take time asking you questions. Back home, in DRC, patients don't have to wait for a long period like they do in these local clinics. When you meet with a doctor he takes time and asks you all questions and he explains to you - something which is totally different from the local clinics where they don't give you time to ask what is wrong with you. In the private clinics, they would communicate with you in the nice manner. They show you love. They don't have a discriminatory attitude like at the public clinic where nurses tell you "rubbish". I am so disappointed with healthcare services at the public clinic."*
(Female, participant 8)

"When I was at home in DRC, I was talking to my friends here (those living in South Africa) about my child who used to suffer from renal problems. They told us in South Africa, healthcare services are high [excellent] but when I arrived here, my main focus was about my child. But for bad luck, my child died. Prior to that I took her to the clinic with the help of one of my friends, I felt abandoned by healthcare workers. I spent more than six hours at the clinic, and no nurse cared to talk to me. It was only after my friend had complained, that they took the temperature [of my child]. We waited again for another two hours before we were able to see the medical doctor. The doctor gave me an appointment to see him again in four days' time. Unfortunately, I lost my child before next appointment. Since then, I have not had any good thing to say about nurses at local clinics." (Female, participant 1)

Some of the participants also indicated that, notwithstanding the negative attitudes of nurses towards refugees in general, they prefer public clinics because of proximity and the fact that the service is free.

"I chose this clinic [public clinic] because the services are free of charge and the clinic is closer to where we live. But I don't like it due to many challenges we are facing at the local clinic. Nurses treat people like 'animals' at the clinic. If you meet the bad or not well-behaved nurse that day at the clinic, you feel like not coming back again - but there are other days when you meet with a good nurse. I cannot choose to go to the private doctor because I don't have money, especially for children whose healthcare services are very expensive. They are so expensive at the private clinics. I have been at the private clinics myself before, so I know how expensive it is - but the services are well organised and of good quality."
(Female, participant 5).

Discussion

The main purpose of this study was to explore refugee caregivers' perceptions of their children's access to healthcare services in South Africa. Our findings showed that the majority of caregivers were not satisfied with healthcare services delivery due to the long waiting hours and the negative attitudes and discriminatory behaviours of healthcare workers, particularly in the public healthcare facilities. The discussion of these key findings is guided by the health access and the household resource models.

Household resources and access to healthcare

The socioeconomic status among refugees is one of the key challenges they face, contributing to their health and well-being vulnerability [8, 27]. Caregivers in the study reported poor housing and living conditions, as well as a relatively low socioeconomic status. The link between poverty and ill health and mental distress is well established [28]. The socioeconomic status of refugees has been found to be one of the major barriers to accessing healthcare services and other support services in the host country [29]. The lack of financial resources is likely to impact negatively on healthcare access [15, 16].

Herein, the material resources of refugee caregivers were very limited. Material resources enable refugees to seek healthcare and pay for transport and medication. Over half of caregivers reported not having enough money for basic needs such as food or clothes, since most are unemployed, and those that do have some form of income obtain this from part-time work and trading. Anecdotal evidence suggests that many refugees work in the informal sector, with little protection, working as car guards, casual labourers in hair salons, and even resort to trading in pirated movies in attempts to keep their families alive [9, 14]. Job opportunities are restricted due to their limited proficiency in English for those living in South Africa. The lack of job opportunities for refugees should be viewed against the high unemployment rate of 25.5% in South Africa [30]. Additionally, the affirmative action legislation and widespread xenophobia among many South Africans may also impede employment opportunities of foreign nationals despite their legal status as refugees [9, 14, 31].

Availability of healthcare services

In this study, caregivers reported having to wait for hours to access healthcare services. These views are likely to contribute to the overall dissatisfaction with the healthcare service and quality of care delivered. It has been reported that, in situations where clients have to wait longer than an hour for healthcare services, this could impact negatively on their beliefs about the quality of the service because of the emotional reactions, including stress and anger [32]. The findings that caregivers had to waste a full day waiting to be seen by a healthcare worker and being aware that they had other household responsibilities, such as preparing meals and caring for their other children, have been previously reported [33]. For full-time caregivers, it seems that spending a full day away from home results in anxiety and anger, which has been reported to impede healthcare seeking behaviour by women in particular [34]. However, waiting in long queues has been a general complaint of the South African public healthcare delivery system [35].

The language barrier due to the limited English proficiency levels among caregivers can be considered as having a negative impact on healthcare service delivery. It has been argued that language barriers contribute to the failure of treating refugees for whom English is not their first language [2]. Not only is it difficult for healthcare workers to render a good quality service if they are unable to communicate with the caregiver of about the child [10, 31, 36], it is also frustrating for caregivers not to be able to raise their concerns and ask questions. The results clearly show that caregivers were dissatisfied with the consultation process as they were not able to ask the necessary questions nor were clear guidelines and explanations given. Language differences have been reported to increase psychological distress and hinder timely healthcare seeking [37, 38].

As the ability to communicate in a shared language is linked to satisfaction with healthcare services [39], the negative views held by caregivers of healthcare delivery could partly stem from the lack of communication between client and health providers, which has previously been reported among refugees in Durban where refugees reported negative views with service delivery in public hospitals partly because of miscommunication and the absence of interpreters [2]. In the absence of professional health interpreters, family members or friends who are able to speak English are often co-opted to translate between client and healthcare worker. This process is also fraught with difficulty and misinterpretation [39–43]. A strong call has therefore been made over the years for the use of professional health interpreters in different parts of the world where there are challenges with delivering a quality service to migrant workers, asylum seekers and refugees [37, 43–45]. Public health clinics that service refugee communities should consider seeking the service of either professional interpreters or, alternatively, training members of the refugee community that have some background in health.

While not investigated herein, it is also likely that healthcare workers do experience frustration at not being able to communicate clearly with their clients. This frustration might be misinterpreted as negative, discriminatory attitudes towards refugees and even xenophobia by refugee clients. However, in the qualitative study, the view was expressed that the negative attitudes of nurses in particular is not linked to language as a barrier, but rather xenophobia directed at refugees in general. A lack of studies among health workers' experiences in delivering healthcare to refugees in South Africa hinders a more balanced understanding of refugee healthcare delivery.

Acceptability of healthcare services

Participants in this study indicated that the services rendered by private doctors are of a higher quality than those provided by the public healthcare system. This finding is supported by existing views of the quality of healthcare services in relation to the divide between those that can afford private healthcare and those that must seek public healthcare [46]. When considering the different levels of work satisfaction among professional nurses in the public and private sector, it has been shown that lower levels of satisfaction among nurses in the public sector negatively impact their client services, including interpersonal relationships [11].

The overall dissatisfaction with public healthcare delivery corroborates previous research findings that have reported negative attitudes of healthcare workers and discrimination against them for foreign citizens [2, 10, 14]. The results pertaining to consultation encounters at public healthcare clinics were negative as the majority of participants who asked questions related to their child's illness was not provided with the necessary information nor felt that enough time had been spent with them during the consultation process. The language barrier in the public healthcare clinics was likely to have contributed to some of the dissatisfaction experienced by caregivers [47]. It has previously been established that refugees' reasons for not returning to a particular clinic include long queues and long waiting times, rudeness of clinic staff and a lack of medication [48]. Therefore, caregivers' dissatisfaction with the public health clinic services for their children seems to be aligned to issues raised by other South African clients about healthcare service delivery in general.

With regards to caregivers' perceptions about xenophobia, it is also possible that, in a context where widespread xenophobia exists, the negative attitudes and rude behaviours of nurses could be interpreted by the caregivers as medical xenophobia [10, 14, 48]. In light of limited research insight into health providers' views about healthcare delivery to migrants and refugees, a deeper understanding of medical xenophobia is not possible; therefore, studies among health workers are required to enhance the quality of healthcare delivery to foreign nationals in South Africa.

Our results further showed that only social networks (a category of household resource) were found to be related to caregiver's satisfaction with child healthcare services. Specifically, caregivers with a higher number of social networks were more satisfied with public healthcare delivery and healthcare services by private doctors. It is likely that social networks help caregivers in identifying possible interpreters to assist them when seeking medical attention at the public health facilities and also assist caregivers in seeking healthcare from particular Congolese doctors, who are likely to improve the consultation experience because of more effective communication, as outlined above. The lack of diverse views about the public healthcare service could also be a consequence of the strong cohesion and seemingly closed networks among members of the DRC refugee community, further enhanced by the generalised xenophobia in South African society [9, 10]. The negative side to social capital therefore results from excessive social cohesion in groups, e.g. families, language and ethnic groups that impact various aspects of society, including economic opportunities [49], as well as 'group think' leading to judgement errors as trust in the group's views inhibits independent thinking [50]. Therefore, sharing negative experiences about public healthcare services is likely to be internalised as their own negative experiences.

Limitations of the study

While the explanatory mixed methods approach attempted to improve the quality of the findings, some limitations should be noted and care should be taken in understanding the results. The study was only conducted in one refugee community, i.e. refugees from the DRC living in Durban. The community's experiences with child healthcare service delivery might be different for other refugee groups in Durban and those living in other parts of South Africa. Care should therefore be taken in generalising the findings to other refugee caregivers. In addition, the relatively small sample size restricts generalisation to all DRC refugee caregivers. The understanding of healthcare delivery to children from the parents' or caregivers' perspective provides only a one-dimensional perspective of service delivery as the view of healthcare workers is absent. Their views might have contributed to a better insight into service delivery challenges faced by healthcare workers within the constraints of current public healthcare delivery. It should be noted that some attempts were initially made to include health workers in the study, but permission to conduct such a study could not be obtained.

Implications for policy and interventions

The findings of this study have implications for health interventions. A better understanding of organisations offering services to refugees within their locality would help them acknowledge and appreciate the work of such organisations. With regards to access to healthcare, f consideration should be first given to the use of translators/interpreters at public healthcare facilities used by refugees to improve healthcare delivery. For example, individuals from the refugee community with a background in health could be trained and employed to assist in translation and interpretation in healthcare contexts. Secondly, healthcare workers should be trained with an emphasis on patient cultural safety and prejudices as well as being made aware of discrimination in healthcare service delivery. Such training would better prepare health workers for the likely challenges they may encounter in the healthcare delivery to foreign nationals, including refugees. Thirdly, the establishment of early day care centres for financially constrained communities within urban areas, where most refugees are located, would not only enable parents and caregivers the opportunity to participate in economic activities but would also assist in the greater integration of refugees into South African society; this is likely to impact positively on the health and well-being of refugees.

Conclusion

This study was conducted to explore refugee parents'/caregivers' perceptions of their children's healthcare problems and challenges regarding accessibility and quality of health service delivery in Durban, South Africa. In summary, caregivers of refugee children reported to be highly dissatisfied with the healthcare services for their children, particularly that in public healthcare facilities. Negative attitudes and discriminatory behaviours by healthcare workers were found to contribute to caregivers' views about the poor quality of the healthcare service. This is one of the first studies to be conducted among parents/caregivers of refugees in Durban pertaining to child healthcare services, thus filling a gap in existing knowledge. These findings underscore the need to address health professionals' attitudes when providing healthcare for refugees. Attitudinal change may improve the relationship between service providers and caregivers of refugee children in South Africa, which may improve the health-related outcomes in refugee children.

Abbreviations

DRC: Democratic Republic of the Congo; NGOs: Non-governmental organizations; UNHCR: United Nations High Commissioner for Refugees; ZAR: the currency of South Africa

Acknowledgements

The authors acknowledge the co-operation and contribution of caregivers of refugee children in Durban, KwaZulu-Natal, South Africa.

Funding

No funding received for this study.

Authors' contribution

BJL designed the study and collected data. KOA was involved in data analysis and drafting of the manuscript. AMW was involved in data analysis and reviewed the manuscript for intellectual content. All authors read, edited and approved the final manuscript.

Competing interests

The authors declare that they have no competing interests.

References

1. UNHCR. Ensuring Access to Health Care: Operational Guidance on Refugee Protection and Solutions in Urban Areas. Geneva: UNHCR; 2015.
2. Apalata T, Kibiribiri ET, Knight S, Lutge E. Refugees' perceptions of their health status and quality of health care services in Durban, South Africa: a community-based survey. Durban: Health Systems Trust; 2007.
3. Burns C, Webster K, Crotty P, Ballinger M, Vincenzo R, Rozman M. Easing the transition: food and nutrition issues of new arrivals. Health Promot J Aust. 2000;10:230–6.
4. Rieder M, Choonara I. Armed conflict and child health. Arch Dis Child. 2012; 97:59–62.
5. World Health Organization. Commission on Social Determinants of Health. Closing the Gap in a Generation. Geneva: WHO; 2015.
6. World Health Organization. World Health Statistics 2011 UN-IGME: Levels and Trends in Child Mortality. 2011. https://data.unicef.org/resources/levels-and-trends-in-child-mortality-report-2011/ . Accessed 20 Dec 2015.
7. Beirens H, Hughes N, Hek R, Spicer N. Preventing social exclusion of refugee and asylum seeking children: building new networks. Soc Policy Society. 2007;6:219–29.
8. Swartz K. Health care for the poor: for whom, what care, and whose responsibility? Focus. 2009;26:1–6.
9. Crush J, DA MD. Transnationalism, African immigration, and new migrant spaces in South Africa: an introduction. Can J Afr Studies. 2000;34:1–19.
10. Zihindula G, Meyer-Weitz A, Akintola O. Lived experiences of Democratic Republic of Congo refugees facing medical xenophobia in Durban, South Africa. J Asian Afr Stud. 2017;52:458–70.
11. Pillay R. Work satisfaction of professional nurses in South Africa: a comparative analysis of the public and private sectors. Hum Resour Health. 2009;7:15.
12. Teagle A. Refugees: Out of the Frying Pan and into the Fire of South Africa's Healthcare System. 2014. http://www.dailymaverick.co.za/article/2014-10-16-refugees-out-of-the-frying-pan-and-into-the-fire-of-south-africas-healthcare-system/#.VrNKi0CWncz. Accessed 15 Dec 2015.
13. Alfaro-Velcamp T. 'Don't send your sick here to be treated, our own people need it more': immigrants access to health care in South Africa. Doctoral Dissertation. University of Cape Town; 2015.
14. Crush J, Tawodzera G. Medical xenophobia and Zimbabwean migrant access to public health services in South Africa. J Ethn Migr Stud. 2014;40:655–70.
15. Peters DH, Garg A, Bloom G, Walker DG, Brieger WR, Hafizur-Rahman M. Poverty and access to health care in developing countries. Ann N Y Acad Sci. 2008;1136:161–71.
16. Wallman S, Baker M. Which resources pay for treatment? A model for estimating the informal economy of health. Soc Sci Med. 1996;42:671–79.
17. Vearey J, Richter M. Challenges to the Successful Implementation of Policy to Protect the Right of Access to Health for All in South Africa. Johannesburg: Report from Migrant Health Forum to Gauteng Department of Health; 2008. http://citeseerx.ist.psu.edu/viewdoc/download?doi=10.1.1.594.2337&rep=rep1&type=pdf. Accessed 20 Dec 2015.
18. Martin P. Economic Integration and Migration: the Mexico-US Case. Paper Presented for the United Nations University world Institute for Development Economics Research (WIDER) Conference in Helsinki; 2002. https://www.econstor.eu/handle/10419/52907. Accessed 18 Oct 2015.
19. Taylor K. Asylum seekers, refugees, and the politics of access to health care: a UK perspective. Brit J Gen Pract. 2009;59:765–72.
20. Creswell JW, Plano-Clark VL. Designing and conducting mixed methods research (2nd Eds.). Thousand Oaks: Sage; 2011.
21. Statistics South Africa. 2014. http://www.statssa.gov.za. Accessed 15 Oct 2014.
22. Lakika D, Kankonde P, Richters A. Violence, suffering and support: Congolese forced migrants' experiences of psychosocial services in Johannesburg. In: Healing and Change in the City of Gold. London: Springer; 2015. p. 101–19.
23. UNHCR. World Refugee Day. 2010. www.unhcr.org. Accessed 18 Dec 2010.
24. Creswell JW. Educational Research: Planning, Conducting and Evaluating Quantitative and Qualitative Approaches to Research. 3rd ed. New Jersey: Pearson Education; 2005.
25. Neuman L. Social Research Methods: Qualitative and Quantitative Approaches. 7th ed. New York: Pearson International; 2011.
26. Braum V, Clarke V. Using thematic analysis in psychology. Qual Res Psychol. 2006;3:77–101.
27. Kirmayer LJ, Narasiah L, Munoz M, Rashid M, Ryder AG, Guzder J, Pottie K. Common mental health problems in immigrants and refugees: general approach in primary care. Can Med Assoc J. 2011;183:E959–67.
28. Yoshikawa H, Aber JL, Beardslee WR. The effects of poverty on the mental, emotional, and behavioural health of children and youth: implications for prevention. Am Psychol. 2012;67:272–84.
29. Payton MPH, Patel MD, Scott MD. Jefferson's Center for Refugee Health: a model of community collaboration. Popul Health Matters. 2015;28:6–9.
30. Statistics South Africa. Employment, Unemployment, Skills and Economic Growth. Pretoria: STATS SA; 2015.
31. Brewer JD. Imagined liberation: xenophobia, citizenship and identity in South Africa, Germany and Canada. Ethnic Racial Stud. 2015;38:1434–5.
32. Bhatia SK, Bhatia SC. Childhood and adolescent depression. Am Fam Physician. 2007;75:73–80.
33. Clough J, Lee S, Chae DH. Barriers to health care among Asian immigrants in the United States: a traditional review. J Health Care Poor Underserved. 2013;24:384–403.
34. Kibiribiri ET, Moodley D, Groves AK, Sebitloane MH. Exploring disparities in prenatal care between refugees and local south African women. Int J Gynaecol Obstet. 2015;132:151–5.
35. Coovadia H, Jewkes R, Barron P, Sanders D, McIntyre D. The health and health system of South Africa: historical roots of current public health challenges. Lancet. 2009;374:817–34.
36. Benson LS, Frost CJ, Gren LH, Jaggi R. Assessing geospatial barriers in refugee resettlement communities: a descriptive exploration about how to identify the health and other resource needs of recently resettled refugee women. Women Health Open J. 2014;1:1–7.
37. Gerrish K, Chau R, Sobowale A, Birks E. Bridging the language barrier: the use of interpreters in primary care nursing. Health Soc Care Comm. 2004;12:407–13.
38. Meuter RF, Gallois C, Segalowitz NS, Ryder AG, Hocking J. Overcoming language barriers in healthcare: a protocol for investigating safe and effective communication when patients or clinicians use a second language. BMC Health Serv Res. 2015;15:371.
39. Morales LS, Cunningham WE, Brown JA, Liu H, Hays RD. Are Latinos less satisfied with communication by health care providers? J Gen Inter Med. 1999;14:409–17.
40. Gany F, Yogendran L, Massie D, Ramirez J, Lee T, Winkel G, Diamod L, Leng J. "Doctor, what do I have?" knowledge of cancer diagnosis among immigrant/migrant minorities. J Cancer Educ. 2013;28:165–70.

41. Wiking E, Saleh-Stattin N, Johansson SE, Sundquist J. Immigrant patients' experiences and reflections pertaining to the consultation: a study on patients from Chile, Iran and Turkey in primary health care in Stockholm, Sweden. Scand J Caring Sci. 2009;23:290–7.

42. Gill PS, Beavan J, Calvert M, Freemantle N. The unmet need for interpreting provision in UK primary care. PLoS One. 2011;6:e20837.

43. O'Donnell C, Higgins M, Chauchan R, Mullen K. Asylum seekers' expectations of and trust in general practice: a qualitative study. Brit J Gen Pract. 2008;58:e1–e11.

44. Bhui K, Abdi A, Abdi M, Pereira S, Dualeh M, Robertson D, Sathyamoorthy G, Ismail H. Traumatic events, migration characteristics and psychiatric symptoms among Somali refugees. Soc Psych Psych Epid. 2003;38:35–43.

45. McColl H, Johnson S. Characteristics and needs of asylum seekers and refugees in contact with London community mental health teams. Soc Psych Psych Epid. 2006;41:789–95.

46. World Health Organization. Trends in maternal trends in maternal mortality: 1990 to 2010. Geneva: WHO; 2010.

47. Mapatano MA, Kayembe K, Piripiri L, Nyandwe K. Immunisation-related knowledge, attitudes and practices of mothers in Kinshasa, Democratic Republic of the Congo. S African Fam Pract. 2008;50:61.

48. Masango-Makgobela AT, Govender I, Ndimande JV. Reasons patients leave their nearest healthcare service to attend Karen Park Clinic, Pretoria North. Afr J Pri Health Care Fam Med. 2013;5:559.

49. Portes A. Downsides of social capital. PNAS. 2014;111:18407–8.

50. Janis I. Group think. In: Lesko WA, editor. Readings in Social Psychology. Boston: Allyn & Bacon; 1997. p. 333–7.

2

Modelling the cost-effectiveness of pay-for-performance in primary care

Ankur Pandya[1,3*], Tim Doran[2], Jinyi Zhu[3], Simon Walker[4], Emily Arntson[5] and Andrew M. Ryan[5]

Abstract

Background: Introduced in 2004, the United Kingdom's (UK) Quality and Outcomes Framework (QOF) is the world's largest primary-care pay-for-performance programme. Given some evidence of the benefits and the substantial costs associated with the QOF, it remains unclear whether the programme is cost-effective. Therefore, we assessed the cost-effectiveness of continuing versus stopping the QOF.

Methods: We developed a lifetime simulation model to estimate quality-adjusted life years (QALYs) and costs for a UK population cohort aged 40–74 years ($n = 27,070,862$) exposed to the QOF and for a counterfactual scenario without exposure. Based on a previous retrospective cross-country analysis using data from 1994 to 2010, we assumed the benefits of the QOF to be a change in age-adjusted mortality of −3.68 per 100,000 population (95% confidence interval −8.16 to 0.80). We used cost-effectiveness thresholds of £30,000/QALY, £20,000/QALY and £13,000/QALY to determine the optimal strategy in base-case and sensitivity analyses.

Results: In the base-case analysis, continuing the QOF increased population-level QALYs and health-care costs yielding an incremental cost-effectiveness ratio (ICER) of £49,362/QALY. The ICER remained >£30,000/QALY in scenarios with and without non-fatal outcomes or increased drug costs, and under differing assumptions about the duration of QOF benefit following its hypothetical discontinuation. The ICER for continuing the programme fell below £30,000/QALY when QOF incentive payments were 36% lower (while preserving QOF mortality benefits), and in scenarios where the QOF resulted in substantial reductions in health-care spending or non-fatal cardiovascular disease events. Continuing the QOF was cost-effective in 18%, 3% and 0% of probabilistic sensitivity analysis iterations using thresholds of £30,000/QALY, £20,000/QALY and £13,000/QALY, respectively.

Conclusions: Compared to stopping the QOF and returning all associated incentive payments to the National Health Service, continuing the QOF is not cost-effective. To improve population health efficiently, the UK should redesign the QOF or pursue alternative interventions.

Background

Introduced in 2004, the United Kingdom's Quality and Outcomes Framework (QOF) is the world's largest primary-care pay-for-performance programme. The QOF links up to 25% of general practitioners' income to performance on a wide range of quality indicators related to clinical management of common chronic conditions, organisation of care and patient experience [1]. This supplements existing payments to practices, which are largely provided through capitation payments. Research on the QOF suggests that the programme accelerated improvement for the incentivised indicators in the 3 years following its implementation [2]. However, this improvement appeared to attenuate over time [3–5]. A recent analysis also found that the QOF did not significantly improve mortality for disease areas targeted under the programme [6].

The QOF is subject to annual review, with changes agreed in negotiations between National Health Service (NHS) Employers and the British Medical Association's General Practitioners Committee, informed by indicator development work conducted by the National Institute for Health and Care Excellence. In 2014/15, 40 indicators—accounting for 35% of the value of total incentive

---

* Correspondence: anpandya@hsph.harvard.edu
[1]Department of Health Policy and Management, Harvard T.H. Chan School of Public Health, 718 Huntington Ave, 2nd Floor, Boston, MA 02115, USA
[3]Center for Health Decision Science, Harvard T.H. Chan School of Public Health, Boston, MA, USA
Full list of author information is available at the end of the article

payments—were removed from the scheme without re-placement, with most of the associated resource used to increase capitation payments [7]. In 2016/17, QOF was discontinued altogether in Scotland and funding was transferred to capitation payments [8]. QOF continues in England, Wales and Northern Ireland, although options for reform or replacement are being considered.

Despite the large costs of the QOF and other pay-for-performance programmes, almost no evidence exists on their cost-effectiveness and how this compares to other system-level interventions to improve longevity [5, 9, 10]. Pay-for-performance programmes introduce additional economic costs to the health-care system, which could have been spent on other health interventions or policies. A cost-effectiveness analysis, the standard method for assessing value for money, can be used to determine whether additional spending on pay-for-performance is worth the health gains produced by these policies. Although a cost-effectiveness analysis has previously been conducted for other pay-for-performance programmes in the UK, decisions on the development or discontinuation of QOF have not been informed by reliable estimates of cost-effectiveness [11]. A systematic review of pay-for-performance programmes found that, despite the promise of cost-effective financial incentives, convincing evidence of the cost-effectiveness of pay-for-performance was lacking [12]. Previous attempts to estimate the cost-effectiveness of pay-for-performance have extrapolated evidence from randomised trials, rather than using direct evidence of its effectiveness on outcomes [4, 9, 13]. These approaches are limited because results from randomised trials may not generalise to the older, sicker patients who are typically excluded from trials [6].

In this study, we address this knowledge gap by evaluating the cost-effectiveness of the QOF under various assumptions around the programme's benefits and costs.

Methods
Overview
We developed a computer-based simulation model to estimate the QOF-related lifetime health effects and costs for a representative UK general population cohort aged 40–74 years ($n = 27,070,862$) exposed to two competing policy alternatives: (1) continuing the QOF and (2) stopping the QOF. We compared the trade-off between lifetime discounted health effects, quantified using quality-adjusted life years (QALYs), and QOF-related health-care costs using an incremental cost-effectiveness analysis from a NHS (health-care payer) perspective. The simulation model discounts health effects and costs using a rate of 3.5% [14]. An overview of our methodology is shown in Fig. 1.

Simulation model and population
The overall goal for our model-based analysis was to estimate the impact of continuing the QOF (compared to stopping the QOF) on lifetime QALYs and costs. The decision of whether or not to continue the QOF will have the most impact on the specific diseases targeted by the QOF. For instance, the lifetime QALYs gained would be greater if the QOF mortality reductions were concentrated in healthy children as opposed to older persons with multiple chronic conditions. Of all the conditions actually included in the QOF, cardiovascular diseases and associated risk conditions (coronary heart disease, stroke, diabetes and hypertension) collectively attract the largest incentives and account for the majority of non-cancer deaths (although cancer is included in the QOF, it only receives weak incentives) [6, 15–17]. In 2005, payments of up to £15,125 were available for the average family practice across 15 ischaemic heart disease and heart failure indicators, but only £1500 was available across two cancer indicators [6]. Therefore, we assumed that the QOF benefits were concentrated in individuals with cardiovascular disease (aged 40–

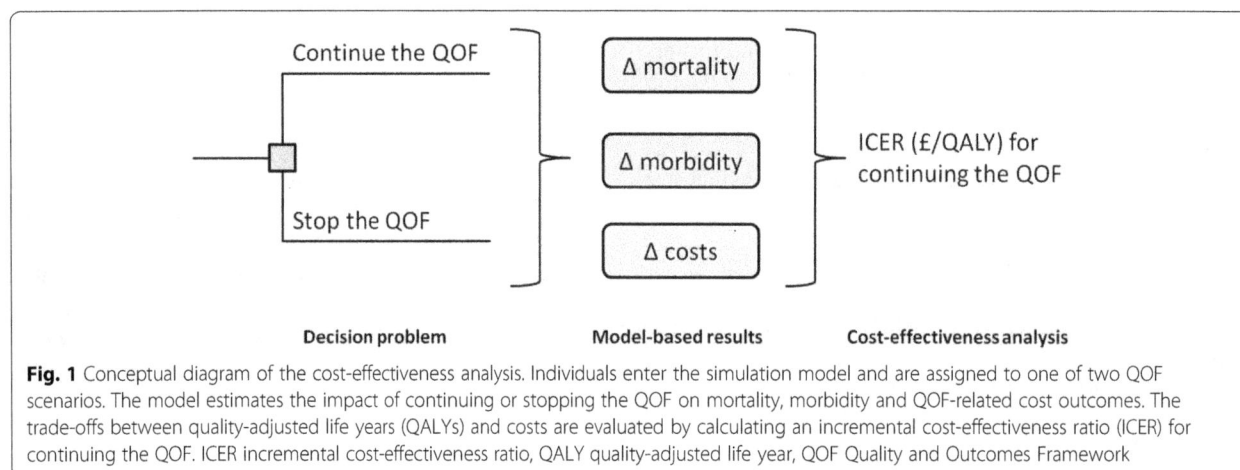

Fig. 1 Conceptual diagram of the cost-effectiveness analysis. Individuals enter the simulation model and are assigned to one of two QOF scenarios. The model estimates the impact of continuing or stopping the QOF on mortality, morbidity and QOF-related cost outcomes. The trade-offs between quality-adjusted life years (QALYs) and costs are evaluated by calculating an incremental cost-effectiveness ratio (ICER) for continuing the QOF. ICER incremental cost-effectiveness ratio, QALY quality-adjusted life year, QOF Quality and Outcomes Framework

74 years at baseline) in our base-case analysis, but relaxed this assumption in sensitivity analyses (including a scenario where the QOF equally benefited all individuals aged 0–74 years with and without disease). We needed to make these assumptions around which population segments would benefit from the QOF because our main effectiveness estimate for the QOF did not specify in whom the mortality benefits were concentrated, but rather reported an overall age-adjusted mortality reduction of 3.68 per 100,000 (across those aged 0–74 years) [6].

We created a hypothetical cohort that would be affected by the QOF using age group- and sex-specific population sizes for the UK, further dividing this population into those with and those without prevalent cardiovascular disease. We used Office for National Statistics data for sex-specific population sizes in 5-year age categories (e.g., 2,255,562 females aged 50–54 years at baseline) and sex- and age-specific cardiovascular disease prevalence estimates from British Heart Foundation data (e.g. 8.4% of females aged 50–54 years at baseline had prevalent cardiovascular disease, ICD-10 codes I00–I99) [15, 16]. Our model uses annual cycles to project the life expectancy, quality-adjusted life expectancy and QOF-related costs for a representative UK cohort until death. Each model population segment faces a risk of death in each model cycle based on the sex, age and cardiovascular disease status of the group being simulated, with additional mortality risk adjustments to account for the absence of the QOF for the non-QOF strategy (i.e. the current life tables include the effects of the QOF, so we increased the risk of death in the life tables when simulating the non-QOF strategy). Those with cardiovascular disease faced higher mortality risks and reduced quality of life compared to those without cardiovascular disease. To estimate mortality risks for those with cardiovascular disease, we multiplied the annual mortality risk all-cause life tables (i.e. the age-specific annual risks of death from any cause) by 1.6 (for men) or 2.1 (for women). These age-adjusted mortality ratios were based on an analysis of linked hospital discharge and 7-year mortality follow-up data from survivors of first acute myocardial infarction in England from 2004 to 2010 [18]. We subtracted cardiovascular disease mortality rates from all-cause life tables to estimate mortality risks for those without cardiovascular disease [18]. The model sums all health effects and costs accrued for each population segment, yielding population-level results. Table 1 shows all model inputs and data sources. The model is programmed in Microsoft Excel with Visual Basic for Applications and is included as Additional file 1.

QOF mortality effects

The mortality increase from stopping the QOF was estimated from a previous difference-in-difference analysis [6]. In their study, Ryan et al. created a synthetic control group as a weighted combination of countries previously characterised as having a high-income epidemiological profile. Based on their study, the QOF programme was associated with a change in age- and sex-adjusted mortality from the major contributors to population mortality targeted by the QOF (ischaemic heart disease, hypertension, stroke, diabetes, chronic kidney disease, asthma and chronic pulmonary disease) of –3.68 per 100,000 population (95% confidence interval of –8.16 to 0.80).

Table 1 Model variables with base-case values and ranges used in sensitivity analyses

Variable	Base-case value	Sensitivity analysis range	Source(s)
QOF mortality benefit (age- and sex-adjusted per 100,000)	−3.68	−8.16 to 0.80	[6]
Adjusted QOF mortality benefit (for those with age > 40 years with CVD)	−58.93	−130.57 to 12.81	Calculated
All-cause age- and sex-specific mortality (and age and sex demographics)	Life table	Not applicable	[45]
CVD prevalence, males (aged 45–64 years, aged 65–74 years)	14.6%, 28.5%	+/− 20%	[16]
CVD prevalence, females (aged 45–64 years, aged 65–74 years)	8.4%, 22.5%	+/− 20%	[16]
CVD mortality multiplier (male, female)	1.6, 2.1	+/−20%	[18]
CVD utility	0.796	+/− 20%	[21]
Non-fatal-to-fatal CVD events averted (ratio)	1.63	0–10	[20]
QOF annual population-level incentive costs	£1,396,843,151	£0–2,000,000,000	Country-specific sources [24, 26, 27]
QOF effect on utilisation costs per £ spent on incentives	£0.011	£1 £1	[29, 30]
Acute CVD event costs (i.e. costs within first year of CVD event)	£10,871	+/−20%	[31]
Chronic CVD event costs (i.e. annual costs for all years after first year)	£3282	+/− 20%	[31]
Average NHS costs by age	Age-based table	£0 to + 100%	[32]
Discount rate	3.5%	0–5%	[14]

QOF Quality and Outcomes Framework, *CVD* cardiovascular disease, *NHS* National Health Service

This estimate was based on age-adjusted mortality rates for populations aged 0–74 years. Since QOF mortality benefits would be concentrated in older individuals with prevalent disease, we adjusted the mortality effect used in our model by back-calculating mortality change (58.9 per 100,000 population) in older individuals (aged 40–74 years, $n = 27,070,862$) with prevalent cardiovascular disease that would result in the Ryan et al. general population result. In other words, a 58.9 per 100,000 mortality decrease concentrated exclusively in individuals aged 40–74 years with cardiovascular disease would result in a 3.68 per 100,000 mortality effect in all individuals (aged 0–74 years among individuals with and without cardiovascular disease, $n = 59,385,341$). We performed a sensitivity analysis using a 3.68 per 100,000 mortality decrease for all individuals (aged 0–74 years) to assess the impact of these two contrasting assumptions (mortality effect concentrated in those aged 40–74 years versus mortality effect spread out among those aged 0–74 years) on the model results. While either assumption had QOF mortality effects stopping at age 74 years (due to our data source [6]), the model cohort was modelled until death in all analyses.

In the base-case analyses, we assumed the QOF-related mortality benefit was immediately lost if the QOF were discontinued. In the sensitivity analyses, we modelled different durations over which the mortality benefit of the QOF waned if the programme were discontinued. In these scenarios, we assumed linear declines in the QOF mortality benefit from first year in the model to a time in the future (1, 3, 5 or 10 years from the model start), at which point the mortality benefit from the QOF would equal zero.

QOF non-fatal effects (i.e. QOF morbidity effects)

Best practice in a cost-effectiveness analysis is to include all health outcomes (fatal and non-fatal) that differ from the choice of a particular strategy over another [19]. While it is likely that the QOF resulted in changes in both fatal and non-fatal outcomes, the Ryan et al. study did not include non-fatal outcomes due to data restrictions. Given the QOF focus on managing cardiovascular disease risk, we applied a ratio of non-fatal cardiovascular disease events averted for every fatal event averted from the QOF based on prevented cardiovascular disease events from a meta-analysis of statin trial data from 90,056 participants [20]. First, we calculated the differences in non-fatal coronary heart disease events between statin and placebo arms in the meta-analysis (1789 – 2460) and divided that difference by the difference in coronary heart disease deaths (1548 – 1960), which resulted in a ratio of non-fatal-to-fatal coronary heart disease events averted of 1.63. We multiplied this ratio by the difference in mortality between the QOF and non-QOF counterfactuals in the model to estimate the number of non-fatal cardiovascular

disease events averted by the QOF in each model cycle. The model incorporates morbidity in the QALY calculation by applying utility values (see *Health-related quality-of-life* section below) to the non-fatal cardiovascular disease events averted by the QOF. We performed sensitivity analyses excluding non-fatal health effects attributable to the QOF in the model in addition to varying the value of the non-fatal-to-fatal ratio used in the model.

Health-related quality of life

The main effectiveness measure for our analysis was life-time cohort-level QALYs. The model calculates QALYs by multiplying the number of individuals alive in a given year by a utility value, which quantifies morbidity. The model assigns utility values ranging between 0 (death) and 1 (perfect health) for each year based on age and cardiovascular disease status. Older individuals and those with cardiovascular disease have lower utility values than younger individuals and those without cardiovascular disease, respectively. Utility values were estimated from the results of the EuroQOL 5 Dimensions (EQ-5D) questionnaire from the Medical Expenditure Panel Survey (US-based descriptive responses to the EQ-5D were combined with UK community-based preference weights to calculate utility values for the UK) [21–23]. For a given age (40–100 years), population segments with cardiovascular disease were assigned the minimum utility for cardiovascular disease (0.796) and age-based utilities (ranging from 0.691–0.848). Population segments without cardiovascular disease were assigned the age-based utility values [23].

QOF costs

We included two major QOF-related cost categories: (1) incentive costs and (2) costs related to changes in health-care utilisation as a result of QOF incentives. We estimated total incentive costs over the first 7 years of the programme at £1,396,843,151 per year based on remuneration data from the four constituent countries of the UK (see Table 4 in the Appendix) [24–27]. These costs include payments for all domains (clinical, organisational and patient experience) and are considered incremental (i.e. new) costs to the health system, as opposed to reallocating existing funds within the health system, as they represent additional resources the UK government committed to primary care in 2004 [28].

Given the focus of the QOF incentives on disease management in the cardiovascular domain, we assumed changes in health-care utilisation driven by the QOF would be concentrated in the utilisation of cardiovascular disease drugs (targeting cholesterol, blood pressure and diabetes). We estimated changes in drug utilisation based on an observational study in Scotland, which reported an average increase in defined daily doses (DDDs) per prescribing unit (PU) per month of QOF-related drugs of 3.79. Among these drugs, cardiovascular disease drugs accounted for 3.47 of the average increase (DDD per PU, 89% of the total increase across all drugs mentioned or implied by the QOF) [29]. For these costs, we used separated DDD per PU per month estimates from that analysis for five cardiovascular disease drug classes (lipid-regulating, renin-angiotensin system, thiazides and related diuretics, oral antidiabetics and antiplatelets) in conjunction with weighted averages of drug class prices (Table 5 in the Appendix) to estimate an overall annual increase in QOF-related drug costs of £15,692,470 (i.e. a ratio of 0.011 of increased drug utilisation per £1 spent on incentives) [30]. We allowed this value to be negative (i.e. a cost saving) in a sensitivity analysis to evaluate the possibility that QOF incentives might result in a net decrease in overall health-care spending from averted disease events and follow-up spending, by varying the ratio from −1 to 1 in a one-way sensitivity analysis. In the model, averted cardiovascular disease events (fatal and non-fatal) resulted in cost savings from averted health-care utilisation. We estimated the costs of averted cardiovascular disease events in the first year of the event (£10,871) and all subsequent years (£3282) from a previous analysis of linked UK cohort datasets with utilisation and cost data [31]. We modelled future average age-based annual health-care costs based on English NHS data and performed separate sensitivity analyses where these costs were excluded and doubled [32]. All costs in our analyses are reported in 2016 pounds sterling (£).

Base-case cost-effectiveness analysis

We used conventional incremental cost-effectiveness analysis methods to calculate an incremental cost-effectiveness ratio (ICER) for continuing the QOF programme compared to stopping the QOF. We used cost-effectiveness thresholds of £30,000/QALY, £20,000/QALY and £13,000/QALY. These thresholds are based on current National Institute for Health and Care Excellence recommendations (£20,000–30,000/QALY) and a 2015 Claxton et al. study that estimated an empirically based opportunity cost for health-care spending (i.e. a cost-effectiveness threshold that estimates the amount of money, at the margin of health-care spending, it would take to produce one additional QALY) in the UK (£13,000/QALY) [33]. We also calculated the opportunity costs of continuing the QOF in terms of population-level incremental net health benefit, which converts incremental costs into QALYs using a cost-effectiveness threshold and subtracts these opportunity costs from QALYs gained as a result of continuing the QOF. In other words, the incremental net health benefit captures the health gains to individuals who benefit from funding being given to an intervention minus the population health forgone as a result of committed resources being unavailable for other individuals' health

care. The health forgone by other individuals was estimated based on the cost-effectiveness thresholds noted above [specifically, the QALYs forgone (incremental net health benefit) equal the incremental costs divided by the cost-effectiveness threshold] [34].

Sensitivity analyses

We performed four types of sensitivity analyses: (1) scenario analyses for the inclusion of non-fatal health effects and increased drug utilisation as a result of the QOF and the duration of the QOF mortality benefit if the QOF were discontinued, (2) one-way sensitivity analyses with high and low values for all model inputs, (3) a two-way sensitivity analysis for different combinations of the levels of QOF incentive payments and the QOF mortality benefit and (4) a probabilistic sensitivity analysis, where we assessed the statistical uncertainty in the QOF mortality benefit (which was based on an estimate that had a 95% confidence interval of −0.80 to 8.16) by drawing 1000 random values for the QOF mortality benefit from a normal probability distribution [35]. The probabilistic sensitivity analysis results for each of the 1000 iterations were used to construct a cost-effectiveness acceptability curve showing the probability that continuing the QOF was cost-effective while varying the cost-effectiveness threshold from £0–200,000/QALY.

Results
Base-case results

Continuing the QOF programme indefinitely would result in more life years, QALYs and QOF-related costs compared to stopping the QOF (Table 2). Compared to stopping the QOF, continuing the QOF had an ICER of £49,362/QALY under base-case assumptions (non-fatal outcomes and increased drug costs included, with instant changes in the QOF mortality benefit if the QOF is discontinued, Table 2). The population opportunity cost of continuing the QOF (i.e. the incremental net health benefit) ranged from 226,109 to 979,917 QALYs lost, assuming cost-effectiveness thresholds of £30,000/QALY to £13,000/QALY, respectively (Table 6 in the Appendix).

Scenario analyses

Table 3 shows the matrix of ICERs for the QOF for every combination of assumptions related to the inclusion of non-fatal outcomes, the inclusion of increased drug costs and waning of the QOF benefit. The ICER remained greater than £30,000/QALY for every combination of assumptions. The ICER for continuing the QOF was £42,296/QALY when we assumed all individuals aged 40–74 years experienced the health benefits of the QOF (as opposed to only those with prevalent cardiovascular disease), and £31,089/QALY when the benefits of the QOF were spread out to all individuals (with and

Table 2 Base-case population-level results and incremental cost-effectiveness analysis of continuing the QOF vs. stopping the QOF

	Undiscounted			Discounted			
	life years	QALYs	QOF-related costs	life years	QALYs	QOF-related costs	ICER (£/QALY)
Stopping the QOF	78,805,931	59,562,301	£0	52,426,797	39,966,375	£0	Reference
Continuing the QOF	79,433,681	60,237,416	£25,881,916,480	52,750,331	40,316,707	£17,293,239,670	49,362
Delta	627,750	675,114	£25,881,916,480	323,534	350,332	£17,293,239,670	–

QOF Quality and Outcomes Framework, *QALY* quality-adjusted life year, *ICER* incremental cost-effectiveness ratio

without disease) aged 0–74 years (these findings can be reproduced using the simulation model attached as Additional file 1).

One-way sensitivity analyses

The ICER was only below alternative National Institute for Health and Care Excellence thresholds of £30,000/QALY, £20,000/QALY and £13,000/QALY when, for every £1 spend on QOF incentives, £0.36, £0.55 or £0.68 were saved as a result of net cost reductions (for example, from averted cardiovascular disease events; Figure 4 in the Appendix). Similarly, the ICER was below the thresholds of £30,000/QALY, £20,000/QALY and £13,000/QALY when the ratios for non-fatal-to-fatal cardiovascular disease events averted were 3.7 (225% of the base-case value), 5.5 (335% of the base-case value) and 7.3 (450% of the base-case value, Figure 5 in the Appendix).

The cost-effectiveness results were robust (ICERs within £40,000–65,000/QALY) in the following sensitivity analyses (with high and low parameter ranges as reported in Table 1, unless otherwise specified): applying the QOF mortality benefit to all individuals aged 0–74 years as opposed to a concentrated (higher) mortality benefit to those with prevalent cardiovascular disease, high and low utility values, high and low cardiovascular disease prevalence and mortality multiplier estimates, and separate scenarios removing and doubling the annual average future health-care costs (Table 7 in the Appendix).

Two-way sensitivity analysis

Fig. 2 shows the ICER as a function of the levels of QOF incentive payments and the QOF mortality benefit

assuming a cost-effectiveness threshold of £30,000/QALY. The ICER was below thresholds of £30,000/QALY, £20,000/QALY and £13,000/QALY with QOF incentive payment levels of £893,979,617 (64% of the base-case value), £628,579,418 (45%) and £446,989,808 (32%), respectively. Similarly, the ICER was below thresholds of £30,000/QALY, £20,000/QALY and £13,000/QALY with QOF age-adjusted mortality reductions of 5.89 (160% of the base-case value), 8.25 (225%) and 11.59 (315%) respectively.

Probabilistic sensitivity analyses

Fig. 3 shows the cost-effectiveness acceptability curve from the probabilistic sensitivity analysis. The QOF was cost-effective in 18.3%, 2.9% and 0.1% of probabilistic sensitivity analysis iterations using thresholds of £30,000/QALY, £20,000/QALY and £13,000/QALY, respectively. The 95% credible interval (i.e. the range where 95% of probabilistic sensitivity analysis results fell) for the ICER was £19,700/QALY to QOF dominated (which means continuing the QOF would result in higher costs and fewer QALYs compared to stopping the QOF).

Discussion

In this study we modelled the cost-effectiveness of continuing the QOF in the UK to evaluate whether the incremental health gains from continuing the pay-for-performance programme would be worth the additional costs to do so. We found that the ICER for continuing the QOF was £49,362/QALY, with an 18% probability of being cost-effective in probabilistic sensitivity analysis

Table 3 Cost-effectiveness ratios (£/QALY) for continuing the QOF versus stopping the QOF under various model scenarios

QOF effects beyond mortality		How long QOF mortality benefit is sustained if QOF discontinued**				
Non-fatal outcomes	Increased drug costs	No waning	1-year waning	3-year waning	5-year waning	10-year waning
Included	Included	49,362*	51,970	57,616	63,765	81,428
Included	Not included	48,768	51,347	56,931	63,011	80,478
Not included	Included	80,515	84,323	92,565	101,535	127,281
Not included	Not included	79,657	83,424	91,575	100,446	125,907

QOF Quality and Outcomes Framework, *QALY* quality-adjusted life year
*Base-case scenario: non-fatal outcomes and increased drug costs included and instant changes in the QOF mortality benefit if the QOF is discontinued
**In waning scenarios, we assumed linear declines in the QOF mortality benefit from the first year in the model to a time in the future (1, 3, 5 or 10 years from the model start), at which point the mortality benefit from the QOF would equal zero

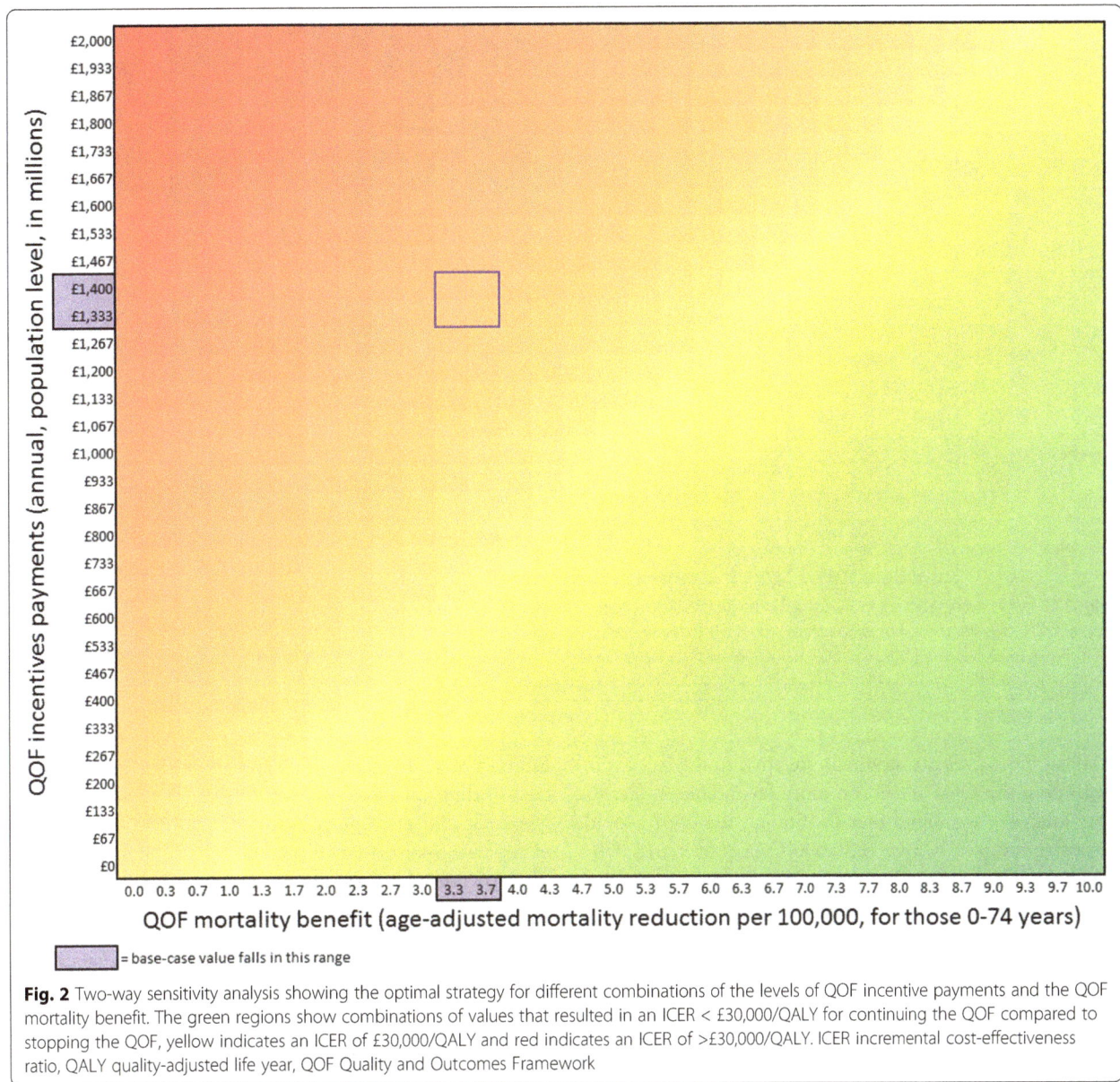

Fig. 2 Two-way sensitivity analysis showing the optimal strategy for different combinations of the levels of QOF incentive payments and the QOF mortality benefit. The green regions show combinations of values that resulted in an ICER < £30,000/QALY for continuing the QOF compared to stopping the QOF, yellow indicates an ICER of £30,000/QALY and red indicates an ICER of >£30,000/QALY. ICER incremental cost-effectiveness ratio, QALY quality-adjusted life year, QOF Quality and Outcomes Framework

using a cost-effectiveness threshold of £30,000/QALY. This estimate was robust to variation in assumptions related to non-fatal outcomes, increased drug costs and waning of benefits from the QOF. A probabilistic sensitivity analysis found that the QOF was cost-effective in only 18% of the scenarios tested. We found that ICERs of the QOF were substantially more favourable only in those scenarios where the QOF was associated with large reductions (beyond our base-case estimates) in (1) costs associated with averted health events or (2) non-fatal cardiovascular disease events. The estimated population opportunity cost of continuing the QOF (in terms of incremental net health benefit) was 226,109–979,917 QALYs lost.

Our estimate of the ICER for the QOF is above the conventional threshold of £20,000–30,000/QALY that is used to determine cost-effectiveness in the UK. This suggests that primary-care pay-for-performance in the United Kingdom has not been a cost-effective strategy to improve health. Nonetheless, our base-case analysis treats QOF incentive costs as incremental to the health system. We assumed that stopping the QOF would return all incentive payments to the NHS. However, if the NHS decided to stop the QOF and return all or some of the QOF payments to providers as increased capitation payments, as has already happened in Scotland, this would maintain the costs for the QOF while losing the benefits (unless the benefits from the QOF remain or wane over time after the

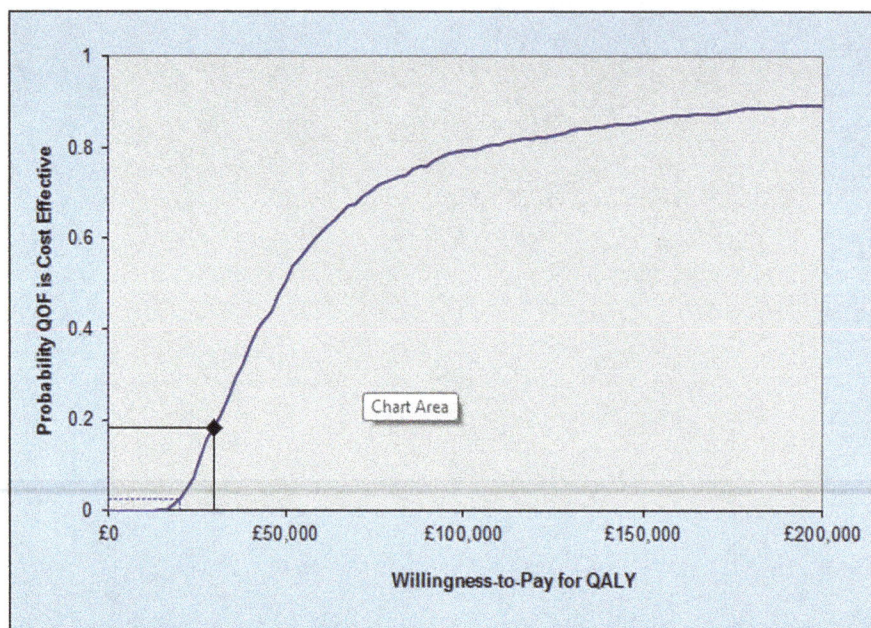

Fig. 3 Cost-effectiveness acceptability curve for the probabilistic sensitivity analysis. The curve shows the probability that the QOF was cost-effective. It was calculated as the proportion of iterations with ICERs that were less than a given cost-effectiveness threshold. The health benefit (base-case value of 3.68 per 100,000 age-adjusted mortality reduction) was randomly drawn from a normal distribution (95% confidence interval −0.80 to 8.16). ICER incremental cost-effectiveness ratio, QALY quality-adjusted life year, QOF Quality and Outcomes Framework

financial incentives are stopped). Relative to this scenario, continuing the QOF would be more favourable. In sensitivity analyses, we found that continuing the QOF would be cost-effective (ICER < £30,000/QALY or < £13,000/QALY) if QOF incentive payments (see Fig. 2) were respectively 32% or 64% lower than our base-case estimate, assuming that the mortality impact of QOF remained unchanged. Our analysis gives policymakers cost-effectiveness information for all joint scenarios of QOF payment and mortality benefit estimates to facilitate decision-making around lower QOF payments considering potential reductions in QOF benefits that would follow from these decisions. Our results were not sensitive to the assumption of concentrating the QOF benefits in those with cardiovascular disease, as shown with an ICER > £30,000/QALY, even if assuming the QOF equally benefited all individuals aged 0–74 years with and without disease.

In general, cost-effectiveness analyses of pay-for-performance policies, especially those that use QALYs as the effectiveness measure (i.e. cost–utility analyses), are rare. In a systematic review of economic evaluations of pay-for-performance policies, Emmert and co-authors found only one cost–utility analysis [10]. That study, by Nahra and co-authors, modelled how hospital process improvements in heart-related care could be used to estimate QALYs via improved medication compliance and found that the pay-for-performance policy was cost-effective [13]. Since the publication of the review by

Emmert et al., Meacock et al. and Walker et al. performed cost–utility analyses of pay-for-performance policies. Meacock and colleagues evaluated the cost-effectiveness of a pay-for-performance scheme for hospitals in the UK (the Advancing Quality programme) using reductions in 30-day mortality (among patients admitted for pneumonia, heart failure or acute myocardial infarction) estimated from a difference-in-difference study and found that the programme was cost-effective using a threshold of £20,000/QALY [11]. Walker and co-authors used previously published literature to estimate the potential cost-effectiveness of the QOF. They found that, for most QOF indicators studied, a less than 1% improvement would be needed for the programme to be cost-effective (using the £20,000–30,000/QALY threshold range). However, this study used estimates from randomised controlled trials to extrapolate the hypothetical effects of incentivising individual activities for which evidence on effectiveness was available, rather than estimating the impact of the overall programme [9].

Our study conflicts with previous attempts to estimate the cost-effectiveness of pay-for-performance policies. Only the Meacock et al. study used effectiveness estimates (reduction in mortality that was translated to QALYs gained) that were directly measured, as opposed to extrapolating intermediate outcomes (such as improvements in medication compliance) to QALYs. The Meacock cost-effectiveness study was based on a difference-in-difference analysis that found no significant impact of a hospital-based pay-for-performance programme on outcomes for two of the incentivised conditions (acute myocardial infarction and heart failure) and a modest improvement for the third (pneumonia) after 18 months [36]. However, this improvement was not sustained and re-analysis of the original data using a synthetic control approach found that the initial improvement for pneumonia was not statistically significant [37, 38]. Unlike the Meacock et al. study, we were not able directly to measure and thus include the administrative costs of running the pay-for-performance programme. Our study is the first to evaluate the cost-effectiveness of the QOF using direct estimates of mortality (as opposed to intermediate outcomes or hospital-based pay-for-performance policies).

Our study has several limitations, including four related to data limitations. First, we could not estimate administrative costs due to data limitations. If administrative cost data become available, these costs could be added to the annual incentive costs in our sensitivity analysis around costs (the horizontal axis in Fig. 2) to estimate the impact of these costs on the cost-effectiveness results. The addition of these administrative costs would increase the ICER for continuing the QOF. Second, although our model cohort was simulated until death, we restricted QOF mortality effects up to age 74 years given the source data [6]. Third, we also had limited information on the effect of the QOF on costs, such as those of additional visits to practices, referrals to secondary care and medication prescriptions. For instance, there are very few studies estimating the impact of the QOF on health-care utilisation, which is why we relied on a 2008 observational study from Scotland to estimate incentivised drug costs despite our model assuming a causal relationship between the QOF incentives and increased utilisation. To address this, we performed a sensitivity analysis around this input value, which showed that cost savings because of the QOF (i.e. averted utilisation costs outweighing the incentive costs) would be necessary to make the QOF cost-effective using a threshold of £30,000/QALY. Fourth, we also had incomplete information about the effects of the QOF on non-fatal outcomes, such as acute myocardial infarction and stroke. To address this, we varied our estimates across a range of assumptions about the effects of the QOF non-fatal outcomes and found that the ratio of fatal-to-non-fatal events would need to be more than doubled from our base-case estimate to make the QOF cost-effective. Fifth, our results from a probabilistic sensitivity analysis showed that there is considerable statistical uncertainty around the cost-effectiveness of continuing the QOF, suggesting that more precise estimates of the effect of the QOF on mortality could reduce the uncertainty around the decision of whether to continue the QOF. We also varied only one parameter (the effectiveness of the

QOF) in the probabilistic sensitivity analysis because it was the only input with a well-estimated 95% confidence interval. Adding other parameters to the probabilistic sensitivity analysis could produce a higher uncertainty in our cost-effectiveness results, but that would not change the overall conclusion of our analysis. Sixth, QOF is subject to annual review and amendment [6–8, 24, 26], and our main estimates for the effectiveness and incentives costs were based on the first 7 years of the programme. Therefore, our analysis is evaluating the decision to continue with incentives contained in QOF from 2004 to 2010 versus discontinuing these incentives. We have not evaluated the most recent versions of the QOF, for which we do not have linked cost and effectiveness data, but incentives for the conditions of interest were retained in these versions.

Despite these limitations, our findings imply that the UK should redesign the QOF or pursue alternative interventions to improve population health efficiently. The QOF is already in transition. The programme was reduced in scope in 2014, with 40 indicators retired to focus on a set of 83 key indicators [7, 39]. In Scotland, the QOF was withdrawn altogether in 2016, with practices continuing to receive payments based on their historical performance without any further need to meet QOF targets. In the future, quality improvement in Scottish practices will be managed by local peer support networks and will rely on clinical governance arrangements rather than financial incentives [40]. NHS England is also now seeking to develop a successor to the QOF [41]. To enable informed decisions on further redesign or replacement of the QOF, future research should compare the cost-effectiveness of the programme with alternative system-level interventions (whether these programmes are different forms of financial incentives for providers or patients, or use other mechanisms to improve quality, costs or access to care). Similar research should be undertaken in other settings where pay-for-performance has been implemented, comparing its cost-effectiveness with other health system-level policies such as value-based insurance design [42], computerised decision support interventions [43] or value-based outcome reporting tools [44]. These future analyses would provide crucial information about whether pay-for-performance in primary care is a cost-effective way to improve population health.

Conclusions

Compared to stopping the QOF and returning all associated incentive payments to the NHS, continuing the QOF is not cost-effective. To improve population health efficiently, the UK should redesign the QOF or pursue alternative interventions.

Appendix

Table 4 Estimates of incentive payments to UK practices under the Quality and Outcomes Framework (inflated to 2016£)

Year	England[a]	Northern Ireland[a]	Scotland[b]	Wales[a]	Total
2004/5	£830,220,692	£36,069,236	£90,923,805	£48,008,831	£1,005,222,565
2005/6	£1,350,199,371	£58,115,719	£155,248,597	£79,707,784	£1,643,271,471
2006/7	£1,237,234,310	£53,602,369	£144,140,152	£73,024,636	£1,508,001,467
2007/8	£1,213,821,483	£52,481,420	£142,189,299	£72,081,589	£1,480,573,791
2008/9	£1,147,372,625	£49,335,331	£135,246,153	£67,898,096	£1,399,852,206
2009/10	£1,128,185,395	£48,508,555	£132,825,069	£66,939,222	£1,376,458,241
2010/11	£1,122,907,420	£46,715,424	£128,483,891	£66,415,581	£1,364,522,315
Total	£8,029,941,295	£344,828,055	£929,056,966	£474,075,739	£9,777,902,056

[a]Based on estimates from the Information Centre for Health and Social Care [24, 26]
[b]Based on payment data from the Information Services Division Scotland [27]

Table 5 Drug classes, changes in utilisation and annual prices

Drug class[a]	DDD/PU/mo[b]	Annual price[c]
Lipid regulating drugs	1.92	61.57
Renin angiotensin	0.84	37.29
Thiazides/diuretics	0.24	5.66
Oral antidiabetic	0.14	42.79
Antiplatelet	0.33	14.77

DDD defined daily dose, *mo* month, *PU* prescribing unit, *QOF* Quality and Outcomes Framework
[a]Cardiovascular disease drug classes from MacBride-Stewart et al. [29]
[b]Increase in defined daily doses (DDDs) per prescribing unit (PU) per month of QOF-related drugs
[c]Weighted average price (weights based on quantity dispensed by specific drugs and doses)
(source: Health and Social Care Information Centre. Prescription cost analysis, England 2012)
https://digital.nhs.uk/data-and-information/publications/statistical/prescription-cost-analysis/prescription-cost-analysis-england-2012

Table 6 Population-level incremental net health benefit results

	Discounted QALYs	Discounted costs	Net health benefit using different cost-effectiveness thresholds (QALYs)		
			£30,000/QALY threshold	£20,000/QALY threshold	£13,000/QALY threshold
Stopping the QOF	39,966,375	£0	39,966,375	39,966,375	39,966,375
Continuing the QOF	40,316,707	£17,293,239,670	39,740,266	39,452,046	38,986,458
Delta	350,332	£17,293,239,670	−226,109	−514,330	−979,917

QOF Quality and Outcomes Framework, *QALY* quality-adjusted life year

Table 7 One-way sensitivity analysis results

Variable	Base-case value	Sensitivity analysis range	ICER at low value	ICER at high value
Adjusted QOF mortality benefit (for those aged > 40 years with CVD)	58.93	−130.57 to 12.81	QOF dominated	£20,044/QALY
CVD prevalence, males (aged 45–64 years, aged 65–74 years)	14.6%, 28.5%	±20%	£49,266/QALY	£49,485/QALY
CVD prevalence, females (aged 45–64 years, aged 65–74 years)	8.4%, 22.5%	±20%	£49,302/QALY	£49,414/QALY
CVD mortality multiplier (male, female)	1.6, 2.1	±20%	£47,246/QALY	£51,249/QALY
CVD utility	0.796	±20%	£43,516/QALY	£64,805/QALY
Acute CVD event costs (i.e. costs within first year of CVD event)	£10,871	±20%	£49,850/QALY	£48,874/QALY
Chronic CVD event costs (i.e. annual costs for all years after first year)	£3282	±20%	£50,350/QALY	£48,375/QALY
Average NHS costs by age	Age-based table	£0 to +100%	£46,270/QALY	£52,455/QALY
Discount rate	3.5%	0–5%	£38,337/QALY	£54,587/QALY

Base-case ICER of £49,362/QALY; base-case values for each variable are reported in Table 1 in the main text
CVD cardiovascular disease, *ICER* incremental cost-effectiveness ratio, *NHS* National Health Service, *QALY* quality-adjusted life year, *QOF* Quality and Outcomes Framework

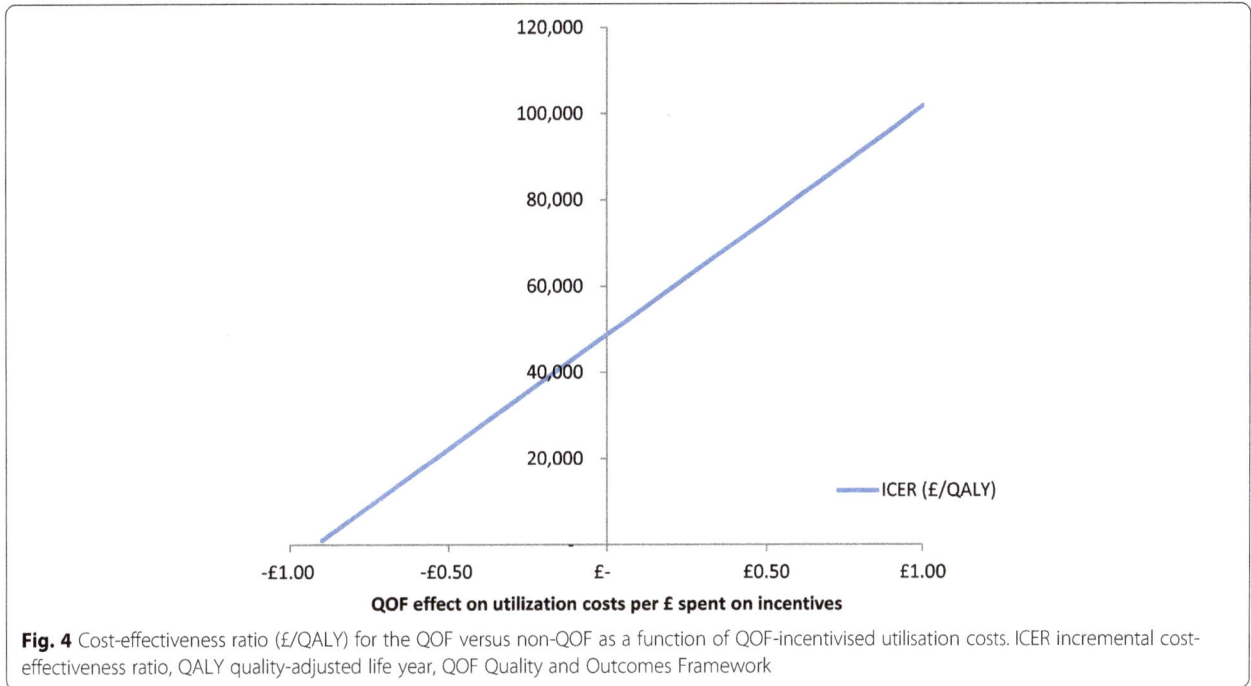

Fig. 4 Cost-effectiveness ratio (£/QALY) for the QOF versus non-QOF as a function of QOF-incentivised utilisation costs. ICER incremental cost-effectiveness ratio, QALY quality-adjusted life year, QOF Quality and Outcomes Framework

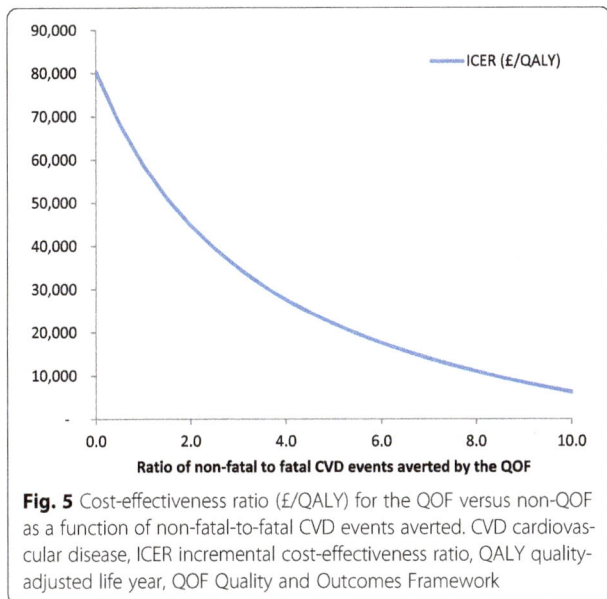

Fig. 5 Cost-effectiveness ratio (£/QALY) for the QOF versus non-QOF as a function of non-fatal-to-fatal CVD events averted. CVD cardiovascular disease, ICER incremental cost-effectiveness ratio, QALY quality-adjusted life year, QOF Quality and Outcomes Framework

Abbreviations

BHF: British heart Foundation; CEAC: Cost-effectiveness acceptability curve; DDD: Defined daily dose; EQ-5D: EuroQOL 5 dimensions; ICD: International classification of diseases; ICER: Incremental cost-effectiveness ratio; NICE: National Institute for health and care excellence; NHS: National health service; PU: Prescribing unit; QALY: Quality-adjusted life year; QOF: Quality and Outcomes Framework; UK: United Kingdom; US: United States

Authors' contributions

AP, TD and AMR conceived the idea of the study. AP, TD, JZ and SW developed the simulation model and estimated model inputs. AP and JZ performed the model-based analyses. AP, EA and AMR wrote the first draft of the manuscript. All authors read and approved the final manuscript.

Competing interests

The authors declare that they have no competing interests.

Author details

[1]Department of Health Policy and Management, Harvard T.H. Chan School of Public Health, 718 Huntington Ave, 2nd Floor, Boston, MA 02115, USA. [2]Department of Health Sciences, University of York, Heslington, York, UK. [3]Center for Health Decision Science, Harvard T.H. Chan School of Public Health, Boston, MA, USA. [4]Centre for Health Economics, University of York, Heslington, York, UK. [5]Department of Health Management and Policy, University of Michigan School of Public Health, Ann Arbor, MI, USA.

References

1. Roland M. Linking physicians' pay to the quality of care--a major experiment in the United Kingdom. N Engl J Med. 2004;351(14):1448–54.
2. Doran T, Kontopantelis E, Valderas JM, Campbell S, Roland M, Salisbury C, Reeves D. Effect of financial incentives on incentivised and non-incentivised clinical activities: longitudinal analysis of data from the UK quality and outcomes framework. BMJ. 2011;342:d3590.
3. Campbell SM, Reeves D, Kontopantelis E, Sibbald B, Roland M. Effects of pay for performance on the quality of primary care in England. N Engl J Med. 2009;361(4):368–78.
4. Fleetcroft R, Parekh-Bhurke S, Howe A, Cookson R, Swift L, Steel N. The UK pay-for-performance programme in primary care: estimation of population mortality reduction. Br J Gen Pract. 2010;60(578):e345–52.
5. Gillam SJ, Siriwardena AN, Steel N. Pay-for-performance in the United Kingdom: impact of the quality and outcomes framework: a systematic review. Ann Fam Med. 2012;10(5):461–8.
6. Ryan AM, Krinsky S, Kontopantelis E, Doran T. Long-term evidence for the effect of pay-for-performance in primary care on mortality in the UK: a population study. Lancet. 2016;388(10041):268–74.

7. Changes to QOF 2014/15: NHS Employers; 2017. http://www.nhsemployers.org/your-workforce/primary-care-contacts/general-medical-services/quality-and-outcomes-framework/changes-to-qof-2014-15.
8. Scotland first to abolish bureaucratic system of GP payments. Government S. 2015. https://news.gov.scot/news/scotland-first-to-abolish-bureaucratic-system-of-gp-payments.
9. Walker S, Mason AR, Claxton K, Cookson R, Fenwick E, Fleetcroft R, Sculpher M. Value for money and the quality and outcomes framework in primary care in the UK NHS. Br J Gen Prac. 2010;60(574):e213–20.
10. Emmert M, Eijkenaar F, Kemter H, Esslinger AS, Schoffski O. Economic evaluation of pay-for-performance in health care: a systematic review. Eur J Health Econ. 2012;13(6):755–67.
11. Meacock R, Kristensen SR, Sutton M. The cost-effectiveness of using financial incentives to improve provider quality: a framework and application. Health Econ. 2014;23(1):1–13.
12. Eijkenaar F, Emmert M, Scheppach M, Schoffski O. Effects of pay for performance in health care: a systematic review of systematic reviews. Health Policy. 2013;110(2–3):115–30.
13. Nahra TA, Reiter KL, Hirth RA, Shermer JE, Wheeler JR. Cost-effectiveness of hospital pay-for-performance incentives. Med Care Res Rev. 2006;63(1 Suppl):49S–72S.
14. Guide to the methods of technology appraisal. National Institute for Health and Care Excellence. 2013. https://www.nice.org.uk/process/pmg9/resources/guide-to-the-methods-of-technology-appraisal-2013-pdf-2007975843781.
15. Population Estimates for UK, England and Wales, Scotland and Northern Ireland: Office for National Statistics. 2016.https://www.ons.gov.uk/peoplepopulationandcommunity/populationandmigration/populationestimates/datasets/populationestimatesforukenglandandwalesscotlandandnorthernireland.
16. Cardiovascular Disease Statistics 2015. British Heart Foundation. 2015.https://www.bhf.org.uk/informationsupport/publications/statistics/cvd-stats-2015.
17. Doran T, Fullwood C, Gravelle H, Reeves D, Kontopantelis E, Hiroeh U, Roland M. Pay-for-performance programs in family practices in the United Kingdom. N Engl J Med. 2006;355(4):375–84.
18. Smolina K, Wright FL, Rayner M, Goldacre MJ. Long-term survival and recurrence after acute myocardial infarction in England, 2004 to 2010. Cir Cardiovas Qual Outcomes. 2012;5(4):532–40.
19. Roberts M, Russell LB, Paltiel AD, Chambers M, McEwan P, Krahn M. Conceptualizing a model: a report of the ISPOR-SMDM modeling good research practices task Force-2. Med Decis Mak. 2012;32(5):678–89.
20. Baigent C, Keech A, Kearney PM, Blackwell L, Buck G, Pollicino C, Kirby A, Sourjina T, Peto R, Collins R, et al. Efficacy and safety of cholesterol-lowering treatment: prospective meta-analysis of data from 90,056 participants in 14 randomised trials of statins. Lancet. 2005;366(9493):1267–78.
21. Sullivan PW, Ghushchyan V. Preference-based EQ-5D index scores for chronic conditions in the United States. Med Decis Mak. 2006;26(4):410–20.
22. Dolan P. Modeling valuations for EuroQol health states. Med Care. 1997;35(11):1095–108.
23. Sullivan PW, Slejko JF, Sculpher MJ, Ghushchyan V. Catalogue of EQ-5D scores for the United Kingdom. Med Decis Mak. 2011;31(6):800–4.
24. Investment in General Practice 2003/04 to 2007/08 England, Wales, and Northern Ireland. National Health Service. 2009. http://webarchive.nationalarchives.gov.uk/20180328130852tf_/http://content.digital.nhs.uk/catalogue/PUB01074/inve-gene-prac-eng-wal-ni-03-08-rep.pdf/.
25. Roland M, Guthrie B. Quality and outcomes framework: what have we learnt? BMJ. 2016;354:i4060.
26. Investment in General Practice 2008/09 to 2012/13 England, Wales, Northern Ireland and Scotland. National Health Service. 2013. http://webarchive.nationalarchives.gov.uk/20180328130852tf_/http://content.digital.nhs.uk/catalogue/PUB11679/inve-gene-prac-eng-wal-ni-scot-08-13.pdf/.
27. Quality and Outcomes Framework. Information Services Division Scotland. 2016. http://www.isdscotland.org/health-Topics/General-Practice/Quality-And-Outcomes-Framework/.
28. Doran T, Roland M. Lessons from major initiatives to improve primary care in the United Kingdom. Health Aff (Millwood). 2010;29(5):1023–9.
29. MacBride-Stewart SP, Elton R, Walley T. Do quality incentives change prescribing patterns in primary care? An observational study in Scotland. Fam Pract. 2008;25(1):27–32.
30. Department of Health. NHS reference costs: financial year 2011 to 2012. 2012.
31. Walker S, Asaria M, Manca A, Palmer S, Gale CP, Shah AD, Abrams KR, Crowther M, Timmis A, Hemingway H, et al. Long-term healthcare use and

costs in patients with stable coronary artery disease: a population-based cohort using linked health records (CALIBER). Eur Heart J Qual Care Clin Outcomes. 2016;2(2):125–40.

32. Asaria M. Health Care Costs in the English NHS: reference tables for average annual NHS. https://www.york.ac.uk/media/che/documents/papers/researchpapers/CHERP147_health_care_costs_NHS.pdf.

33. Claxton K, Martin S, Soares M, Rice N, Spackman E, Hinde S, Devlin N, Smith PC, Sculpher M. Methods for the estimation of the National Institute for health and care excellence cost-effectiveness threshold. Health Technol Assess. 2015;19(14):1–503. v-vi

34. Stinnett AA, Mullahy J. Net health benefits: a new framework for the analysis of uncertainty in cost-effectiveness analysis. Med Decis Mak. 1998;18(2 Suppl):S68–80.

35. Doubilet P, Begg CB, Weinstein MC, Braun P, McNeil BJ. Probabilistic sensitivity analysis using Monte Carlo simulation. A practical approach. Med Decis Making. 1985;5(2):157–77.

36. Sutton M, Nikolova S, Boaden R, Lester H, McDonald R, Roland M. Reduced mortality with hospital pay for performance in England. N Engl J Med. 2012;367(19):1821–8.

37. Kreif N, Grieve R, Hangartner D, Turner AJ, Nikolova S, Sutton M. Examination of the synthetic control method for evaluating health policies with multiple treated units. Health Econ. 2016;25(12):1514–28.

38. Kristensen SR, Meacock R, Turner AJ, Boaden R, McDonald R, Roland M, Sutton M. Long-term effect of hospital pay for performance on mortality in England. N Engl J Med. 2014;371(6):540–8.

39. Doran T, Kontopantelis E, Reeves D, Sutton M, Ryan AM. Setting performance targets in pay for performance programmes: what can we learn from QOF? Bmj. 2014;348:g1595.

40. Improving together. A national framework for quality and GP clusters in Scotland. Scottish Government. 2017. http://www.gov.scot/Resource/0051/00512739.pdf.

41. NHS five year forward view: national health service England; 2017.https://www.england.nhs.uk/five-year-forward-view/next-steps-on-the-nhs-five-year-forward-view/primary-care/.

42. Braithwaite RS, Omokaro C, Justice AC, Nucifora K, Roberts MS. Can broader diffusion of value-based insurance design increase benefits from US health care without increasing costs? Evidence from a computer simulation model. PLoS Med. 2010;7(2):e1000234.

43. O'Reilly D, Holbrook A, Blackhouse G, Troyan S, Goeree R. Cost-effectiveness of a shared computerized decision support system for diabetes linked to electronic medical records. J Am Med Inform Assoc. 2012;19(3):341–5.

44. Lee VS, Kawamoto K, Hess R, Park C, Young J, Hunter C, Johnson S, Gulbransen S, Pelt CE, Horton DJ, et al. Implementation of a value-driven outcomes program to identify high variability in clinical costs and outcomes and association with reduced cost and improved quality. JAMA. 2016;316(10):1061–72.

45. National jife tbles. United Kingdom: Office for national statistics; 2016. https://www.ons.gov.uk/peoplepopulationandcommunity/birthsdeathsandmarriages/lifeexpectancies/datasets/nationallifetablesunitedkingdomreferencetables.

3

Serum magnesium levels and risk of coronary artery disease: Mendelian randomisation study

Susanna C. Larsson[1*], Stephen Burgess[2,3] and Karl Michaëlsson[4]

Abstract

Background: Observational studies have shown that serum magnesium levels are inversely associated with risk of cardiovascular disease, but whether this association is causal is unknown. We conducted a Mendelian randomisation study to investigate whether serum magnesium levels may be causally associated with coronary artery disease (CAD).

Methods: This Mendelian randomisation analysis is based on summary-level data from the CARDIoGRAMplusC4D consortium's 1000 Genomes-based genome-wide association meta-analysis of 48 studies with a total of 60,801 CAD cases and 123,504 non-cases. Six single-nucleotide polymorphisms associated with serum magnesium levels at genome-wide significance were used as instrumental variables.

Results: A genetic predisposition to higher serum magnesium levels was inversely associated with CAD. In conventional Mendelian randomisation analysis, the odds ratio of CAD was 0.88 (95% confidence interval [CI] 0.78 to 0.99; $P = 0.03$) per 0.1-mmol/L (about 1 standard deviation) increase in genetically predicted serum magnesium levels. Results were consistent in sensitivity analyses using the weighted median and heterogeneity-penalised model averaging methods, with odds ratios of 0.84 (95% CI 0.72 to 0.98; $P = 0.03$) and 0.83 (95% CI 0.71 to 0.96; $P = 0.02$), respectively.

Conclusions: This study based on genetics provides evidence that serum magnesium levels are inversely associated with risk of CAD. Randomised controlled trials elucidating whether magnesium supplementation lowers the risk of CAD, preferably in a setting at higher risk of hypomagnesaemia, are warranted.

Keywords: Coronary artery disease, Magnesium, Mendelian randomisation, Single-nucleotide polymorphisms

Background

Magnesium is the second most abundant intracellular cation. It plays a crucial role in many processes regulating cardiovascular function, such as vascular tone, endothelial function and myocardial excitability, and it is involved in regulation of glucose and insulin metabolism [1, 2]. Experimental evidence indicates that magnesium insufficiency promotes atherosclerosis and that magnesium fortification attenuates atherogenesis [2–7]. Moreover, randomised controlled trials have shown that magnesium supplementation improves endothelial function [8, 9] and reduces blood pressure [8, 10–12], arterial stiffness [13], fasting glucose [12, 14], insulin resistance [15] and postoperative arrhythmias [16, 17]. Randomised controlled trials assessing whether magnesium supplementation may prevent cardiovascular events are lacking.

Evidence from observational studies indicates that high circulating magnesium levels and magnesium intake are associated with a modest reduction in risk of cardiovascular disease, including coronary heart disease [18, 19], but the causality of these associations is unknown. The observed inverse association between magnesium and cardiovascular disease may be due to confounding by other potentially cardioprotective nutrients in magnesium-rich foods or by health behaviours adopted by individuals consuming these foods. Rich food sources of magnesium include green leafy vegetables, legumes, nuts, seeds, avocados, dark chocolate, whole grains, yoghurt and fish. It has been estimated that magnesium intake from a normal Western diet is often inadequate. In the USA, two-thirds

* Correspondence: susanna.larsson@ki.se
[1]Unit of Nutritional Epidemiology, Institute of Environmental Medicine, Karolinska Institutet, 171 77 Stockholm, Sweden
Full list of author information is available at the end of the article

of the adult population has a magnesium intake below the estimated average requirement [20].

Exploiting genetic variants as instrumental variables of an exposure can strengthen causal inference regarding an exposure-outcome relationship. This technique, known as Mendelian randomisation (MR), reduces confounding because genetic variants are randomly allocated at meiosis and thus should be unrelated to self-selected lifestyle factors and behaviours. It also overcomes reverse causation bias since allelic randomisation always precedes the onset of disease. Causal inference from an MR study relies on the instrumental variable assumptions, which require that the genetic variant is robustly associated with the exposure; independent of confounders of the exposure-outcome relationship; and influences the outcome through the exposure only and not through any alternative causal pathway (Fig. 1) [21].

We applied a two-sample MR framework to determine the causal association between serum magnesium levels and coronary artery disease (CAD).

Methods
Genetic variants and data sources
We used an MR study design based on publicly available summary-level data from genome-wide association studies (GWASs) (Table 1). As instrumental variables for the MR analyses, we selected all single-nucleotide polymorphisms (SNPs) associated with serum magnesium levels at genome-wide significance ($P < 5 \times 10^{-8}$) in the largest available GWAS on serum magnesium levels [22]. We selected all six SNPs that achieved genome-wide significance in the joint analysis of the discovery ($n = 15,366$ individuals) and replication ($n = 8463$ individuals) cohorts [22]. All the SNPs were in different genomic regions and in linkage equilibrium.

Summary-level data (beta coefficients and standard errors) for the associations of the six magnesium-associated

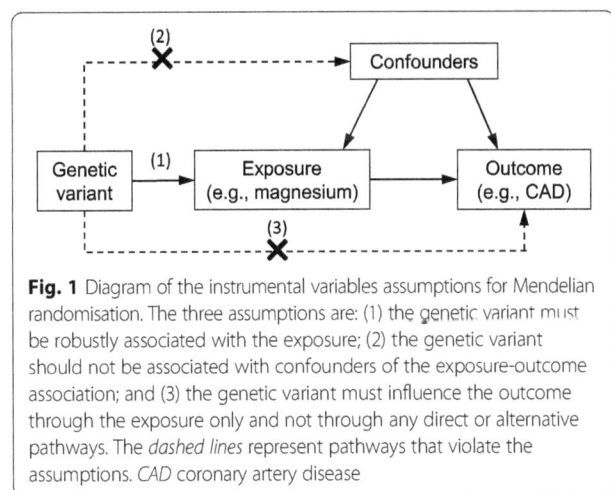

Fig. 1 Diagram of the instrumental variables assumptions for Mendelian randomisation. The three assumptions are: (1) the genetic variant must be robustly associated with the exposure; (2) the genetic variant should not be associated with confounders of the exposure-outcome association; and (3) the genetic variant must influence the outcome through the exposure only and not through any direct or alternative pathways. The *dashed lines* represent pathways that violate the assumptions. *CAD* coronary artery disease

SNPs with CAD were acquired from the CARDIoGRAMplusC4D consortium's 1000 Genomes-based genome-wide association meta-analysis of 60,801 CAD cases and 123,504 non-cases from 48 studies [23]. One SNP (rs7965584) was not part of the CARDIoGRAMplusC4D dataset and was replaced by a linked SNP (rs10858938; $r^2 = 0.96$ in Europeans). In the CARDIoGRAMplusC4D consortium, CAD was defined using a broad definition that included myocardial infarction (about 70% of the total number of cases), acute coronary syndrome, chronic stable angina or coronary artery stenosis of at least 50% [23]. Ethical approval was not sought, because this study involved analysis of publicly available summary-level data (beta coefficients and standard errors) from GWASs, and no individual-level data were used.

Statistical analysis
The main analysis was conducted using the conventional inverse-variance weighted method [24] (hereafter referred to as conventional MR analysis). Several sensitivity analyses were carried out, including (1) the leave-one-out analysis, in which one SNP in turn was removed to evaluate the impact of outlying SNPs; (2) the weighted median method, which gives accurate estimates if at least 50% of the instrumental variables are valid [24]; (3) the heterogeneity-penalised model averaging method, which provides consistent estimates if a plurality of the instrumental variables are valid [25]; and (4) MR-Egger regression, which can detect and adjust for pleiotropy [24, 26]. MR-Egger is disposed to effect estimate dilution due to the NO Measurement Error (NOME) assumption for the instrument-exposure associations. The NOME assumption was tested using the I^2_{GX} statistic, and the MR-Egger estimate was adjusted for dilution using the simulation extrapolation (SIMEX) method [27]. The strength of the instrumental variables was assessed using the F-statistic [28].

To investigate potential pleiotropy and mediating pathways from serum magnesium to CAD, we performed conventional MR analyses of the association of serum magnesium levels with cardiometabolic risk factors, using publicly available GWAS data [29–34] (Table 1).

All reported odds ratios (ORs) with their 95% confidence intervals (CIs) are scaled to a 0.1-mmol/L (about one standard deviation [SD]) increase in serum magnesium levels. All statistical tests were two-sided and considered statistically significant at $P < 0.05$. The analyses were conducted using the mrrobust [35] and MendelianRandomization [36] packages.

Results
The six magnesium-associated SNPs explained 1.62% of the variance in serum magnesium levels, and the mean F-statistic was 64 (Table 2). Five of the SNPs were

Table 1 Details of studies and datasets used for analyses

Exposure/outcome	Consortium	Participants	Web source if publicly available
Serum magnesium	CHARGE and replication studies [22]	23,829 individuals of European ancestry	Not available
Coronary artery disease	CARDIoGRAMplusC4D consortium's 1000 Genomes-based GWAS [23]	184,305 individuals (60,801 CAD cases and 123,504 non-cases) of mainly European (77%) and Asian (19%) ancestry	www.cardiogramplusc4d.org/
Blood pressure	ICBP [29]	69,395 individuals of European ancestry	www.ncbi.nlm.nih.gov/projects/gap/cgi-bin/study.cgi?study_id=phs000585.v1.p1
Lipids	GLGC [30]	188,577 individuals of European ancestry	csg.sph.umich.edu/abecasis/public/lipids2013/
Glycaemic traits	MAGIC [31]	46,186 non-diabetic individuals of European ancestry	www.magicinvestigators.org/
Body mass index	GIANT [32]	339,224 individuals of mainly European (95%) ancestry	portals.broadinstitute.org/collaboration/giant/index.php/GIANT_consortium
Waist-to-hip ratio	GIANT [33]	224,459 individuals of mainly European (94%) ancestry	portals.broadinstitute.org/collaboration/giant/index.php/GIANT_consortium
Smoking	TAGC [34]	74,053 individuals of European ancestry	www.med.unc.edu/pgc/results-and-downloads

CHARGE Cohorts for Heart and Aging Research in Genomic Epidemiology Consortium, *GIANT* Genetic Investigation of Anthropometric Traits, *GLGC* Global Lipids Genetics Consortium, *ICBP* International Consortium for Blood Pressure, *MAGIC* Meta-Analyses of Glucose and Insulin-related traits Consortium, *TAGC* Tobacco and Genetics Consortium

inversely, albeit non-statistically significantly, associated with CAD (Table 2). In conventional MR analysis, genetically predicted serum magnesium was inversely associated with CAD, but there was evidence of heterogeneity between estimates from individual SNPs ($P_{\text{heterogeneity}} = 0.06$). The ORs of CAD per a 0.1-mmol/L (about one SD) increase in genetically predicted serum magnesium levels were 0.88 (95% CI, 0.78–0.99; $P = 0.03$) and 0.88 (95% CI, 0.74–1.05; $P = 0.14$) when standard errors were calculated using fixed-effects and random-effects models, respectively (Fig. 2). In the leave-one-out analysis, it was found that rs11144134 in the *TRPM6* gene region was responsible for the heterogeneity among estimates from individual SNPs. After exclusion of this SNP, there was no heterogeneity between estimates ($P_{\text{heterogeneity}} = 0.73$), and the OR was

0.82 (95% CI, 0.72–0.93; $P = 0.002$) in both fixed-effects and random-effects models (Fig. 2).

Results were consistent in sensitivity analyses using the weighted median (OR, 0.84; 95% CI, 0.72–0.98; $P = 0.03$) and heterogeneity-penalised model averaging (OR, 0.83; 95% CI, 0.71–0.96; $P = 0.02$) methods (Additional file 1: Table S1). The MR-Egger analysis did not provide evidence of either directional pleiotropy (intercept −0.023; $P = 0.21$) or a causal association (OR = 1.19; 95% CI, 0.72–1.98; $P = 0.50$), but the precision of the estimates was low (Additional file 1: Table S1). I^2_{GX} was 0.87 (relative bias of 13% towards the null), and adjusting for dilution bias using the SIMEX method did not materially change the MR-Egger estimate (Additional file 1: Table S1).

Table 2 Characteristics of the single-nucleotide polymorphisms associated with serum magnesium levels

SNP	Closest gene	Chr	EA[b]	EAF[c]	% variance explained	F-statistic	Association with magnesium[a]			Association with CAD[a]		
							Beta (mmol/L)	SE	P	Beta[d]	SE	P
rs4072037	*MUC1*	1	T	0.54	0.57	136	0.010	0.001	2.0×10^{-36}	−0.015	0.010	0.11
rs7965584[e]	*ATP2B1*	12	A	0.71	0.25	60	0.007	0.001	1.1×10^{-16}	−0.016	0.011	0.13
rs3925584	*DCDC5*	11	T	0.55	0.25	60	0.006	0.001	5.2×10^{-16}	−0.016	0.010	0.09
rs11144134	*TRPM6*	9	C	0.08	0.23	55	0.011	0.001	8.2×10^{-15}	0.039	0.019	0.04
rs13146355	*SHROOM3*	4	A	0.44	0.19	45	0.005	0.001	6.3×10^{-13}	−0.003	0.010	0.76
rs448378	*MDS1*	3	A	0.53	0.13	30	0.004	0.001	1.3×10^{-8}	−0.017	0.009	0.06

CAD coronary artery disease, *Chr* chromosome, *EA* effect allele, *EAF* effect allele frequency, *SE* standard error, *SNP* single-nucleotide polymorphism
[a]Beta coefficients and standard errors were obtained from genome-wide association studies on serum magnesium (23,829 individuals) [22] and CAD (60,801 cases and 123,504 non-cases) [23]
[b]Allele associated with higher serum magnesium levels
[c]Frequency of the magnesium-raising allele in the magnesium genome-wide association study [22]
[d]Log odds ratio of CAD for each additional magnesium-increasing allele
[e]Proxy (rs10858938; $r^2 = 0.96$ in European descent individuals) was used in the CAD data

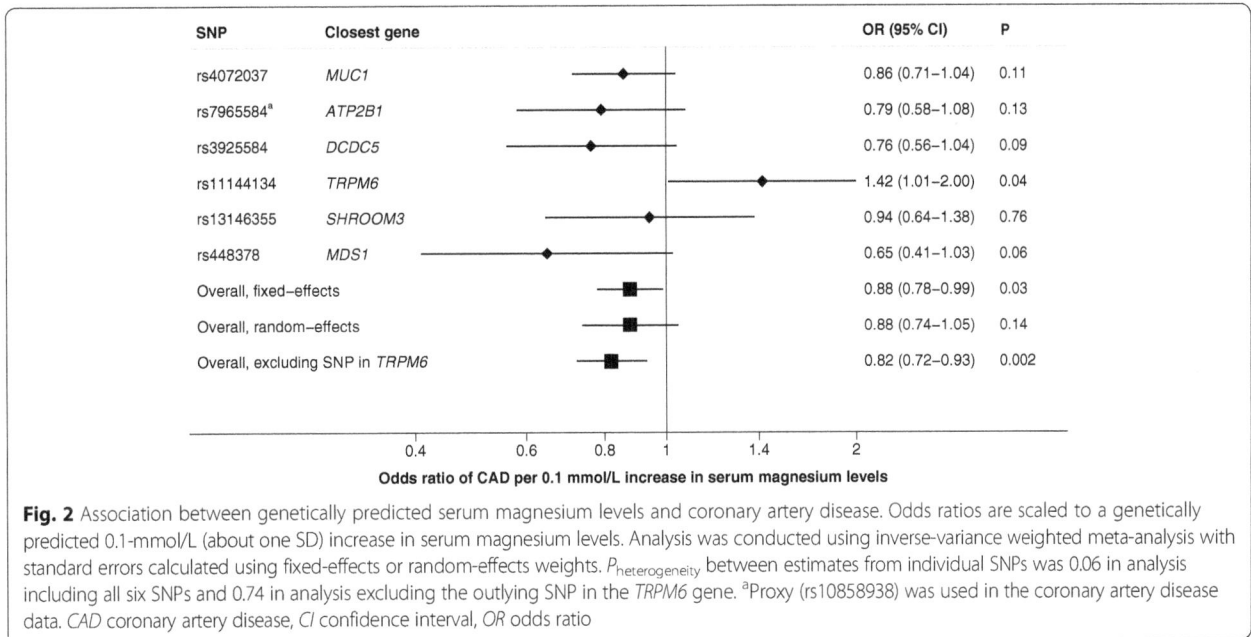

Fig. 2 Association between genetically predicted serum magnesium levels and coronary artery disease. Odds ratios are scaled to a genetically predicted 0.1-mmol/L (about one SD) increase in serum magnesium levels. Analysis was conducted using inverse-variance weighted meta-analysis with standard errors calculated using fixed-effects or random-effects weights. $P_{heterogeneity}$ between estimates from individual SNPs was 0.06 in analysis including all six SNPs and 0.74 in analysis excluding the outlying SNP in the *TRPM6* gene. [a]Proxy (rs10858938) was used in the coronary artery disease data. *CAD* coronary artery disease, *CI* confidence interval, *OR* odds ratio

In conventional MR analyses, genetic predisposition to higher serum magnesium levels was weakly associated with higher systolic blood pressure ($P = 0.04$) and triglycerides ($P = 0.04$), but was not associated with diastolic blood pressure, cholesterol, fasting glucose, fasting insulin, insulin resistance, body mass index, waist-to-hip ratio or smoking (Table 3).

Discussion

The main result of this study is that genetic variants predisposing to higher serum magnesium levels may confer a decreased risk of CAD. A genetically predicted 0.1-mmol/L (about one SD) increase in serum magnesium levels was associated with 12% lower odds of CAD in the primary analysis. This finding corroborates the results from observational prospective studies showing inverse associations of circulating magnesium levels and dietary magnesium intake with risk of coronary heart disease and cardiovascular disease [18] (Fig. 3).

There is no gold standard MR analysis method. Available methods have advantages and limitations that balance precision and adjustment for bias. In the present study, several MR approaches were applied to evaluate the robustness of the causal association between serum magnesium levels and CAD. Although we cannot entirely rule out pleiotropy, we observed a consistent inverse association between serum magnesium levels and CAD in conventional MR analysis and sensitivity analyses using the weighted median and heterogeneity-penalised model averaging methods. MR-Egger analysis, which has lower statistical power compared with the other methods, suggested no bias due to pleiotropy (i.e. when a genetic variant affects more than one phenotype) and did not detect a

causal association, but the confidence interval was wide. The I^2_{GX} and *F*-statistics were high, suggesting that violation of the NOME assumption was limited and that weak instrument bias due to dilution did not materially affect the results. As in any MR study, we cannot entirely

Table 3 Associations between genetically predicted serum magnesium levels and cardiometabolic risk factors

Outcome	Estimate[a]	P value
Continuous outcomes	Beta (95% CI)	
Diastolic blood pressure	0.46 (−0.34 to 1.26) mm Hg	0.26
Systolic blood pressure	1.31 (0.05 to 2.57) mm Hg	0.04
Low-density lipoprotein cholesterol	0.06 (−0.00 to 0.13) SD	0.07
High-density lipoprotein cholesterol	−0.03 (−0.09 to 0.03) SD	0.34
Triglycerides	0.06 (0.00 to 0.12) SD	0.04
Fasting glucose	0.02 (−0.03 to 0.07) mmol/L	0.35
Fasting insulin	0.02 (−0.03 to 0.07) log pmol/L	0.43
HOMA-IR	0.01 (−0.04 to 0.06)	0.67
BMI	−0.02 (−0.07 to 0.02) SD	0.34
Waist-to-hip ratio adjusted for BMI	0.02 (−0.03 to 0.07) SD	0.50
Cigarettes per day	−0.59 (−1.66 to 0.49) cigarettes/day	0.29
Binary outcomes	OR (95% CI)	
Ever smoker	1.00 (0.98 to 1.01)	0.62
Former smoker	1.00 (0.98 to 1.02)	0.78

BMI body mass index, *CI* confidence interval, *HOMA-IR* homeostatic model assessment of insulin resistance, *OR* odds ratio, *SD* standard deviation
[a]Estimates correspond to a 0.1-mmol/L (about one SD) increase in genetically predicted serum magnesium levels

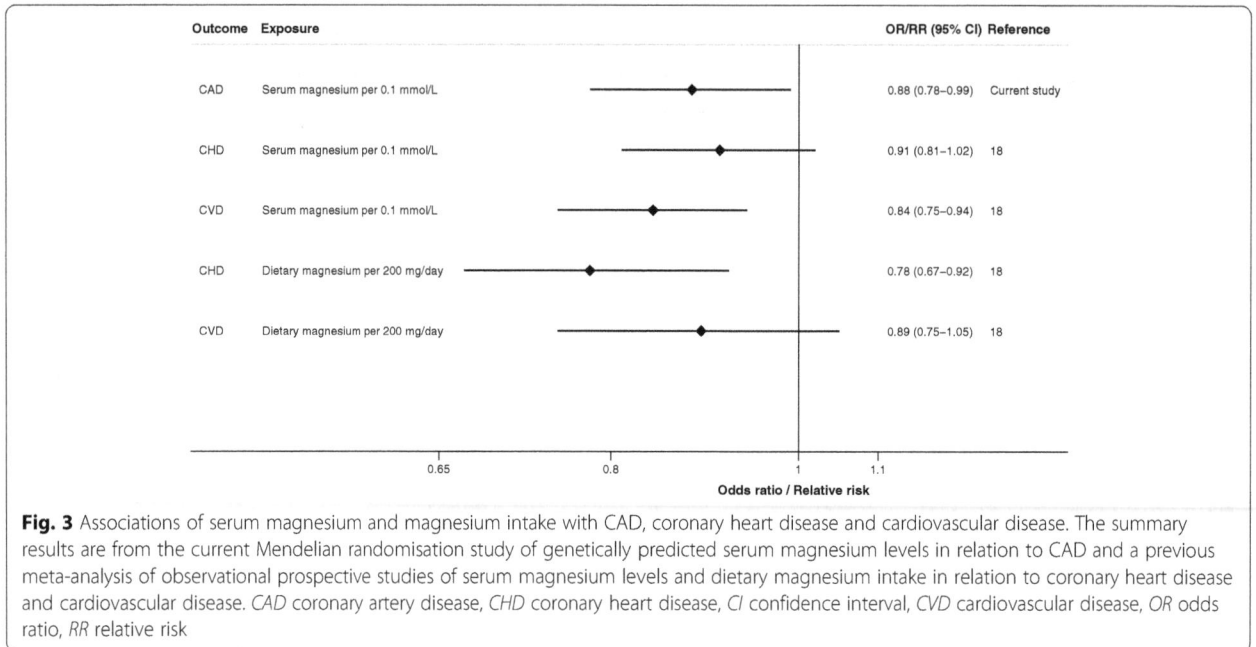

Fig. 3 Associations of serum magnesium and magnesium intake with CAD, coronary heart disease and cardiovascular disease. The summary results are from the current Mendelian randomisation study of genetically predicted serum magnesium levels in relation to CAD and a previous meta-analysis of observational prospective studies of serum magnesium levels and dietary magnesium intake in relation to coronary heart disease and cardiovascular disease. *CAD* coronary artery disease, *CHD* coronary heart disease, *CI* confidence interval, *CVD* cardiovascular disease, *OR* odds ratio, *RR* relative risk

exclude population stratification as a source of bias in this study. However, the GWAS datasets used for the present analyses largely comprised individuals of European ancestry and adjustment was made for ancestry within the contributing studies, reducing possible bias due to population stratification.

There are several plausible mechanisms whereby magnesium may affect the risk of CAD. Magnesium is involved in blood pressure regulation and in glucose and insulin metabolism [1, 2]. Meta-analyses of randomised controlled trials have shown that magnesium supplementation may modestly reduce blood pressure [8, 10–12], fasting glucose [12, 14] and insulin resistance [15]. However, we found no evidence that genetically higher magnesium levels were associated with lower blood pressure or glycaemic traits, suggesting that these risk factors are not likely mediators or confounders of the magnesium-CAD relationship. In addition, the inverse association between serum magnesium levels and CAD is unlikely explained by major lipids, as genetically higher magnesium levels were not associated with cholesterol but were weakly associated with higher triglycerides, which increase CAD risk [37].

Magnesium could potentially confer protection against CAD by enhancing endothelium-dependent vasodilation and reducing vascular resistance, oxidative stress and oxidised lipids, inflammation and thrombosis, and by anti-arrhythmic effects [2, 4, 7, 16, 17]. Several [8, 9, 13] but not all [38, 39] randomised trials have shown that magnesium supplementation improves endothelial function and reduces arterial stiffness. The inconsistent results may be related to magnesium status among study participants, as improvement in endothelial function

with magnesium supplementation was observed in trials involving patients with low serum magnesium levels [9] and patients using diuretics [8], which often cause hypomagnesaemia. Both extracellular and intracellular free magnesium can modulate vascular smooth muscle tone [2]. Extracellular magnesium is considered to be a calcium antagonist, because it inhibits many of the physiological actions of calcium [2, 40]. Magnesium decreases calcium release from and into the sarcoplasmic reticulum and protects the cells against calcium overload during myocardial ischaemia [2, 40]. Multiple lines of evidence indicate that a modestly elevated serum calcium level increases CAD risk [41–43]. In this context, mutations in *TRPM6* (encoding a transient receptor potential cation channel) cause hypomagnesaemia with secondary hypocalcaemia [44, 45]. Hence, the observed positive association between the magnesium-raising allele of the genetic variant in *TRPM6* and CAD might be mediated by calcium. Another magnesium-associated genetic variant is located nearby the *ATP2B1* gene, which encodes plasma-membrane calcium ATPase responsible for removal of calcium ions from cells [22].

A limitation of this study is that the specific biological functions of most of the genetic variants associated with serum magnesium levels are unknown (Additional file 1: Table S2). However, the magnesium-associated SNPs have shown association with hypomagnesaemia and with phenotypes related to serum magnesium levels, such as fasting glucose (SNP in *MUC1*), bone mineral density (SNPs in *MUC1* and *TRPM6*) and kidney function (SNPs in *SHROOM3* and *DCDC5*) [22]. Kidney function has been associated with cardiovascular disease risk in observational studies [46], but there was little support for a causal association between kidney function and coronary heart disease in a recent MR analysis [47], suggesting that the observed association between magnesium levels and CAD in the present study is unlikely mediated by kidney function. Further research is needed to better understand the role of the genetic variants and their link to circulating and intracellular magnesium levels.

Conclusions

This study based on genetics provides evidence that serum magnesium levels are inversely associated with risk of CAD. Randomised controlled trials elucidating whether magnesium supplementation reduces the risk of CAD are warranted. As magnesium supplementation is expected to be most beneficial in individuals with an inadequate magnesium status, such a trial may preferably involve a setting with persons at higher risk of hypomagnesaemia.

Abbreviations

CAD: Coronary artery disease; CI: Confidence interval; GWAS: Genome-wide association study; NOME: NO Measurement Error; OR: Odds ratio; SD: Standard deviation; SIMEX: Simulation extrapolation; SNP: Single-nucleotide polymorphism

Acknowledgements

Data on genetic associations with CAD have been contributed by CARDIoGRAMplusC4D investigators and have been downloaded from www.cardiogramplusc4d.org/. Data on genetic associations with glycaemic traits have been contributed by the Meta-Analyses of Glucose and Insulin-related traits Consortium (MAGIC) investigators and have been downloaded from www.magicinvestigators.org. The authors also wish to thank the Tobacco and Genetics Consortium (TAGC), the International Consortium for Blood Pressure (ICBP) Genome-Wide Association Studies (dbGaP accession phs000585.v1.p1), the Global Lipids Genetics Consortium (GLGC) and the Genetic Investigation of Anthropometric Traits (GIANT) Consortium for access to their data.

Authors' contributions

SCL had full access to all of the data in the study and takes responsibility for the integrity of the data and the accuracy of the data analysis. SCL, SB and KM conceived and designed the study. SCL acquired the data and performed the statistical analysis. SCL, SB and KM interpreted the data. SCL drafted the manuscript. SCL, SB and KM critically revised the manuscript for important intellectual content. All authors read and approved the final manuscript.

Competing interests

The authors declare that they have no competing interests.

Author details

[1]Unit of Nutritional Epidemiology, Institute of Environmental Medicine, Karolinska Institutet, 171 77 Stockholm, Sweden. [2]MRC Biostatistics Unit, University of Cambridge, Cambridge, UK. [3]Department of Public Health and Primary Care, University of Cambridge, Cambridge, UK. [4]Department of Surgical Sciences, Uppsala University, Uppsala, Sweden.

References

1. Volpe SL. Magnesium, the metabolic syndrome, insulin resistance, and type 2 diabetes mellitus. Crit Rev Food Sci Nutr. 2008;48:293–300.
2. Kolte D, Vijayaraghavan K, Khera S, Sica DA, Frishman WH. Role of magnesium in cardiovascular diseases. Cardiol Rev. 2014;22:182–92.
3. Maier JA. Endothelial cells and magnesium: implications in atherosclerosis. Clin Sci (Lond). 2012;122:397–407.
4. Zheltova AA, Kharitonova MV, Iezhitsa IN, Spasov AA. Magnesium deficiency and oxidative stress: an update. Biomedicine (Taipei). 2016;6:20.
5. Chaudhary DP, Boparai RK, Bansal DD. Implications of oxidative stress in high sucrose low magnesium diet fed rats. Eur J Nutr. 2007;46:383–90.
6. Adrian M, Chanut E, Laurant P, Gaume V, Berthelot A. A long-term moderate magnesium-deficient diet aggravates cardiovascular risks associated with aging and increases mortality in rats. J Hypertens. 2008;26:44–52.
7. Morais JB, Severo JS, Santos LR, de Sousa Melo SR, de Oliveira SR, de Oliveira AR, et al. Role of magnesium in oxidative stress in individuals with obesity. Biol Trace Elem Res. 2017;176:20–6.
8. Cunha AR, D'El-Rei J, Medeiros F, Umbelino B, Oigman W, Touyz RM, et al. Oral magnesium supplementation improves endothelial function and attenuates subclinical atherosclerosis in thiazide-treated hypertensive women. J Hypertens. 2017;35:89–97.
9. Shechter M, Sharir M, Labrador MJ, Forrester J, Silver B, Bairey Merz CN. Oral magnesium therapy improves endothelial function in patients with coronary artery disease. Circulation. 2000;102:2353–8.
10. Zhang X, Li Y, Del Gobbo LC, Rosanoff A, Wang J, Zhang W, et al. Effects of magnesium supplementation on blood pressure: a meta-analysis of randomized double-blind placebo-controlled trials. Hypertension. 2016;68:324–33.
11. Dibaba DT, Xun P, Song Y, Rosanoff A, Shechter M, He K. The effect of magnesium supplementation on blood pressure in individuals with insulin resistance, prediabetes, or noncommunicable chronic diseases: a meta-analysis of randomized controlled trials. Am J Clin Nutr. 2017;106:921–9.
12. Verma H, Garg R. Effect of magnesium supplementation on type 2 diabetes associated cardiovascular risk factors: a systematic review and meta-analysis. J Hum Nutr Diet. 2017;30:621–33.
13. Joris PJ, Plat J, Bakker SJ, Mensink RP. Long-term magnesium supplementation improves arterial stiffness in overweight and obese adults: results of a randomized, double-blind, placebo-controlled intervention trial. Am J Clin Nutr. 2016;103:1260–6.
14. Song Y, He K, Levitan EB, Manson JE, Liu S. Effects of oral magnesium supplementation on glycaemic control in Type 2 diabetes: a meta-analysis of randomized double-blind controlled trials. Diabet Med. 2006;23:1050–6.
15. Simental-Mendia LE, Sahebkar A, Rodriguez-Moran M, Guerrero-Romero F. A systematic review and meta-analysis of randomized controlled trials on the effects of magnesium supplementation on insulin sensitivity and glucose control. Pharmacol Res. 2016;111:272–82.
16. Lee HY, Ghimire S, Kim EY. Magnesium supplementation reduces postoperative arrhythmias after cardiopulmonary bypass in pediatrics: a metaanalysis of randomized controlled trials. Pediatr Cardiol. 2013;34:1396–403.
17. Shiga T, Wajima Z, Inoue T, Ogawa R. Magnesium prophylaxis for arrhythmias after cardiac surgery: a meta-analysis of randomized controlled trials. Am J Med. 2004;117:325–33.
18. Del Gobbo LC, Imamura F, Wu JH, de Oliveira Otto MC, Chiuve SE, Mozaffarian D. Circulating and dietary magnesium and risk of cardiovascular disease: a systematic review and meta-analysis of prospective studies. Am J Clin Nutr. 2013;98:160–73.

19. Fang X, Liang C, Li M, Montgomery S, Fall K, Aaseth J, et al. Dose-response relationship between dietary magnesium intake and cardiovascular mortality: a systematic review and dose-based meta-regression analysis of prospective studies. J Trace Elem Med Biol. 2016;38:64–73.

20. Moshfegh AJ, Goldmand JD, Ahuja JKC, LaComb RP. What we eat in America, NHANES 2005–2006: usual nutrient intakes from food and water compared to 1997 dietary references intakes for vitamin D, calcium, phosphorus, and magnesium. US: Department of Agriculture, Agricultural Research Service; 2009.

21. Burgess S, Thompson SG: Mendelian randomization: methods for using genetic variants in causal estimation. London: Chapman & Hall; 2015.

22. Meyer TE, Verwoert GC, Hwang SJ, Glazer NL, Smith AV, van Rooij FJ, et al. Genome-wide association studies of serum magnesium, potassium, and sodium concentrations identify six loci influencing serum magnesium levels. PLoS Genet. 2010;6:e1001045.

23. Nikpay M, Goel A, Won HH, Hall LM, Willenborg C, Kanoni S, et al. A comprehensive 1,000 Genomes-based genome-wide association meta-analysis of coronary artery disease. Nat Genet. 2015;47:1121–30.

24. Burgess S, Bowden J, Fall T, Ingelsson E, Thompson SG. Sensitivity analyses for robust causal inference from Mendelian randomization analyses with multiple genetic variants. Epidemiology. 2017;28:30–42.

25. Burgess S, Zuber V, Gkatzionis A, Rees JMB, Foley C. Improving on a modal-based estimation method: model averaging for consistent and efficient estimation in Mendelian randomization when a plurality of candidate instruments are valid. BioRxiv https://doi.org/10.1101/175372. 2017.

26. Burgess S, Thompson SG. Interpreting findings from Mendelian randomization using the MR-Egger method. Eur J Epidemiol. 2017;32:377–89.

27. Bowden J, Del Greco MF, Minelli C, Davey Smith G, Sheehan NA, Thompson JR. Assessing the suitability of summary data for two-sample Mendelian randomization analyses using MR-Egger regression: the role of the I2 statistic. Int J Epidemiol. 2016;45:1961–74.

28. Burgess S, Thompson SG. Avoiding bias from weak instruments in Mendelian randomization studies. Int J Epidemiol. 2011;40:755–64.

29. Ehret GB, Munroe PB, Rice KM, Bochud M, Johnson AD, Chasman DI, et al. Genetic variants in novel pathways influence blood pressure and cardiovascular disease risk. Nature. 2011;478:103–9.

30. Willer CJ, Schmidt EM, Sengupta S, Peloso GM, Gustafsson S, Kanoni S, et al. Discovery and refinement of loci associated with lipid levels. Nat Genet. 2013;45:1274–83.

31. Dupuis J, Langenberg C, Prokopenko I, Saxena R, Soranzo N, Jackson AU, et al. New genetic loci implicated in fasting glucose homeostasis and their impact on type 2 diabetes risk. Nat Genet. 2010;42:105–16.

32. Locke AE, Kahali B, Berndt SI, Justice AE, Pers TH, Day FR, et al. Genetic studies of body mass index yield new insights for obesity biology. Nature. 2015;518:197–206.

33. Shungin D, Winkler TW, Croteau-Chonka DC, Ferreira T, Locke AE, Magi R, et al. New genetic loci link adipose and insulin biology to body fat distribution. Nature. 2015;518:187–96.

34. Tobacco and Genetics Consortium. Genome-wide meta-analyses identify multiple loci associated with smoking behavior. Nat Genet. 2010;42:441–7.

35. Spiller W, Davies NM, Palmer TM. Software application profile: mrrobust — a tool for performing two-sample summary Mendelian randomization analyses. BioRxiv https://doi.org/10.1101/142125. 2017.

36. Yavorska OO, Burgess S. MendelianRandomization: an R package for performing Mendelian randomization analyses using summarized data. Int J Epidemiol. 2017; https://doi.org/10.1093/ije/dyx034. [Epub ahead of print].

37. Holmes MV, Asselbergs FW, Palmer TM, Drenos F, Lanktree MB, Nelson CP, et al. Mendelian randomization of blood lipids for coronary heart disease. Eur Heart J. 2015;36:539–50.

38. Joris PJ, Plat J, Bakker SJ, Mensink RP. Effects of long-term magnesium supplementation on endothelial function and cardiometabolic risk markers: a randomized controlled trial in overweight/obese adults. Sci Rep. 2017;7:106.

39. Cosaro E, Bonafini S, Montagnana M, Danese E, Trettene MS, Minuz P, et al. Effects of magnesium supplements on blood pressure, endothelial function and metabolic parameters in healthy young men with a family history of metabolic syndrome. Nutr Metab Cardiovasc Dis. 2014;24:1213–20.

40. Iseri LT, French JH. Magnesium: nature's physiologic calcium blocker. Am Heart J. 1984;108:188–93.

41. Larsson SC, Burgess S, Michaelsson K. Association of genetic variants related to serum calcium levels with coronary artery disease and myocardial infarction. JAMA. 2017;318:371–80.

42. Bolland MJ, Grey A, Avenell A, Gamble GD, Reid IR. Calcium supplements with or without vitamin D and risk of cardiovascular events: reanalysis of the Women's Health Initiative limited access dataset and meta-analysis. BMJ. 2011;342:d2040.

43. Reid IR, Gamble GD, Bolland MJ. Circulating calcium concentrations, vascular disease and mortality: a systematic review. J Intern Med. 2016;279:524–40.

44. Schlingmann KP, Weber S, Peters M, Niemann Nejsum L, Vitzthum H, Klingel K, et al. Hypomagnesemia with secondary hypocalcemia is caused by mutations in TRPM6, a new member of the TRPM gene family. Nat Genet. 2002;31:166–70.

45. Lainez S, Schlingmann KP, van der Wijst J, Dworniczak B, van Zeeland F, Konrad M, et al. New TRPM6 missense mutations linked to hypomagnesemia with secondary hypocalcemia. Eur J Hum Genet. 2014;22:497–504.

46. Pattaro C, Teumer A, Gorski M, Chu AY, Li M, Mijatovic V, et al. Genetic associations at 53 loci highlight cell types and biological pathways relevant for kidney function. Nat Commun. 2016;7:10023.

47. Charoen P, Nitsch D, Engmann J, Shah T, White J, Zabaneh D, et al. Mendelian randomisation study of the influence of eGFR on coronary heart disease. Sci Rep. 2016;6:28514.

4

Neighbourhood level real-time forecasting of dengue cases

Yirong Chen[1] [iD], Janet Hui Yi Ong[2], Jayanthi Rajarethinam[2], Grace Yap[2], Lee Ching Ng[2*] and Alex R. Cook[1]

Abstract

Background: Dengue, a vector-borne infectious disease caused by the dengue virus, has spread through tropical and subtropical regions of the world. All four serotypes of dengue viruses are endemic in the equatorial city state of Singapore, and frequent localised outbreaks occur, sometimes leading to national epidemics. Vector control remains the primary and most effective measure for dengue control and prevention. The objective of this study is to develop a novel framework for producing a spatio-temporal dengue forecast at a neighbourhood level spatial resolution that can be routinely used by Singapore's government agencies for planning of vector control for best efficiency.

Methods: The forecasting algorithm uses a mixture of purely spatial, purely temporal and spatio-temporal data to derive dynamic risk maps for dengue transmission. LASSO-based regression was used for the prediction models and separate sub-models were constructed for each forecast window. Data were divided into training and testing sets for out-of-sample validation. Neighbourhoods were categorised as high or low risk based on the forecast number of cases within the cell. The predictive accuracy of the categorisation was measured.

Results: Close concordance between the projections and the eventual incidence of dengue were observed. The average Matthew's correlation coefficient for a classification of the upper risk decile (operational capacity) is similar to the predictive performance at the optimal 30% cut-off. The quality of the spatial predictive algorithm as a classifier shows areas under the curve at all forecast windows being above 0.75 and above 0.80 within the next month.

Conclusions: Spatially resolved forecasts of geographically structured diseases like dengue can be obtained at a neighbourhood level in highly urban environments at a precision that is suitable for guiding control efforts. The same method can be adapted to other urban and even rural areas, with appropriate adjustment to the grid size and shape.

Keywords: Spatio-temporal prediction, Dengue forecast, LASSO, Control and prevention

Background

Dengue, a vector-borne infectious disease caused by the dengue virus (DENV, four serotypes DENV1–4), has spread through tropical and subtropical regions of the world in recent decades [1]. It is transmitted by the *Aedes* mosquitoes, and in urban areas, primarily by the anthropophilic *Aedes aegypti*. The total number of dengue infections globally has been estimated to be 390 million per year [2], of which 96 million manifest clinically, the majority of which (70%) are found in Asia. It has been estimated that 3.97 billion people from 128 countries are at risk of dengue infection [3], and as urbanisation continues across much of Asia [4], the incidence is liable to grow [5]. Dengue fever usually leads to self-limiting symptoms including fever, headaches, pain behind the eyes, nausea, vomiting, swollen glands, rash, and joint, bone, or muscle pains [6]. However, when dengue fever develops into severe dengue, then plasma leakage, severe bleeding, severe organ impairment, and even death

* Correspondence: NG_Lee_Ching@nea.gov.sg
[2]Environmental Health Institute, 11 Biopolis Way, Singapore 138667, Singapore

may occur [7], making dengue control an important public health problem.

In the equatorial city state of Singapore, since the 1990s there has been a dramatic increase in the number of notified dengue cases, and all four serotypes are endemic [8]. Singapore's favourable climatic condition (average monthly temperature varying from 26 to 28 °C), its highly urbanised environment and its being a hub for international travel and transition [9] make it ideal for the breeding of *Aedes* mosquitoes and transmission of dengue. Since 2013, a dengue incidence of more than 150 per 100,000 population has been reported [10] and this has been related to a sizable disease burden to Singapore [11]. Although a new dengue vaccine, Dengvaxia® (CYD-TDV), first licensed in Mexico in 2015 [12], has been approved by the Health Science Authority in Singapore for persons aged 12 to 45, and has been available commercially since 2017, the vaccine is primarily effective against DENV3 and DENV4 but less so against DENV1 and DENV2 [13], which are the predominant serotypes in Singapore [14]. The vaccine is more effective for individuals with a prior exposure to dengue virus [12], but increases the risk of severity in subsequent infection for immune naïve individuals [15]. It is, thus, not recommended for Singapore where endemicity and seroprevalence are low [16, 17].

At present, vector control remains the primary and most effective measure for dengue control and prevention [18]. The National Environment Agency (NEA) of Singapore deploys officers to inspect premises, eliminate potential breeding grounds and outreach to remind residents to remove sources of stagnant water. Such resource-intensive vector control measures could be optimised by targeting areas with a greater risk of transmission.

As well as providing an indication of where dengue transmission is ongoing, incident case data also foreshadow where future outbreaks are most likely, and hence provide a guide to which areas could be prioritised for preventive efforts. To do so requires quantifying the likely number of cases in different areal units, which can be addressed through short-term forecasting.

In the literature, various models have been proposed for the prediction of dengue cases. Machine learning methods (including the support vector regression algorithm, gradient boosted regression tree algorithm, and regression or auto-regression models) have been used at national [19], sub-national [20] and urban levels [21], using incidence and climatic variables, including temperature, relative humidity, rainfall and solar radiation. Examples from Singapore [22–24] have provided forecasts at a national level, with the Environment Health Institute in Singapore currently relying on least absolute shrinkage and selection operator (LASSO) based models, incorporating recent case data, meteorological data, vector surveillance data

and population-based national statistics, to derive up to 3-month national forecasts to guide vector control [24]. In the past 5 years, extensive work has been done in many dengue-affected areas in the world on dengue forecasting, including Thailand, Indonesia, Ecuador and Pakistan [25–29], to create early warnings of potential dengue outbreaks. In addition to the conventionally used meteorological or disease epidemiological information as predictors [23, 30, 31], recent forecast models have begun to incorporate human mobility information [32, 33], land use [34], frequency of social media mentions and appearances on online search engines [35, 36], and spatial dynamics [37–39] to provide additional information for accurate predictions.

Even within a small city state such as Singapore, spatial variations in risk may be profound, reflecting differences in urban density, the presence of natural areas (such as rainforest and reservoirs) and differential age profiles of different housing estates, and as such, a finer resolution forecast, if one were available, would potentially allow better targeting of the response. The objective of this study is, therefore, to develop a new approach for spatio-temporal dengue forecasting at a finer spatial resolution that can be routinely used by Singapore's government agencies for planning of vector control for best efficiency, and which may potentially be adapted to other settings.

Methods
Modelling objectives
Our objective is to develop a suite of models, each of which will make a forecast for one specified time window, based on the data available at the time the forecast is made. Each model will predict for each neighbourhood the number of cases within a 1-week interval, which will then be used to rank neighbourhoods according to projected risk. This ranking can then be used to identify those areas to be prioritised for interventions, subject to resource availability. Accuracy will be assessed by correlating observed and actual numbers of cases and calculating the receiver operating characteristics when neighbourhoods are classified as high or low risk.

Source of data
The forecasting algorithm uses a mixture of purely spatial, purely temporal and spatio-temporal data to derive dynamic risk maps for dengue transmission.

Spatio-temporal
The Ministry of Health, Singapore, continuously monitors the incidence of dengue through mandatory notification of virologically confirmed or laboratory-confirmed cases. The residential address and date of onset of each case in Singapore are recorded. We aggregated individual-level

data into weekly number of cases in 315 spatial units of size 1 km × 1 km (henceforth, *neighbourhoods*), from 2010 to 2016, spanning the major residential areas of the country.

The movement patterns of mobile subscribers were derived by analysing their cell phones' network activities among subscribers of Starhub Ltd, one of the three major mobile telephone companies (telcos) in Singapore. These data were aggregated and used to determine the connectivity between different neighbourhoods, which was subsequently used to derive a variable we called the *connectivity-weighted transmission potential*, which captures the future risk to a neighbourhood from other neighbourhoods with current dengue cases, based on the amount of movement from one neighbourhood to the other. A detailed description of these data is provided in Additional file 1.

Building age was obtained from the Housing Development Board and the Urban Redevelopment Authority and averaged over all buildings within a neighbourhood. Previous studies have shown that the quality of buildings can impact the presence of potential breeding habitats [40], thus increasing the risk of dengue transmission. Because building practices have evolved over time and newer buildings are designed to reduce vector breeding sites, building age is a plausible risk factor for transmission, and as preliminary analyses showed a high association with both *Aedes* mosquito and dengue incidence, this was used as a predictor in the model.

Meteorological data are incorporated to account for the important role that climate has in the mosquito life cycle. Despite Singapore's small size, there are some systematic differences in climate across the country [41], and to accommodate that, meteorological data were estimated for each neighbourhood using weekly mean, maximum and minimum temperature, and average relative humidity from the nearest (of 21) weather stations across the island managed by the Meteorological Services Singapore.

Temporal

Other than weekly incidence in the cells, individual-level dengue incidence data were aggregated into weekly national cases as a proxy for the general epidemic level.

Spatial

The vegetation index refers to the Normalised Difference Vegetation Index (NDVI), which is an index of plant viridescence or photosynthetic activity. NDVI is based on the observation that different surfaces reflect different types of light differently. NDVI data were obtained from the Centre for Remote Imaging, Sensing and Processing in the National University of Singapore from a processed satellite image. Travel history data derived

from trips made using EZLink cards (a card to pay for public transport fares in Singapore) were used to measure how connected each neighbourhood is to other parts of the country by public transport. These were processed and aggregated by the provider, prior to analysis, which derived a connectivity ranking based on the number of trips in and out of each cell (as described in the Additional file 1). The cells were ranked by percentile to form the connectivity ranking. In contrast to the telco data, this data source captures short transits through neighbourhoods.

The Institutional Review Board of the National University of Singapore provided the ethical approval for this study.

Statistical analysis

LASSO regression was used for the prediction models [42]. In contrast to standard linear regression in which parameters are estimated by minimising the sum of squares of residuals, LASSO regression imposes an extra constraint that the sum of the absolute value of the regression coefficients be less than a fixed value, which is selected for optimal out-of-sample predictive performance. This algorithm shrinks coefficients towards zero, with some becoming exactly zero, and hence, the covariates associated with these coefficients are not associated with the outcome variable in the model. Compared to a simple regression, which estimates coefficients for a pre-specified set of predictors, a LASSO regression allows all covariates, at multiple lags, to be included as potential predictors, despite the usual concerns about the size of the variable space or the presence of collinearities. The optimal balance between model accuracy and complexity is obtained by varying the constraint and optimising out-of-sample predictive accuracy over the data not used in the model building process, which is inherently well suited to the problem of forecasting, as described in earlier non-spatial work [24, 43].

Separate LASSO sub-models were constructed for each forecast window, which were defined as the number of weeks ahead the sub-model is predicting. All 315 (approximate) squares of size 1 km × 1 km covering residential areas of Singapore were included in each sub-model. For each sub-model, information for all 315 grid neighbourhoods at all time points in the training set were included. Each candidate predictor appeared several times in each sub-model, at different historical lags. To allow for contagion and typical epidemic duration, we used past incidence of up to 8 weeks. To accommodate non-linearities, we also used past incidence squared, cubic, and square root, up to 8 weeks in the past. Polynomials are commonly used to approximate any non-linearity in the relationship between the covariate and outcome, and thus, we allow (but do not force) polynomial terms to account for potential non-linearities between future number of cases and autoregressive terms. In addition, the total number of cases in nearby areas were included at up to 8 weeks lag. Two tiers of nearby areas were used: within 1 km radius and within a ring from 1 km to 2 km from the centroid of the neighbourhood of interest. These are depicted in Additional file 2: Figure S1. Climatic variables (average, minimum and maximum temperature, and humidity) of up to 5 weeks' lag were included. Cells were included in the analysis if the centroid falls within a residential area of Singapore; some cells near the boundary are truncated to the part on the main island, Pulau Ujong.

For each forecast window (from $k = 1$ to 12 weeks), a separate LASSO sub-model was developed, which used data available at the time of the forecast only. Each LASSO sub-model is as follows:

$$
\begin{aligned}
y_{t+k,i} = \alpha_k &+ \sum_{l=0}^{7} \beta_{k_1,l} y_{t-l,i} + \sum_{l=0}^{7} \beta_{k_2,l} y_{t-l,i}^2 \\
&+ \sum_{l=0}^{7} \beta_{k_3,l} y_{t-l,i}^3 + \sum_{l=0}^{7} \beta_{k_4,l} \sqrt{y_{t-l,i}} \\
&+ \sum_{r=1}^{2} \sum_{l=0}^{7} \phi_{k_r,l} n_{t-l,i,r} \\
&+ \sum_{c=1}^{4} \sum_{l=0}^{4} \gamma_{k_c,l} W_{t-l,i,c} + \lambda_k T_{t,\ i} + \theta_k A_{t,\ i} \\
&+ \delta_k N_t + \omega_k V_i + + \rho_k U_i + \varepsilon_k,
\end{aligned}
$$

where $y_{t,\ i}$ is the number of cases (natural log-transformed, with 1 added to avoid logging 0) in neighbourhood i in week t. The terms $y_{t,i}^2$, $y_{t,i}^3$ and $\sqrt{y_{t,i}}$ are the square, cubic and square root of the number of cases. Similarly, $n_{t,\ i,\ 1}$ and $n_{t,\ i,\ 2}$ are the total number of cases (similarly, natural log-transformed, with 1 added to avoid logging 0) from all neighbourhoods whose centroids are within 1 km radius and within a ring from 1 km to 2 km from the centroid of neighbourhood i, in week t, respectively. $W_{t,\ i,\ c}$ represents the climatic variable (average, minimum and maximum temperature, and average relative humidity) at time t in neighbourhood i. $T_{t,\ i}$ measures the number of cases moving into neighbourhood i in week t, derived from a one-time telco dataset on the movement of users. $A_{t,i}$ measures average building age in neighbourhood i in week t. N_t is the national total number of cases (natural log-transformed, with 1 added) in week t. V_i and U_i measure the vegetation and connectivity index of neighbourhood i. Detailed information on the type of each set of variables are documented in Additional file 3: Table S1. Covariates in the LASSO regression were z-scored prior to estimation and the coefficients were rescaled afterwards.

Parameter estimation was subject to the LASSO constraint: $\sum_{j=1}^{4} \sum_{l=0}^{7} |\beta_{k_j,l}| + \sum_{r=1}^{2} \sum_{l=0}^{7} |\phi_{k_r,l}| + \sum_{c=1}^{4} \sum_{l=0}^{4} |\gamma_{k_c,l}| + |\lambda_k| + |\theta_k| + |\delta_k| + |\omega_k| + |\rho_k| \le p$. Ten-fold cross validation was performed and the constraint term that optimised the out-of-sample performance was chosen as the optimal p for the forecast model.

As the models were built separately for each forecast window, the variables included in the final forecast model and their lags and parameter magnitude and sign may differ substantially.

LASSO models were built using all the data from the training dataset, which comprised information from 2010 to 2015. Out-of-sample validation was performed on the testing dataset consisting of data from 2016.

Effect size

The effect size of each predictor at different time lags and for different forecast windows and the corresponding 95% confidence intervals were derived by taking 1000 bootstrap samples and fitting LASSO models to them. We used a standard bootstrap algorithm to derive 95% confidence intervals from the lower and upper 2.5 percentiles of the bootstrap sampling distribution of the LASSO estimates. The ranges and distributions of all predictor values were derived based on the training set and the effect size obtained by multiplying the LASSO coefficient and values within the range.

Forecast

As well as the forecast number of cases per neighbourhood, we categorised neighbourhoods as being low or high risk, as follows. The predicted number of cases for each neighbourhood was derived using information only up to when the predictions were made. Model parameters were derived from model fitting using only the training dataset. At each forecast time point, neighbourhoods were ordered by the predicted number of cases and categorised as high risk if they were in the upper decile (i.e. top 32 neighbourhoods out of 315 residential areas) for that time point. The choice of dichotomising at 10% was taken considering the operating capacity of the NEA for vector control. Predicted cases during the validation period (2016) constitute a genuine out-of-sample forecast. During the training period (2010–2015), the full time span was used to estimate parameters, but only covariates available at the time of the forecast were used to make the forecast. As such, predictive accuracy may be slightly overstated for the training period.

Accuracy

In the model building, predictive accuracy was measured using the root-mean-square error. Subsequently, we assessed the predictive accuracy by evaluating the accuracy of their categorisation of high-risk areas for the validation dataset. For each forecast window, a receiver operating characteristic (ROC) curve —frequently used to evaluate classifiers' performance—was derived [44]. Predictions and classifications at all 40 prediction time points were aggregated to derive one ROC curve for each forecast window. Given the actual classification of high- and low-risk neighbourhoods based on observed actual incidences (i.e. the 10% of neighbourhoods with the greatest number of cases were classified as high risk) and our forecast models, the ROC curve demonstrates relative trade-offs between true positives and false positives. The area under the ROC curve (AUC), a commonly used measurement to summarise the two-dimensional ROC performance as a single value between 0 and 1 [45], was derived for each forecast window. ROC, AUC and their respective confidence intervals were obtained using 50 bootstrap samples. A baseline level AUC was also derived using the temporal average of the number of cases from all previous years as the prediction for all 40 prediction time points, and we computed the AUC by comparing this "prediction" with the actual observed distribution of cases.

To assess the robustness of the findings to the choice of the 10% cut-off we currently adopted for the categorisation, an average Matthew's correlation coefficient was calculated for each forecast window at 14 different cut-off points (1%, 3%, 5%, 10%, 15%, 20%, 25%, 30%, 40%, 50%, 60%, 70%, 80% and 90%). This measures the

correlation coefficient between the observed and predicted binary classification, and thus the quality of binary classifications [46], and takes a value from −1 to 1 with 1 indicating perfect agreement, 0 indicating no better than random and −1 indicating total disagreement. Matthew's correlation coefficient was computed for each forecast window at all prediction time points and averaged over time to derive an average coefficient for each forecast window.

All statistical analysis were performed using statistical software R [47].

Results

Selected independent variables in the prediction model are presented in Fig. 1. A mix of spatial and temporal variables are shown (other independent variables are presented in Additional file 4: Figure S2, Additional file 5: Figure S3, Additional file 6: Figure S4, Additional file 7: Figure S5, Additional file 8: Figure S6, Additional file 9: Figure S7, Additional file 10: Figure S8, Additional file 11: Figure S9 and Additional file 12: Figure S10). There are

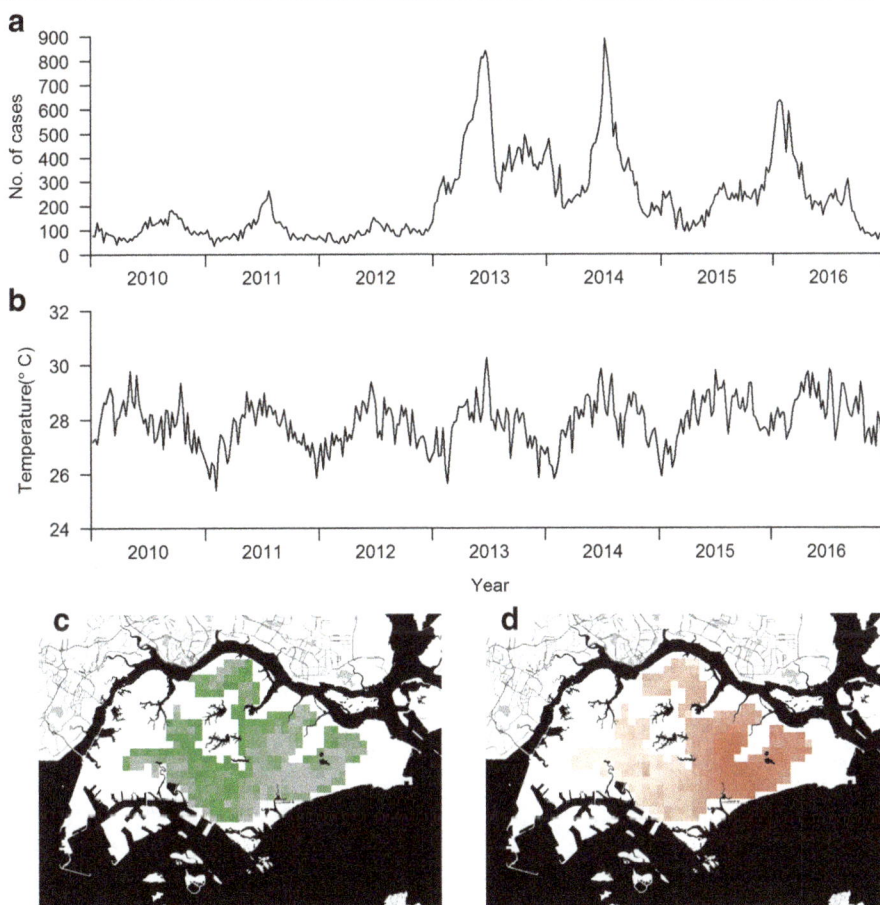

Fig. 1 Time series and spatial density of selected predictors in the LASSO model. **a** Time series of weekly national number of cases from 2010 to 2016. **b** Time series of average temperature for one arbitrarily selected residential neighbourhood from 2010 to 2016. **c, d** Density of vegetation and movement for one arbitrarily selected time point for all 315 residential neighbourhoods

no strong annual cycles in either case counts (Fig. 1a) or climatic variables (Fig. 1b, Additional file 7: Figure S5, Additional file 8: Figure S6, Additional file 9: Figure S7 and Additional file 10: Figure S8). The geographic distribution of greenery is shown in Fig. 1c, while case movement data for a random week derived from the telco information on movement of the general population is shown similarly on a heat map in Fig. 1d.

Figure 2 shows the forecast and actual distribution of dengue incidence at four distinct time points (epidemiological weeks 1, 14, 27 and 40 for 2016) for 4-week ahead forecasts (predictions at other time points are presented in Additional file 13: Video S1, Additional file 14: Video S2, Additional file 15: Video S3, Additional file 16: Video S4, Additional file 17: Video S5, Additional file 18: Video S6, Additional file 19: Video S7, Additional file 20: Video S8, Additional file 21: Video S9, Additional file 22: Video S10, Additional file 23: Video S11 and Additional file 24: Video S12 for forecast windows 1 to 12). These demonstrate the close concordance between the projections and the eventual incidence. The average Matthew's correlation coefficient for all 12 forecast windows at 14 different risk classification cut-offs are shown in Fig. 3 (and tabulated in Additional file 25: Table S2). For most of the forecast windows, a classification of the upper risk decile—the operational capacity—as high risk had similar predictive performance as the optimal (30%).

The quality of the spatial predictive algorithm as a classifier is measured by ROC curves and the respective

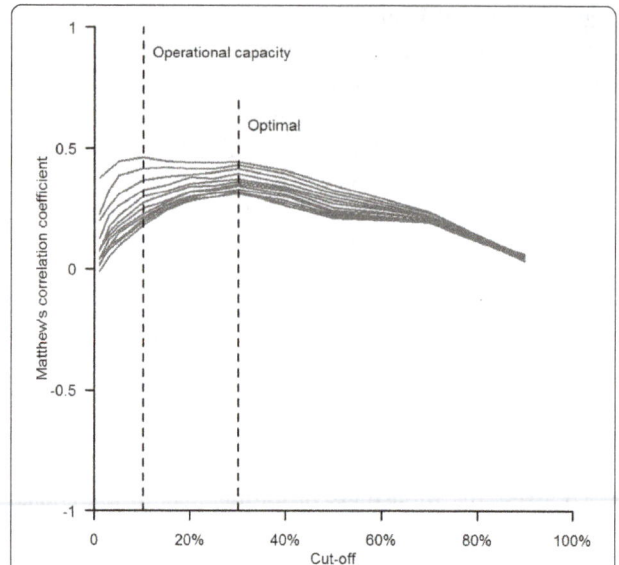

Fig. 3 Average Mathew's correlation coefficient for all 12 forecast windows at 14 different cut-offs (1%, 3%, 5%, 10%, 15%, 20%, 25%, 30%, 40%, 50%, 60%, 70%, 80% and 90%). Cut-off are set at different levels so that different percentages of the neighbourhoods are classified as higher risk areas

AUCs. ROC curves for prediction windows at 1, 2, 4, 8 and 12 weeks are presented in Fig. 4 (bootstrap confidence intervals are very narrow and are not shown in the figure). All AUCs at forecast windows up to 12 weeks are above 0.75 and within 5 weeks, AUCs are above

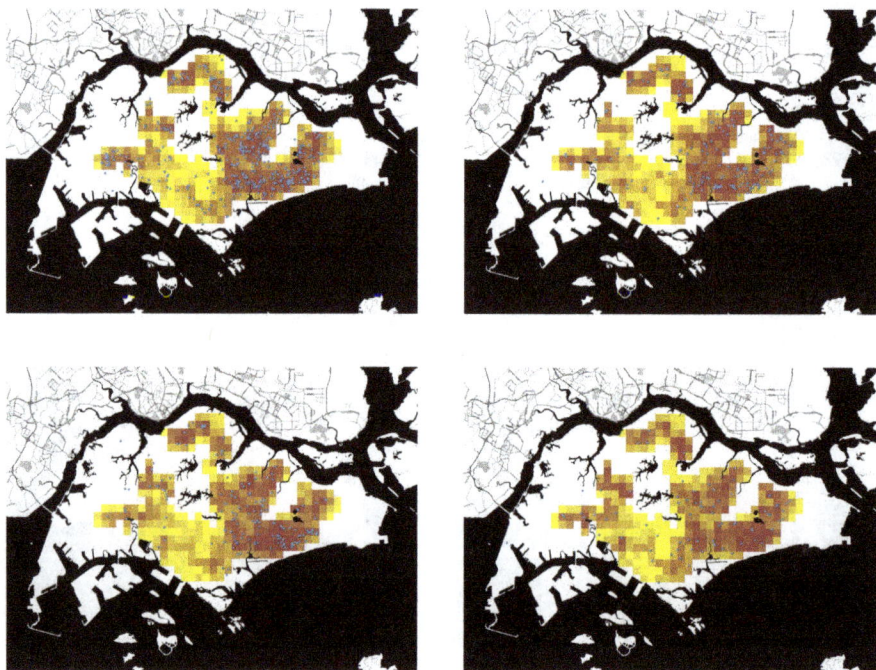

Fig. 2 Actual distribution of cases (dark blue dots) and 4-week ahead forecasts of density at four time points (epidemiological weeks 1, 14, 27 and 40 for 2016). Yellow indicates neighbourhoods with relatively fewer predicted cases and dark red indicates those with relatively more predicted cases

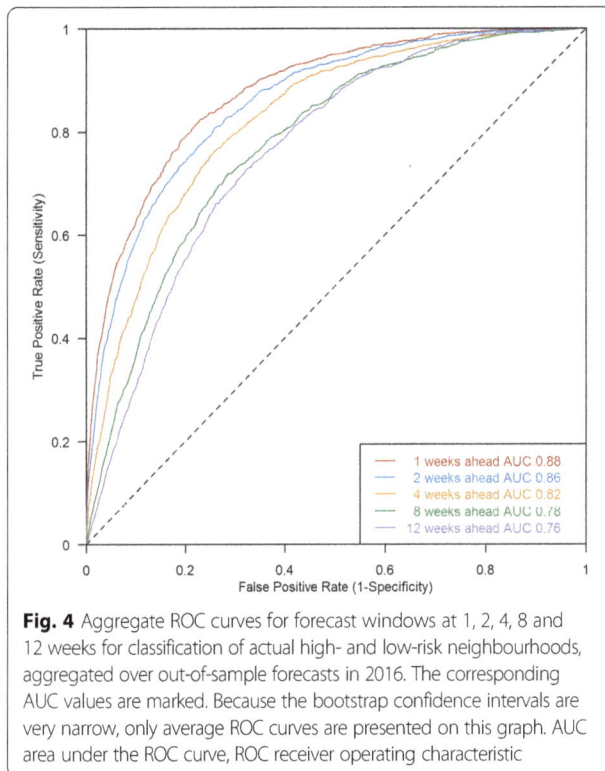

Fig. 4 Aggregate ROC curves for forecast windows at 1, 2, 4, 8 and 12 weeks for classification of actual high- and low-risk neighbourhoods, aggregated over out-of-sample forecasts in 2016. The corresponding AUC values are marked. Because the bootstrap confidence intervals are very narrow, only average ROC curves are presented on this graph. AUC area under the ROC curve, ROC receiver operating characteristic

0.80, indicating adequate performance in attributing neighbourhoods to be at high risk of imminent or on-going transmission. The baseline AUC that uses the average of all past years' cases as the prediction for the out-of-sample forecast is derived to be 0.78, which is better than guessing (i.e. the AUC is greater than 0.5) but which demonstrates that there are substantial gains in short-term predictive performance resulting from using updated data streams within our framework. Predictions for 6 weeks ahead and beyond revert to baseline risk.

The effect of risk factors on local dengue risk are shown in Figs. 5, 6 and 7. Figure 5 shows the effects of case counts within the neighbourhood and in proximate neighbourhoods for the 1-week ahead forecast model at three different time lags. The number of cases in a neighbourhood has a larger effect over short time lags compared to longer time lags, while the number of proximate cases has an effect size close to 0 at all lags. Although the relationship can be non-linear through the polynomial terms, the estimated effect is approximately linear. Climatic variables and their effects are shown in Fig. 6 (at time lags 2 and 4 for the 1-week ahead forecast). Maximum temperature, minimum temperature and relative humidity had a larger effect at longer time lags than the week immediately preceding the prediction, but relative to incidence, the effect is negligible. Figure 7 shows the effects of parameters without time

lags. As expected, an increasing number of national weekly cases, less greenery, older buildings, greater connectivity to other areas and more incoming travellers to the area implied more cases. These parameters generally had a bigger effect than climatic variables, after adjusting for incidence and all other independent variables in the model. For each forecast window, the probability of each parameter being included in the final model, the estimated parameter coefficient and respective confidence interval are shown in Additional file 26: Tables S3 to S14 based on 1000 bootstrap samples. Incidence and neighbouring incidence at shorter lags were more likely to be included in the final model while climatic variables had a relatively smaller probability of being included and a smaller effect size.

An overall view of the 1-week ahead prediction model is shown in Fig. 8 (summaries for other all other forecast windows are shown in Additional file 27: Figure S11, Additional file 28: Figure S12, Additional file 29: Figure S13, Additional file 30: Figure S14, Additional file 31: Figure S15, Additional file 32: Figure S16, Additional file 33: Figure S17, Additional file 34: Figure S18, Additional file 35: Figure S19, Additional file 36: Figure S20 and Additional file 37: Figure S21). Panels Fig. 8(a) show the yearly sum of the 1-week ahead predicted number of cases and actual observed number of cases in all neighbourhoods. The relative sizes of the discrepancies were generally larger for smaller numbers, where accuracy may be less important, but the majority of predictions were accurate. Panels Fig. 8(b) show the average risk over all prediction points for the 1-week ahead forecast. Neighbourhoods in the east of Singapore had a higher risk than the other regions.

Discussion

In Singapore, the average annual economic impact of dengue has been estimated to be around US$100 million, of which 42–59% is attributable to the cost of control [11]. Routine surveillance identifies residential and workplace addresses for all notified cases, which leads to dengue clusters being identified, namely localities with putatively active transmission where NEA's vector control intervention is targeted [48]. A cluster is formed when two or more cases have onset within 14 days and are located within 150 m of each other based on the addresses as well as movement history. Three alert levels, depending on the number of cases in the cluster, lead to efforts to mobilise the community to check their premises for mosquito breeding, and guide the extent of NEA's vector control intervention. However, these alert levels are based on current or recent infections, rather than the areas most likely to see further transmission. Being able to focus control on where new cases are most likely to arise, rather than where they are currently,

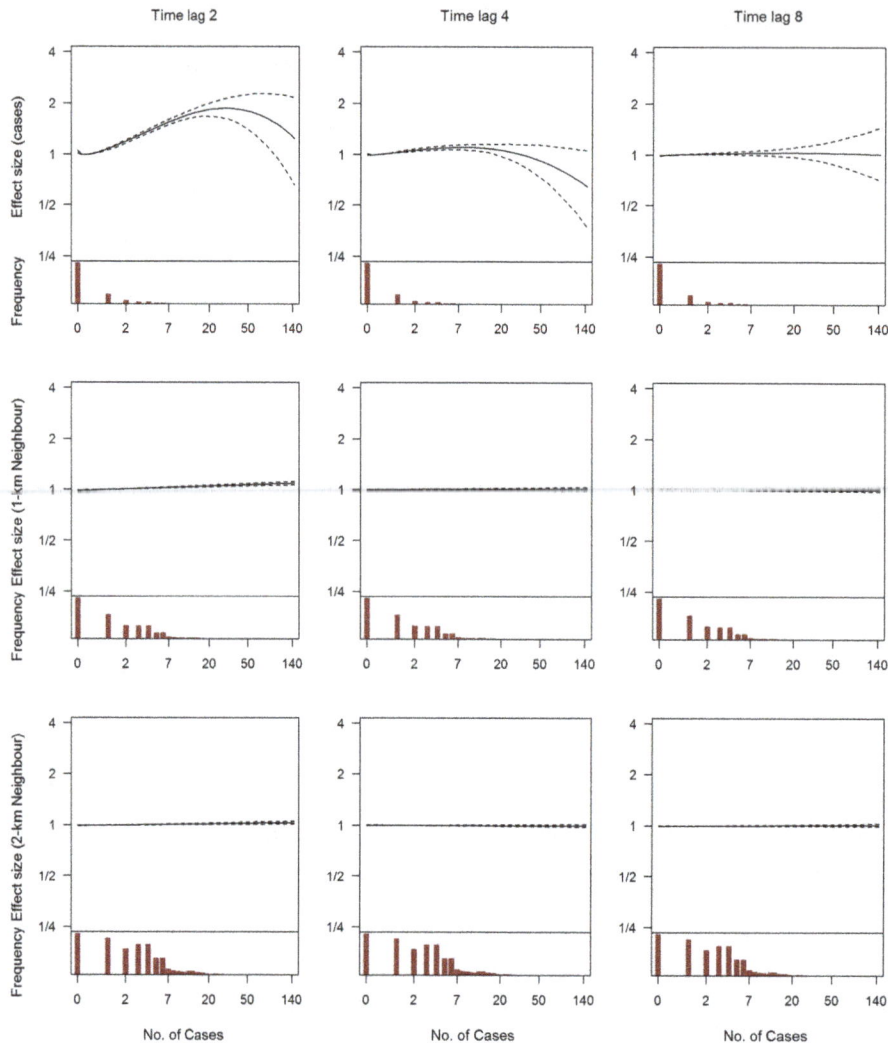

Fig. 5 Histogram of the distribution and effect size on 1-week ahead forecast of dengue cases per neighbourhood. Recent case counts in neighbourhoods and total number of cases in the immediate vicinity are shown, at three time lags (2, 4 and 8). Histograms of the distribution are shown in the lower panes. The effects of covariates compared to the mean for that covariate are shown in the upper panes. Confidence intervals were derived using bootstrap sampling and are 95% equal tailed intervals

could allow preemptive mitigation and potentially yield greater efficiencies and reduce costs accordingly.

Thus, in this study we developed a novel method to forecast spatial risk within an urban environment at a neighbourhood resolution up to 3 months in advance, using a LASSO-based prediction model. The method gave rather accurate forecasts (AUCs > 0.8 within the next month), with a high correlation with the subsequent incidence data. However, for longer forecast windows, the risk reverted to a baseline risk profile for the neighbourhood. By implementing it as part of our standing vector control programme, the spatio-temporal prediction model can potentially change the current dengue control paradigm into a dengue prevention approach by forecasting dengue risk at a finer resolution in the urbanised environments in which the dengue vectors proliferate. This would allow

targeted public health control measures that would use resources most efficiently. The system was robust to changes in the baseline incidence over time (illustrated in Fig. 1a), as demonstrated in the high correlation between observed and predicted incidence (Fig. 8a). As such, secular changes in the detection rates due to better diagnosis or in incidence due to changes in immunity or dominant serotypes may not matter unless the change is large.

This approach can readily be automated to run on routinely collected notification data, but the accuracy of the prediction is dependent on the timeliness at which notification data become available and the accuracy of such data. The approach does not require that all infections be notified or confirmed by a lab—the low rate of symptomatic dengue presentation is well known [49]— as long as the rate remains relatively stable over space

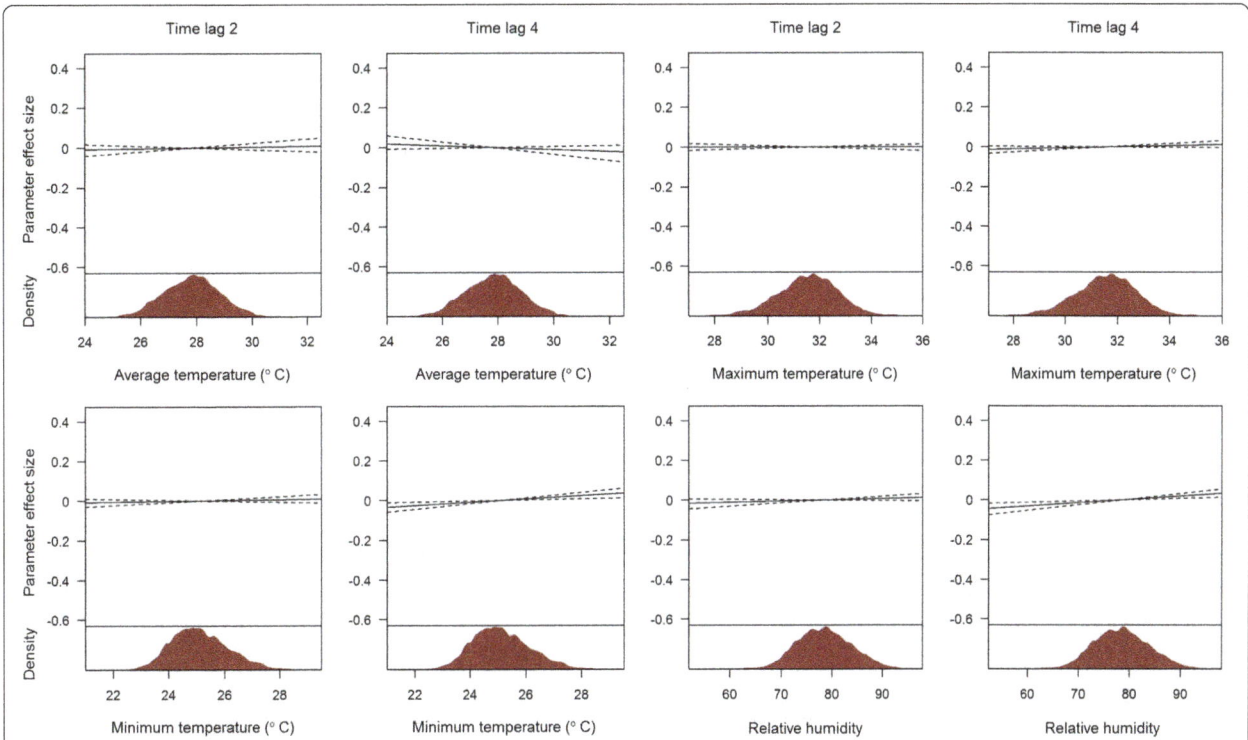

Fig. 6 Distribution of climatic parameter and parameter effect in excess of the mean effect at two different time lags (2 and 4) for 1-week ahead forecasts. Upper panes show the effect and lower panes show the distribution of parameters. Confidence intervals were derived using bootstrap sampling

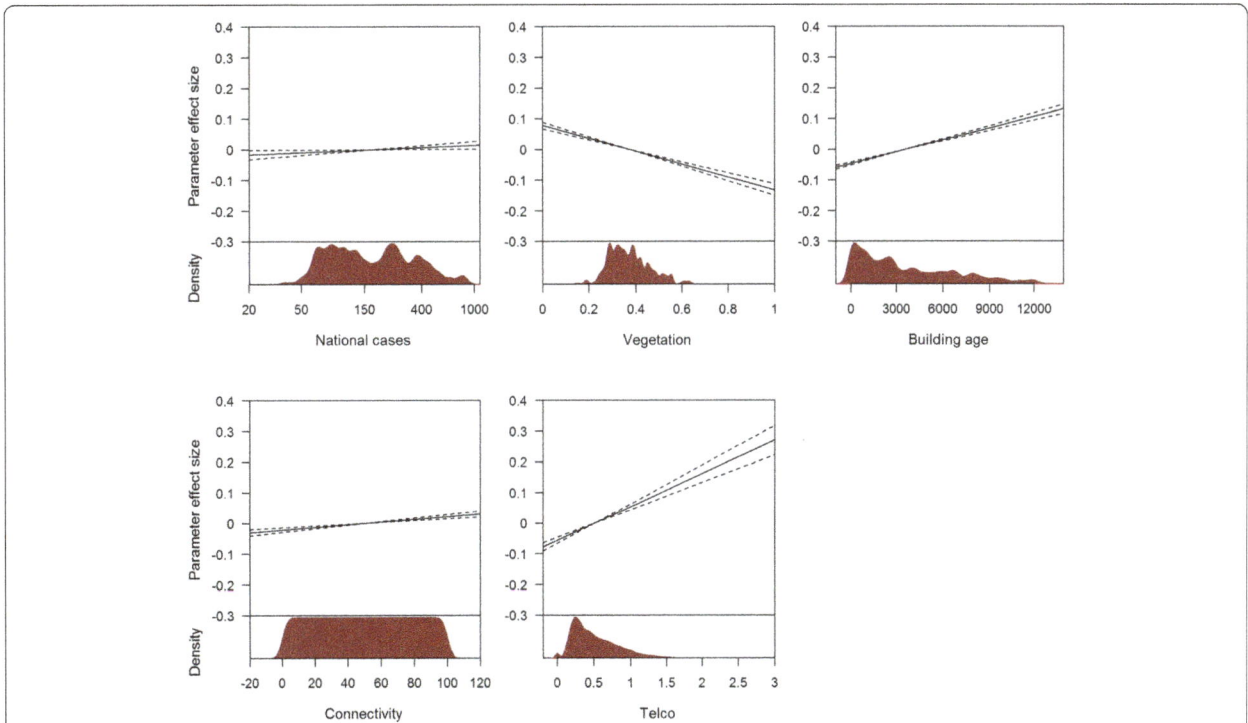

Fig. 7 Distribution of parameters without time lags and parameter effect in excess of the mean effect. Upper panes show the effect and lower panes show the distribution of the parameters. Confidence intervals were derived using bootstrap sampling

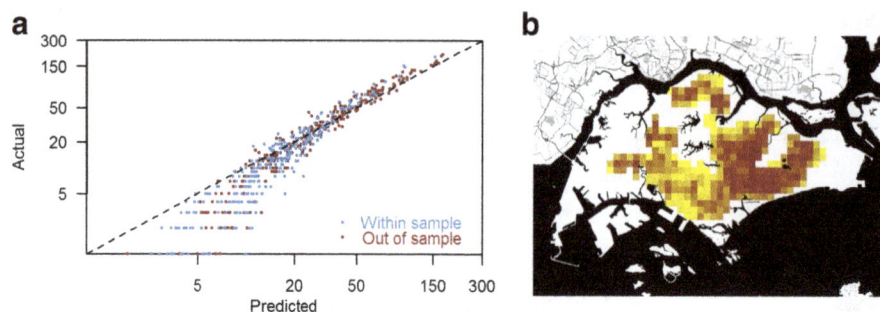

Fig. 8 Comparisons of forecast and actual scenario for 1-week ahead forecast model. **a** Actual and predicted yearly total number of cases for all neighbourhoods for both within-sample prediction (blue dots) and out-of-sample prediction (dark red dots). **b** Average risk over all prediction points (both within-sample and out-of-sample) for the 1-week ahead forecast

and time. The training dataset used in this modelling framework, however, may need to be updated regularly. In the current approach, the performance for 2016 (the data for which were not used in training) was good (AUC above 0.75 for all forecast windows), and so we recommend retraining the algorithm every year.

Through regular evaluation of all the parameter effect sizes, variables with a constant minimal effect in the forecast model may be eliminated, reducing the cost of obtaining them. Other potential parameters may be added to the model in a similar way. The frequent modification of the model to allow additional data streams to be incorporated will ensure the model continues to enjoy high predictive performance.

We expect that the same method can be adapted to other urban and even rural areas, though in the latter, the grid size determining neighbourhoods may need to be adjusted. We used a regular grid, but the framework lends itself to other tessellations, for instance, administrative boundaries. We anticipate that such regional or neighbourhood-level forecasts will have improved accuracy and utility than predictions of aggregate national-level data streams.

There are several limitations of the approach outlined herein. The forecast is phenomenological rather than mechanistic, and as such may break down in the presence of changes to the underlying epidemic process and changes to interventions. A previous non-spatial forecast (described in Ref. [24]) struggled to reproduce the magnitude of the record-breaking outbreak of 2013, for instance, although it was able to herald the timing of the outbreak in advance. Fundamental changes, such as vaccination or the introduction of a new serotype to the population, may require the retraining of the algorithm if the accuracy is not to be deleteriously affected. Further mechanistic modelling could be valuable in providing additional insight into the spatial structure of dengue transmission in Singapore, if challenges about non-notified infections and the paucity of data on historic exposures to

each serotype could be overcome. The multiple lags and forecast windows allows highly predictive combinations of variables to be selected, but have the effect of obscuring relationships, and as a result, the approach is not suitable for identifying why particular neighbourhoods are predicted to be at risk of future or imminent transmission. The most important limitation to the work is its high reliance on a rich dataset of georeferenced case identifications being available in near real time. This is possible in Singapore's comprehensive case notification system but may be less feasible in jurisdictions that do not enjoy Singapore's small size and the clear demarcation of the city population. The effectiveness of vector control measures based on the forecast is not evaluated in the current model, and to predict the impact would require additional data streams that capture the details of the ongoing vector control efforts. This would be an avenue for further work.

Conclusions

In conclusion, this report demonstrates that spatially resolved forecasts of geographically structured diseases like dengue can be obtained at a neighbourhood-level in highly urban environments at a precision that is suitable for guiding control efforts.

Additional files

Additional file 1: Supplementary information. (DOCX 19 kb)

Additional file 2: Figure S1. Demonstration of the two tiers of neighbouring cells in the study. (PNG 338 kb)

Additional file 3: Table S1. Groups of variables and their respective types that are included in the LASSO model. (DOCX 11 kb)

Additional file 4: Figure S2. Temporal and spatial average of the weekly number of cases in all grid cells from 2010 to 2016. (PNG 200 kb)

Additional file 5: Figure S3. Temporal and spatial average of the sum of the weekly number of cases in all first-tier neighbouring cells (within 1 km) from 2010 to 2016. (PNG 199 kb)

Additional file 6: Figure S4. Temporal and spatial average of the sum of the weekly number of cases in all second-tier neighbouring cells (between 1 km and 2 km) from 2010 to 2016. (PNG 198 kb)

Additional file 7: Figure S5. Temporal and spatial average of the average temperature in all grid cells from 2010 to 2016. (PNG 202 kb)

Additional file 8: Figure S6. Temporal and spatial average of the maximum temperature in all grid cells from 2010 to 2016. (PNG 200 kb)

Additional file 9: Figure S7. Temporal and spatial average of the minimum temperature in all grid cells from 2010 to 2016. (PNG 201 kb)

Additional file 10: Figure S8. Temporal and spatial average of the average humidity in all grid cells from 2010 to 2016. (PNG 201 kb)

Additional file 11: Figure S9. Temporal and spatial average of the movement of incoming incidences in all grid cells from 2010 to 2016. (PNG 198 kb)

Additional file 12: Figure S10. Temporal and spatial average of the average building age in all grid cells from 2010 to 2016. (PNG 197 kb)

Additional file 13: Video S1. Video of 1-week ahead forecast and actual distribution of dengue incidence in 2016. (MP4 1177 kb)

Additional file 14: Video S2. Video of 2-week ahead forecast and actual distribution of dengue incidence in 2016. (MP4 1159 kb)

Additional file 15: Video S3. Video of 3-week ahead forecast and actual distribution of dengue incidence in 2016. (MP4 1148 kb)

Additional file 16: Video S4. Video of 4-week ahead forecast and actual distribution of dengue incidence in 2016. (MP4 1125 kb)

Additional file 17: Video S5. Video of 5-week ahead forecast and actual distribution of dengue incidence in 2016. (MP4 1107 kb)

Additional file 18: Video S6. Video of 6-week ahead forecast and actual distribution of dengue incidence in 2016. (MP4 1097 kb)

Additional file 19: Video S7. Video of 7-week ahead forecast and actual distribution of dengue incidence in 2016. (MP4 1071 kb)

Additional file 20: Video S8. Video of 8-week ahead forecast and actual distribution of dengue incidence in 2016. (MP4 1057 kb)

Additional file 21: Video S9. Video of 9-week ahead forecast and actual distribution of dengue incidence in 2016. (MP4 1037 kb)

Additional file 22: Video S10. Video of 10-week ahead forecast and actual distribution of dengue incidence in 2016. (MP4 1019 kb)

Additional file 23: Video S11. Video of 11-week ahead forecast and actual distribution of dengue incidence in 2016. (MP4 1008 kb)

Additional file 24: Video S12. Video of 12-week ahead forecast and actual distribution of dengue incidence in 2016. (MP4 992 kb)

Additional file 25: Table S2. Average Matthew's correlation coefficient for all 12 forecast windows at 14 different cut-offs. Cut-off are set at different levels so that different percentages of the cells are classified as higher risk areas. (DOCX 12 kb)

Additional file 26: Table S3. Summary of parameters included in LASSO forecast model for the 1-week ahead forecast. **Table S4.** Summary of parameters included in LASSO forecast model for the 2-week ahead forecast. **Table S5.** Summary of parameters included in LASSO forecast model for the 3-week ahead forecast. **Table S6.** Summary of parameters included in LASSO forecast model for the 4-week ahead forecast. **Table S7.** Summary of parameters included in LASSO forecast model for the 5-week ahead forecast. **Table S8.** Summary of parameters included in LASSO forecast model for the 6-week ahead forecast. **Table S9.** Summary of parameters included in LASSO forecast model for the 7-week ahead forecast. **Table S10.** Summary of parameters included in LASSO forecast model for the 8-week ahead forecast. **Table S11.** Summary of parameters included in LASSO forecast model for the 9-week ahead forecast. **Table S12.** Summary of parameters included in LASSO forecast model for the 10-week ahead forecast. **Table S13.** Summary of parameters included in LASSO forecast model for the 11-week ahead forecast. **Table S14.** Summary of parameters included in LASSO forecast model for the 12-week ahead forecast. (DOCX 37 kb)

Additional file 27: Figure S11. Comparisons of forecast and actual scenario for the 2-week ahead forecast model. **a** Actual and predicted yearly total number of cases for all neighbourhoods for both within-sample prediction (blue dots) and out-of-sample prediction (dark red dots). **b** Average risk over all prediction points (both within-sample and out-of-sample) for the 1-week ahead forecast. (PNG 189 kb)

Additional file 28: Figure S12. Comparisons of forecast and actual scenario for the 3-week ahead forecast model. **a** Actual and predicted yearly total number of cases for all neighbourhoods for both within-sample prediction (blue dots) and out-of-sample prediction (dark red dots). **b** Average risk over all prediction points (both within-sample and out-of-sample) for the 1-week ahead forecast. (PNG 189 kb)

Additional file 29: Figure S13. Comparisons of forecast and actual scenario for the 4-week ahead forecast model. **a** Actual and predicted yearly total number of cases for all neighbourhoods for both within-sample prediction (blue dots) and out-of-sample prediction (dark red dots). **b** Average risk over all prediction points (both within-sample and out-of-sample) for the 1-week ahead forecast. (PNG 189 kb)

Additional file 30: Figure S14. Comparisons of forecast and actual scenario for the 5-week ahead forecast model. **a** Actual and predicted yearly total number of cases for all neighbourhoods for both within-sample prediction (blue dots) and out-of-sample prediction (dark red dots). **b** Average risk over all prediction points (both within-sample and out-of-sample) for the 1-week ahead forecast. (PNG 190 kb)

Additional file 31: Figure S15. Comparisons of forecast and actual scenario for the 6-week ahead forecast model. **a** Actual and predicted yearly total number of cases for all neighbourhoods for both within-sample prediction (blue dots) and out-of-sample prediction (dark red dots). **b** Average risk over all prediction points (both within-sample and out-of-sample) for the 1-week ahead forecast. (PNG 190 kb)

Additional file 32: Figure S16. Comparisons of forecast and actual scenario for the 7-week ahead forecast model. **a** Actual and predicted yearly total number of cases for all neighbourhoods for both within-sample prediction (blue dots) and out-of-sample prediction (dark red dots). **b** Average risk over all prediction points (both within-sample and out-of-sample) for the 1-week ahead forecast. (PNG 190 kb)

Additional file 33: Figure S17. Comparisons of forecast and actual scenario for the 8-week ahead forecast model. **a** Actual and predicted yearly total number of cases for all neighbourhoods for both within-sample prediction (blue dots) and out-of-sample prediction (dark red dots). **b** Average risk over all prediction points (both within-sample and out-of-sample) for the 1-week ahead forecast. (PNG 190 kb)

Additional file 34: Figure S18. Comparisons of forecast and actual scenario for the 9-week ahead forecast model. **a** Actual and predicted yearly total number of cases for all neighbourhoods for both within-sample prediction (blue dots) and out-of-sample prediction (dark red dots). **b** Average risk over all prediction points (both within-sample and out-of-sample) for the 1-week ahead forecast. (PNG 190 kb)

Additional file 35: Figure S19. Comparisons of forecast and actual scenario for the 10-week ahead forecast model. **a** Actual and predicted yearly total number of cases for all neighbourhoods for both within-sample prediction (blue dots) and out-of-sample prediction (dark red dots). **b** Average risk over all prediction points (both within-sample and out-of-sample) for the 1-week ahead forecast. (PNG 190 kb)

Additional file 36: Figure S20. Comparisons of forecast and actual scenario for the 11-week ahead forecast model. **a** Actual and predicted yearly total number of cases for all neighbourhoods for both within-sample prediction (blue dots) and out-of-sample prediction (dark red dots). **b** Average risk over all prediction points (both within-sample and out-of-sample) for the 1-week ahead forecast. (PNG 190 kb)

Additional file 37: Figure S21. Comparisons of forecast and actual scenario for the 12-week ahead forecast model. **a** Actual and predicted yearly total number of cases for all neighbourhoods for both within-sample prediction (blue dots) and out-of-sample prediction (dark red dots). **b** Average risk over all prediction points (both within-sample and out-of-sample) for the 1-week ahead forecast. (PNG 190 kb)

Abbreviations
AUC: Area under the ROC curve; DENV: Dengue virus; LASSO: Least absolute shrinkage and selection operator; NDVI: Normalised difference vegetation

index; NEA: National Environment Agency; ROC: Receiver operating characteristic; Telco: Mobile telephone company

Acknowledgements
The authors would like to thank the Communicable Disease Division of the Ministry of Health, Singapore; the Meteorological Service Singapore of the NEA; the Housing Development Board, Singapore; the Urban Redevelopment Authority, Singapore; the Centre for Remote Imaging, Sensing and Processing, National University of Singapore and Starhub Ltd for providing the data used in this project.

Funding
YC is funded by the Saw Swee Hock School of Public Health, National University of Singapore. ARC is supported by the Singapore Ministry of Health's National Medical Research Council under the Centre Grant Programme - Singapore Population Health Improvement Centre (NMRC/CG/C026/2017_NUHS). We thank the Ministry of Finance for its reinvestment funding to NEA.

Authors' contributions
YC, GY, LCN and ARC conceptualised the study. YC, JHYO and JR analysed the data. YC and ARC interpreted the results. YC, JHYO, JR and ARC drafted the manuscript. All authors read and approved the final manuscript.

Competing interests
The authors declare that they have no competing interests.

Author details
[1]Saw Swee Hock School of Public Health, National University of Singapore and National University Health System, 12 Science Drive 2, Singapore 117549, Singapore. [2]Environmental Health Institute, 11 Biopolis Way, Singapore 138667, Singapore.

References
1. WHO | Dengue. WHO. Available from: http://www.who.int/immunization/diseases/dengue/en/. [cited 2017 Oct 25].
2. Bhatt S, Gething PW, Brady OJ, Messina JP, Farlow AW, Moyes CL, et al. The global distribution and burden of dengue. Nature. 2013;496:504–7.
3. Brady OJ, Gething PW, Bhatt S, Messina JP, Brownstein JS, Hoen AG, et al. Refining the global spatial limits of dengue virus transmission by evidence-based consensus. PLoS Negl Trop Dis. 2012;6:e1760.
4. United Nations. World Urbanization Prospects The 2014 Revision. 2014. Available from: https://esa.un.org/unpd/wup/Publications/Files/WUP2014-Highlights.pdf
5. Struchiner CJ, Rocklöv J, Wilder-Smith A, Massad E. Increasing dengue incidence in Singapore over the past 40 years: population growth, climate and mobility. PLoS One. 2015;10:e0136286.
6. Symptoms and What To Do If You Think You Have Dengue | Dengue | CDC. 2017. Available from: https://www.cdc.gov/dengue/symptoms/index.html. [cited 2018 Feb 20]
7. WHO | Dengue/Severe dengue frequently asked questions. WHO. Available from: http://www.who.int/denguecontrol/faq/en/. [cited 2017 Oct 26]
8. Lee K-S, Lo S, Tan SS-Y, Chua R, Tan L-K, Xu H, et al. Dengue virus surveillance in Singapore reveals high viral diversity through multiple introductions and in situ evolution. Infect Genet Evol. 2012;12:77–85.
9. Gubler DJ. Dengue, urbanization and globalization: the unholy trinity of the 21st century. Trop Med Health. 2011;39:3–11.
10. Vector Control Data - Dengue Outbreak Statistics. Data.gov.sg. Available from: https://data.gov.sg/dataset/vector-control-data-dengue-outbreak-statistics?view_id%3D581ef702-e3aa-4c34-ba18-a3ca931d9fc3%26resource_id%3D0e185366-f2a0-489f-bce8-17b4a24ea339. [cited 2017 Nov 1]
11. Carrasco LR, Lee LK, Lee VJ, Ooi EE, Shepard DS, Thein TL, et al. Economic impact of dengue illness and the cost-effectiveness of future vaccination programs in Singapore. Halstead SB, editor. PLoS Negl Trop Dis. 2011;5:e1426.
12. WHO | Questions and Answers on Dengue Vaccines. WHO. Available from: http://www.who.int/immunization/research/development/dengue_q_and_a/en/. [cited 2017 Nov 1]
13. Malisheni M, Khaiboullina SF, Rizvanov AA, Takah N, Murewanhema G, Bates M. Clinical Efficacy, Safety, and Immunogenicity of a Live Attenuated Tetravalent Dengue Vaccine (CYD-TDV) in Children: A Systematic Review with Meta-analysis. Front Immunol. 2017;8. https://doi.org/10.3389/fimmu.2017.00863.
14. Hapuarachchi HC, Koo C, Rajarethinam J, Chong C-S, Lin C, Yap G, et al. Epidemic resurgence of dengue fever in Singapore in 2013-2014: a virological and entomological perspective. BMC Infect Dis. 2016;16:300.
15. Dans AL, Dans LF, Lansang MAD, Silvestre MAA, Guyatt GH. Controversy and debate on dengue vaccine series-paper 1: review of a licensed dengue vaccine: inappropriate subgroup analyses and selective reporting may cause harm in mass vaccination programs. J Clin Epidemiol. 2018;95:137–9.
16. Low S-L, Lam S, Wong W-Y, Teo D, Ng L-C, Tan L-K. Dengue Seroprevalence of healthy adults in Singapore: Serosurvey among blood donors, 2009. Am J Trop Med Hyg. 2015;93:40–5.
17. World Health Organization. Dengue vaccine: WHO position paper - July 2016. 2016.
18. Ooi E-E, Goh K-T, Gubler DJ. Dengue prevention and 35 years of vector control in Singapore. Emerg Infect Dis. 2006;12:887–93.
19. Johansson MA, Reich NG, Hota A, Brownstein JS, Santillana M. Evaluating the performance of infectious disease forecasts: a comparison of climate-driven and seasonal dengue forecasts for Mexico. Sci Rep. 2016;6:33707.
20. Guo P, Liu T, Zhang Q, Wang L, Xiao J, Zhang Q, et al. Developing a dengue forecast model using machine learning: a case study in China. PLoS Negl Trop Dis. 2017;11:e0005973.
21. Martínez-Bello DA, López-Quílez A, Torres-Prieto A. Bayesian dynamic modeling of time series of dengue disease case counts. PLoS Negl Trop Dis. 2017;11. https://doi.org/10.1371/journal.pntd.0005696.
22. Earnest A, Tan SB, Wilder-Smith A, Machin D. Comparing Statistical Models to Predict Dengue Fever Notifications. Comput Math Methods Med. 2012; 2012:758674.
23. Hii YL, Zhu H, Ng N, Ng LC, Rocklöv J. Forecast of dengue incidence using temperature and rainfall. PLoS Negl Trop Dis. 2012;6:e1908.
24. Shi Y, Liu X, Kok S-Y, Rajarethinam J, Liang S, Yap G, et al. Three-Month Real-Time Dengue Forecast Models: An Early Warning System for Outbreak Alerts and Policy Decision Support in Singapore. Environ Health Perspect. 2016; 124:1369–75.
25. Lauer SA, Sakrejda K, Ray EL, Keegan LT, Bi Q, Suangtho P, et al. Prospective forecasts of annual dengue hemorrhagic fever incidence in Thailand, 2010–2014. Proc Natl Acad Sci. 2018;115(10):E2175–82.
26. Ramadona AL, Lazuardi L, Hii YL, Holmner Å, Kusnanto H, Rocklöv J. Prediction of dengue outbreaks based on disease surveillance and meteorological data. PLoS One. 2016;11:e0152688.
27. Lowe R, Stewart-Ibarra AM, Petrova D, García-Díez M, Borbor-Cordova MJ, Mejía R, et al. Climate services for health: predicting the evolution of the 2016 dengue season in Machala, Ecuador. Lancet Planet Health. 2017;1: e142–51.
28. Rehman NA, Kalyanaraman S, Ahmad T, Pervaiz F, Saif U, Subramanian L. Fine-grained dengue forecasting using telephone triage services. Sci Adv. 2016;2:e1501215.
29. Cortes F, Turchi Martelli CM, Arraes de Alencar Ximenes R, Montarroyos UR, Siqueira Junior JB, Gonçalves Cruz O, et al. Time series analysis of dengue surveillance data in two Brazilian cities. Acta Trop. 2018;182:190–7.
30. Sirisena P, Noordeen F, Kurukulasuriya H, Romesh TA, Fernando L. Effect of climatic factors and population density on the distribution of dengue in Sri

Lanka: a GIS based evaluation for prediction of outbreaks. PLoS One. 2017; 12. https://doi.org/10.1371/journal.pone.0166806.

31. Baquero OS, Santana LMR, Chiaravalloti-Neto F. Dengue forecasting in São Paulo city with generalized additive models, artificial neural networks and seasonal autoregressive integrated moving average models. PLoS One. 2018;13:e0195065.

32. Zhu G, Liu J, Tan Q, Shi B. Inferring the Spatio-temporal patterns of dengue transmission from surveillance data in Guangzhou, China. PLoS Negl Trop Dis. 2016;10. Available from: https://doi.org/10.1371/journal.pntd.0004633.

33. Wesolowski A, Qureshi T, Boni MF, Sundsøy PR, Johansson MA, Rasheed SB, et al. Impact of human mobility on the emergence of dengue epidemics in Pakistan. Proc Natl Acad Sci U S A. 2015;112:11887–92.

34. Cheong YL, Leitão PJ, Lakes T. Assessment of land use factors associated with dengue cases in Malaysia using boosted regression trees. Spat Spatio-Temporal Epidemiol. 2014;10:75–84.

35. Marques-Toledo CA, Degener CM, Vinhal L, Coelho G, Meira W, Codeço CT, et al. Dengue prediction by the web: tweets are a useful tool for estimating and forecasting dengue at country and city level. PLoS Negl Trop Dis. 2017; 11:e0005729.

36. Anggraeni W, Aristiani L. Using Google trend data in forecasting number of dengue fever cases with ARIMAX method case study: Surabaya, Indonesia, 2016 Int Conf Inf Commun Technol Syst ICTS; 2016. p. 114–8.

37. Li Q, Cao W, Ren H, Ji Z, Jiang H. Spatiotemporal responses of dengue fever transmission to the road network in an urban area. Acta Trop. 2018;183:8–13.

38. Liu K, Zhu Y, Xia Y, Zhang Y, Huang X, Huang J, et al. Dynamic spatiotemporal analysis of indigenous dengue fever at street-level in Guangzhou city, China. PLoS Negl Trop Dis. 2018;12. https://doi.org/10.1371/journal.pntd.0006318.

39. Zhu G, Xiao J, Zhang B, Liu T, Lin H, Li X, et al. The spatiotemporal transmission of dengue and its driving mechanism: a case study on the 2014 dengue outbreak in Guangdong, China. Sci Total Environ. 2018;622–623:252–9.

40. Van Benthem BHB, Vanwambeke SO, Khantikul N, Burghoorn-Maas C, Panart K, Oskam L, et al. Spatial patterns of and risk factors for seropositivity for dengue infection. Am J Trop Med Hyg. 2005;72:201–8.

41. Meteorological Service Singapore. Climate of Singapore. Available from: http://www.weather.gov.sg/climate-climate-of-singapore/. [cited 2018 May 7]

42. Tibshirani R. Regression Shrinkage and Selection via the Lasso. J R Stat Soc Ser B Methodol. 1996;58:267–88.

43. Chen Y, Chu CW, Chen MIC, Cook AR. The utility of LASSO-based models for real time forecasts of endemic infectious diseases: a cross country comparison. 2018;81:16–30.

44. Fawcett T. An introduction to ROC analysis. Pattern Recogn Lett. 2006;27: 861–74.

45. Bradley AP. The use of the area under the ROC curve in the evaluation of machine learning algorithms. Pattern Recogn. 1997;30:1145–59.

46. Matthews BW. Comparison of the predicted and observed secondary structure of T4 phage lysozyme. Biochim Biophys Acta BBA - Protein Struct. 1975;405:442–51.

47. R Core Team. R: A language and environment for statistical computing. Vienna: R Foundation for Statistical Computing; 2017. Available from: https://www.R-project.org/

48. Dengue Clusters. Available from: http://www.nea.gov.sg/public-health/dengue/dengue-clusters. [cited 2018 Jan 3]

49. Endy TP, Chunsuttiwat S, Nisalak A, Libraty DH, Green S, Rothman AL, et al. Epidemiology of Inapparent and symptomatic acute dengue virus infection: a prospective study of primary school children in Kamphaeng Phet, Thailand. Am J Epidemiol. 2002;156:40–51.

5

Global incidence of suicide among Indigenous peoples

Nathaniel J. Pollock[1,2]* (iD), Kiyuri Naicker[3], Alex Loro[3], Shree Mulay[1] and Ian Colman[3]

Abstract

Background: Suicide is the second leading cause of death among adolescents worldwide, and is a major driver of health inequity among Indigenous people in high-income countries. However, little is known about the burden of suicide among Indigenous populations in low- and middle-income nations, and no synthesis of the global data is currently available. Our objective was to examine the global incidence of suicide among Indigenous peoples and assess disparities through comparisons with non-Indigenous populations.

Methods: We conducted a systematic review of suicide rates among Indigenous peoples worldwide and assessed disparities between Indigenous and non-Indigenous populations. We performed text word and Medical Subject Headings searches in PubMed, MEDLINE, Embase, Cumulative Index of Nursing and Allied Health (CINAHL), PsycINFO, Latin American and Caribbean Health Sciences Literature (LILACS), and Scientific Electronic Library Online (SciELO) for observational studies in any language, indexed from database inception until June 1, 2017. Eligible studies examined crude or standardized suicide rates in Indigenous populations at national, regional, or local levels, and examined rate ratios for comparisons to non-Indigenous populations.

Results: The search identified 13,736 papers and we included 99. Eligible studies examined suicide rates among Indigenous peoples in 30 countries and territories, though the majority focused on populations in high-income nations. Results showed that suicide rates are elevated in many Indigenous populations worldwide, though rate variation is common, and suicide incidence ranges from 0 to 187.5 suicide deaths per 100,000 population. We found evidence of suicide rate parity between Indigenous and non-Indigenous populations in some contexts, while elsewhere rates were more than 20 times higher among Indigenous peoples.

Conclusions: This review showed that suicide rates in Indigenous populations vary globally, and that suicide rate disparities between Indigenous and non-Indigenous populations are substantial in some settings but not universal. Including Indigenous identifiers and disaggregating national suicide mortality data by geography and ethnicity will improve the quality and relevance of evidence that informs community, clinical, and public health practice in Indigenous suicide prevention.

Keywords: Indigenous, First peoples, Inuit, Health disparities, Suicide, Mortality, Surveillance, Epidemiology

Background

Globally, suicide accounts for approximately 800,000 deaths annually [1] and is the second leading cause of mortality among adolescents [2]. According to the World Health Organization (WHO), low- and middle-income countries and high-income countries have similar annual age-standardized suicide rates at 11.2 and 12.7 per 100,000 respectively; however, low- and middle-income countries account for 75% of suicide deaths worldwide [1]. National suicide rates range from less than one to 44 per 100,000 population, though there is often a disproportionate burden among specific subgroups within countries, such as Indigenous peoples [1]. Studies from high-income countries including Australia [3, 4], New Zealand [5], the USA [6, 7], Canada [8–10], and other Arctic nations [11–14] consistently find elevated suicide rates among Indigenous

* Correspondence: nathaniel.pollock@med.mun.ca
[1]Division of Community Health and Humanities, Faculty of Medicine, Memorial University, Prince Philip Drive, St. John's, Newfoundland and Labrador A1B 3V6, Canada
[2]Labrador Institute of Memorial University, P.O. Box 490, Stn. B, 219 Hamilton River Road, Happy Valley-Goose Bay, ,Newfoundland and Labrador A0P 1E0, Canada
Full list of author information is available at the end of the article

populations, with substantial rate disparities compared to non-Indigenous populations. Several studies have shown that regional suicide rates vary greatly among Indigenous peoples, and that some Indigenous populations have low rates or no incidence of suicide [15, 16].

Indigenous peoples and nations differ vastly in culture, language, political autonomy, and relative wealth, yet many face similar social disadvantages and health disparities as a result of colonization [17–19]. Colonial governments have used discriminatory legislation and policies to deny rights and economic opportunities, and have attempted to acculturate Indigenous people into non-Indigenous societies [17, 19, 20]. Structural violence meted out by governments has taken many forms including dispossessing Indigenous peoples from traditional and sovereign lands, forced settlement and relocation, and outlawing cultural practices and languages [17–21]. This violence is grossly evident in the twentieth century assimilationist policies of former British colonies such as Canada and Australia. Indigenous children were systematically removed from their communities and placed in non-Indigenous institutions or families with the policy mandate to "weaken family ties and cultural linkages, and to indoctrinate children into a new culture" ([20], p. v). The contemporary legacy of this type of social engineering manifests in differential exposures to health threats and in inequitable outcomes that show up across generations [20, 22]. Intergenerational trauma from institutionalized abuse and racism experienced by Indigenous peoples has been linked to persistent social and mental health problems in some communities [19, 20, 23].

Although evidence has shown a disproportionate burden of suicide among Indigenous populations in national and regional studies, a global and systematic investigation of this topic has not been undertaken to date. Previous reviews of suicide epidemiology among Indigenous populations have tended to be less comprehensive or not systematic, and have often focused on subpopulations such as youth [24, 25], high-income countries [9, 26], or regions such as Oceania [27] or the Arctic [24, 28]. Given that approximately 80% of the world's more than 300 million Indigenous people live in Asia, Latin America, and Africa [17, 18], a comprehensive study of global suicide rates that includes low- and middle-income countries is needed. Our aim was to examine the published findings on the incidence of suicide among Indigenous peoples worldwide, and to compare rates with non-Indigenous or general populations to assess relative disparities.

Methods

Search strategy

We systematically reviewed findings on the incidence of suicide in Indigenous populations worldwide. We searched for studies that analyzed population-based data on suicide deaths, and included papers that reported crude or standardized mortality rates. Health science librarians were consulted about the design of the search strategy with the aim to capture all peer-reviewed literature. The search combined terms related to three concept areas: population (Indigenous), outcome (suicide mortality rates), and study design (observational). Term selection was based on previous systematic reviews and combined key terms adapted for each database and also Medical Subject Headings (MeSH) as applicable. The study protocol is available in Additional file 1: Supplement 1. Additional details about the methods are reported in Additional file 1: Supplement 2, including citations for previous reviews, a list of included terms, a description of the procedures used for study selection and eligibility criteria, and a complete list of databases and hand-searched review articles.

One author (NJP) performed online text word and MeSH searches for articles indexed in PubMed, MEDLINE, Embase, Cumulative Index of Nursing and Allied Health (CINAHL), PsycINFO, Latin American and Caribbean Health Sciences Literature (LILACS), and Scientific Electronic Library Online (SCiELO). A second author (KN) replicated the search in PubMed and obtained the same number of articles as the first author. We searched for studies in any language, indexed from database inception until June 1, 2017. We conducted a secondary search with a comprehensive list of terms for specific tribal groups, nations, and populations identified in previous reviews. As no additional studies were identified, this approach validated the primary search. We also searched the WHO's regional medical literature indexes, Indigenous-specific online research portals, and journals focused on Indigenous health. We hand-searched the reference lists of included articles and previous reviews to identify other eligible studies. Additional file 1: Supplement 2 includes a list of all databases and hand-searched sources.

One author (NJP) imported the results into a reference management program and removed duplicates. Two authors (NJP and KN) read the abstracts and screened in papers if they (1) reported a population-based crude and/or standardized suicide rate, or count and population data; (2) reported a rate for an Indigenous population; and (3) used an observational design. We excluded articles that did not include an Indigenous population, focused only on a specific age, gender, clinical subgroup, or deaths from a specific cause (for example, firearms), or were not peer-reviewed. Articles were also excluded if they were iterations, program evaluations or experimental studies, not primary studies, from the gray literature, or used identical data sources as prior studies.

Although there is no international consensus on the definition of Indigenous, we used the United Nation's working definition to assess study population eligibility

[17, 18]. The UN's conceptualization of Indigenous involves self and group identification; a special attachment to and use of traditional land, distinct knowledge, language, and culture; distinct social, economic, and political systems; common ancestry with original territorial occupants; participation in maintenance and reproduction of distinct ethnic identity; and a non-dominant socio-political status [17, 18]. A paper was eligible based on this criterion if it reported an outcome for an Indigenous population, tribe, community, nation, or group, including papers that used the geographic proxy method. For the proxy method, census data is used to detect areas where Indigenous people are a majority population [29, 30]. We considered an area to be a proxy identifier if 80% or more of the population self-identified as Indigenous.

Two authors reviewed the full text of each paper and assessed eligibility based on inclusion criteria. At this stage, we excluded papers that did not report rates for the majority of the population (aged 15–65 years), did not conduct the primary data analysis, or provided rates in figures only and did not report count and population data. If two eligible articles used the same data source with a period of overlap, we included the article with the longer study period. During screening, full text review, and data extraction, we resolved disagreements through discussion or consultation with a third author. Translators helped assess non-English language articles and assisted with data extraction for four included studies. The following data was independently extracted by two authors (AL and NJP), then compared: citation, study design, country and region/community, Indigenous population, data source, standard population, number of suicide deaths, population count, crude and standardized suicide rates (overall and by gender and age group), comparative rates for a non-Indigenous or general population, and the measure of relative effect (incidence rate ratio).

Data analysis

We summarized all included studies in a table and reported counts, population, crude and standardized suicide mortality rates, and rate ratios. We calculated crude suicide mortality incidence rates for articles that reported only count and population data, and we estimated rate ratios when not otherwise reported by dividing the Indigenous population rate by the comparison population rate. To identify global patterns, we presented rates and rate ratios in tables and figures grouped by WHO region, country, population, and gender; we did not pool the data due to heterogeneity. We also reported on trends in suicide mortality over time and by age group; reported time trends reflect results from included studies, not pooled and recalculated rates. We modified the Newcastle-Ottawa Scale and used it to

assess the quality of included articles. Additional file 1: Supplement 2 includes a description of the quality assessment procedures and scoring, and the Preferred Reporting Items for Systematic Reviews and Meta-Analyses (PRISMA) checklist is provided in Additional file 1: Supplement 4 [31].

Results

The search identified 13,736 papers; after removing duplicates, screening abstracts, and full text review, we included 99 in our analysis (Fig. 1). Included studies examined suicide rates in Indigenous populations in 30 countries and territories across six decades (Table 1), though the majority focused on those in high-income countries such as American Indian and Alaska Natives in the USA ($n = 35$) and Inuit and First Nations in Canada ($n = 14$). Studies in low- and middle-income countries ($n = 22$) were mostly from Brazil ($n = 4$), China and Taiwan ($n = 6$), and Fiji ($n = 5$). Coverage included circumpolar Indigenous peoples such as Sámi ($n = 3$) and Nenets ($n = 1$), and populations from the Western Pacific region including Aboriginal and Torres Strait Islanders in Australia ($n = 6$) and Māori and other Pacific peoples ($n = 16$). Four studies were transnational comparisons [32–35], though numerous papers included multiple Indigenous groups within a single country. Studies were mostly of moderate quality (mean 2.79 on a 4-point scale) based on our assessment of study characteristics, as reported in Additional file 1: Supplement 3, Tables S1 and S2.

Incidence

We extracted population-based suicide mortality rates from 93 papers (Table 2) and included gender-specific incidence data from six additional studies [5, 10, 36–39]. Overall, suicide rates among Indigenous peoples varied at all levels of aggregation in both high-income and low- and middle-income countries, and spanned from zero to 187.5 deaths per 100,000 person-years (PY; Table 2). In high-income countries, national and provincial suicide rates among Indigenous peoples ranged from 1.7 per 100,000 in Brunei Darussalam [40] to 50.4 per 100,000 among Aboriginal and Torres Strait Islanders in Northern Territory, Australia [41]. Rates in high-income countries were highest among rural Indigenous populations and in sparsely populated regions such as the Arctic. Among low- and middle-income countries, Palawan communities in the Philippines had the highest crude suicide rates (134 per 100,000) [42], while Indigenous peoples in Malaysia [43] and some Pacific small island states such as Fiji had crude rates under 7 per 100,000 population. The number of suicide deaths used for rate calculations ranged from zero to 4219 (Table 2).

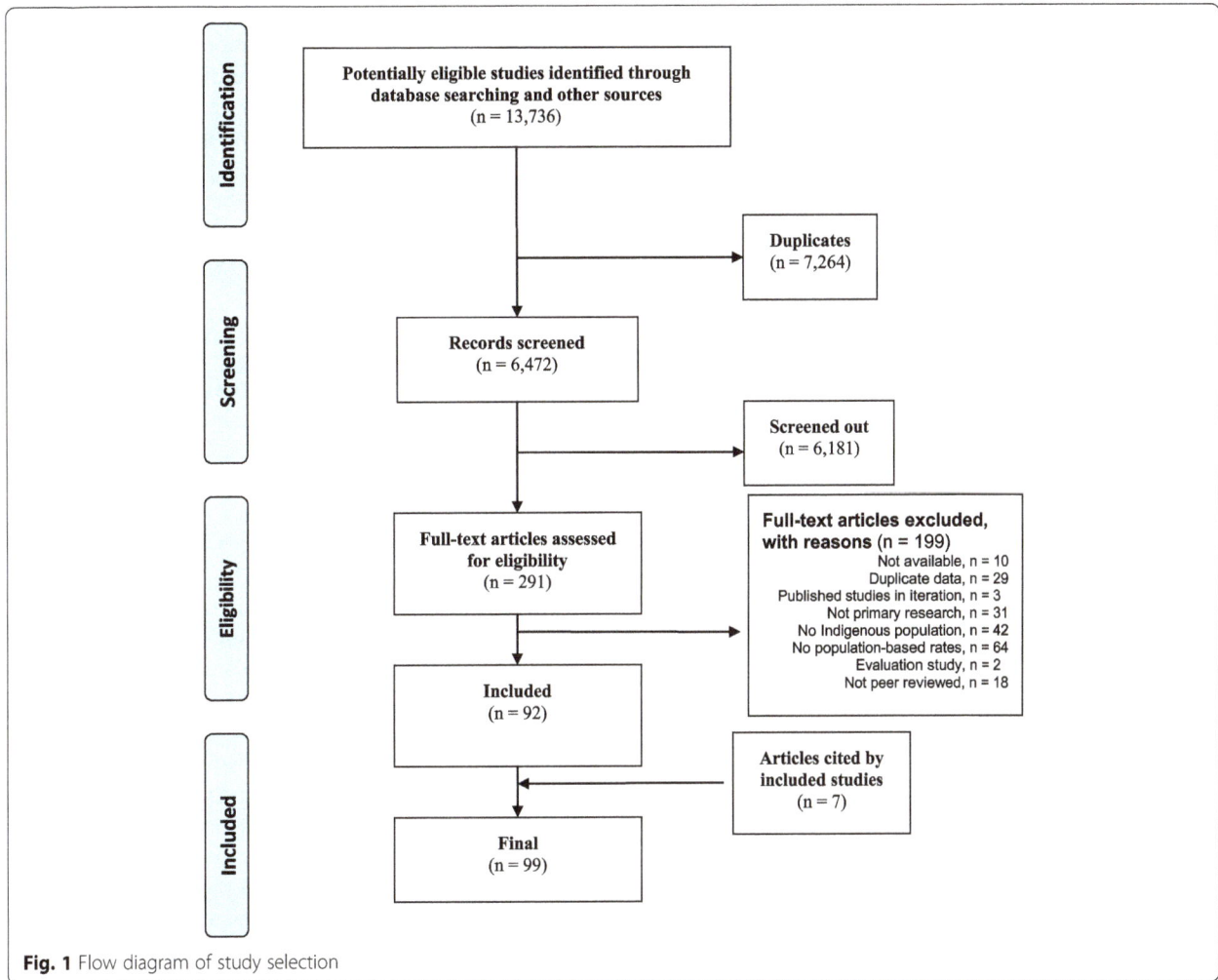

Fig. 1 Flow diagram of study selection

Measure of relative effect

Incidence rate ratios were reported or calculated for 102 Indigenous populations in 69 studies. The results showed rate disparities in the majority of studies (Fig. 2), though 22 reported rate ratios below one. The rate ratios ranged from 0.04 in China [44] to more than 20 in Brazil [45] and Canada [30] (Additional file 1: Supplement 3, Table S4). Most Indigenous populations had higher suicide rates than comparison groups; disparities were widest in studies with small populations. One study reported a suicide rate of zero for an urban Indigenous population in Brazil compared the general population rate of 4.8 per 100,000 in the same city [46].

Time trends

Suicide rates appeared to increase over time, especially in the latter half of the twentieth century, though reports were limited. Among studies with reported time series (*n* = 24), most (83%, *n* = 20) had fewer than 10 data points and covered an average of

19 years. A study in Greenland was the exception; it reported longitudinal data that showed a steady suicide rate increase among Inuit that began with the near absence of suicide in the early part of the twentieth century (2.4 per 100,000) and climbed exponentially to a rate of 110.4 per 100,000 in 2010–2011; the average number of suicides per year changed from less than one to 55 during this period [12]. Aboriginal and Torres Strait Islanders in Northern Territory, Australia experienced similar rate accelerations (6.1 per 100,000 in 1981 to 50.4 per 100,000 in 2002) [41], while incidence among Alaska Natives was relatively stable, though high, from the 1980s to the early 2000s [47, 48]. Indigenous peoples in the Micronesian islands experienced a sixfold increase in suicide rates between the 1960s and the late 1980s (from 4.3 to 25.8 per 100,000) [35], and one study reported slight rate declines for both Māori and non-Māori in New Zealand from 1996 to 2002 [5]. Annual rates tended to fluctuate in studies with small populations.

Table 1 Overview of included studies

	No. of studies (*N*)	% of total (*n*/99)
Decade of publication		
1960–1979	12	12.1%
1980s	23	23.2%
1990s	25	25.3%
2000s	17	17.2%
2010s	22	22.2%
World Bank income		
High-income	76	76.8%
Low- and middle-income	22	22.2%
Multiple	1	1.0%
WHO Region		
Western Pacific	33	33.3%
European	8	8.1%
Region of the Americas	56	56.6%
Multiple regions	2	2.0%
Total Indigenous population		
Less than 10,000	17	17.2%
10,000–99,999	32	32.3%
100,000–999,999	12	12.1%
1,000,000+	4	4.0%
Not reported	34	34.3%
Number of suicide deaths among Indigenous population		
Less than 20	18	18.2%
21–99	23	23.2%
100–999	23	23.2%
1000+	4	4.0%
Not reported	31	31.3%

Age differences

Age-specific rates were reported in 39 studies; various age categories were used, and rates were often only available for select strata. Youth less than 30 years old, especially those aged 15–24 years old, had the highest suicide rates of any age group in 89% of studies (*n* = 34) that reported age-specific rates. In the larger studies (> 100 total suicides) with age-specific incidence, youth suicide rates ranged from 15.9 to 108 per 100,000 population. Very few studies reported deaths or rate estimates for adults more than 60 years old.

Gender differences

Men accounted for the majority of suicide deaths in all but four studies; only two of these four studies reported a greater number of suicide deaths among women [49, 50]. Studies with gender-specific crude and age-standardized rates (*n* = 35) ranged from zero to 75.5 per 100,000 among Indigenous women (Additional file 1: Supplement 3, Table S3). Suicide rates were higher among Indigenous men compared to Indigenous women, though rate differences were marginal among some Pacific populations [33, 51]. Suicide rates were also higher among Indigenous men than for men in comparison populations in all countries except Israel and Fiji. Outside of the relatively low rates among Indigenous men in these countries, estimates ranged from 19.5 among Sámi [13] to 248.7 per 100,000 among Inuit [30].

Discussion

This study showed that the rate of suicide is elevated in many Indigenous populations globally, but that rate variation is common (Fig. 1). The evidence of substantial rate disparities for Indigenous peoples in Australia, Brazil, Taiwan, and circumpolar countries is notable. Equally important, we found that disparities were marginal or non-existent in some US territories and Pacific nations; we also identified 21 studies in which Indigenous populations had lower suicide rates than non-Indigenous populations. These results demonstrate that the high incidence of suicide and large rate disparities are not universal among Indigenous peoples. This confirms and extends findings from prior research that reported variation in localized estimates in the USA [52] and Canada [16].

Worldwide variation in the incidence of suicide among Indigenous peoples has complex and place-based social origins. These origins are traceable to regional differences in the impact of colonization, which is widely recognized as a major determinant of Indigenous health [17–19, 53]. Colonial governments have historically threatened the well-being of Indigenous peoples through chronic and often state-sanctioned discrimination and human rights abuses, and continue to do so in many countries [18, 20, 23]. Until 2016, several high-income countries had not ratified the United Nations Declaration on the Rights of Indigenous Peoples, and therefore legislative reforms to recognize Indigenous self-determination lagged. As a result, many Indigenous nations have yet to attain political sovereignty over lands and natural resources, education, or health care.

Globally, Indigenous peoples commonly experience social and economic marginalization and, as a consequence, some of the most disparate health outcomes [17, 18, 53]. In this context, the extent and the persistence of high suicide rates and rate disparities reveal a striking deficit in the global effort to prevent suicide and achieve social and health equity. This is further challenged by overlapping barriers to accessing health care and community supports, especially in rural areas and low- and middle-income countries. Barriers include fragmented care networks, lack of access to services due to geography, discriminatory attitudes from health care providers, and services that are not culturally safe or provided in the necessary language [18, 54, 55]. In resource-

Table 2 Suicide mortality rates among Indigenous populations by WHO region and country

WHO Region	Country	Indigenous peoples[a]	Population	Period	Deaths	CSIR	SSIR
European Region							
Soininen (2008) [14]	Finland (Northern region)	Sámi	2091	1979–2005	24	50.0	–
Thorslund (1989) [70]	Greenland	Kalaallit (Inuit)	–	1986	57	129	–
Bjerregaard (2015) [72]	Greenland	Kalaallit (Inuit)	57,000	1970–2011	1678	87.7	–
	East/north regions	Kalaallit (Inuit)	–	1970–2011	–307	187.5	–
	Nuuk	Kalaallit (Inuit)	–	1970–2011	–303	86.6	–
	Towns in Western region	Kalaallit (Inuit)	–	1970–2011	–837	81.2	–
	Villages in Western region	Kalaallit (Inuit)	–	1970–2011	–222	61.4	–
Klomek (2016) [71]	Israel	Bedouin	–	1999–2011	39	4.4	3.2
Silviken (2009) [11]	Norway (Northern region)	Sámi	19,801	1970–1998	89	18.9	–
Sumarokov (2014) [72]	Russia (Nenets Autonomous Okrug)	Nenets	7504	2002–2012	67	79.8	72.7
Hassler (2005) [13]	Sweden	Sámi	41,721	1961–2000	114	11.7	–
		Sámi (non-herding)	–	1961–2000	76	9.8	–
		Sámi (reindeer herding)	–	1961–2000	38	19.6	–
Western Pacific Region (Australia)							
Clayer (1991) [73]	Australia (South Australia)	Aboriginal and Torres Strait Islander	13,298	1988	14	105.3	–
Cantor (1997) [74]	Australia (Queensland)	Aboriginal and Torres Strait Islander	–	1990–1992	–	–	17.1
Stevenson (1998) [34]	Australia	Aboriginal and Torres Strait Islander	–	1990–1992	67	–	11.1
Bramley (2004) [32]	Australia	Aboriginal and Torres Strait Islander	–	1999	–	–	19.4
De Leo (2011) [4]	Australia (Queensland)	Aboriginal and Torres Strait Islander	–	1994–2007	544	–	27.2
Measey (2006) [41]	Australia (Northern Territory)	Aboriginal and Torres Strait Islander	–	2002	–	–	50.4
Pridmore (2009) [3]	Australia (Northern Territory)	Aboriginal and Torres Strait Islander	–	2001–2006	130	–	36.7
Campbell (2016) [75]	Australia (Kimberley)	Aboriginal and Torres Strait Islander	11,550	2005–2014	102	–	74
Western Pacific Region (Oceania)							
Booth (1999) [33]	American Samoa	Samoan	54,800	1990–1991	–	18	–
Hezel (1984) [76]	FSM (Chuuk)	Chuukese	37,488	1971–1983	129	30	–
Hezel (1989) [35]	Federated States of Micronesia	Pacific peoples	142,298	1984–1987	134	25.8	–
	Chuuk	Chuukese	44,000	1984–1987	51	28.3	–
	Kosrae	Kosraen	6448	1984–1987	6	25.9	–
	Pohnpei	Pohnpeian	28,879	1984–1987	18	16.7	–
	Yap	Yapese	10,139	1984–1987	5	20.2	–
Booth (1999) [33]	Federated States of Micronesia	Pacific peoples	105,700	1988–1992	–	31	–
	Chuuk	Chuukese	–	1988–1992	–	35	–

Table 2 Suicide mortality rates among Indigenous populations by WHO region and country (Continued)

WHO Region	Country	Indigenous peoples[a]	Population	Period	Deaths	CSIR	SSIR
	Kosrae	Kosraen	–	1988–1992	–	48	–
	Pohnpei	Pohnpeian	–	1988–1992	–	20	–
	Yap	Yapese	–	1988–1992	–	48	–
Ree (1971) [77]	Fiji (Macuata)	iTaukei	9950	1962–1968	4	5.7	–
Price (1975) [51]	Fiji	iTaukei	–	1971–1972	6	1.3	–
Haynes (1984) [78]	Fiji (Macuata)	iTaukei	8111	1979–1982	2	6.7	–
Pridmore (1994) [79]	Fiji (Western Division)	iTaukei	–	1986–1992	–	2	–
Pridmore (1995) [80]	Fiji	iTaukei	–	1969–1989	–	3.6	–
Booth (1999) [33]	Fiji	iTaukei	–	1982–1983	–	3	3
Booth (1999) [33]	French Polynesia	Polynesian	218,000	1988–1992	–	9	9
Booth (2010) [81]	Guam	Chamorro	–	1998–2000	–	21	–
Hezel (1989) [35]	Marshall Islands	Marshallese	39,060	1984–1987	39	26.5	–
Booth (1999) [33]	Marshall Islands	Marshallese	54,700	1988–1992	–	26	–
Langley (1990) [82]	Aotearoa/New Zealand	Māori	–	1984	22	–	8
Langley (2000) [83]	Aotearoa/New Zealand	Māori	–	1985–1994	271	8.8	–
Bramley (2004) [32]	Aotearoa/New Zealand	Māori	–	1999	–	–	12.9
Hezel (1989) [35]	Palau	Palauan	13,772	1984–1987	15	28.8	–
Booth (1999) [33]	Palau	Palauan	16,500	1988–1992	–	29	–
Parker (1966) [84]	Papua New Guinea	Pacific peoples	–	1961–1965	41	0.7	–
Smith (1981) [50]	Papua New Guinea (Southern Highlands)	Huli	50,000	1971–1976	26	17	–
Booth (1999) [33]	Papua New Guinea	Pacific peoples	4,216,100	1990	–	<1	–
Booth (1999) [33]	Samoa	Samoan	163,400	1981	–	31	34
Pridmore (1997) [49]	Solomon Islands (Honiara area)	Pacific peoples	75,000	1989–1993	13	3.9	–
Vivili (1999) [85]	Tonga	Tongan	98,200	1982–1997	43	2.9	–
Booth (1999) [33]	Vanuatu	ni-Vanuatu	164,100	1990–1992	–	3	–
De Leo (2013) [86]	Vanuatu	ni-Vanuatu	245,619	2010	2	0.8	–
Western Pacific Region (East Asia)							
Telisinghe (2014) [40]	Brunei Darussalam	Indigenous peoples (7 tribes)[b]	14,000	1991–2010	4	1.7	–
Wang (1997) [87]	China (Hohhot, Inner Mongolia)	Meng	27,000	1986–1991	–	2.4	–
		Hui	21,600	1986–1991	–	1.2	–
Lu (2013) [44]	China (Yunnan Province)	Dai	325,126	2004–2005	–	12	–
		Yi	582,596	2004–2005	–	20.8	–
		Li su	147,794	2004–2005	–	50.8	–

Table 2 Suicide mortality rates among Indigenous populations by WHO region and country (Continued)

WHO Region	Country	Indigenous peoples[a]	Population	Period	Deaths	CSIR	SSIR
		Other ethnic minorities	1,922,430	2004–2005	—	0.96–36.4[c]	—
Ali (2014) [43]	Malaysia (Sabah and Sarawak)	Bumiputera	2,981,300	2009	11	0.4	—
Jollant (2014) [42]	Philippines	Palawan	1192	2002–2012	16	134	—
Cheng (1992) [88]	Taiwan	Atayal	—	1981–1985	—	46.3	—
		Ami	—	1981–1985	—	5.3	—
		Bunun	—	1981–1985	—	64.8	—
		Paiwan	—	1981–1985	—	16.3	—
Hsieh (1994) [89]	Taiwan	Indigenous peoples	200,000	1971–1990	1597	40.1	—
		Atayal	—	1971–1990	928	57.6	—
		Bunun	—	1971–1990	222	44.7	—
		Paiwan	—	1971–1990	204	21.3	—
Wen (2004) [90]	Taiwan	Indigenous peoples	200,537	1998–2000	128	21.9	—
Liu (2011) [91]	Taiwan (East region)	Ami	—	1979–1981	30	15.6	—
		Atayal	—	1979–1981	30	68.2	—
Region of the Americas (Brazil and Canada)							
Coloma (2006) [45]	Brazil (Mato Grosso do Sul)	Indigenous peoples (6 tribes)[d]	53,325	2000–2003	194	96.2	—
Souza (2013) [46]	Brazil (Amazonas)	Indigenous peoples	184,764	2006–2010	131	—	18.4
	Manaus	Indigenous peoples	—	2006–2010		—	0
	Sao Gabriel da Cachoeira	Indigenous peoples	—	2006–2010		—	41.9
	Tabatinga	Indigenous peoples	—	2006–2010		—	75.8
Machado (2015) [92]	Brazil	Indigenous peoples	—	2012		14.4	—
Orellana (2016) [21]	Brazil (Mato Grosso do Sul)	Indigenous peoples (3 tribes)[e]	75,000	2009–2011		—	65.2
Butler (1965) [93]	Canada (NWT/Nunavut)	Inuit	7949	1959–1964	9	18.8	—
	NWT	First Nation	5284	1959–1964	0	0	—
	Yukon	First Nation	2207	1959–1964	5	37.7	—
Young (1983) [94]	Canada (Northwestern Ontario)	Cree and Ojibway	10,000	1972–1981	17	16.1	—
Fox (1984) [95]	Canada (Wikwemikong, Ontario)	Anishinaabe	3000	1976–1980	—	26.7	—
Wotton (1985) [96]	Canada (Labrador)	Innu and Inuit	2500	1979–1983	8	65.5	—
Spaulding (1985) [97]	Canada (Northern Ontario)	Ojibway	3005	1975–1982	14	61.7	—
Mao (1986) [98]	Canada (7 provinces)	First Nation (on reserve)	168,529	1977–1982	344	34	—
Ross (1986) [68]	Canada	Cree	2822	1981–1984	7	83	—
Garro (1988) [99]	Canada (Manitoba)	First Nation (Status Indians)	43,000	1973–1982	174	40.2	—
		Dene	—	1973–1982	—	13	—

Table 2 Suicide mortality rates among Indigenous populations by WHO region and country (*Continued*)

WHO Region	Country	Indigenous peoples[a]	Population	Period	Deaths	CSIR	SSIR
		Ojibway (Northern)	–	1973–1982	–	5	–
		Cree	–	1973–1982	–	22	–
		Saulteaux	–	1973–1982	–	48	–
		Dakota	–	1973–1982	–	80	31.8
Malchy (1997) [100]	Canada (Manitoba)	First Nation and Métis	–	1988–1994	227	38	–
Chandler (1998) [16]	Canada (British Colombia)	First Nation	–	1987–1992	220	45.2	–
Isaacs (1998) [101]	Canada (NWT)	Dene	–	1994–1996	–	29	–
	NWT/Nunavut	Inuit	–	1994–1996	–	79	–
Bramley (2004) [32]	Canada	First Nation	–	1999	–	–	27.8
Macaulay (2004) [8]	Canada (Kivalliq, Nunavut)	Inuit	7131	1987–1996	31	–	45.1
Penney (2009) [102]	Canada (Nunavut)	Inuit	20,489	1999–2003	–	–	95.6
	Canada (Nunavik)	Inuit	7628	1999–2003	–	–	159.8
Pollock (2016) [30]	Canada (Labrador)	Innu	1815	1993–2009	28	–137.0	114
	Canada (Labrador)	Inuit	2415	1993–2009	64	–186.8	165.6
Region of the Americas (USA, National)							
Ogden (1970) [103]	USA (24 Western states)	American Indian and Alaska Native	630,000	1967	94	17	23.1
Young (1993) [104]	USA (IHSA)	American Indian and Alaska Native	–	1979–1981	–	18.6	–
Lester (1994) [105]	USA	American Indian and Alaska Native	–	1980	–	13.3	–
Lester (1995) [106]	USA (48 states)	American Indian and Alaska Native	984–166,464¶	1980	–	0.0–64.7[f]	15.5
Stevenson (1998) [34]	USA	American Indian	–	1990–1992	572	–	15.5
Bramley (2004) [32]	USA	American Indian and Alaska Native	–	1999	–	–	12
Howard (2014) [107]	USA	American Indian and Alaska Native	2,439,419	1999–2010	4219	–	14.2
Herne (2014) [6]	USA (IHSA)	American Indian and Alaska Native	–	1999–2009	3600	–	21.1
	Pacific Coast IHSA	American Indian and Alaska Native	–	1999–2009	532	–	18.2
	Southwest IHSA	American Indian and Alaska Native	–	1999–2009	1066	–	19.9
	South Plains IHSA	American Indian & Alaska Native	–	1999–2009	626	–	18.7
	North Plains IHSA	American Indian and Alaska Native	–	1999–2009	755	–	26.2
	East IHSA	American Indian and Alaska Native	–	1999–2009	93	–	8.4
	Alaska IHSA	American Indian and Alaska Native	–	1999–2009	528	–	42.5
Region of the Americas (USA, Alaska)							
Kraus (1979) [108]	USA (Alaska)	Alaska Native	56,477	1970	–	29.6	–
Travis (1983) [109]	USA (Alaska)	Alaska Native	–	1975–1979	–	15.8–52.6[g]	–
Travis (1984) [110]	USA (NANA, Alaska)	Inupiat	7345	1974–1980	–	106	–

Table 2 Suicide mortality rates among Indigenous populations by WHO region and country (*Continued*)

WHO Region	Country	Indigenous peoples[a]	Population	Period	Deaths	CSIR	SSIR
	USA (Arctic Slope, Alaska)	Inupiat	-	1974–1980	-	19.2	-
Hlady (1988) [111]	USA (Alaska)	Alaska Native	-	1983–1984	65	-	42.9
Forbes (1988) [112]	USA (Alaska)	Alaska Native	-	1985	47	64.9	68.8
Kettl (1991) [113]	USA (Alaska)	Alaska Native	-	1979–1984	90	23.4	-
Andon (1997) [114]	USA (Alaska)	Athabascan	6041	1977–1987	40	55.1	-
Marshall (1998) [115]	USA (Alaska)	Alaska Native	25,000	1979–1990	186	49	-
		Yupik	-	1979–1990	103	53	-
		Inupiat	-	1979–1990	60	89	-
		Athabascan	-	1979–1990	23	147	-
Day (2003) [47]	USA (Alaska)	Alaska Native	91,300	1989–1998	-	-	49.7
Day (2009) [116]	USA (Alaska)	Alaska Native	97,012	1999–2003	204	-	36.1
Wexler (2012) [7]	USA (Northwestern Alaska)	Alaska Native	7965	2001–2009	38	60	-
Holck (2013) [48]	USA (Alaska)	Alaska Native	138,312	2004–2008	252	-	42.4
Region of the Americas (USA, Lower 48 States + Hawaii)							
Levy (1965) [117]	USA (New Mexico)	Navajo	87,000	1954–1963	59	8.3	-
Kalish (1968) [118]	USA (Hawai'i)	Kānaka Maoli (Native Hawaiian)	-	1959–1965	-	17.8	-
		Other Pacific peoples	-	1959–1965	-	6.8	-
Conrad (1974) [119]	USA (Arizona)	Tohono O'odham	12,179	1967–1971	10	-	18
Shore (1975) [120]	USA (Pacific Northwest)	American Indian	23,921	1969–1971	20	27.8	-
Sievers (1975) [121]	USA (Arizona)	American Indian	40,361	1971–1973	17	16.8	-
		Apache	-	1971–1973	-	40	-
		Akimel O'odham	-	1971–1973	-	7	-
		Other American Indian tribes	-	1971–1973	-	26	-
Miller (1979) [122]	USA (Southwest)	American Indian	-	1977	-	57.8	-
Humphrey (1982) [123]	USA (North Carolina)	Cherokee	-	1974–1976	-	31.1	-
		Lumbee	-	1974–1976	-	10.3	-
Broudy (1983) [124]	USA (Mexico and Arizona)	American Indian	162,303	1975–1977	-	-	28.5
Simpson (1983) [125]	USA (Northeastern Arizona)	Hopi	9406	1979–1980	5	27	-
Levy (1987) [126]	USA (Northern Arizona)	American Indian	7600	1981	-	23.7	-
Copeland (1989) [127]	USA (Florida)	American Indian	11,050	1982–1986	1	11	-
Sievers (1990) [128]	USA (Arizona)	Akimel O'odham	4915	1975–1984	26	53	51
Van Winkle (1993) [15]	USA (New Mexico)	Apache	-	1980–1987	179[h]	-	48.8
		Navajo	58,936	1980–1987	-	-	18.2

Table 2 Suicide mortality rates among Indigenous populations by WHO region and country (*Continued*)

WHO Region	Country	Indigenous peoples[a]	Population	Period	Deaths	CSIR	SSIR
		Pueblo	–	1980–1987	–	–	32.2
Wissow (2001) [129]	USA (Southwest)	American Indian	12,000	1985–1996	–	30.7	24.6
Mullany (2009) [130]	USA (Arizona)	White Mountain Apache	15,500	2001–2006	41	45.5	40
Martin (2010) [131]	USA (North Carolina)	American Indian	–	2004–2007	39	8.5	–
Christensen (2013) [132]	USA (South Dakota)	American Indian	82,073	2000–2010	236	29	28

WHO World Health Organization, *CSIR* crude suicide incidence rate, *SSIR* standardized suicide incidence rate, *FSM* Federated States of Micronesia, *NWT* Northwest Territories, *IHSA* Indian Health Services Area

Standardized rates were adjusted with various populations; therefore they are not directly comparable. Population *n* are based on reported estimates in each article, but may not reflect denominators used to calculate incidence

[a]General terms such as Indigenous, Pacific Peoples, or First Nation were used when a specific nation or tribe was not identifiable

[b]Indigenous tribes in Brunei Darussalam included Kedayan, Belait, Tutong, Bisya, Murut, Dusun, and Iban

[c]Rate range for 10 ethnic minority groups in Yunnan Province, China: Hui, Ha ni, A chang, Pumi, Bai, Yao, Zhuang, Miao, Meng gu, and Jing po minorities

[d]Indigenous tribes in Mato Grosso do Sul, Brazil included Kadiwe'u, Guato, Ofaié-Xavante, Guarani-Kaiowá, Guarani-Ñandeva, and Terena

[e]Indigenous tribes included Guarani-Kaiowá, Guarani-Ñandeva, and Terena

[f]Population and rate range included 48 states

[g]Rate range for 9 Native regional corporations in Northwest Alaska: Athna, Bering Straits, Bristol Bay, Calista, Chugach, Cook Inlet, Doyon, Koniag, and Sealaska (NANA and Arctic Slope not extracted due to duplicate data with Travis, 1984 [110])

[h]Total number of deaths for Apache, Navajo, and Pueblo populations combined

limited and conflict settings in particular, mental health services are inadequate in scope and quality, chronically under-funded, and in some places non-existent [18, 54].

Challenges in accessing mental health care are compounded by the limited relevance and generalizability of some "best practice" interventions in Indigenous contexts [56, 57]. Recent clinical trials with gatekeeper training [57], hospital-based interventions [58], and mobile self-help applications [59] reported adverse and limited effects on suicide-related outcomes for Indigenous peoples. Overall, intervention studies with Indigenous populations are rare, and community-based programs are often not evaluated or have weak study designs [60–63]. These challenges point to a need to expand efforts to generate Indigenous-specific evidence [23, 56, 60]. Indeed, many communities have developed contextualized and complex approaches to suicide prevention that respond to local priorities. There is emergent evidence that such programs increase protective factors and reduce suicide-related behavior [63–65]. However, knowledge about programs' effectiveness, implementation, and capacity to scale up is limited, and many programs are not sustainably funded [56, 60–62].

Indigenous organizations and governments in New Zealand, Canada, and several Arctic states have moved beyond programmatic approaches and designed Indigenous-specific suicide prevention strategies [23, 55, 66]. These strategies integrate evidence-based public health and clinical interventions with Indigenous knowledge about the consequences of colonization, institutionalized violence and racism, and the value of culture. They also recognize that social conditions have an important role in shaping mental health, especially during the early years of life, and that improving these conditions can have a positive impact on population mental health and suicide-related outcomes. The path to lowering the incidence of suicide among Indigenous peoples and achieving health equity requires broader social transformation both within states and globally. This transformation must be collaborative, with Indigenous organizations and communities as leaders and rights-holders in knowledge production and decision-making [23, 29, 53, 56, 66, 67]. Public health systems can also enhance capacity for Indigenous suicide prevention with efforts to increase the visibility of community-level differences in health status and by accurately tracking changes in suicide mortality over time.

Limitations

This study is a comprehensive synthesis of the published evidence on the global epidemiology of suicide among Indigenous peoples. Although it is the first review of this scale, our study has several important limitations. First, included studies varied their methods of identifying Indigenous populations. Self-identification is the gold standard in administrative and registry data [67]. However, this is a recent benchmark. Its uptake has varied internationally, and some countries do not identify Indigenous populations in health data at all [53, 67]. The majority of included studies relied on linkages with census or registry data, geographic proxies, or observer-determined assessments. These procedures are useful approximations, but they use varied definitions and tend to under-count Indigenous people, especially groups without legal recognition [29, 53, 67]. This can lead to ascertainment bias and underestimation of inequities [53, 67]. A second and related limitation is the under-representation of studies from low- and middle-income countries. In our review, we may have missed studies, particularly from the Global South, due to the conceptualization of Indigenous and the search terms used, which do not necessarily apply in all contexts. We attempted to limit this bias by searching databases focused on low- and middle-income countries and including non-English language papers.

The third limitation was that it was difficult to compare suicide rates between countries. Included studies were heterogeneous in population size, number of cases, aggregation, data source and outcome assessment, method of identifying Indigenous peoples, and coverage period. Many papers provided crude estimates only and did not report numerator and denominator data by age group, gender, or ethnicity. For studies with adjusted rates, different standard populations were used, and confidence intervals were rarely reported. Differences in analytic and reporting practices made it challenging to directly and reliably compare suicide rates across studies. To address this, we examined rate ratios to assess relative differences between Indigenous and non-Indigenous/general populations. This allowed us to estimate rate disparities, which were compared globally.

The fourth limitation was that studies reporting low suicide rates may be under-represented, which is a potential publication bias. It is unclear whether the lack of low incidence populations is related to the common finding of elevated rates of suicide among Indigenous peoples compared to non-Indigenous populations or, as we suspect is more likely, to the possibility that suicide rates are rarely studied when they are low. Additional low incidence reports may exist outside of peer-reviewed studies; however, these were not identified because we did not search the gray literature. The primary reason for excluding gray literature reports was the extensive volume of sources with variable quality and also the risk of over-including data from high-income nations where public reporting of mortality data is common and vital statistics infrastructure is of high quality. Nonetheless, we identified 23 papers that reported rate parity or had a rate ratio below one, but these tended to use older data. A related problem is that case studies tended to examine suicide clusters in small populations [42, 68]. The

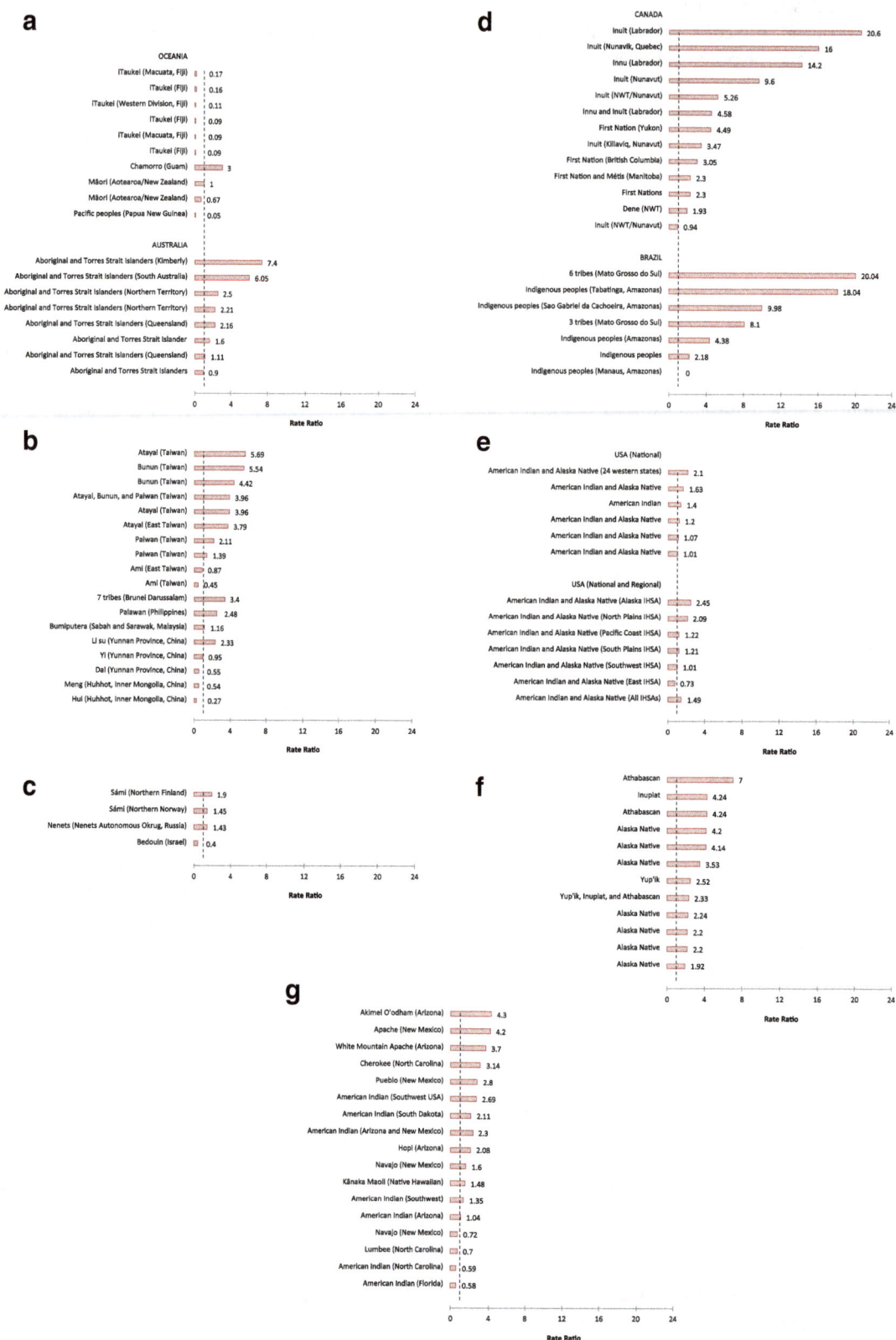

a

OCEANIA

ITaukei (Macuata, Fiji)	0.17
ITaukei (Fiji)	0.16
ITaukei (Western Division, Fiji)	0.11
ITaukei (Fiji)	0.09
ITaukei (Macuata, Fiji)	0.09
ITaukei (Fiji)	0.09
Chamorro (Guam)	3
Māori (Aotearoa/New Zealand)	1
Māori (Aotearoa/New Zealand)	0.67
Pacific peoples (Papua New Guinea)	0.05

AUSTRALIA

Aboriginal and Torres Strait Islanders (Kimberly)	7.4
Aboriginal and Torres Strait Islanders (South Australia)	6.05
Aboriginal and Torres Strait Islanders (Northern Territory)	2.5
Aboriginal and Torres Strait Islanders (Northern Territory)	2.21
Aboriginal and Torres Strait Islanders (Queensland)	2.16
Aboriginal and Torres Strait Islander	1.6
Aboriginal and Torres Strait Islanders (Queensland)	1.11
Aboriginal and Torres Strait Islanders	0.9

b

Atayal (Taiwan)	5.69
Bunun (Taiwan)	5.54
Bunun (Taiwan)	4.42
Atayal, Bunun, and Palwan (Taiwan)	3.96
Atayal (Taiwan)	3.96
Atayal (East Taiwan)	3.79
Palwan (Taiwan)	2.11
Palwan (Taiwan)	1.39
Ami (East Taiwan)	0.87
Ami (Taiwan)	0.45
7 tribes (Brunei Darussalam)	3.4
Palawan (Philippines)	2.48
Bumiputera (Sabah and Sarawak, Malaysia)	1.16
Li su (Yunnan Province, China)	2.33
Yi (Yunnan Province, China)	0.95
Dai (Yunnan Province, China)	0.55
Meng (Huhhot, Inner Mongolia, China)	0.54
Hui (Huhhot, Inner Mongolia, China)	0.27

c

Sámi (Northern Finland)	1.9
Sámi (Northern Norway)	1.45
Nenets (Nenets Autonomous Okrug, Russia)	1.43
Bedouin (Israel)	0.4

d

CANADA

Inuit (Labrador)	20.6
Inuit (Nunavik, Quebec)	16
Innu (Labrador)	14.2
Inuit (Nunavut)	9.6
Inuit (NWT/Nunavut)	5.26
Innu and Inuit (Labrador)	4.58
First Nation (Yukon)	4.49
Inuit (Kitlaviq, Nunavut)	3.47
First Nation (British Columbia)	3.05
First Nation and Métis (Manitoba)	2.3
First Nations	2.3
Dene (NWT)	1.93
Inuit (NWT/Nunavut)	0.94

BRAZIL

6 tribes (Mato Grosso do Sul)	20.04
Indigenous peoples (Tabatinga, Amazonas)	18.04
Indigenous peoples (Sao Gabriel da Cachoeira, Amazonas)	9.98
3 tribes (Mato Grosso do Sul)	8.1
Indigenous peoples (Amazonas)	4.38
Indigenous peoples	2.18
Indigenous peoples (Manaus, Amazonas)	0

e

USA (National)

American Indian and Alaska Native (24 western states)	2.1
American Indian and Alaska Native	1.63
American Indian	1.4
American Indian and Alaska Native	1.2
American Indian and Alaska Native	1.07
American Indian and Alaska Native	1.01

USA (National and Regional)

American Indian and Alaska Native (Alaska IHSA)	2.45
American Indian and Alaska Native (North Plains IHSA)	2.09
American Indian and Alaska Native (Pacific Coast IHSA)	1.22
American Indian and Alaska Native (South Plains IHSA)	1.21
American Indian and Alaska Native (Southwest IHSA)	1.01
American Indian and Alaska Native (East IHSA)	0.73
American Indian and Alaska Native (All IHSAs)	1.49

f

Athabascan	7
Inupiat	4.24
Athabascan	4.24
Alaska Native	4.2
Alaska Native	4.14
Alaska Native	3.53
Yup'ik	2.52
Yup'ik, Inupiat, and Athabascan	2.33
Alaska Native	2.24
Alaska Native	2.2
Alaska Native	2.2
Alaska Native	1.92

g

Akimel O'odham (Arizona)	4.3
Apache (New Mexico)	4.2
White Mountain Apache (Arizona)	3.7
Cherokee (North Carolina)	3.14
Pueblo (New Mexico)	2.8
American Indian (Southwest USA)	2.69
American Indian (South Dakota)	2.11
American Indian (Arizona and New Mexico)	2.3
Hopi (Arizona)	2.08
Navajo (New Mexico)	1.6
Kānaka Maoli (Native Hawaiian)	1.48
American Indian (Southwest)	1.35
American Indian (Arizona)	1.04
Navajo (New Mexico)	0.72
Lumbee (North Carolina)	0.7
American Indian (North Carolina)	0.59
American Indian (Florida)	0.58

Fig. 2 (See legend on next page.)

(See figure on previous page.)
Fig. 2 Global suicide mortality incidence rate ratios among Indigenous and comparison populations. **a** Western Pacific Region (Oceania and Australia). **b** Western Pacific Region (East Asia). **c** European Region. **d** Region of the Americas (Canada and Brazil). **e** Region of the Americas (USA, National). **f** Region of the Americas (USA, Alaska). **g** Region of the Americas (Lower 48 states and Hawaii). *NWT* Northwest Territories, *IHSA* Indian Health Services Area. The *dotted line* indicates a rate ratio of one (RR = 1). This means that there is rate parity (no difference) between the incidence of suicide in Indigenous and comparative populations. Rate ratios to the left of the dotted line (RR < 1) indicate that rates are comparatively higher in the non-Indigenous population. Conversely, rate ratios to the right of the dotted line (RR > 1) show that the Indigenous population has a comparatively higher rate. Citations for each study are reported in Additional file 1: Supplement 3, Table S4

advantage of using localized data is the ability to contextualize a complex health issue. The disadvantage is that the potential to compare health status between multiple groups, across regions, and over time is reduced.

Strengthening surveillance in Indigenous suicide prevention

Our results substantiate previous work [16, 52] to demonstrate that elevated suicide rates are not universal among Indigenous people and debunk notions that Indigeneity increases risk for suicide. Our results also point to several gaps in knowledge about the epidemiology of suicide in Indigenous populations globally. The lack of published suicide data on Indigenous populations in low- and middle-income countries is a glaring absence. Previous studies noted a scarcity of Indigenous-specific data in the Global South overall [18, 53]. Poor infrastructure for death registration is a key limitation [1]. In the context of suicide, this is especially problematic, because countries in Asia, Africa, and Latin and South America are the homelands for the majority of the world's Indigenous populations [18] and, at a national level, account for more than three quarters of all suicide deaths [1]. Suicide data in high-income countries tends to be of better quality than that in low- and middle-income countries; however, many governments do not include Indigenous or other ethnic identifiers in administrative health data, and do not routinely link census or Indigenous registries with national health datasets such as vital statistics. In Canada for example, the federal government does not know how many Indigenous people die by suicide in a given year. Globally, there is a critical need to strengthen capacity for surveillance in Indigenous suicide prevention.

National governments can take several steps to improve suicide surveillance in Indigenous populations. Actions should include efforts to enhance suicide data quality and standardized classification by improving vital registration infrastructure, especially in low- and middle-income countries, and integrating mortality data with monitoring of suicide attempts [1]. Countries should adopt an equity-based approach to data collection that includes Indigenous identifiers derived from self-reported sources and linked to registries or census data to address gaps in identification, and align Indigenous identification procedures

with recommendations from the International Group for Indigenous Health Measurement, adapted for each national context [1, 53, 56, 67, 69]. Building inclusive, Indigenous-centered models of data governance in suicide prevention will be a critical element of strengthened surveillance. To achieve this will require national statistical agencies to not only consult Indigenous communities, organizations, and leaders about priorities, but to respect Indigenous rights to determine the parameters of data ownership, custodianship, access, and use [29, 32, 67].

Future research and global suicide surveillance efforts will be further strengthened with longitudinal and up-to-date national and state-level datasets that allow disaggregation and comparisons of outcomes in small areas and subpopulations by ethnicity [1, 17, 53, 56]. Overall, these actions will help maintain robust public health surveillance systems in order to monitor health status, increase knowledge about the social determinants of suicide, target interventions, and evaluate strategies aimed at reducing the incidence of suicide among Indigenous peoples worldwide [1, 56]. Increasing the visibility of populations that bear the greatest burden from suicide can help drive efforts to achieve the WHO and Sustainable Development Goals of reducing national suicide rates by up to 30% [1, 69].

Conclusions

Suicide among Indigenous peoples is not a universal or intractable problem. Our study showed substantial global rate variation, with striking disparities in some countries. Efforts to understand these differences and to continue to build the knowledge base for effective interventions will require sustained political and financial investments in Indigenous communities, health systems, and governments. Across sectors and countries, Indigenous peoples have called for suicide prevention strategies that are community-led, strengths-based, and trauma-informed, and that redress intersecting forms of structural discrimination, social inequity, and their downstream consequences. Global efforts to reduce suicide rates among Indigenous peoples must include actions focused on communities that experience the most profound disparities, while also seeking to promote population mental health and improve health equity.

Abbreviations

CI: Confidence interval; CSIR: Crude suicide incidence rate; FSM: Federated States of Micronesia; IHSA: Indian Health Services Area (USA); NWT: Northwest Territories (Canada); SSIR: Standardized suicide incidence rate; UN: United Nations; USA: United States of America; WHO: World Health Organization

Acknowledgements

Work on this study was conducted while the authors resided in communities in Newfoundland and Labrador, Canada situated on the homelands of the Innu, Inuit, Mi'kmaq, and Beothuk peoples, and in communities in Ontario, Canada situated on the traditional and unceded territory of the Algonquin Nation. We respectfully acknowledge their ancestral and continued ties to the lands and waters.

We wish to thank the health science librarians who contributed their expertise to the design of this study: Janice Linton, University of Manitoba; Lindsay Alcock, Memorial University; and Lindsey Sikora, University of Ottawa. Thank you as well to our colleagues who assisted with translation, data extraction, and article access, and provided feedback on previous versions of this manuscript: Dr. Marina Sokolova, University of Ottawa; Dr. Albert Formanek, Laval University; Dr. Joseph Murray, University of Pelotas; Dr. Peter Bjerregaard, University of Southern Denmark; Dr. Yanqing Yi, Memorial University; Christopher Penney, Indigenous and Northern Affairs Canada, Government of Canada; Dr. Joyce Law, Labrador-Grenfell Health; Michele Wood, Department of Health and Social Development, Nunatsiavut Government; and Morgon Mills, Labrador Institute, Memorial University. We also recognize and are grateful for ongoing partnerships and research collaborations with the Nunatsiavut Government, Innu Nation, NunatuKavut Community Council, and Labrador-Grenfell Regional Health Authority, and for administrative support from the Labrador Institute and Faculty of Medicine at Memorial University, and the University of Ottawa.

Funding

NJP was supported by doctoral scholarships from the Canadian Institutes of Health Research and is a research associate at the Labrador Institute of Memorial University with salary funding from the Government of Canada's Atlantic Canada Opportunities Agency. KN was supported by a studentship from the Ontario Mental Health Foundation. IC is an associate professor at the University of Ottawa and received salary support through the Canada Research Chairs program. SM is a professor in the Faculty of Medicine at Memorial University. There was no direct funding source for this study. All authors had full access to all the data in the study, take responsibility for the integrity and accuracy of the data, and had the final responsibility for the decision to submit for publication.

Authors' contributions

NJP, KN, AL, SM, and IC met the International Committee of Medical Journal Editors criteria for authorship, and no individual who met these criteria was excluded. NJP, IC, KN, SM, and AL conceived and designed the review; NJP and KN conducted the searches and screened titles and abstracts; NJP, IC, KN, and SM reviewed full text articles; AL, NJP, and KN extracted and cleaned the data; NP and IC analyzed the data; and NJP and IC planned and drafted the manuscript. All authors interpreted the results, revised the manuscript, and approved the final version of the article. NJP is the guarantor.

Competing interests

The authors declare that they have no competing interests.

Author details

[1]Division of Community Health and Humanities, Faculty of Medicine, Memorial University, Prince Philip Drive, St. John's, Newfoundland and Labrador A1B 3V6, Canada. [2]Labrador Institute of Memorial University, P.O. Box 490, Stn. B, 219 Hamilton River Road, Happy Valley-Goose Bay, ,Newfoundland and Labrador A0P 1E0, Canada. [3]School of Epidemiology and Public Health, Faculty of Medicine, University of Ottawa, 600 Peter Morand Cr, Room 308C, Ottawa, ON K1G 5Z3, Canada.

References

1. World Health Organization. Preventing suicide: A global imperative; 2014. http://www.who.int/mental_health/suicide-prevention/world_report_2014/en/. Accessed 17 Nov 2017.
2. Patton GC, Coffey C, Sawyer SM, et al. Global patterns of mortality in young people: a systematic analysis of population health data. Lancet. 2009; 374(9693):881–92.
3. Pridmore S, Fujiyama H. Suicide in the Northern Territory, 2001-2006. Aust N Z J Psychiatry. 2009;43(12):1126–30.
4. De Leo D, Sveticic J, Milner A. Suicide in Indigenous people in Queensland, Australia: trends and methods, 1994-2007. Aust N Z J Psychiatry. 2011;45(7):532–8.
5. Beautrais AL, Fergusson DM. Indigenous suicide in New Zealand. Arch Suicide Res. 2006;10(2):159–68.
6. Herne MA, Bartholomew ML, Weahkee RL. Suicide mortality among American Indians and Alaska Natives, 1999-2009. Am J Public Health. 2014; 104(S3):S336–42.
7. Wexler L, Silveira ML. Bertone–Johnson E. Factors associated with Alaska Native fatal and nonfatal suicidal behaviors 2001-2009: trends and implications for prevention. Arch Suicide Res. 2012;16(4):273–86.
8. Macaulay A, Orr P, Macdonald S, et al. Mortality in the Kivalliq Region of Nunavut, 1987-1996. Int J Circumpolar Health. 2004;63(Suppl 2):80–5.
9. Kirmayer LJ. Suicide among Canadian Aboriginal peoples. Transcult Psychiatry. 1994;31(1):3–58.
10. Mao Y, Moloughney BW, Semenciw RM, Morrison HI. Indian reserve and registered Indian mortality in Canada. Can J Public Health. 1992;83(5):350–3.
11. Silviken A. Prevalence of suicidal behaviour among indigenous Sámi in northern Norway. Int J Circumpolar Health. 2009;68(3):204–11.
12. Bjerregaard P, Larsen CVL. Time trend by region of suicides and suicidal thoughts among Greenland Inuit. Int J Circumpolar Health. 2015;74 https://doi.org/10.3402/ijch.v74.26053.
13. Hassler S, Johansson R, Sjölander P, Grönberg H, Damber L. Causes of death in the Sámi population of Sweden, 1961-2000. Int J Epidemiol. 2005;34(3):623–9.
14. Soininen L, Pukkala E. Mortality of the Sámi in northern Finland 1979-2005. Int J Circumpolar Health. 2008;67(1):43–55.
15. Van Winkle N, May PA. An update on American Indian suicide in New Mexico, 1980-1987. Hum Organ. 1993;52(3):304–15.
16. Chandler MJ, Lalonde C. Cultural continuity as a hedge against suicide in Canada's First Nations. Transcultural Psychiatry. 1998;35(2):191–219.
17. Gracey M, King M. Indigenous health part 1: determinants and disease patterns. Lancet. 2009;374(9683):65–75.
18. United Nations Department of Economic and Social Development. State of the world's Indigenous Peoples: indigenous people's access to health services, 2015. http://www.un.org/esa/socdev/unpfii/documents/2016/Docs-updates/The-State-of-The-Worlds-Indigenous-Peoples-2-WEB.pdf. Accessed 13 June 2017.
19. Kirmayer LJ, Brass GM, Tait CL. The mental health of Aboriginal peoples: transformations of identity and community. Can J Psychiatr. 2000;45(7):607–16.
20. Truth and Reconciliation Commission of Canada. Honouring the truth, reconciling for the future: Summary of the final report of the Truth and Reconciliation Commission of Canada, 2015. http://www.trc.ca/websites/trcinstitution/File/2015/Findings/Exec_Summary_2015_05_31_web_o.pdf. Accessed 17 November 2017.

21. Orellana JD, Balieiro AA, Fonseca FR, Basta PC, Souza ML. Spatial-temporal trends and risk of suicide in Central Brazil: an ecological study contrasting indigenous and non-indigenous populations. Rev Bras Psiquiatr. 2016;38(3):222–30.

22. McQuaid RJ, Bombay A, McInnis OA, Humeny C, Matheson K, Anisman H. Suicide Ideation and Attempts among First Nations Peoples Living On-Reserve in Canada: The Intergenerational and Cumulative Effects of Indian Residential Schools. Can J Psy. 2017;62(6):422–30.

23. Inuit Tapiriit Kanatami. National Inuit Suicide Prevention Strategy. Ottawa: Inuit Tapiriit Kanatami; 2016. https://www.itk.ca/wp-content/uploads/2016/07/ITK-National-Inuit-Suicide-Prevention-Strategy-2016.pdf. Accessed 17 Nov 2017

24. Lehti V, Niemelä S, Hoven C, Mandell D, Sourander A. Mental health, substance use and suicidal behaviour among young indigenous people in the Arctic: a systematic review. Soc Sci Med. 2009;69(8):1194–203.

25. Harder HG, Rash J, Holyk T, Jovel E, Harder K. Indigenous Youth Suicide: A Systematic Review of the Literature. Pimatisiwin. 2012;10(1):125.

26. Hunter E, Harvey D. Indigenous suicide in Australia, New Zealand, Canada and the United States. Emerg Med. 2002;14(1):14–23.

27. Else IRN, Andrade NN, Nahulu LB. Suicide and suicidal-related behaviors among indigenous Pacific Islanders in the United States. Death Stud. 2007;31(5):479–501.

28. Kue Young T, Revich B, Soininen L. Suicide in circumpolar regions: an introduction and overview. Inter J Circu Health. 2015;74(1):27349.

29. Smylie JK, Firestone M. Back to the basics: identifying and addressing underlying challenges in achieving high quality and relevant health statistics for Indigenous populations in Canada. Statistical J IAOS. 2015;31(1):67–87.

30. Pollock NJ, Mulay S, Valcour J, Jong M. Suicide rates in Aboriginal communities in Labrador, Canada. Am J Public Health. 2016;106(7):1309–15.

31. Moher D, Liberati A, Tetzlaff J, Altman DG, The PRISMA Group. Preferred Reporting Items for Systematic Reviews and Meta-Analyses: the PRISMA statement. PLoS Med. 2009;6(7):e1000097.

32. Bramley D, Hebert P, Jackson R, Chassin M. Indigenous disparities in disease-specific mortality, a cross-country comparison: New Zealand, Australia, Canada, and the United States. N Z Med J. 2004;117(1207):U1215.

33. Booth H. Pacific Island suicide in comparative perspective. J Biosoc Sci. 1999;31(4):433–48.

34. Stevenson MR, Wallace LJD, Harrison J, Moller J, Smith RJ. At risk in two worlds: injury mortality among indigenous people in the US and Australia, 1990–92. Aust N Z J Public Health. 1998;22(6):641–4.

35. Hezel FX. Suicide and the Micronesian family. Contemp Pac. 1989;1(1):43–74.

36. Becker TM, Samet JM, Wiggins CL, Key CR. Violent death in the west: suicide and homicide in New Mexico, 1958-1987. Suicide Life Threat Behav. 1990;20(4):324–34.

37. Bjorksten KS, Bjerregaard P, Kripke DF. Suicides in the midnight sun — a study of seasonality in suicides in West Greenland. Psychiatry Res. 2005;133(2–3):205–13.

38. Hislop TG, Threlfall WJ, Gallagher RP, Band PR. Accidental and intentional violent deaths among British Columbia Native Indians. Can J Public Health. 1987;78(4):271–4.

39. Rubinstein DH. Epidemic suicide among Micronesian adolescents. Soc Sci Med. 1983;17(10):657–65.

40. Telisinghe PU, Colombage SM. Patterns of suicide in Brunei Darussalam and comparison with neighbouring countries in South East Asia. J Forensic Legal Med. 2014;22:16–9.

41. Measey MAL, Li SQ, Parker R, Wang Z. Suicide in the Northern Territory, 1981-2002. Med J Aust. 2006;185(6):315–9.

42. Jollant F, Malafosse A, Docto R, Macdonald C. A pocket of very high suicide rates in a non-violent, egalitarian and cooperative population of South–East Asia. Psychol Med. 2014;44(11):2323–9.

43. Ali NH, Zainun KA, Bahar N, et al. Pattern of suicides in 2009: data from the National Suicide Registry Malaysia. Asia–Pacific Psychiatry. 2014;6(2):217–25.

44. Lu J, Xiao Y, Xu X, Shi Q, Yang Y. The suicide rates in the Yunnan Province, a multi-ethnic province in southwestern China. Int J Psychiatry Med. 2013;45(1):83–96.

45. Coloma C, Hoffman JS, Crosby A. Suicide among Guarani Kaiowa and Nandeva youth in Mato Grosso do Sul, Brazil. Arch Suicide Res. 2006;10(2):191–207.

46. Souza MLP, Orellana JDY. Inequalities in suicide mortality between Indigenous and non-Indigenous people in the state of Amazonas, Brazil. J Brasileiro de Psiquiatria. 2013;62(4):245–52.

47. Day GE, Lanier AP. Alaska Native mortality, 1979-1998. Public Health Rep. 2003;118(6):518–30.

48. Holck P, Day GE, Provost E. Mortality trends among Alaska Native people: successes and challenges. Int J Circumpolar Health. 2013;72:21185.

49. Pridmore S. Suicidal behavior in the Honiara area of the Solomon Islands. Int J Ment Health. 1997;25(4):33–8.

50. Smith D. Suicide in a remote preliterate society in the highlands of Papua New Guinea. P N Guinea Med J. 1981;24(4):242–6.

51. Price J, Karim I. Suicide in Fiji: a two year survey. Acta Psychiatr Scand. 1975;52(3):153–9.

52. Van Winkle N, May P. Native American suicide in New Mexico, 1957-1979: a comparative study. Hum Organ. 1986;45(4):296–309.

53. Anderson I, Robson B, Connolly M, et al. Indigenous and tribal peoples' health (the Lancet–Lowitja Institute Global Collaboration): a population study. Lancet. 2016;388(10040):131–57.

54. Incayawar M, Bouchard L, Maldonado-Bouchard S. Living without psychiatrists in the Andes: plight and resilience of the Quichua (Inca) people. Asia–Pacific Psychiatry. 2010;2(3):119–25.

55. Sami Norwegian National Advisory Unit on Mental Health and Substance Abuse, Saami Council. Plan for suicide prevention among the Sami people in Norway, Sweden, and Finland. Norway: SANKS; 2017. http://www.saamicouncil.net/fileadmin/user_upload/Documents/Eara_dokumeanttat/Suicide_plan_EN.pdf. Accessed 17 Nov 2017

56. Wexler L, Chandler M, Gone JP, et al. Advancing suicide prevention research with rural American Indian and Alaska Native populations. Am J Public Health. 2015;105(5):891–9.

57. Sareen J, Isaak C, Bolton S-L, et al. Gatekeeper training for suicide prevention in First Nations community members: a randomized controlled trial. Depress Anxiety. 2013;30(10):1021–9.

58. Hatcher S, Coupe N, Wikiriwhi K, Durie SM, Pillai A. Te Ira Tangata: a Zelen randomised controlled trial of a culturally informed treatment compared to treatment as usual in Māori who present to hospital after self-harm. Soc Psychiatry Psychiatr Epidemiol. 2016;51(6):885–94.

59. Tighe J, Shand F, Ridani R, Mackinnon A, De La Mata N, Christensen H. Ibobbly mobile health intervention for suicide prevention in Australian Indigenous youth: a pilot randomised controlled trial. BMJ Open. 2017;7(1):e013518.

60. Clifford AC, Doran CM, Tsey K. A systematic review of suicide prevention interventions targeting indigenous peoples in Australia, United States, Canada and New Zealand. BMC Public Health. 2013;13(1):463.

61. Redvers J, Bjerregaard P, Eriksen H, et al. A scoping review of Indigenous suicide prevention in circumpolar regions. Int J Circumpolar Health. 2015;74:27509.

62. Harlow AF, Bohanna I, Clough A. A systematic review of evaluated suicide prevention programs targeting indigenous youth. Crisis. 2014;35(5):310–21.

63. Mamakwa S, Kahan M, Kanate D, et al. Evaluation of 6 remote First Nations community-based buprenorphine programs in northwestern Ontario. Can Fam Physician. 2017;63(2):137–45.

64. Cwik MF, Tingey L, Maschino A, et al. Decreases in suicide deaths and attempts linked to the White Mountain Apache suicide surveillance and prevention system, 2001–2012. Am J Public Health. 2016;106(12):2183–9.

65. Allen J, Rasmus SM, Fok CCT, Charles B, Henry D, Team Q. Multi-level cultural intervention for the prevention of suicide and alcohol use risk with Alaska Native youth: a nonrandomized comparison of treatment intensity. Prev Sci. 2018;19:174–85.

66. McClintock K, McClintock R. Hoea te waka: indigenous suicide prevention outcomes framework and evaluation processes - Part 1. J Indigenous Wellbeing – Te Mauri: Pimatisiwin. 2017;2(2):68–72.

67. Coleman C, Elias B, Lee V, et al. International Group for Indigenous Health Measurement: recommendations for best practice for estimation of Indigenous mortality. Stat J IAOS. 2016;32:729–38.

68. Ross CA, Davis B. Suicide and parasuicide in a northern Canadian native community. Can J Psychiatr. 1986;31(4):331–4.

69. World Health Organization. World Health Statistics 2016: Monitoring health for the Sustainable Development Goals 2016. http://www.who.int/gho/publications/world_health_statistics/2016/en/. Accessed 17 Nov 2017).

70. Thorslund J, Misfeldt J. On suicide statistics. Arctic Med Res. 1989;48(3):124–30.

71. Klomek AB, Nakash O, Goldberger N, et al. Completed suicide and suicide attempts in the Arab population in Israel. Soc Psychiatry Psychiatr Epidemiol. 2016;51(6):869–76.

72. Sumarokov YA, Brenn T, Kudryavtsev AV, Nilssen O. Suicides in the indigenous and non-indigenous populations in the Nenets Autonomous Okrug, northwestern Russia, and associated socio-demographic characteristics. Int J Circumpolar Health. 2014;73:24308.

73. Clayer JR, Czechowicz AS. Suicide with Aboriginal people in South Australia: comparison with suicide deaths in the total urban and rural populations. Med J Aust. 1991;154(10):683–5.

74. Cantor CH, Slater PJ. A regional profile of suicide in Queensland. Aust N Z J Public Health. 1997;21(2):181–6.

75. Campbell A, Chapman M, McHugh C, Sng A, Balaratnasingam S. Rising indigenous suicide rates in Kimberley and implications for suicide prevention. Australasian Psychiatry. 2016;24(6):561–4.

76. Hezel FX. Cultural patterns in Trukese suicide. Ethnology. 1984;23(3):193–206.

77. Ree GH. Suicide in Macuata province, Fiji: a review of 73 cases. Pract. 1971; 207(241):669–71.

78. Haynes RH. Suicide in Fiji: a preliminary study. Br J Psychiatry. 1984;145:433–8.

79. Pridmore S, Ryan K. The influence of race and sex on the method of suicide in the western division of Fiji. Fiji Med J. 1994;20:9–12.

80. Pridmore S, Ryan K, Blizzard L. Victims of violence in Fiji. Aust N Z J Psychiatry. 1995;29(4):666–70.

81. Booth H. The evolution of epidemic suicide on Guam: context and contagion. Suicide Life Threat Behav. 2010;40(1):1–13.

82. Langley JD, Johnston SE. Purposely self-inflicted injury resulting in death and hospitalisation in New Zealand. Community Health Stud. 1990;14(2): 190–9.

83. Langley J, Broughton J. Injury to Maori I: fatalities. N Z Med J. 2000; 113(1123):508–10.

84. Parker N, Suicide in Papua B-BB, Guinea N. Med J Aust. 1966;2(24):1125.

85. Vivili P, Finau S, Finau E. Suicide in Tonga, 1982-1997. Pac Health Dialog. 1999;6(2):211–2.

86. De Leo D, Milner A, Fleischmann A, et al. The WHO START study: suicidal behaviors across different areas of the world. Crisis. 2013;34(3):156–63.

87. Wang D, Wang YT, Wang XY. Suicide in three ethnic groups in Huhhot, Inner Mongolia. Crisis. 1997;18(3):112–4.

88. Cheng TA, Hsu M. A community study of mental disorders among four Aboriginal groups in Taiwan. Psychol Med. 1992;22(1):255–63.

89. Hsieh SF, Liu BH, Pan BJ, Chang SJ, Ko YC. Mortality patterns of Taiwan Aborigines due to accidents. Kaohsiung J Med Sci. 1994;10(7):367–78.

90. Wen CP, Tsai SP, Shih YT, Chung WSI. Bridging the gap in life expectancy of the aborigines in Taiwan. Int J Epidemiol. 2004;33(2):320–7.

91. Liu IC, Liao SF, Lee WC, Kao CY, Jenkins R, Cheng ATA. A cross-ethnic comparison on incidence of suicide. Psychol Med. 2011;41(6):1213–21.

92. Machado DB. dos Santos DN. Suicide in Brazil, from 2000 to 2012. J Bras Psiquiatr. 2015;64(1):45–54.

93. Butler GC. Incidence of suicide among the ethnic groups of the Northwest Territories and Yukon Territory. Med Serv J Can. 1965;21(4):252–6.

94. Young TK. Mortality pattern of isolated Indians in northwestern Ontario: a 10-year review. Public Health Rep. 1983;98(5):467.

95. Fox J, Manitowabi D, Ward JA. An Indian community with a high suicide rate: 5 years after. Can J Psychiatr. 1984;29(5):425–7.

96. Wotton K. Mortality of Labrador Innu and Inuit, 1971–1982. In: Fortuine R, editor. Circumpolar Health 84: Proceedings of the Sixth International Symposium on Circumpolar Health; 1985 May 13–18, 1984. Anchorage: University of Washington Press; 1985. p. 139–42.

97. Spaulding JM. Recent suicide rates among ten Ojibwa Indian bands in northwestern Ontario. Omega. 1985;16(4):347–54.

98. Mao Y, Morrison H, Semenciw R, Wigle D. Mortality on Canadian Indian reserves 1977-1982. Can J Public Health. 1986;77(4):263–8.

99. Garro LC. Suicides by status Indians in Manitoba. Arctic Med Res. 1988; 47(Suppl 1):590–2.

100. Malchy B, Enns MW, Young TK, Cox BJ. Suicide among Manitoba's aboriginal people, 1988 to 1994. Can Med Assoc J. 1997;156(8):1133–8.

101. Isaacs S, Keogh S, Menard C, Hockin J. Suicide in the Northwest Territories: a descriptive review. Chronic Dis Can. 1998;19(4):152–6.

102. Penney C, Bobet E, Guimond E, Senécal S. Effect of community-level factors on suicide in Inuit Nunangat. Can Divers. 2009;7(3):77–84.

103. Ogden M, Spector MI, Hill CA Jr. Suicides and homicides among Indians. Public Health Rep. 1970;85(1):75–80.

104. Young TJ, French LA. Suicide and social status among Native Americans. Psychol Rep. 1993;73(2):461–2.

105. Lester D. Differences in the epidemiology of suicide in Asian Americans by nation of origin. Omega. 1994;29(2):89–93.

106. Lester D. Social correlates of American Indian suicide and homicide rates. Am Indian Alsk Native Ment Health Res. 1995;6(3):46–55.

107. Howard G, Peace F, Howard VJ. The contributions of selected diseases to disparities in death rates and years of life lost for racial/ethnic minorities in the United States, 1999-2010. Prev Chronic Dis. 2014;11:E129.

108. Kraus RF, Buffler PA. Sociocultural stress and the American native in Alaska: an analysis of changing patterns of psychiatric illness and alcohol abuse among Alaska natives. Cult Med Psychiatry. 1979;3(2):111–51.

109. Travis R. Suicide in Northwest Alaska. White Cloud J Am Indian Ment Health. 1983;3(1):23–30.

110. Travis R. Suicide and economic development among the Inupiat Eskimo. White Cloud J Am Indian. Ment Health. 1984;3(3):14–21.

111. Hlady WG, Middaugh JP. Suicides in Alaska: firearms and alcohol. Am J Public Health. 1988;78(2):179–80.

112. Forbes N, Van der Hyde V. Suicide in Alaska from 1978 to 1985: updated data from state files. Am Indian Alsk Native Ment Health Res. 1988;1(3):36–55.

113. Kettl PA, Bixler EO. Suicide in Alaska natives, 1979-1984. Psychiatry. 1991; 54(1):55–63.

114. Andon HB. Patterns of injury mortality among Athabascan Indians in interior Alaska 1977–1987. Am Indian Alsk Native Ment Health Res. 1997;7(3):11–33.

115. Marshall D, Soule S. Accidental deaths and suicides among Alaska natives, 1979-1994. Int J Circumpolar Health. 1998;57(Suppl 1):497–502.

116. Day GE, Provost E, Lanier AP. Alaska native mortality rates and trends. Public Health Rep. 2009;124(1):54–64.

117. Levy J. Navajo suicide. Hum Organ. 1965;24(4):308–18.

118. Kalish RA. Suicide: an ethnic comparison in Hawaii. Bull Suicidology. 1968; 1968:37–43.

119. Conrad RD, Kahn MW. An epidemiological study of suicide among the Papago Indians. Am J Psychiatr. 1974;131(1):69–72.

120. Shore JH. American Indian suicide: fact and fantasy. Psychiatry. 1975;38(1): 86–91.

121. Sievers ML, Cynamon MH, Bittker TE. Intentional isoniazid overdosage among southwestern American Indians. Am J Psychiatr. 1975;132(6):662–5.

122. Miller M. Suicides on a southwestern American Indian reservation. White Cloud J Am Indian. Ment Health. 1979;1(3):14–8.

123. Humphrey JA, Kupferer HJ. Homicide and suicide among the Cherokee and Lumbee Indians of North Carolina. Int J Soc Psychiatry. 1982;28(2):121–8.

124. Broudy DW, May PA. Demographic and epidemiologic transition among the Navajo Indians. Soc Biol. 1983;30(1):1–16.

125. Simpson SG, Reid R, Baker SP, Teret S. Injuries among the Hopi Indians: a population-based survey. J Am Med Assoc. 1983;249(14):1873–6.

126. Levy JE, Kunitz SJ. A suicide prevention program for Hopi youth. Soc Sci Med. 1987;25(8):931–40.

127. Copeland AR. Suicide among nonwhites. The metro Dade county experience, 1982-1986. Am J Forensic Med Pathol. 1989;10(1):10–3.

128. Sievers ML, Nelson RG, Bennett PH. Adverse mortality experience of a southwestern American Indian community: overall death rates and underlying causes of death in Pima Indians. J Clin Epidemiol. 1990;43(11): 1231–42.

129. Wissow LS, Walkup J, Barlow A, Reid R, Kane S. Cluster and regional influences on suicide in a southwestern American Indian tribe. Soc Sci Med. 2001;53(9):1115–24.

130. Mullany B, Barlow A, Goklish N, et al. Toward understanding suicide among youths: results from the White Mountain Apache tribally mandated suicide surveillance system, 2001-2006. Am J Public Health. 2009;99(10):1840–8.

131. Martin SL, Proescholdbell S, Norwood T, Kupper LL. Suicide and homicide in North Carolina: initial findings from the North Carolina Violent Death Reporting System, 2004-2007. N C Med J. 2010;71(6):519–25.

132. Christensen M, Kightlinger L. Premature mortality patterns among American Indians in South Dakota, 2000-2010. Am J Prev Med. 2013;44(5):465–71.

6

Switching to dual/monotherapy determines an increase in CD8+ in HIV-infected individuals

Cristina Mussini[1*], Patrizia Lorenzini[2], Alessandro Cozzi-Lepri[3], Giulia Marchetti[4], Stefano Rusconi[4], Andrea Gori[4], Silvia Nozza[5], Miriam Lichtner[6], Andrea Antinori[2], Andrea Cossarizza[7], Antonella d'Arminio Monforte[4] and for the Icona Foundation Study Group

Abstract

Background: The CD4/CD8 ratio has been associated with the risk of AIDS and non-AIDS events. We describe trends in immunological parameters in people who underwent a switch to monotherapy or dual therapy, compared to a control group remaining on triple antiretroviral therapy (ART).

Methods: We included patients in Icona who started a three-drug combination ART regimen from an ART-naïve status and achieved a viral load ≤ 50 copies/mL; they were subsequently switched to another triple or to a mono or double regimen. Standard linear regression at fixed points in time (12-24 months after the switch) and linear mixed model analysis with random intercepts and slopes were used to compare CD4 and CD8 counts and their ratio over time according to regimen types (triple vs. dual and vs. mono).

Results: A total of 1241 patients were included; 1073 switched to triple regimens, 104 to dual (72 with 1 nucleoside reverse transcriptase inhibitor (NRTI), 32 NRTI-sparing), and 64 to monotherapy. At 12 months after the switch, for the multivariable linear regression the mean change in the $\log_{10}$ CD4/CD8 ratio for patients on dual therapy was −0.03 (95% confidence interval (CI) −0.05, −0.0002), and the mean change in CD8 count was +99 (95% CI +12.1, +186.3), taking those on triple therapy as reference. In contrast, there was no evidence for a difference in CD4 count change. When using all counts, there was evidence for a significant difference in the slope of the ratio and CD8 count between people who were switched to triple (points/year change ratio = +0.056, CD8 = −25.7) and those to dual regimen (ratio = −0.029, CD8 = +110.4).

Conclusions: We found an increase in CD8 lymphocytes in people who were switched to dual regimens compared to those who were switched to triple. Patients on monotherapy did not show significant differences. The long-term implications of this difference should be ascertained.

Keywords: CD8, CD4/CD8 ratio, Chronic inflammation, Monotherapy, Dual therapy

Background

Long-term side effects of antiretroviral therapy (ART) drugs have led to the introduction in clinical practice of nucleoside reverse transcriptase inhibitor (NRTI)-sparing regimens as double or monotherapy, and their use is now recommended in specific populations according to international guidelines

* Correspondence: crimuss@unimore.it
Work partially presented at the IXth IAS Conference on HIV Science 23–26 July Paris, France Abstract MOPEB0323.
[1]Clinic of Infectious Diseases, University Hospital, University of Modena and Reggio Emilia, Via del Pozzo, 71, 41124 Modena, Italy
Full list of author information is available at the end of the article

[1, 2]. Indeed, based on the monitoring of surrogate markers of ART efficacy, most of these unconventional regimens, when used in switch studies, have been shown to have a non-inferior virological efficacy and a good CD4 recovery compared to standard triple drug-based therapy [3–8]. The results of these studies were so encouraging that dual combinations are currently being tested in randomized clinical trials of ART-naïve patients [9, 10]. The results of the GEM-INI 1-2 international trials on ART-naïve patients with a baseline plasma viremia < 500,000 copies/mL randomized to receive either tenofovir/emtricitabine or lamivudine both

combined with dolutegravir are also ongoing [11]. If dual regimes are going to be proved non-inferior to triple combination therapy in the ART-naïve population, a single tablet of this dual regimen will likely be developed. Thus, as a consequence of the publication of the results of these studies, in order to save toxicities and resources, we could see a shift in drug production and clinical use of dual therapies [12, 13]. However, it has been recently shown that virological suppression and CD4 cell count fail to protect from the major causes of death of persons living with HIV (PLWHIV), which are mainly non-AIDS-related events, also known as serious non-AIDS events (SNAEs) [14]. At present, the best marker to evaluate the risk of developing SNAEs has not been determined. Interestingly, the analysis of the data of our and other cohorts have shown that, in contrast with recent data from the Antiretroviral Therapy Cohort Collaboration (ART-CC) [15], a low CD4/CD8 ratio is a predictor of non-AIDS-related events independently from CD4 cell count [16, 17], while other studies have shown an association of this marker with non-AIDS-defining cancers [18] or, more recently, with pulmonary emphysema [19].

Therefore, we hereby aimed to compare CD4/CD8 ratio changes in a group of patients who, in the presence of undetectable plasma HIV viremia, were switched to a protease inhibitor monotherapy (mono) or a dual ART, to a control group who was switched to a standard triple drug-based treatment.

Methods

Study design and participants

The Icona Foundation Study is a cohort of HIV-infected patients; this study superseded the original I.Co.N.A. (Italian Cohort of Antiretroviral-Naïve Patients) study (a detailed description of this cohort is given elsewhere [20]), recruiting HIV-positive patients when they are still ART-naïve regardless of the reason. CD4 and CD8 cell counts and viral load are measured every 4–6 months together with other laboratory parameters (e.g., liver and kidney function, lipids, etc.) as well as clinical and therapy data. All patients signed consent forms to participate in the Icona Foundation Study, locally in each of the participating clinical sites, and the research study protocol has been approved by local institutional review boards. The accuracy of non-AIDS events diagnoses is checked by both central and in situ monitoring, by HIV Cohorts Data Exchange Protocol (HICDEP) coding. Central monitoring is done every 6 months to check the accuracy of the data entered. A data monitor goes to each center annually and controls 10–25% of the clinical charts. In case of discordances, the percentage of checked clinical charts increases to 50%, according to the procedure of the D:A:D study, in which Icona participates.

All analyses were restricted to patients in the cohort who did the following: started a combination ART (cART) regimen including three antiretrovirals from being ART-naïve; had reached a confirmed HIV RNA ≤ 50 copies/mL; had switched to either another triple regimen or to double or monotherapy for any reason and at any time after achieving suppression, had maintained virological suppression after 12 months on this same regimen which had been switched to and had in the time window [−3; +3] around 12 months from the switch at least one CD4 and CD8 measurement available (only the first switch episode after achieving suppression was included). Those who switched to triple therapies were considered as the control group in order to have a more uniform population and to avoid, if possible, biases.

If more measurements were available in the defined time window, the nearest to 12 months was selected. We included only patients with a date of switch that occurred after January 2006, because this was the first year in which the switch to mono/dual therapy in people with suppressed HIV RNA was introduced in clinical practice in Italy. We also selected a subgroup of patients for whom at least a CD4 and a CD8 count were available in the window [−3; +3] around 24 months from the switch and the same regimen and the virological suppression were still maintained. Four patients who switched to a dual therapy including maraviroc were excluded from the analyses, as exposure to this drug is believed to increase the CD8 count [21].

The follow-up was interrupted at the date of discontinuation of at least one drug in the regimen started after the switch or at the date of the first of two consecutive HIV RNA levels > 50 or at the date of the CD4/CD8 ratio at 24 months, whichever occurred first.

During the follow-up, the total number of single viral blips, where a blip is defined as (1) a single value of HIV RNA ≥ 50 copies/mL followed by a value < 50 with no treatment switch and (2) a single value of HIV RNA ≥ 200 copies/mL followed by a value < 200, was evaluated and described.

Statistical analyses

The characteristics of the study population at the time of the switch, stratified by treatment strategy, were compared using the non-parametric Kruskal-Wallis test for continuous parameters and the chi-square test for categorical variables.

Endpoints of the analysis were the change in CD4/CD8 ratio, in CD8, and in CD4 from the switch to 12 and 24 months. Multivariable linear regressions were used to evaluate the association between endpoints and type of regimen, adjusting for main confounders. A linear mixed model with random intercepts and random slopes for repeated measurements of ratio, CD8, and CD4 change was used to compare the course over time of these markers according to regimen strategies. The follow-up started at the date of ART switch and ended at first virological rebound defined by the first of two consecutive HIV RNA measures > 50 copies/mL or a stop/change of at least one drug of the regimen or the date of the last CD4/CD8 count at 24 months from the switch, whichever came first. The sample size of the mono/dual therapy group became too small after 24 months to yield accurate estimates.

The comparison between mono/dual and triple switch was controlled for a number of potential time-fixed confounders measured at the time of the switch or at previous times: age, gender, nation of birth, mode of HIV transmission, hepatitis C virus (HCV) co-infection, AIDS diagnosis, CD4 counts and HIV RNA at ART initiation, years of HIV infection, duration of viral suppression before switch, CD4 and CD8 counts at switch, and reasons for switch. The analysis was not controlled for time-dependent confounders.

Results

Study population

A total of 1241 patients were included in the analysis; 1073 switched to triple regimens, 104 to dual regimens, and 64 to monotherapy. Concerning the baseline regimens, almost all patients were receiving tenofovir + emtricitabine, 935 (75.3%), while the third agents are described in Additional file 1: Table S1.

Figure 1 presents a flowchart with the distribution of the various regimens to which participants were switched.

No differences in age, gender, nationality, duration of HIV infection, HCV co-infection, or virological condition at the time of first starting ART were observed among the three groups who switched to triple, mono, or dual therapy (Table 1). The CD4 count before cART initiation was more frequently lower than 350 and less frequently more than 500 cells/uL in patients who switched to a triple regimen compared to those on mono or double therapy. The median duration of the first line regimen and of viral suppression before the switch was similar for the three groups. The CD8 cell counts at the switch were similar, while the median of the CD4/CD8 ratio and the CD4 count at the switch were slightly higher in patients who switched to monotherapy. Patients who were switched to a triple regimen were more likely to have acquired HIV via heterosexual contacts and less frequently through homosexual contacts and were more frequently in Centers for Disease Control and Prevention (CDC) stage C compared to patients with lower drug regimens.

The switch to monotherapy compared to those who switched to triple or dual therapy less frequently was made for simplification and more frequently for toxicity, in particular, kidney toxicity (3.8% vs. 14.4%, $p < 0.001$).

The three groups of patients showed a similar length of follow-up after the date of switch (22.1, 21.9, and 22.7 months respectively for the triple, dual, and mono regimens, $p = 0.084$). Over a median follow-up of 22 months (interquartile range (IQR) 21–24) the total numbers of single blips of HIV RNA > 200 and > 50 copies/mL during the follow-up period were similar for the three groups: 7.0% for the triple, 6.7% for the dual, and 5.9% for the mono regimen ($p = 0.837$) and 1.9%, 0%, and 0% ($p = 0.120$) respectively.

Univariable analysis: change from baseline to 12 and 24 months

At 12 months from the date of switching, patients on the triple regimen showed a higher mean CD4/CD8 ratio ($\log_{10}$) increase +0.12 vs. +0.04 ($p = 0.017$) compared

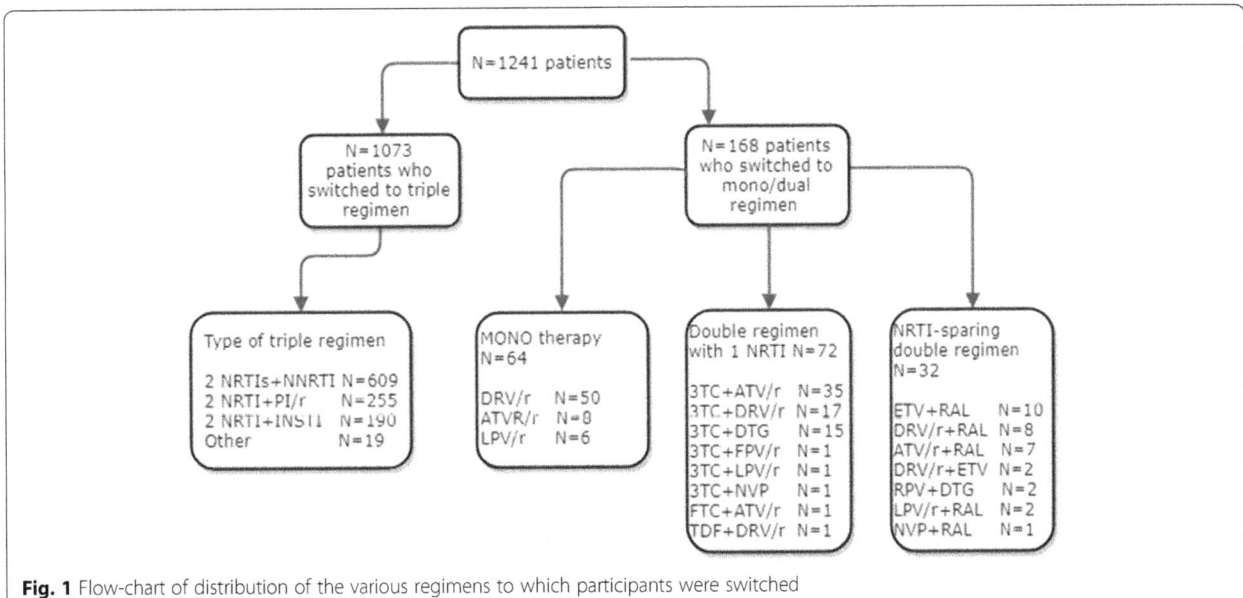

Fig. 1 Flow-chart of distribution of the various regimens to which participants were switched

Table 1 Main characteristics of study population according to regimen started after switch

Patients' characteristics	All study population (n = 1241)	Triple (n = 1073)	Dual (n = 104)	Mono (n = 64)	p value –
Male gender, n (%)	988 (79.6%)	853 (79.5%)	86 (82.7%)	49 (76.6%)	0.612
Age, median (IQR)	43 (36–50)	42 (35–50)	45 (38–51)	44 (38–49)	0.065
Mode of HIV transmission, n (%)					
Heterosexual	534 (43.0%)	474 (44.2%)	40 (38.5%)	20 (31.3%)	0.025
Injection drug use	100 (8.1%)	92 (8.6%)	5 (4.8%)	3 (4.7%)	
Men who have sex with men	533 (42.9%)	440 (41.0%)	54 (51.9%)	39 (60.9%)	
Other/unknown	74 (6.0%)	67 (6.2%)	5 (4.8%)	2 (3.1%)	
Migrants, n (%)	151 (12.2%)	136 (12.7%)	8 (7.7%)	7 (10.9%)	0.317
Previous AIDS event, n (%)	161 (130%)	152 (14.2%)	8 (7.7%)	1 (1.6%)	0.004
Years of HIV infection, median (IQR)	3.4 (1.6–6.3)	3.3 (1.6–6.3)	3.3 (1.6–6.5)	4.2 (2.1–6.1)	0.472
HCV Ab, n (%)					
Negative	1057 (85.2%)	908 (84.6%)	88 (84.6%)	61 (95.3%)	0.197
Positive	120 (9.7%)	109 (10.2%)	10 (9.6%)	1 (1.6%)	
Unknown	64 (5.1%)	56 (5.2%)	6 (5.8%)	2 (3.1%)	
CD4 before cART start, n (%)					
< 200	368 (29.7%)	334 (31.1%)	24 (23.1%)	10 (15.6%)	0.047
201–350	399 (32.2%)	344 (32.1%)	29 (27.9%)	26 (40.6%)	
351–500	307 (24.7%)	258 (24.0%)	30 (28.9%)	19 (29.7%)	
500+	143 (11.5%)	116 (10.8%)	18 (17.3%)	9 (14.1%)	
Missing	24 (1.9%)	21 (2.0%)	3 (2.8%)	–	
HIV RNA before cART start, n (%)					
< 20,000	337 (27.2%)	279 (26.0%)	37 (35.5%)	21 (32.8%)	0.385
20,000–100,000	410 (33.0%)	358 (33.3%)	30 (28.9%)	22 (34.4%)	
100,000–250,000	235 (18.9%)	207 (19.3%)	18 (17.3%)	10 (15.6%)	
250,000+	233 (18.8%)	208 (19.4%)	15 (14.4%)	10 (15.6%)	
Missing	26 (2.1%)	21 (2.0%)	4 (3.9%)	1 (1.6%)	
CD4 at switch, median (IQR)					
< 350	219 (17.7%)	199 (18.6%)	14 (13.5%)	6 (9.4%)	0.008
350–500	285 (23.0%)	255 (23.8%)	23 (22.1%)	7 (10.9%)	
500+	737 (59.3)	619 (57.6%)	67 (64.4%)	51 (79.7%)	
CD4 at switch, median (IQR)	554 (402–740)	547 (394–729)	600 (426–819)	614 (506–807)	0.012
CD8 at switch, median (IQR)	824 (600–1118)	832 (601–1121)	797 (587–1124)	768 (597–1009)	0.467
CD4/CD8 ratio at switch, median (IQR)	0.69 (0.45–0.98)	0.67 (0.44–0.97)	0.78 (0.51–1.10)	0.83 (0.58–1.09)	0.008
CD4/CD8 ratio at switch > = 1, n (%)	303 (24.4%)	256 (23.9%)	29 (27.9%)	18 (28.1%)	0.513
Months of antiretroviral exposure, median (IQR)	18 (9–34)	17 (8–35)	18 (12–36)	20 (12–31)	0.184
Months of viral suppression, median (IQR)	21 (11–39)	21 (10–39)	20 (12–37)	20 (13–34)	0.824
Reason for switch, n (%)					
Toxicity	330 (26.6%)	294 (27.4%)	27 (26.0%)	9 (14.1%)	< 0.001
Simplification	493 (39.6%)	407 (38.0%)	42 (40.4%)	44 (68.7%)	
Patient's decision	18 (1.5%)	17 (1.6%)	0 (0.0%)	1 (1.6%)	
Other	387 (31.2%)	346 (32.2%)	31 (29.8%)	10 (15.6%)	
Missing	13 (1.1%)	9 (0.8%)	4 (3.8%)	0 (0.0%)	

to patients on the dual therapy and +0.07 ($p = 0.079$) compared to patients on the monotherapy (Table 2). We found that 30.6% of patients on the triple regimen had a CD4/CD8 ratio ≥ 1 vs. 36.5% of patients on the dual therapy and 35.9% of patients on the monotherapy ($p = 0.328$).

The same comparison was performed after restricting to 724 patients who had data at 24 months available (622 triple, 57 dual, and 45 mono), and again in this analysis the triple regimens showed higher mean ratio increase compared to the dual therapy patients (+0.17 vs. +0.08, $p = 0.024$), but not compared to the monotherapy patients (+0.12, $p = 0.786$) (Table 3). However, the percentage of patients with ratio ≥ 1 at 24 months was still not different among patients who switched to triple, dual, and mono regimens (34.4%, 34.3%, 40.0% respectively, $p = 0.696$).

Interestingly, the mean change of CD4 count from baseline to 12 months was not different between the groups: +66 for the switch to triple, +86 for the switch to dual, and +59 for the switch to mono at 12 months and +95, +89, and +141 at 24 months respectively. Conversely, the mean change of CD8 count was different among the three groups. In patients who were switched to dual therapy, at 12 months the mean change was +62 cells/mm^3, and it was +34 in those who switched to monotherapy, while in the group who switched to triple therapy the mean change was –28 cells. This difference was observed and again was more pronounced at 24 months: patients on the triple regimen had a mean reduction of CD8 of –45 cells, patients switched to the dual regimen presented a mean increase of +28 cells, and there was an increase of +101 for those who switched to the monotherapy.

Factors associated with the change of CD4/CD8 ratio and of CD8: simple linear regression analysis of marker change

In the multivariable analysis, the type of switch strategy was associated with the change in CD4/CD8 ratio from the switch to (1) 12 months and (2) 24 months, when analyzed as continuous outcomes (Table 4). After adjusting for age, gender, mode of HIV transmission, nationality, previous AIDS event, years of HIV infection, HCV co-infection, HIV RNA and CD4 at cART initiation, CD4 and CD8 count at switch, reason for switch, and months of viral suppression before switch, patients on dual therapy showed a gain in log$_{10}$ ratio at 12 months and at 24 months lower than that seen in patients on the triple regimen. Patients switched to monotherapy showed a change not significantly different compared to the reference group on triple therapy.

From multivariable models with the change of CD8 at 12 and 24 months as the outcome, patients on dual therapy showed a higher mean change than that seen in people on triple therapy. Patients on monotherapy showed a mean change of CD8 not different compared to that for subjects on the triple regimen. No difference was found for the CD4 change between the two types of regimen.

Mixed models

Our 1241 patients contributed 6528 CD4/CD8 ratio measurements over a period of 24 months. A median number of 5 (IQR 4–7) CD4/CD8 ratio values/patient were recorded. In the univariable analysis, the estimate of the overall increase in the log$_{10}$ ratio was +0.040 points/year (95% confidence interval (CI) +0.036, +0.044; $p < 0.001$). Points/year change in the log$_{10}$ ratio were +0.042 (95% CI +0.037, +0.047) for patients on the triple regimen and –0.013 (95% CI –0.029, –0.003) for subjects who switched to dual

Table 2 Comparison of mean value and standard deviation (SD) of CD4/CD8 ratio, CD8, and CD4 at switch and 12 months after switch between triple and dual and between triple and monotherapy

	Triple ($N = 1073$)	Dual ($N = 104$)	p value	Mono ($N = 64$)	p value
CD4/CD8 ratio					
At switch, mean (SD)	0.76 (0.46)	0.85 (0.51)	0.054	0.89 (0.50)	0.009
12 months after switch, mean (SD)	0.88 (0.63)	0.89 (0.52)	0.666	0.97 (0.55)	0.091
Change, mean (SD)	+0.12 (0.48)	+0.04 (0.15)	0.004	+0.07 (0.21)	0.079
CD8 cell count					
At switch, mean (SD)	912 (454)	924 (504)	0.778	825 (345)	0.220
12 months after switch, mean (SD)	884 (506)	986 (558)	0.197	860 (410)	0.576
Change, mean (SD)	−28 (471)	+62 (321)	0.010	+34 (222)	0.096
CD4 cell count					
At switch, mean (SD)	588 (289)	652 (320)	0.039	646 (260)	0.022
12 months after switch, mean (SD)	654 (294)	738 (338)	0.012	705 (223)	0.017
Change, mean (SD)	+66 (184)	+86 (180)	0.251	+59 (197)	0.757

Table 3 Comparison of mean value and standard deviation (SD) of CD4/CD8 ratio, CD8, and CD4 at switch and 24 months after switch between triple and dual and between triple and monotherapy in two different regimens in 724 patients who had available data at 24 months

	Triple (N = 622)	Dual (N = 57)	p value	Mono (N = 45)	p value
CD4/CD8 ratio					
At switch, mean (SD)	0.76 (0.45)	0.80 (0.37)	0.167	0.90 (0.48)	0.025
24 months after switch, mean (SD)	0.93 (0.71)	0.88 (0.43)	0.824	1.02 (0.50)	0.105
Change, mean (SD)	+0.17 (0.58)	+0.08 (0.19)	0.024	+0.12 (0.22)	0.786
CD8 cell count					
At switch, mean (SD)	912 (458)	882 (471)	0.396	812 (363)	0.173
24 months after switch, mean (SD)	867 (451)	911 (411)	0.337	913 (575)	0.870
Change, mean (SD)	−45 (401)	+28 (256)	0.017	+101 (404)	0.012
CD4 cell count					
At switch, mean (SD)	588 (285)	614 (269)	0.402	654 (274)	0.040
24 months after switch, mean (SD)	683 (294)	703 (272)	0.285	795 (332)	0.006
Change, mean (SD)	+95 (181)	+89 (175)	0.943	+141 (229)	0.205

therapy (Table 5). After adjustment for baseline values in the intercept, changes for the triple regimen were +0.056 (95% CI +0.047, +0.064), while for the dual regimen they were −0.029 (95% CI −0.056, −0.002). There was evidence for a significant difference in slope between the triple and dual regimens (interaction test, $p = 0.033$).

The overall observed trend for CD8 count was −7.2 cells/year (95% CI −31, +17; $p = 0.559$). In the univariable analysis, subjects on the triple regimen showed a change of −22.2 (95% CI −48.0, +3.7) CD8 cells/year, while patients on dual therapy had a mean change of +114.9 (95% CI −32.9, +197.0) CD8 cells/year. In the multivariable analysis the CD8 counts of patients on the triple regimen were reduced by −25.7 (95% CI −51.6, +0.28), while CD8 counts for the dual regimen showed a significant increase of +110.4 cells/year (95% CI +27.3, +193.6). There was evidence for a significant difference in slope between the triple and dual regimens (interaction test $p = 0.009$). Neither the CD4/CD8 ratio nor the CD8 count showed a significant linear trend in the group of patients on monotherapy.

Discussion

The main result of our study is that when comparing three groups of patients undergoing different switch strategies in the presence of undetectable HIV RNA, those who were switched to dual regimens showed a stabilization of the CD4/CD8 ratio, while the CD4/C8 ratio of those who were switched to a three-drug-based regimen continued to improve after the switch. This result appears not to be due to the CD4 increase, since no significant difference in the CD4 count trajectory between the two groups could be detected, but to a specific increase in CD8 lymphocyte count in participants switching to dual therapy. More importantly, because

CD4 count continued to increase and plasma viral load continued by analysis design to be undetectable in all subjects, this difference in the ratio would possibly go undetected by standard monitoring of HIV RNA and CD4 count alone.

A lower CD4/CD8 ratio can be interpreted as a measure of dysregulation of a patient's immune system, known as immunological risk phenotype, in the general population and has been clearly associated with a higher risk of AIDS and non-AIDS events in HIV-infected patients [16, 17]. Therefore, more and more frequently, in people with undetectable HIV RNA, chronic inflammation is becoming an important long-term prognosis issue, and measuring the CD4/CD8 ratio could clinically represent a reliable tool to monitor this phenomenon.

Indeed, despite successful cART, there is evidence for continuous quantitative, qualitative, and functional defects in the CD8 compartments, although some of these defects in some cases could be reversed by early treatment [22]. However, during chronic HIV infection, peripheral CD8 T cells persistently maintain several defects which are reflected in continuous maintenance of the immune activation parameters. It has been shown that this activation contributes to immunologic exhaustion, hyporesponsiveness of specific T cells, and perturbations in the T cell receptor repertoire. However, reasons for the persistence of elevated CD8 T cells during treatment have not been fully elucidated. Long-term therapy usually determines a significant CD4 recovery, contrasting with, despite a decrease from baseline, persistently elevated CD8 T cell counts [23]. Previous analyses of cohort data have shown that elevated CD8 T lymphocytes at cART initiation were associated with a poor increase in the CD4 T cell count, even if the studies showed no data on CD8 activation [22, 23].

Table 4 Two separate multivariable linear models to test the association of the dependent variable with the type of regimen started after switch. Every model is adjusted for: age, gender, mode of HIV transmission, Italian nationality, previous AIDS event, years of HIV infection, HCV co-infection, HIV RNA and CD4 at cART initiation, CD4 and CD8 count at switch, reason for switch, months of viral suppression

a) Multivariable linear regression with changes at 12 months

	Coefficient	95% CI	p value
Dependent variable: CD4/CD8 ratio ($\log_{10}$) change at 12 months			
Regimen after switch			
Triple	Ref.		
Dual	−0.03	−0.05, −0.0002	0.049
Mono	−0.007	−0.04, +0.03	0.685
Dependent variable: CD8 change at 12 months			
Regimen after switch			
Triple	Ref.		
Dual	+99.2	+12.1, +186.3	0.026
Mono	+24.7	−84.1, +133.5	0.656
Dependent variable: CD4 change at 12 months			
Regimen after switch			
Triple	Ref.		
Dual	+28.8	−8.0, +65.6	0.125
Mono	−4.8	−50.8, +41.1	0.837

b) Multivariable linear regression with changes at 24 months

	Coefficient	95% CI	p value
Dependent variable: CD4/CD8 ratio ($\log_{10}$) change at 24 months			
Regimen after switch			
Triple	Ref.		
Dual	−0.06	−0.10, −0.02	0.003
Mono	−0.01	−0.06, +0.03	0.549
Dependent variable: CD8 change at 24 months			
Regimen after switch			
Triple	Ref.		
Dual	+192.0	−8.4, +392.3	0.060
Mono	+29.3	−200.7, +259.4	0.802
Dependent variable: CD4 change at 24 months			
Regimen after switch			
Triple	Ref.		
Dual	+2.1	−48.9, +53.1	0.936
Mono	+51.2	−7.3, +109.8	0.086

Indeed, in Caby's study, 50% of individuals with a ratio < 1 despite a normalized CD4 count (> 500 cells/uL) still displayed a CD8 count that remained abnormally high (> 1000 cells/uL) [24]. Moreover, only individuals with a ratio ≥ 1.5 achieved an apparently normal median CD8 count when compared to healthy HIV-seronegative individuals [24]. Furthermore, after 8 years of suppressive cART, only one-third of patients of the French Hospital Database on HIV cohort achieved CD4/CD8 restoration [23]. Encouragingly, Saracino et al. have shown that patients with more than 15 years of cART had a progressive increase in the CD4/CD8 ratio which never reached a plateau, but patients included in that analysis were receiving triple therapy [25]. Our data suggest that treating patients with less than three drugs might lead to a stop of this virtuous trend.

What could explain the CD8 increase observed in our patients who were switched to dual therapies? One possible explanation is that two drugs could not suppress HIV as well as three drugs can. A small residual viremia, probably in lymphoid tissues, could thus trigger the production of proinflammatory and/or homeostatic cytokines that, in turn, would stimulate and/or maintain CD8 T cell proliferation/activation. In our analysis, everybody had an HIV RNA ≤ 50 copies, but we could not create a finer classification below this threshold with the available information on the assays used. In addition, we have shown that viral blips > 50 copies/mL were rare, and their rate of occurrence was similar between the mono, dual, and triple regimen groups, while those > 200 copies/mL were actually more frequent among those who were in the triple regimen. Moreover, it has been previously described that even more sophisticated markers of residual HIV replication, such as HIV -DNA, did not differ between patients switched to dual or monotherapy compared to those continuing triple therapy [26, 27]. However, it is possible that viral replication restarts in lymphoid tissues, and it could be detected by new sophisticated techniques like digital droplet polymerase chain reaction (PCR) or functional virological assays [28] or by analyzing cells resident in those anatomic districts—assays that typically are not available in routine clinical studies. Indeed, recent data from the Collaboration of Observational HIV Epidemiological Research in Europe (COHERE) have shown that, in HIV controllers, the decrease of the ratio and the increase in CD8 lymphocyte counts preceded by 5 years the end of virological control. Moreover, CD8 lymphocyte counts increased significantly in those who experienced loss of virological control, whereas they remained stable in the other groups [29]. Currently it is very unlikely to see randomized clinical trials which last longer than 144 weeks, which is too short a time to verify the COHERE observation in the context of randomized data. Moreover, very rarely are CD8 lymphocyte count data reported in clinical trials. Helleberg et al. have shown that in patients receiving cART for 10 years a value of CD8 lymphocyte count which stays above 1500 cells/uL is

Table 5 Unadjusted and adjusted coefficients from linear mixed model regression analysis to test the association between the dependent variable and type of regimen started after switch. Every model is adjusted for: age, gender, mode of HIV transmission, Italian nationality, previous AIDS event, years of HIV infection, HCV co-infection, HIV RNA and CD4 at cART initiation, CD4 and CD8 count at switch, reason for switch, months of viral suppression

	Unadjusted coefficient	95% CI	Adjusted coefficient	95% CI
CD4/CD8 ratio ($\log_{10}$)				
Regimen after switch				
Triple	+0.042	(+0.037, +0.047)	+0.056	(+0.047, +0.064)
Dual	−0.013	(−0.029, −0.003)	−0.029	(−0.056, −0.002)
Mono	−0.013	(−0.030, +0.005)	−0.011	(−0.044, +0.021)
CD8, cells/mm^3				
Regimen after switch				
Triple	−22.2	(−48.0, +3.7)	−25.7	(−51.6, +0.28)
Dual	+114.9	(−32.9, +197.0)	+110.4	(+27.3, +193.6)
Mono	+73.5	(−25.4, +172.5)	+64.7	(−35.6, +165.0)
CD4, cells/mm^3				
Regimen after switch				
Triple	+46.7	(+40.3, +53.1)	+45.2	(+30.7, +59.6)
Dual	+7.6	(−13.5, +28.8)	+32.1	(−13.1, +77.3)
Mono	+23.6	(−1.40, +48.7)	+18.0	(−36.9, +72.9)

associated with increased non-AIDS-related mortality (mortality rate ratio 1.82; CI 1.09–3.22) [22].

The changes in ratio and in CD8 were not detected in subjects switched to monotherapy. Indeed, although there was a trend in the univariable analysis, it was not confirmed with the multivariable linear regression and mixed models analysis. One possible explanation could be the lower number of subjects who were switched to monotherapy, but another could be that their better immunological profile was definitively better at baseline.

We are well aware of the limitations of our study. First, among dual therapies we could not examine protease inhibitor (PI) and integrase strand transfer inhibitor (INSTI)-based combinations separately (not many people received dolutegravir either); second, a median follow-up of 2 years could not allow us to evaluate either the persistence of this phenomenon or the impact of the strategies on the onset of non-AIDS events; third, we did not have more detailed immunological data than the counts themselves, and it would be extremely relevant to stratify the analysis according to specific CD8 subpopulations and CD38/HLDR+ expression. Finally, since our analysis is retrospective and non-randomized, it only accounts for measured fixed confounders at the time of the therapy switch. Thus, we cannot rule out bias being introduced by unmeasured confounders or time-dependent confounders that have not been appropriately controlled for. In particular, even in the controlled setting of undetectable HIV RNA, patients

switching to a reduced drug regimen (less than three) instead of another three-drug regimen might be determined by the factors that we did not measure.

After more than 20 years since the introduction of cART because of the use in clinic of new potent and better tolerated drugs, there is now interest in reassessing the ideal number of antiretroviral drugs which need to be prescribed. In the absence of data from randomized studies, our results appear to be relevant to this debate. Current research on the clinical effectiveness of dual cART regimens is focused on non-inferiority of the virological outcome and on saving toxicity due to reducing drugs in the regimens. Nevertheless, it is possible that dual regimens have an unfavorable impact on the CD4/CD8 ratio, and this possibility must be thoroughly investigated before implementing novel drug treatment strategies including less than three drugs.

At present, there is evidence supporting CD8 count monitoring as optional in patients with satisfactory virological and immunological control during ART [30], and this is currently taken into account by international guidelines [2]. However, immunological monitoring based only on the predictive role of a low CD4 count on the risk of developing clinical events may underestimate the role of the CD8 count as a surrogate of a proinflammatory state.

Conclusions

In this cohort of treated and virologically suppressed HIV-positive patients, the CD4/CD8 ratio continued to increase in those who switched to triple regimens, whereas it stabilized due to a selective increase in CD8 cells among those who switched to dual therapy. Our results suggest that, before dual therapy may eventually become a standard of care in patients with HIV infection, the impact of this strategy on the immune system should be further assessed and considered.

Abbreviations
ART: antiviral therapy; cART: combination antiviral therapy; NRTI: nucleoside reverse transcriptase inhibitor; SNAEs: serious non-AIDS events; ART-CC: Antiretroviral Therapy Cohort Collaboration; I.Co.N.A.: Italian Cohort of Antiretroviral-Naïve Patients; HICDEP: HIV Cohorts Data Exchange Protocol; CDC: Centers for Disease Control and Prevention

Acknowledgements
We acknowledge the following regarding this research:
Icona Foundation Study Group.
Board of directors
A d'Arminio Monforte (President), A Antinori, A Castagna, F Castelli, R Cauda, G Di Perri, M Galli, R Iardino, G Ippolito, A Lazzarin, GC Marchetti, CF Perno, G Rezza, F von Schloesser, P Viale.
Scientific secretary
A d'Arminio Monforte, A Antinori, A Castagna, F Ceccherini-Silberstein, A Cozzi-Lepri, E Girardi, S Lo Caputo, C Mussini, M Puoti.
Steering committee
M Andreoni, A Ammassari, A Antinori, C Balotta, A Bandera, P Bonfanti, S Bonora, M Borderi, A Calcagno, L Calza, MR Capobianchi, A Castagna, F Ceccherini-Silberstein, A Cingolani, P Cinque, A Cozzi-Lepri, A d'Arminio Monforte, A De Luca, A Di Biagio, E Girardi, N Gianotti, A Gori, G Guaraldi, G Lapadula, M Lichtner, S Lo Caputo, G Madeddu, F Maggiolo, G Marchetti, S Marcotullio, L Monno, C Mussini, S Nozza, M Puoti, E Quiros Roldan, R Rossotti, S Rusconi, MM Santoro, A Saracino, M Zaccarelli.
Statistical and monitoring team
A Cozzi-Lepri, I Fanti, L Galli, P Lorenzini, A Rodano, M Shanyinde, A Tavelli.
Biological bank INMI
F Carletti, S Carrara, A Di Caro, S Graziano, F Petrone, G Prota, S Quartu, S Truffa.
Participating physicians and centers
Italy: A Giacometti, A Costantini, V Barocci (Ancona); G Angarano, L Monno, C Santoro (Bari); F Maggiolo, C Suardi (Bergamo); P Viale, V Donati, G Verucchi (Bologna); F Castelli, C Minardi, E Quiros Roldan (Brescia); T Quirino, C Abeli (Busto Arsizio); PE Manconi, P Piano (Cagliari); B Cacopardo, B Celesia (Catania); J Vecchiet, K Falasca (Chieti); L Sighinolfi, D Segala (Ferrara); P Blanc, F Vichi (Firenze); G Cassola, C Viscoli, A Alessandrini, N Bobbio, G Mazzarello (Genova); C Mastroianni, I Pozzetto (Latina); P Bonfanti, I Caramma (Lecco); A Chiodera, P Milini (Macerata); A d'Arminio Monforte, M Galli, A Lazzarin, G Rizzardini, M Puoti, A Castagna, G Marchetti, MC Moioli, R Piolini, AL Ridolfo, S Salpietro, C Tincati, (Milano); C Mussini, C Puzzolante (Modena); A Gori, G Lapadula (Monza); N Abrescia, A Chirianni, G Borgia, R Orlando, G Bonadies, F Di Martino, I Gentile, L Maddaloni (Napoli); AM Cattelan, S Marinello (Padova); A Cascio, C Colomba (Palermo); F Baldelli, E Schiaroli (Perugia); G Parruti, F Sozio (Pescara); G Magnani, MA Ursitti (Reggio Emilia); M Andreoni, A Antinori, R Cauda, A Cristaudo, V Vullo, R Acinapura, G Baldin, M Capozzi, S Cicalini, A Cingolani, L Fontanelli Sulekova, G Iaiani, A Latini, I Mastrorosa, MM Plazzi, S Savinelli, A Vergori (Roma); M Cecchetto, F Viviani (Rovigo); G Madeddu, P Bagella (Sassari); A De Luca, B Rossetti (Siena); A Franco, R Fontana Del Vecchio (Siracusa); D Francisci, C Di Giuli (Terni); P Caramello, G Di Perri, S Bonora, GC Orofino, M Sciandra (Torino); M Bassetti, A Londero (Udine); G Pellizzer, V Manfrin (Vicenza); G Starnini, A Ialungo (Viterbo).

Funding
The Icona Foundation cohort is supported by unrestricted grants from several companies: ViiV, Gilead, Janssen, and Merck Sharp & Dohme (MSD). The financial support does not interfere with any of the activities or the research of the Icona Foundation.

Authors' contributions
CM co-conceived the research and wrote the manuscript. PL performed the statistical analyses. ACL co-planned and supervised the statistical analyses. GM co-conceived the research and wrote the manuscript. SR co-conceived the research and wrote the manuscript. AG wrote and revised the manuscript. SN revised the manuscript. AA and ML revised the manuscript. AC co-conceived the research and wrote the manuscript. AAM coordinates the Icona cohort, contributed to ideation of the paper, and revised the manuscript. All authors read and approved the final manuscript.

Competing interests
The authors declare that they have no competing interests.

Author details
[1]Clinic of Infectious Diseases, University Hospital, University of Modena and Reggio Emilia, Via del Pozzo, 71, 41124 Modena, Italy. [2]National Institute for Infectious Diseases L. Spallanzani, Rome, Italy. [3]Department of Infection and Population Health Division of Population Health, University College London, Hampstead Campus, London, UK. [4]Clinic of Infectious Diseases, Department of Health Sciences San Paolo Hospital, DIBIC Luigi Sacco, University of Milan, Milan, Italy. [5]Clinic of Infectious Diseases, San Raffaele Hospital, University Vita e Salute, Milan, Italy. [6]Department of Public Health and Infectious Diseases, Sapienza University of Rome, Polo Pontino, Italy. [7]Pathology and Immunology, University of Modena and Reggio Emilia, Modena, Italy.

References
1. European AIDS Clinical Society Guidelines 2017. www.eacsociety.org/files/guidelines_8.2-english.pdf. Accessed Jan 2017.
2. DHHS Guidelines for the Use of Antiretroviral Agents in Adults and Adolescents Living with HIV. https://aidsinfo.nih.gov/guidelines. Accessed 27 Mar 2018.
3. Arribas JR, Clumeck N, Nelson M, Hill A, van Delft Y, Moecklinghoff C. The MONET trial: week 144 analysis of the efficacy of darunavir/ritonavir (DRV/r) monotherapy versus DRV/r plus two nucleoside reverse transcriptase inhibitors, for patients with viral load <50 HIV-1 RNA copies/mL at baseline. HIV Med. 2012;13:398–405.
4. Valantin MA, Lambert-Niclot S, Flandre P, et al. Long-term efficacy of darunavir/ritonavir monotherapy in patients with HIV-1 viral suppression: week 96 results from the MONOI ANRS 136 study. J Antimicrob Chemother. 2012;67:691–5.
5. Raffi F, Babiker AG, Richert L, et al. Ritonavir-boosted darunavir combined with raltegravir or tenofovir-emtricitabine in antiretroviral-naive adults infected with HIV-1: 96 week results from the NEAT001/ANRS143 randomised non-inferiority trial. Lancet. 2014;384:1942–51.
6. Perez-Molina JA, Rubio R, Rivero A, et al. Dual treatment with atazanavir-ritonavir plus lamivudine versus triple treatment with atazanavir-ritonavir plus two nucleos(t)ides in virologically stable patients with HIV-1 (SALT): 48

week results from a randomised, open-label, non-inferiority trial. Lancet Infect Dis. 2015;15:775–84.

7. Di Giambenedetto S, Fabbiani M, Quiros Roldan E, et al. Treatment simplification to atazanavir/ritonavir + lamivudine versus maintenance of atazanavir/ritonavir + two NRTIs in virologically suppressed HIV-1-infected patients: 48 week results from a randomized trial (ATLAS-M). J Antimicrob Chemother. 2017;72:1163–71.

8. Libre JM, Hung CC, Brinson C, et al. Efficacy, safety, and tolerability of dolutegravir-rilpivirine for the maintenance of virological suppression in adults with HIV-1: phase 3, randomised, non-inferiority SWORD-1 and SWORD-2 studies. Lancet. 2018;391:839–49. https://doi.org/10.1016/S0140-6736(17)33095-7.

9. Cahn P, Andrade-Villanueva J, Arribas JR, et al. Dual therapy with lopinavir and ritonavir plus lamivudine versus triple therapy with lopinavir and ritonavir plus two nucleoside reverse transcriptase inhibitors in antiretroviral-therapy-naive adults with HIV-1 infection: 48 week results of the randomised, open label, non-inferiority GARDEL trial. Lancet Infect Dis. 2014;14:572–80.

10. Cahn P, Rolòn MJ, Figueroa MI, Gun A, Paerson P, Sued O. Dolutegravir-lamivudine as initial therapy in HIV-infected, ARV naive patients: 48 week results of the PADDLE study. J Int AIDS Soc. 2017;20:21678.

11. An Efficacy, Safety, and Tolerability Study Comparing Dolutegravir Plus Lamivudine with Dolutegravir Plus Tenofovir/Emtricitabine in Treatment naïve HIV Infected Subjects (Gemini 1). ClinicalTrials.gov identifier: NCT02831673. https://clinicaltrials.gov/ct2/show/NCT02831673.

12. Restelli U, Fabbiani M, Di Giambenedetto S, Nappi C, Croce D. Budget impact analysis of the simplification to atazanavir + ritonavir + lamivudine dual therapy of HIV-positive patients receiving atazanavir-based triple therapies in Italy starting from data of the Atlas-M trial. Clinicoecon Outcomes Res. 2017;9:173–9.

13. Oddershede L, Walker S, Stöhr W, Dunn DT, Arenas-Pinto A, Paton NI, Sculpher M. Protease Inhibitor monotherapy Versus Ongoing Triple therapy (PIVOT) Trial Team. Cost effectiveness of protease inhibitor monotherapy versus standard triple therapy in the long-term management of HIV patients: analysis using evidence from the PIVOT trial. PharmacoEconomics. 2016;34:795–804.

14. Smith CJ, Ryom L, Weber R, et al. Trends in underlying causes of death in people with HIV from 1999 to 2011 (D:A:D): a multicohort collaboration. Lancet. 2014;384:241–8.

15. Trickey A, May MT, Schommers P, et al. CD4:CD8 ratio and CD8 count as prognostic markers for mortality in human immunodeficiency virus-infected patients on antiretroviral therapy: the Antiretroviral Therapy Cohort Collaboration (ART-CC). Clin Infect Dis. 2017;65:959–66.

16. Mussini C, Lorenzini P, Cozzi-Lepri A, et al. CD4/CD8 ratio normalization and non-AIDS related events in individuals with HIV who achieved viral load suppression on antiretroviral therapy: an observational cohort study. Lancet HIV. 2015;2:e98–106.

17. Serrano-Villar S, Saiz T, Sulggi AL, et al. HIV infected individuals with low CD4/CD8 ratio despite effective antiretroviral therapy exhibit altered T cell subsets, heightened CD8+T cell activation and increased risk of non-AIDS morbidity and mortality. PLoS Pathog. 2014;10:e1004078.

18. Hema MN, Ferry T, Dupon M, et al. Low CD4/CD8 ratio is associated with non-AIDS-defining cancers in patients on antiretroviral therapy: ANRS CO8(Aproco/copilote) prospective cohort study. PLoS One. 2016;11:e0161594.

19. Triplette M, Attia EF, Akgun KM, et al. A low peripheral blood CD4/CD8 ratio is associated with pulmonary emphysema in HIV. PLoS One. 2017;12:e0170857.

20. d'Arminio Monforte A, Cozzi-Lepri A, Rezza G, et al. Insights into the reasons for discontinuation of the first highly active antiretroviral therapy (HAART) regimen in a cohort of antiretroviral naive patients. I.CO.N.A. Study Group. Italian Cohort of Antiretroviral-Naive Patients. AIDS. 2000;14:499–507.

21. Rusconi S, Vitiello P, Adorni F, et al. Maraviroc as intensification strategy in HIV-1 positive patients with deficient immunological response: an Italian randomized clinical trial. PLoS One. 2013;8:e80157.

22. Helleberg M, Kronborg G, Ullum H, Ryder LP, Obel N, Gerstoft J. Course and clinical significance of CD8+T-cell counts in a large cohort of HIV-infected individuals. J Infect Dis. 2015;211:1726–34.

23. Writing committee of the CD4/CD8 Ratio Working Group of the French Hospital Database on HIV (FHDH-ANRS CO4). CD4/CD8 ratio restoration in long-term treated HIV-1-infected individuals: incidence and determinants. AIDS. 2017;31:1685–95.

24. Caby F, Guihot A, Lambert-Niclot S, et al. Determinants of a low CD4/CD8 ratio in HIV-1-infected individuals despite long-term viral suppression. Clin Infect Dis. 2016;62:1297–303.

25. Saracino A, Bruno G, Scudeller L, et al. Chronic inflammation in a long-term cohort of HIV-infected patients according to the normalization of the CD4:CD8 ratio. AIDS Res Hum Retrovir. 2014;30:1178–84.

26. Lambert-Niclot S, Flandre P, Valantin MA, et al. Similar evolution of cellular HIV-1 DNA level in darunavir/ritonavir monotherapy versus triple therapy in MONOI-ANRS136 trial over 96 weeks. PLoS One. 2012;7:e41390.

27. Lombardi F, Belmonti S, Quiros-Roldan E, et al. Evolution of blood-associated HIV-1 DNA levels after 48 weeks of switching to atazanavir/ritonavir+lamivudine dual therapy versus continuing triple therapy in the randomized AtLaS-M trial. J Antimicrob Chemother. 2017;72:2055–9.

28. Gibellini L, Pecorini S, De Biasi S, et al. HIV-DNA content in different CD4+ T-cell subsets correlates with CD4+ cell: CD8+ cell ratio or length of efficient treatment. AIDS. 2017;31:1387–92.

29. Chereau F, Madec Y, Sabin C, et al. Impact of CD4 and CD8 dynamics and viral rebound on loss of virological control in HIV controllers. PLoS One. 2017;12:e0173893.

30. Gianotti N, Marchetti G, Antinori A, et al. Brief report: drop in CD4+ counts below 200 cells/μL after reaching (or starting from) values higher than 350 cells/μL in HIV-infected patients with virological suppression. J Acquir Immune Defic Syndr. 2017;76:417–22.

7

Bayesian adaptive algorithms for locating HIV mobile testing services

Gregg S. Gonsalves[1*] ⓘ, J. Tyler Copple[1,2], Tyler Johnson[1], A. David Paltiel[3] and Joshua L. Warren[4]

Abstract

Background: We have previously conducted computer-based tournaments to compare the yield of alternative approaches to deploying mobile HIV testing services in settings where the prevalence of undetected infection may be characterized by 'hotspots'. We report here on three refinements to our prior assessments and their implications for decision-making. Specifically, (1) enlarging the number of geographic zones; (2) including spatial correlation in the prevalence of undetected infection; and (3) evaluating a prospective search algorithm that accounts for such correlation.

Methods: Building on our prior work, we used a simulation model to create a hypothetical city consisting of up to 100 contiguous geographic zones. Each zone was randomly assigned a prevalence of undetected HIV infection. We employed a user-defined weighting scheme to correlate infection levels between adjacent zones. Over 180 days, search algorithms selected a zone in which to conduct a fixed number of HIV tests. Algorithms were permitted to observe the results of their own prior testing activities and to use that information in choosing where to test in subsequent rounds. The algorithms were (1) Thompson sampling (TS), an adaptive Bayesian search strategy; (2) Besag York Mollié (BYM), a Bayesian hierarchical model; and (3) Clairvoyance, a benchmarking strategy with access to perfect information.

Results: Over 250 tournament runs, BYM detected 65.3% (compared to 55.1% for TS) of the cases identified by Clairvoyance. BYM outperformed TS in all sensitivity analyses, except when there was a small number of zones (i.e., 16 zones in a 4 × 4 grid), wherein there was no significant difference in the yield of the two strategies. Though settings of no, low, medium, and high spatial correlation in the data were examined, differences in these levels did not have a significant effect on the relative performance of BYM versus TS.

Conclusions: BYM narrowly outperformed TS in our simulation, suggesting that small improvements in yield can be achieved by accounting for spatial correlation. However, the comparative simplicity with which TS can be implemented makes a field evaluation critical to understanding the practical value of either of these algorithms as an alternative to existing approaches for deploying HIV testing resources.

Background

Of the estimated 37 million people currently infected with the human immunodeficiency virus (HIV) worldwide, as many as 14 million remain unaware of their infection and unable to avail themselves of the antiretroviral therapy that could both prolong their lives and prevent the further spread of the virus to their sexual or needle-sharing partners [1]. Rates of undetected HIV infection are highly variable from one setting to the next, exceeding 60% in many

parts of Africa, Eastern Europe, and the Middle East [2]. These sobering facts justify continued investigation of novel, cost-effective strategies to focus HIV screening efforts where they will maximize the yield of newly detected cases and to identify areas of concentrated recent infection (so-called HIV 'hotspots').

As we have described in previous work, the deployment of scarce resources to optimize the return on investment in HIV screening can be portrayed as an 'explore-versus-exploit' problem [3]. This canonical formulation, which emerges from the field of statistical decision theory, adopts the perspective of a decision-maker whose long-term objective is to maximize yield by

* Correspondence: gregg.gonsalves@yale.edu
[1]Department of Epidemiology of Microbial Diseases, Yale School of Public Health, 60 College Street, New Haven, CT, USA
Full list of author information is available at the end of the article

making a sequence of short-term choices either to acquire better information about the prevailing state of a system (i.e., to explore) or to make the best possible decision based on the information already at hand (i.e., to exploit) [4, 5]. Under highly stylized conditions simulating a mobile HIV testing service, we have demonstrated that a simple, adaptive search algorithm consistently outperforms more traditional approaches used to deploy disease screening resources.

In this paper, we once again conduct a computer-based tournament to compare the performance of different approaches to targeted mobile HIV testing in a hypothetical city of geographic zones with differing rates of undetected HIV infection. As in our prior work [3], our aim is to understand the circumstances under which different search algorithms may or may not outperform one another. We report here on three important refinements to our prior assessment and their implications for decision-making. First, we have greatly enlarged the number of geographic zones considered. Second, we have admitted the possibility of spatial correlation in the prevalence of undetected HIV infection between adjacent zones. Finally, we have introduced and evaluated a new search algorithm that accounts for and capitalizes upon spatial correlation between zones.

Methods

Analytic overview

We used a computer simulation to compare the performance of three strategies for targeting mobile HIV testing services. We created a hypothetical city consisting of contiguous geographic zones, each with its own (unobserved) prevalence of undetected HIV infection.

Over each of 180 sequential rounds of play, hereafter referred to as days or days of testing, strategies were required to choose a single geographic zone in which to conduct a fixed number of HIV tests. Strategies were permitted to observe and remember the results of their own prior testing activities and to use that information in choosing where to test in subsequent rounds.

We define a 'tournament run' as a fixed number of sequential days. In the main analysis, all outcome measures used to evaluate the relative performance of one strategy against another are reported over a tournament run length of 180 days. Stable estimates of these performance measures and their variance are obtained by repeating each 180-day tournament run 250 times.

HIV infection, hotspots, and spatial correlation

We constructed a hypothetical city consisting of geographic zones on a $n \times n$ grid. For the main analysis, consisting of the base case assumptions, we assumed that there were 36 zones ($i \in \{1, ..., 36\}$) on a 6×6 grid. In sensitivity analyses considering alternative data

simulation settings, we varied the total number of zones between 16 and 100.

The prevalence of undetected HIV infection, establishing the initial number of infected and uninfected persons, in a given zone was simulated using the following model:

$$\text{logit}(p_i) = \beta_0 + \phi_i, \quad i = 1, ..., n^2$$

where p_i is the prevalence for zone i, β_0 is an intercept term that describes the center of the distribution of all prevalences, and ϕ_i is a value specific to zone i that determines how much zone i's prevalence differs from the center of the distribution (large values indicate hotspots while lower values indicate cool spots or non-hotspots). For all data simulation settings, we fixed β_0 to be -5.00, centering the distribution of prevalences on 0.007. The ϕ_i values were simulated from a multivariate normal distribution, centered at zero, with a covariance matrix that allowed for the possibility of spatial correlation depending on the choice of an associated correlation parameter (large value indicates spatial independence while small value indicates high spatial correlation). Once the ϕ_i values were generated, we standardized them (the vector centered at zero with a standard deviation of one) in order to create a distribution of prevalence values with similar center/variability across all data simulation settings and, therefore, allowing us to more accurately attribute differences in the performance of each method to changes in the underlying data assumptions. We then multiplied each ϕ_i value by an inflation factor in order to create greater/fewer hotspots depending on the data simulation setting. Finally, once ϕ_i and β_0 were selected, we calculated p_i for each zone using the inverse logit transformation and set all prevalences larger than 0.03 (the maximum hotspot value) equal to 0.03. Recognizing that not all persons with undetected HIV infection will be amenable to the offer of HIV testing, we capped the maximum prevalence of detectable HIV infection at 3%. This is slightly below the estimated prevalence of undetected HIV infection in high-risk African settings (e.g., Lusaka, Zambia). A new set of zone prevalences was generated using this framework for each of the 250 tournament runs of a given data simulation setting. Populations for each zone, m_i, were drawn from a lognormal distribution based on the population of districts in the same representative African urban area (Lusaka, Zambia). Based on these final starting values for HIV prevalence of undetected HIV infection for each zone and the populations assigned initially to them, each zone thus began the simulation with a fixed number, rounded up to integer values, of infected ($p_i \times m_i$) and uninfected persons ($m_i - [p_i \times m_i]$).

The main analysis was run over 180 days of testing and is meant to reflect the real-world potential use of these methods in the daily decision-making of HIV testing providers. We used the following notation to denote some useful population levels:

- $U_i(t)$, the number of uninfected persons in zone i on day t. This was given by the sum of $OU_i(t)$ and $UU_i(t)$, namely the number of observed and unobserved uninfected persons.
- $I_i(t)$, the number of infected persons in zone i on day t. This was given by the sum of $OI_i(t)$ and $UI_i(t)$, namely the number of observed and unobserved infected persons.
- $\frac{I_i(t)}{I_i(t)+U_i(t)}$, the prevalence of HIV infection in zone i on day t;
- $UP_i(t)$, the prevalence of HIV infection among persons whose HIV infection status is unknown in zone i on day t. This was given by $\frac{UI_i(t)}{UI_i(t)+UU_i(t)}$
- $X_i(t)$, the number of previously undetected cases identified by screening in zone i on day t.

The yield of HIV testing, $X_i(t)$, follows a binomial distribution with success probability $UP_i(t)$. Implicit in this formulation was the assumption that HIV tests are conducted only on persons with unknown HIV infection. In reality, a great deal of HIV testing takes place among persons whose infection status is already known. Our simplifying assumption could be relaxed to include repeat testing and to produce an across-the-board reduction in the effectiveness of screening; however, this would have no impact on the relative yield of different strategies (our performance measure of interest). We also assumed that the population in a given zone greatly exceeds the number of HIV tests that can be performed in that zone in a single day. This permitted us to make the additional simplifying assumption that sampling for HIV on any given day occurs 'with replacement'. This assumption too could be relaxed without overly complicating the analysis but would not likely have a material impact on the performance results of interest.

At the end of each day, the prevalence of HIV infection among persons whose status is unknown, $UP_i(t)$, was updated to account for three different considerations. First, 'shelf life', where the reliability and relevance of a negative result declines with the passage of time. We assumed that observed uninfected individuals eventually return to the pool of unobserved uninfected individuals. Second, 'new arrivals', where, as described above, we permitted the arrival of persons with unobserved HIV infection status (both infected and uninfected). Finally, 'new HIV testing', through which, if m HIV tests were conducted in

zone i on day t, the unknown prevalence the following day was updated as follows:

$$UP_i(t+1) = \frac{UI_i(t)-X_i(t)}{[UI_i(t)-X_i(t)] + [UU_i(t)-(m-X_i(t))]}.$$

Strategy 1: Thompson sampling (TS)

TS is an adaptive algorithm whose actions aim to maximize expected value based on random sampling from prior probability distributions on the prevalence of undetected HIV in each zone. These prior distributions are themselves the ex post result of updates based on previous rounds of observation. The user seeds the algorithm with initial probability distributions for the prevalence of undetected HIV in each zone at time 0. At the start of each day, TS samples randomly from its current probability distribution for each zone. It then elects to conduct testing in whichever zone yields the largest realized value (note that the zone selection process is based on random sampling from prior probability distributions – the algorithm's 'belief structure' – and not from any actual HIV testing in a zone; this indirect selection mechanism ensures that every zone has a non-zero probability of being chosen for testing on any given day while, at the same time, ensuring that a zone will be selected with a probability that is proportional to the strength of the algorithm's beliefs about how much undetected HIV infection exists in that zone). If a zone is selected for testing on a given day, the results of those testing activities will be employed to update the algorithm's prior beliefs for that zone; the posterior distribution that results from that updating process will become the sampling distribution for zone selection on the subsequent day.

We used a $Beta(\alpha_i, \beta_i)$ distribution to describe TS's beliefs about the prevalence of undetected HIV infection in zone i. The $Beta$, a continuous distribution on the interval $(0, 1)$, is a natural choice for this purpose; first, because it is conjugate to the binomial distribution (i.e., a $Beta$ prior and $Binomial$ likelihood will yield a $Beta$ posterior) and, second, because its two parameters are easily interpreted as 'total observed positive HIV tests' and 'total observed negative HIV tests', respectively. Thus, if m new HIV tests yield x new cases detected in zone i, the posterior probability will follow a $Beta(\alpha_i + x, \beta_i + (m-x))$ distribution (see Additional file 1 for more details).

Strategy 2: Besag York Mollié model (BYM)

Conditional autoregressive (CAR) models are used to account for spatial correlation in areal data when what is observed in neighboring regions is assumed to be more similar than observations occurring at larger distances

[6]. They can be incorporated into Bayesian hierarchical models and the Besag York Mollié (BYM) framework used here employs an intrinsic CAR (ICAR) distribution (improper version of the CAR model) for the spatial random effects and exchangeable, normally distributed random effects to account for non-spatial heterogeneity in the data [7].

Similar to TS, our BYM modeling strategy begins the sampling process by assuming independent $Beta(\alpha_i, \beta_i)$ prior distributions for the prevalence of undetected HIV infection in each of the zones. During an initial 'learning' period, the BYM model proceeds in the same way as TS, selecting a zone for testing on a given day by sampling from its current probability distribution for each zone's prevalence of undetected HIV prevalence and then choosing the zone that yields the largest realized value. Using TS, when the number of completed days is low, zones are selected almost at random. This is because TS assumes an uninformative, independent $Beta(1, 1)$ prior distribution for the prevalence of undetected HIV infection in each zone and little new information across all zones is collected at the beginning of the simulations. As a result, on average, we observe a mix of low and high prevalence zones that are used to fit the BYM model for the first time. At the end of the learning period, the BYM model is fitted to the total set of collected data from each individual zone (number of identified infected individuals versus total number of sampled individuals in each zone). The choice of 10 zones for the initial learning period was made to ensure we had a reasonable number of spatial data points with which to fit the BYM model. For instance, it would be impossible to learn about the spatial correlation in the data using only data from a single spatial region. Once the BYM model is fitted to the current set of observed data, the marginal posterior predictive distribution of the underlying prevalence of undetected HIV cases at each zone is obtained via Markov chain Monte Carlo (MCMC) posterior sampling. We then randomly select a single value from each of these zone-specific distributions and identify the zone that corresponds to the largest value. This zone is selected for sampling on the subsequent day. This process is then repeated until the end of the simulation time period.

Unlike TS, which only gathers information as it visits a given individual zone, the BYM model can leverage inter-zone correlation to take what it observes in one zone and use that information to draw useful inferences about the prevalence of undetected HIV in neighboring zones. The model for the underlying prevalence at each zone is a function of a shared intercept, a spatially correlated random effect (ICAR distribution), and an exchangeable, normally distributed random effect (logistic regression model assumed). Because the intercept is shared across all zones, as data are gathered about a particular zone, the model is simultaneously learning about the value of the intercept and, therefore, about all zone prevalences. Similarly, because the spatial random effect assumes similarity between neighboring zones a priori, as data are gathered on a particular zone, the model is also learning about that zone's neighbors (and beyond). The exchangeable random effect ensures that all variability in the prevalences is not attributed to spatial similarity and therefore prevents the model from oversmoothing the data. In the case of no spatially correlated variability and complete independence between data from the different zones, the BYM model will collapse to something very similar to TS (see Additional file 1 for more details).

Strategy 3: Clairvoyance

For purposes of benchmarking, we sought to establish a credible upper-bound on the number of new HIV cases that any search strategy could possibly detect. To that end, we developed the Clairvoyance strategy, an algorithm that chooses to test in whichever zone has the greatest underlying prevalence of undetected HIV infection on any given day. Clairvoyance has access to perfect current information about new arrivals/departures, about individuals whose previous test results have exceeded their shelf life, and about the results of its previous testing activities. This permits it to select the most promising zone for testing on any given day. We emphasize, however, that it has no special knowledge about the HIV-infection status of any individuals selected for testing within that zone. Like any other strategy, it samples with replacement within whichever zone it selects.

Parameter estimates, main analysis, and sensitivity analyses

Initial parameter values as well as those used in the sensitivity analyses are described in Tables 1 and 2. Our goal was to understand the performance of strategies under a broad variety of plausible data simulation settings. We therefore defined parameter ranges that reflected observations drawn from a multiplicity of international settings. Areas differ in terms of population size. Numbers of infected and uninfected persons in a zone were assigned via random realizations from a lognormal distribution (rounded to the nearest integer) that was itself estimated using 2010 census data on the number of adults aged 15–59 years living in urban wards of Lusaka, Zambia [8]. We explored values ranging from less than 0.5% to 3.0%, for the underlying prevalence of undetected HIV infection, reflecting zones with lower numbers of undetected individuals and zones that can be considered hotspots. The prevalence of undiagnosed

Table 1 Parameter main analysis values

Parameters	Values
Overall population	Simulate from lognormal distribution based on 2010 Lusaka, Zambia census
Grid dimensions	6×6
Level of correlation, percentage of hotspots in grid	Low, 20% (on average)
Percentage of new infections (times zone population divided by 365 days)	0.66%
Percentage of new HIV-negative arrivals (times zone population divided 365 days)	3.4%
Days until return to unobserved, uninfected pool	45
Initial observed HIV^+/HIV^- (priors for TS)	$Beta(1, 1)$
Initial observed HIV^+/HIV^- (priors for ICAR/BYM during learning period)	$Beta(1, 1)$
Intercept (priors for ICAR/BYM)	$Normal(0, 2.85)$
Priors for ICAR and exchangeable random effects	$Inverse\text{-}Gamma(3, 2)$
Days of testing	180
Tests per day	25

BYM Besag York Mollié, *ICAR* intrinsic conditional autoregressive, *TS* Thompson sampling

Table 2 Parameter values for sensitivity analysis

Parameters	Values
Grid dimensions	4×4; 5×5; 10×10
Percentage of new HIV-negative arrivals (times zone population divided 365 days)	0, 1.7%, 6.8%
Percentage of new infections (times zone population divided by 365 days)	0, 0.33%, 1.32%
No arrivals or infections	0
Level of correlation, percentage of hotspots in grid	None, 20% (on average)
Level of correlation, percentage of hotspots in grid	Low, 10% (on average)
Level of correlation, percentage of hotspots in grid	Low, 30% (on average)
Level of correlation, percentage of hotspots in grid	Medium, 20% (on average)
Level of correlation, percentage of hotspots in grid	High, 20% (on average)
Days until return to unobserved, uninfected pool	10, 90
Days of testing	90, 365
Tests per day	10, 40

HIV infection in some settings, including sub-Saharan Africa, can be larger than 3%. For instance, 12.3% of Zambian adults (15–59) are HIV positive, but 32.7% of them do not know their serostatus, and thus 4% of adults are still undiagnosed [9, 10]. However, we chose the 3% ceiling of undetected HIV prevalence in this simulation to represent a fraction of this population, as not all undiagnosed individuals will necessarily come forward for testing.

We considered different rates of population movement, setting in-migration of new HIV-negative individuals at an annual 3.4% of a zone's population in the main analysis, so that the daily number of new HIV-negative individuals entering a zone was 3.4% times the zone's population divided by 365 days. The main analysis data simulation setting was derived from projections from the 2010 Zambian census for Lusaka [8]. In the sensitivity analyses, we doubled this number in each zone to reflect fast-growing settings but we also considered a case with half of the base case values and with no in-migration in sensitivity analyses. In the main analysis, zones were assigned HIV incidence rates based on annual incidence rates for Lusaka and daily new infections took the annual incidence figure (0.66%), multiplied it by the population of each zone and divided it by 365 days [9]. In the sensitivity analyses, we doubled this figure to represent faster growing epidemics, and also considered a case with half of the base case values and with no new infections. Finally, we also examined the case where no new HIV-negative and no new HIV infections occurred daily in each zone.

Other HIV testing program parameter ranges were selected to correspond roughly to values reported in the literature. We relied on two South African studies to assume that a mobile testing service could conduct $m = 25$ tests in a given zone on a given day; daily values ranging from 10 to 40 tests were considered in sensitivity analyses [11, 12]. We further assumed that individuals who are found to be uninfected return to the unobserved uninfected pool after 45 days, with values ranging from 10 to 90 days in the sensitivity analysis [13, 14]. Finally, we conducted the main analysis over 180 days (sensitivity analyses range, 90–365 days), reflecting our assumption that decision-makers might devote a half year to experimenting with new approaches to deploying HIV testing resources.

In the main analysis, the spatial correlation was set in the 'low' setting, where we defined 'low' as the correlation between prevalences from the two closest zones (i.e., based on distance between zone centroids) equal to 0.20. Spatial correlation was defined as a function of distance between zone centroids, with increasing distance leading to decreasing correlation. In subsequent sensitivity analyses, we varied the spatial correlation as follows:

1. None: Maximum correlation capped at 1×10^{-100} (independence);
2. Low: Maximum correlation capped at 0.20;
3. Medium: Maximum correlation capped at 0.50;
4. High: Maximum correlation capped at 0.90.

In addition, for the main analysis, we scaled the ϕ_i value by 1.80 (on average 20% of the zones were hotspots) while, for sensitivity analyses, we increased this value to 2.90 (30% hotspots) to create more extreme prevalence values and decreased it to 1.20 (10% hotspots) to create less variability (i.e., fewer hotspots) in the distribution of prevalences across all zones.

Both the TS and BYM strategies require the user to specify their 'initial beliefs' – that is, the probability distributions for the prevalence of undetected HIV infection in each zone at $t = 0$. For TS, we applied uniform(0, 1), uninformative $Beta(1, 1)$ distributions to all zones. This reflected the highly conservative assumptions that virtually nothing is known about the starting prevalence of HIV infection in any of the zones. For the BYM strategy, we also assumed $Beta(1, 1)$ prior distributions for the zone prevalences at the outset of the learning period. The intercept term was given a $N(0, 2.85)$ prior distribution while the variance parameters associated with the ICAR and exchangeable random effects were each assigned inverse-gamma(3, 2) prior distributions. The prior distribution for the intercept resulted in an approximately uniform(0, 1) prior distribution for zone prevalences under the assumption of no additional variability.

To ensure we could statistically differentiate the performance of each of the methods, the tournament was run 250 times for each of the data simulation settings. Performance statistics reported in the Results section below represent averages across these 250 tournament runs as well as an examination of the absolute number of new diagnoses (minimum, first quartile, median, third quartile, and maximum) detected during these 250 tournament runs by each strategy. A strategy was deemed to have outperformed another in a head-to-head comparison if it detected a greater number of new cases in at least 55.25% of the 250 tournament runs. This significance value represents the threshold for a difference in proportions with $p < 0.05$ in a one-sided Z-test. We also examined the difference in the mean number of cases detected by each strategy, assessing significance with a one-side Welch's t test.

Results
Main analysis
Figure 1 shows a representative 6×6 grid from the main analysis, consisting of 36 zones with low spatial correlation in the data and with 30% of the zones being hotspots. Across the 250 tournament runs, the average

proportion of hotspots was roughly 20%. While a new grid of prevalences for the zones is generated for each set of 250 tournament runs of a given data simulation setting, Fig. 1 is meant to offer an example of what the underlying structure of probabilities looks like at $t = 0$ before the 180 days of testing begin. In each of the 250 tournament runs, all strategies begin with the same underlying grid of prevalences. Figure 2 shows the estimated prevalence of undetected HIV infection assumed by each strategy in the main analysis at five time-points ($t = 5, 45, 90, 135$, and 180 days). Figure 2 shows that the TS and BYM estimates of the underlying prevalence of undetected HIV infection shifts over time but in different ways. BYM's estimation of the underlying prevalence of undetected HIV infection among the zones declines over time, but the algorithm maintains estimates that are higher than those of TS across all 180 days of testing in more zones than TS. With TS, estimates of prevalences among the zones, particularly non-hotspots, declines earlier on. This can be seen in the shift from reds to blues in the top panel (TS) of Fig. 2 in contrast to the middle panel where reds still predominate (BYM) as the number of days of testing in the simulation mounts. The Clairvoyance strategy in Fig. 2 has perfect information on the prevalence of undetected HIV infection on each day and thus its 'estimate' represents the actual values on the grid and impact over time of new, incident HIV infections, new HIV-negative in-migration, the 'shelf life' of HIV-negative test results, and its own success at finding new cases of HIV infection. Figure 3 shows the aggregate visits to each zone up until each of the same five time-points for all strategies. BYM visits and exploits hotspots more often than TS over time (conversely spending less time in non-hotspots than TS), while TS continues to explore more zones, even those that are non-hotspots, over the course of the 180 days. Clairvoyance visits all the hotspots of 3.00% prevalence in rotation throughout the 180 days and spends no time elsewhere. Clairvoyance does not even visit hotspots with slightly lower prevalence values (e.g., 2.70%). We provide versions of these three figures for data simulation settings with medium and high spatial correlation as additional files for readers interested in seeing the performance of the three strategies under these conditions (Additional file 2: Figure S1–S6).

Figure 4 shows the key results for the main analysis, indicating the absolute number of new diagnoses detected by each strategy over 180 days (minimum, first quartile, median, third quartile, and maximum) in 250 tournament runs of the simulation. Clairvoyance outperformed all other strategies in overall mean number of new HIV diagnoses detected, identifying 141.87 (SD 11.83) new cases over the course of the 250 tournament runs, while TS uncovered 78.24 (SD 11.44) and BYM

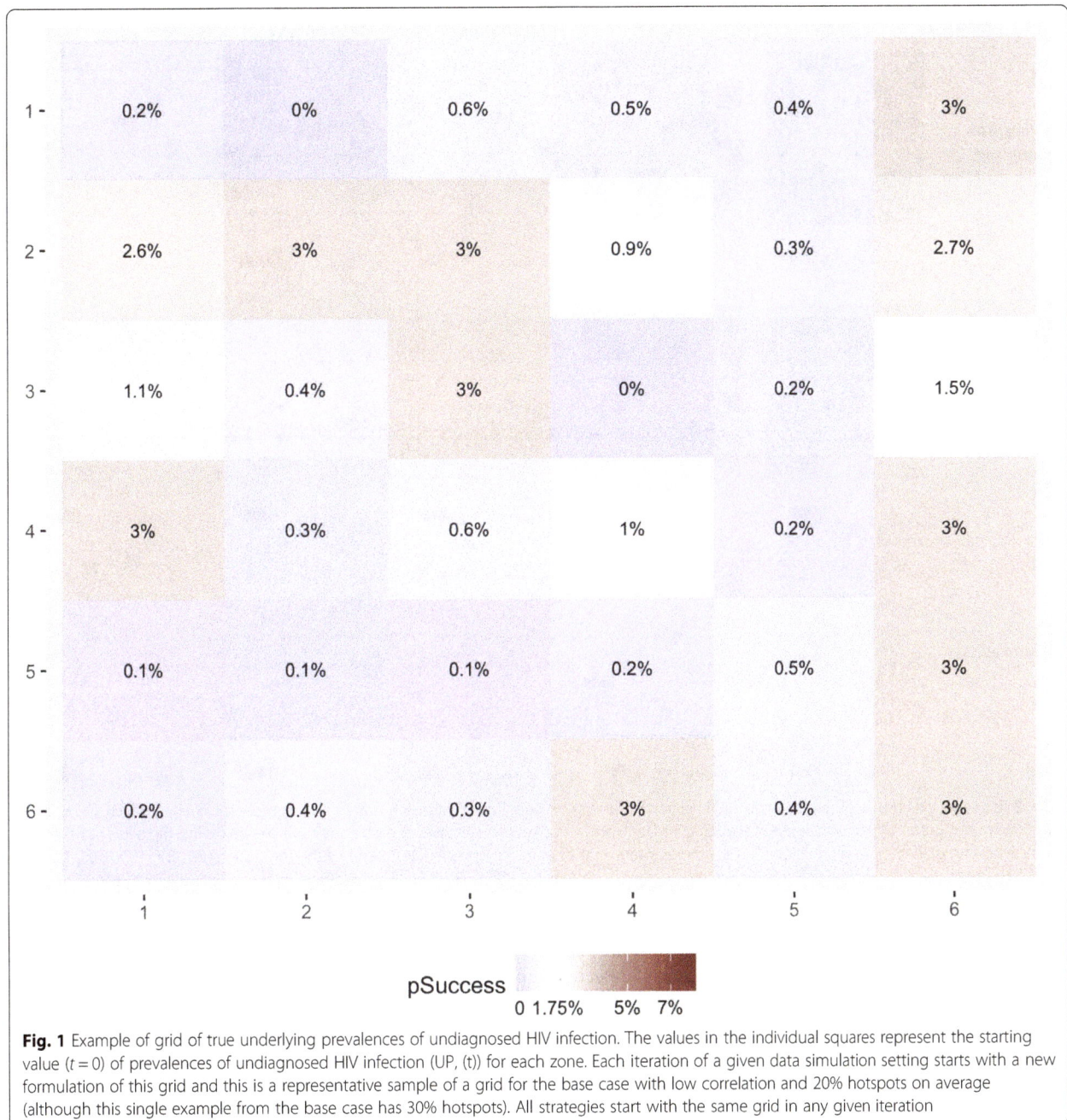

Fig. 1 Example of grid of true underlying prevalences of undiagnosed HIV infection. The values in the individual squares represent the starting value (t = 0) of prevalences of undiagnosed HIV infection (UP, (t)) for each zone. Each iteration of a given data simulation setting starts with a new formulation of this grid and this is a representative sample of a grid for the base case with low correlation and 20% hotspots on average (although this single example from the base case has 30% hotspots). All strategies start with the same grid in any given iteration

found 92.59 (SD 12.37). These results are also shown in Table 3 and Additional file 3: Table S1. The differences in the mean number of cases detected over 250 tournament runs between TS and BYM, TS and Clairvoyance, and BYM and Clairvoyance were all significant by Welch's t test ($p < 0.0001$). This indicates that TS and BYM identified 55.1% and 65.3%, respectively, of the total infections detected by the Clairvoyance strategy. Finally, over the course of 250 tournament runs in the main analysis in pairwise head-to-head competition, BYM won 80% of the time over TS, with Clairvoyance winning 100% of the time against TS and BYM. These

results are significant by a one-sided Z-test of a difference in proportions ($p < 0.0001$).

Sensitivity analyses

We re-evaluated all findings using the settings specified in Tables 1 and 2. The mean number (and SD) of new diagnoses detected by TS and BYM in the main analysis and in all sensitivity analyses are described in Table 3. Under every scenario we examined in sensitivity analysis, Clairvoyance detected the greatest number of new HIV-positive cases (see Additional file 3: Table S1 for mean number of new diagnoses detected by Clairvoyance

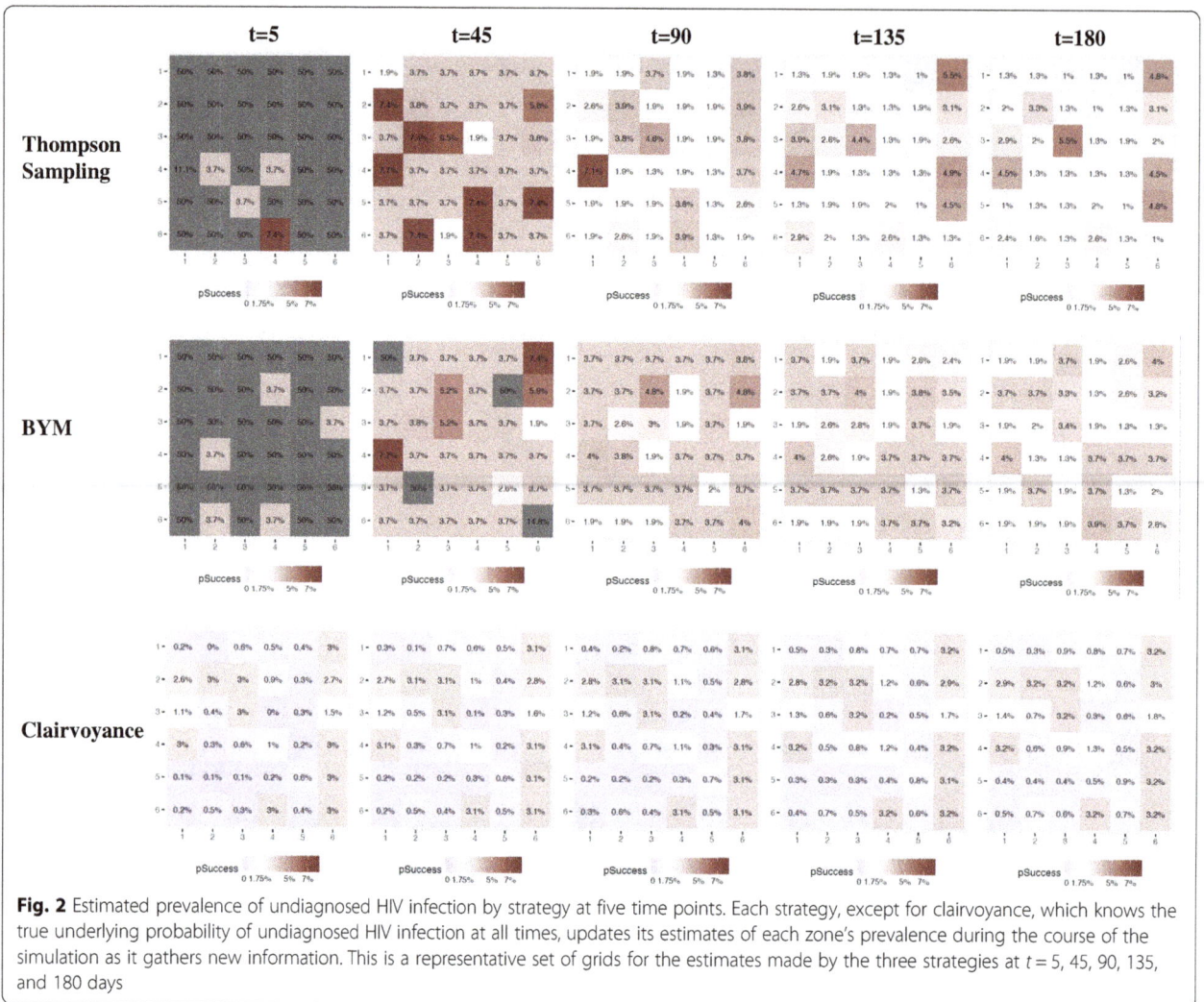

Fig. 2 Estimated prevalence of undiagnosed HIV infection by strategy at five time points. Each strategy, except for clairvoyance, which knows the true underlying probability of undiagnosed HIV infection at all times, updates its estimates of each zone's prevalence during the course of the simulation as it gathers new information. This is a representative set of grids for the estimates made by the three strategies at $t = 5$, 45, 90, 135, and 180 days

in the main analysis and in all sensitivity analyses). BYM almost always outperformed TS. TS narrowly defeated BYM when we considered a smaller grid size (e.g., 4 × 4) but this margin of victory (i.e., differences in the number of new diagnoses) was not statistically significant.

Sensitivity analysis revealed that the margin of victory between TS and BYM remains small under almost all circumstances. Averaging across all sensitivity analyses, the difference in the number of cases detected between TS and BYM was just over 12 cases. By contrast, Clairvoyance's average margin of victory over its competitors exceeded 50 cases.

Discussion

In our previous work, we introduced TS as a potential method for more efficiently deploying mobile HIV testing services and suggested that this algorithm could be useful in improving the detection and diagnosis of other infectious or chronic diseases [3]. In that study, TS was pitted against, and consistently outperformed, a winner-take-all strategy that

sampled each geographic zone consecutively before deciding, based upon the zone with the largest yield of new diagnoses, where to devote all of its remaining testing resources. This winner-take-all strategy will not work for a larger collection of zones since a stepwise approach is time-consuming, with initial sampling periods quickly exceeding number of days of testing in the simulation. Thus, we were interested in finding other algorithms that could be compared against TS in an expanded setting and in particular where spatial correlation may exist in terms of the probability of finding new cases of undetected HIV infection in neighboring zones.

While BYM is a widely used method in spatial statistics and epidemiology, used to map disease occurrence and to predict outbreaks, it has not generally been deployed in public health as a spatial sequential decision-making tool and we can consider this a novel potential use for it [15, 16]. In other settings, particularly environmental management and commercial applications such as oil exploration, related methods have been used to model space-structured sequential decision-making under uncertainty [17–19].

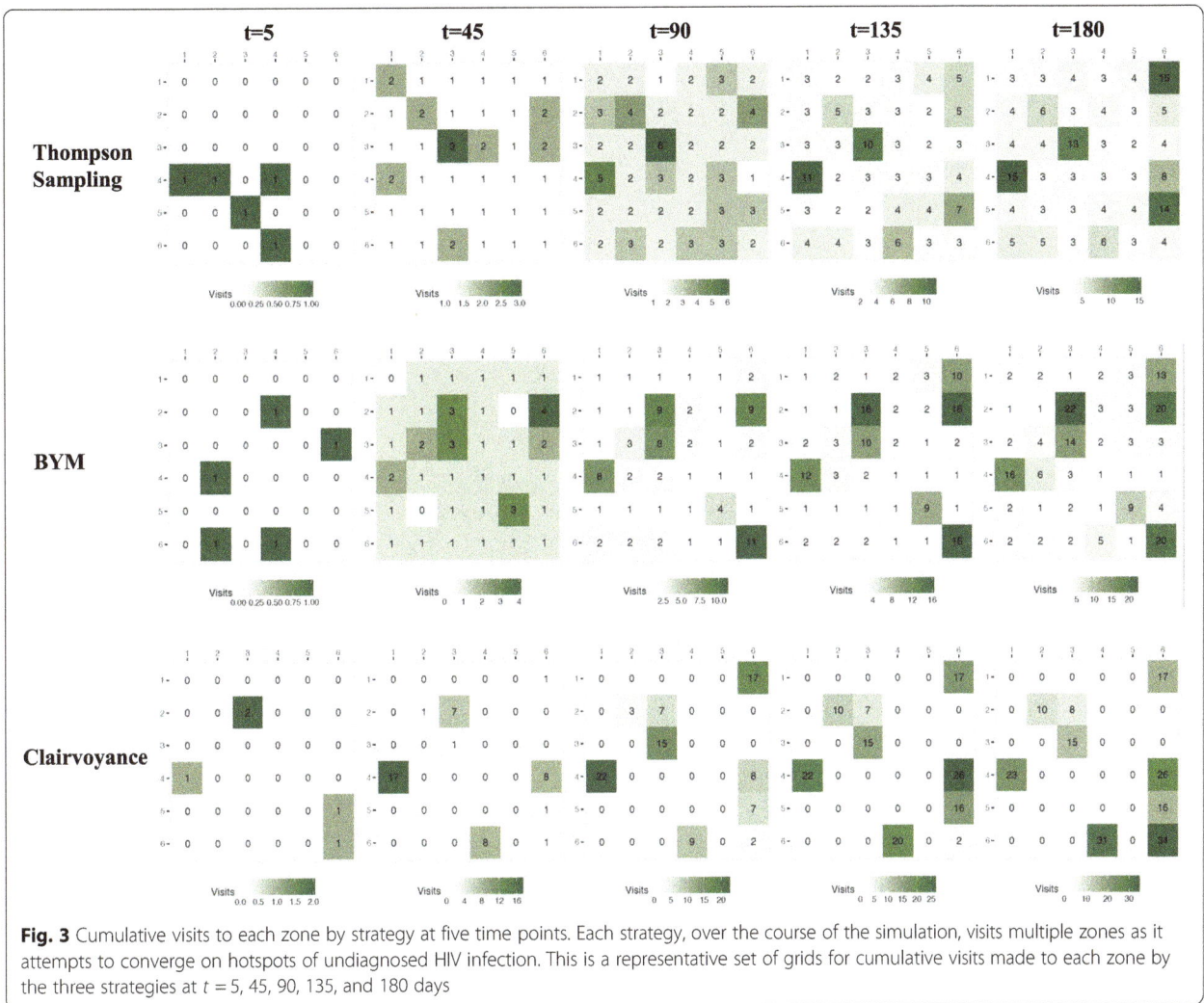

Fig. 3 Cumulative visits to each zone by strategy at five time points. Each strategy, over the course of the simulation, visits multiple zones as it attempts to converge on hotspots of undiagnosed HIV infection. This is a representative set of grids for cumulative visits made to each zone by the three strategies at $t = 5$, 45, 90, 135, and 180 days

The BYM model deployed here represents an improvement on the yield of new diagnoses over TS in our tournament. In almost all cases it outperforms TS, except when the number of zones is smaller (i.e., when the grid size is 4×4). This is not surprising as during the BYM model's learning period (up until 10 zones), the algorithm is following the same procedural steps as TS. With 16 zones, BYM has only just begun to incorporate information about neighboring zones into its decision-making process.

What is surprising is that, while BYM outperforms TS in all other settings, there does not seem to be an advantage for BYM in settings with higher spatial correlation in the data. This may be because the number of zones considered in this work is too small to fully exploit the benefits of modeling the spatial correlation. In cases where there is a larger number of zones and fewer hotspots, it may be more important to model the spatial correlation to avoid spending excess time in low prevalence areas. However, BYM's stronger performance overall may be due to the fact that BYM continues to

incorporate information across zones during estimation even in the absence of spatial correlation. The intercept parameter and exchangeable random effect variance parameter are shared across all zones. This should allow the BYM model to quickly learn about low prevalence areas and avoid spending time in them. In fact, this is demonstrated in Fig. 3, as BYM makes fewer visits to lower prevalence areas than TS.

There are several implications of these findings. First, the BYM model in simulation is a better tool for detecting new cases of undetected HIV infection in most settings than TS. Second, because it is difficult to make assumptions about whether there is indeed correlation in the data (is the probability of finding new cases of undetected HIV infection from one zone to another linked neighbor-to-neighbor?) there is a strong rationale to rely on BYM as it is functionally similar to TS in the absence of spatial variability.

However, there are operational complexities with BYM that might make it less attractive as a tool for use in the

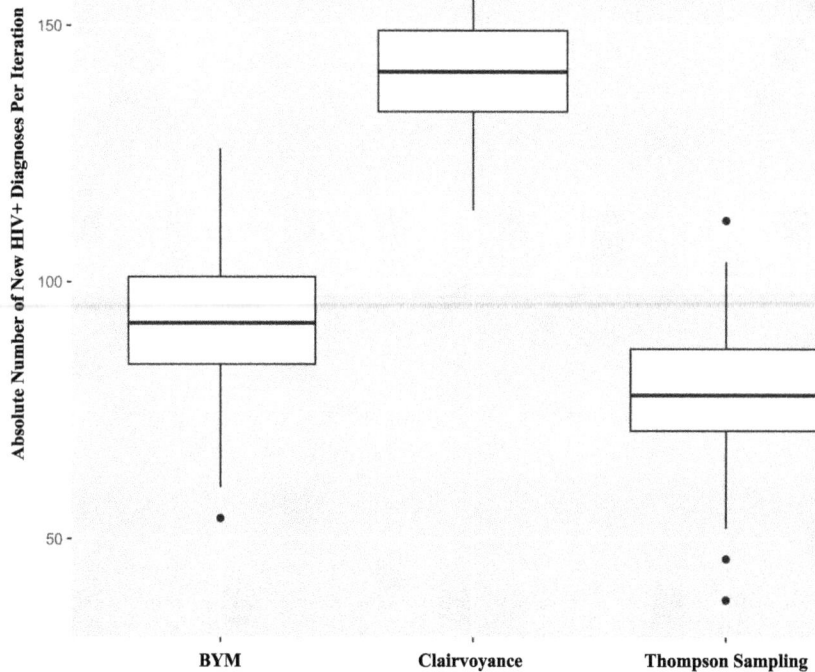

Fig. 4 Basic statistics for yield of new HIV diagnoses by strategy. The minimum, first quartile, median, third quartile, and maximum number of new diagnoses detected by each strategy over 180 days in 250 iterations of the simulation for the main analysis

field. TS is a simple algorithm that can be implemented in a spreadsheet with a few formulas and requires only a daily report of new HIV-positive and HIV-negative diagnoses for the Bayesian updating process. By contrast, the BYM model can be computationally demanding in comparison to TS (depending on the number of zones) because of its reliance on MCMC model fitting techniques; the convergence of the MCMC algorithm must be assessed, it requires the ability to determine the neighborhood structure of the data (e.g., shapefiles for different regions are needed) and a certain number of zones need to be visited before estimation stabilizes [20, 21]. Integrated Nested Laplace Approximation often represents a computationally convenient alternative to Bayesian model fitting and provides approximations to marginal posterior distributions for model parameters. It can also be used to fit the BYM model if MCMC techniques become computationally difficult due to an extremely large number of zones in a particular application. However, both MCMC and Integrated Nested Laplace Approximation still remain more complex to utilize than TS, which can be implemented using a spreadsheet program or by hand [22, 23].

While BYM performs better than TS in simulation, its modest margin of victory (~ 10%) in yield of new infections diagnosed must be weighed against these practical difficulties. In resource-poor settings (in fact, any settings without sufficient computing infrastructure and statistical support) the logistical simplicity of implementation might commend TS as the preferred tool for locating HIV testing services.

Because TS and BYM only detected 55.1% and 65.3%, respectively, of the total infections detected by Clairvoyance there may be room for improvement in the yield of new diagnoses. This work represents a bridging of several different fields, including sequential decision-making, reinforcement learning, spatial statistics, and epidemiology, all in a Bayesian context. However, thus far, only two algorithms from these fields, TS and BYM, have been tested in simulation in the context of mobile HIV testing. The current simulation code allows for the addition of new strategies as modules on top of the larger evaluative framework; therefore, exploring additional algorithms can be easily undertaken in future work, which may allow us to identify new strategies that preserve simplicity of implementation and offer greater yields of new diagnoses.

Table 3 Results for main analysis and sensitivity analyses

Parameters	Values	Thompson sampling			Besag York Mollié		
		Win percentage	New diagnoses Mean	New diagnoses Std Dev	Win percentage	New diagnoses Mean	New diagnoses Std dev
Main analysis	N/A	20%	78.24	11.44	80%	92.59	12.37
percentage of new HIV-negative arrivals (times zone population divided 365 days)	0	17%	79.75	12.02	83%	96.40	11.50
percentage of new HIV-negative arrivals (times zone population divided 365 days)	1.7%	19%	79.07	11.21	81%	92.88	11.52
percentage of new HIV-negative arrivals (times zone population divided 365 days)	6.8%	16%	77.53	12.10	84%	93.17	10.85
Grid dimensions	4 × 4	54%	94.94	13.73	46%	93.18	13.85
Grid dimensions	5 × 5	38%	85.70	13.30	62%	91.98	11.84
Grid dimension	10 × 10	28%	65.81	9.52	72%	74.69	11.40
Percentage of new infections (times zone population divided by 365 days)	0	13%	71.99	11.19	87%	88.34	11.40
Percentage of new infections (times zone population divided by 365 days)	0.33%	14%	74.52	10.72	86%	89.88	10.21
Percentage of new infections (times zone population divided by 365 days)	1.32%	20%	85.46	11.30	80%	99.84	12.63
No arrivals or infections	N/A	20%	78.24	11.44	80%	92.59	12.37
Level of correlation, percentage of hotspots in grid	None, 20% (on average)	18%	78.20	12.07	82%	93.97	12.57
Level of correlation, percentage of hotspots in grid	Low, 10% (on average)	16%	68.13	9.70	84%	82.93	13.29
Level of correlation, percentage of hotspots in grid	Low, 30% (on average)	23%	88.59	11.89	77%	100.56	11.82
Level of correlation, percentage of hotspots in grid	Medium, 20% (on average)	18%	78.83	11.31	82%	93.62	11.86
Level of correlation, percentage of hotspots in grid	High, 20% (on average)	14%	78.41	11.56	86%	95.86	11.38
Days until return to unobserved, uninfected pool	10	23%	79.46	12.34	77%	92.54	12.00
Days until return to unobserved, uninfected pool	90	16%	78.28	10.90	84%	93.58	12.05
Days of testing	90	27%	33.17	6.84	73%	39.81	7.83
Days of testing	365	30%	193.79	20.24	70%	206.10	21.31
Tests per day	10	27%	27.55	6.07	73%	32.53	6.83
Tests per day	40	29%	137.54	15.17	71%	148.91	16.43

Our study has several limitations. While we have expanded the number of zones in this paper to explore the performance of these algorithms beyond the small set of uncorrelated geographic locations in the earlier toy model, we have not yet included a temporal component to our analyses. Hotspots for detecting new cases of undetected HIV infection may shift, not only in space, but in time, both in the short-term (e.g., with opening and closing of social venues) and the longer term (e.g., as neighborhood demographics change). In addition, the ICAR prior in the BYM model requires an assumption about contiguous zones, namely that observations in immediate neighbors will be correlated [24]. However, this correlation by virtue of adjacency in the setting of HIV testing may not hold. For instance, a gay bar may exist in the context of a neighborhood that does not share the demographic characteristics of its patrons. This problem where geographic proximity exists among zones but the probability of finding undetected cases of HIV infection among them may be disparate can be addressed by spatial boundary detection methods, but a discussion of them is beyond the scope of this paper [25]. Finally, the simulation study results suggest that the choice of 10 unique zones for the initial learning strategy for the BYM strategy works well in comparison to TS under our specific HIV testing data settings. However, in future applications of the model, these choices may need to be revisited based on problem-specific prevalences and zonal geography.

Our portrayal of the epidemiology of HIV infection and the mechanics of HIV testing is, admittedly, simplistic. Among the many details that it omits are the use of testing services by people who already know their infection status; the possibility that infection risk may influence an individual's decision to obtain an HIV test; the costs of moving a mobile testing facility from one location to another; more complicated forms of immigration and emigration, including daily travel between zones, via either public or private transportation, for work or other activities; and the possibility that even a few HIV tests on a single day might have a material influence on the prevalence of infection and the success of continued testing in a given zone on a given day. Each of these simplifications can be accommodated within the current analytic framework if circumstances suggest that they are more important than we have argued here.

Conclusions

TS and the BYM algorithm both offer ways to manage the exploration−exploitation trade-off in deciding where to locate mobile HIV testing services from day to day. TS may be more suitable for settings where there are resource constraints in terms of computing power and statistical support. Spatial algorithms could be important tools, particularly if their execution could be simplified for use by non-experts in the field.

Abbreviations
BYM: Besag York Mollié; CAR: Conditional autoregressive; HIV: Human immunodeficiency virus; ICAR: Intrinsic conditional autoregressive; MCMC: Markov chain Monte Carlo; TS: Thompson sampling

Acknowledgements
The authors thank Forrest W. Crawford, PhD, for helpful discussions on the manuscript.

Funding
Financial support for this study was provided in part by the National Institute on Drug Abuse (R01 DA015612) and the National Institutes of Mental Health (R01MH105203).
GSG acknowledges support from the National Institutes of Mental Health (R01MH105203), the National Institute on Drug Abuse (R01 DA015612), and the Laura and John Arnold Foundation.
ADP acknowledges the support of a sabbatical leave from the Yale School of Public Health and a visiting appointment at SciencesPo, Paris, supported by a public grant overseen by the French National Research Agency (ANR) as part of the "Investissements d'Avenir" program within the framework of the Laboratory for Interdisciplinary Evaluation of Public Policies (LIEPP) center of excellence (ANR11LABX0091, ANR 11 IDEX000502). JLW acknowledges support from CTSA Grant Number UL1 TR001863 and KL2 TR001862 from the National Center for Advancing Translational Science (NCATS), components of the National Institutes of Health (NIH), and NIH roadmap for Medical Research.

Authors' contributions
GSG, JTC, ADP, and JLW contributed to the conception of the study design. JLW developed and provided code for the BYM algorithm and the underlying starting grids. JTC coded the simulation. GSG, TJ, and JLW acquired data and developed parameter estimates. GSG, JTC, and JLW conducted the analysis. GSG, JTC, TJ, ADP, and JLW analyzed and interpreted the results. GSG wrote the first manuscript draft. GSG, JTC, TJ, ADP, and JLW edited the manuscript. All authors read and approved the final manuscript.

Competing interests
The authors declare that they have no competing interests.

Author details
[1]Department of Epidemiology of Microbial Diseases, Yale School of Public Health, 60 College Street, New Haven, CT, USA. [2]Independent Consultant, Yale School of Public Health, 60 College Street, New Haven, CT, USA. [3]Department of Health Policy and Management, Yale School of Public Health, 60 College Street, New Haven, CT, USA. [4]Department of Biostatistics, Yale School of Public Health, 60 College Street, New Haven, CT, USA.

References

1. HIV.gov. The Global AIDS Epidemic. Global HIV/AIDS Overview. 2017. https://www.hiv.gov/federal-response/pepfar-global-aids/global-hiv-aids-overview. Accessed 19 Mar 2018.
2. Joint United Nations Programme on HIV/AIDS (UNAIDS). UNAIDS Data 2017. Geneva: UNAIDS; 2017. http://www.unaids.org/sites/default/files/media_asset/20170720_Data_book_2017_en.pdf. Accessed 19 Mar 2018
3. Gonsalves GS, Crawford FW, Cleary PD, Kaplan EH, Paltiel AD. An adaptive approach to locating mobile HIV testing services. Med Decis Mak. 2018;38:262.
4. Gigerenzer G, Todd PM, The ABC Research Group. Simple Heuristics that Make us Smart. Oxford: Oxford University Press; 1999.
5. Robbins H. Some Aspects of the Sequential Design of Experiments. New York: Springer; 1985. p. 169–177.
6. MacNab YC. Hierarchical Bayesian modeling of spatially correlated health service outcome and utilization rates. Biometrics. 2003;59:305–15.
7. Besag J, York J, Mollié A. Bayesian image restoration, with two applications in spatial statistics. Ann Inst Stat Math. 1991;43:1–20.
8. Zambia - Census of Population and Housing 2010 - IPUMS Subset. http://microdata.worldbank.org/index.php/catalog/2124. Accessed 19 Mar 2018.
9. The PHIA Project. The Zambia Population-Based HIV Impact Assessment. http://phia.icap.columbia.edu/countries/zambia/. Accessed 2 Mar 2018.
10. New PHIA Survey Data Show Critical Progress Towards Global HIV Targets. 2017. https://www.cdc.gov/globalhivtb/who-we-are/events/world-aids-day/phia-surveys.html. Accessed 19 Mar 2018.
11. Bassett IV, Govindasamy D, Erlwanger AS, Hyle EP, Kranzer K, van Schaik N, et al. Mobile HIV screening in Cape Town, South Africa: clinical impact, cost and cost-effectiveness. PLoS One. 2014;9:e85197.
12. Maheswaran H, Thulare H, Stanistreet D, Tanser F, Newell M-L. Starting a home and mobile HIV testing service in a rural area of South Africa. J Acquir Immune Defic Syndr. 2012;59:e43–6.
13. Taylor D, Durigon M, Davis H, Archibald C, Konrad B, Coombs D, et al. Probability of a false-negative HIV antibody test result during the window period: a tool for pre- and post-test counselling. Int J STD AIDS. 2015;26:215–24.
14. Webster DP, Donati M, Geretti AM, Waters LJ, Gazzard B, Radcliffe K. BASHH/EAGA position statement on the HIV window period. Int J STD AIDS. 2015;26:760–1.
15. Corberán-Vallet A. Prospective surveillance of multivariate spatial disease data. Stat Methods Med Res. 2012;21:457–77.
16. Best N, Richardson S, Thomson A. A comparison of Bayesian spatial models for disease mapping. Stat Methods Med Res. 2005;14:35–59.
17. Martinelli G, Eidsvik J, Hauge R. Dynamic decision making for graphical models applied to oil exploration. Eur J Oper Res. 2013;230:688–702.
18. Moore CT, Shaffer TL, Gannon JJ. Spatial education: improving conservation delivery through space-structured decision making. J Fish Wildl Manag. 2013;4:199–210.
19. Peyrard N, Sabbadin R, Spring D, Brook B, Mac NR. Model-based adaptive spatial sampling for occurrence map construction. Stat Comput. 2013;23:29–42.
20. Gelman A, Shirley K. Inference from simulations and monitoring convergence. Handbook for Markov Chain Monte Carlo. Boca Raton: CRC Press; 2011. p. 163–74.
21. Lawson AB. Bayesian disease mapping: hierarchical modeling in spatial epidemiology. 2nd ed. Boca Raton: CRC Press; 2013.
22. Rue H, Martino S, Chopin N. Approximate Bayesian inference for latent Gaussian models by using integrated nested Laplace approximations (with discussion). J R Statist Soc B. 2009;71:319–92.
23. Martins TG, Simpson D, Lindgren F, Rue H. Bayesian computing with INLA: new features. Computnl Statist Data Anal. 2013;67:68–83.
24. Lee D. A comparison of conditional autoregressive models used in Bayesian disease mapping. Spat Spatio-Temporal Epidemiol. 2011;2:79–89.
25. Lee D, Mitchell R. Boundary detection in disease mapping studies. Biostat Oxf Engl. 2012;13:415–26.

8

Investigating spillover of multidrug-resistant tuberculosis from a prison: a spatial and molecular epidemiological analysis

Joshua L. Warren[1*], Louis Grandjean[2,3], David A. J. Moore[3,4], Anna Lithgow[4], Jorge Coronel[3], Patricia Sheen[3], Jonathan L. Zelner[5], Jason R. Andrews[6] and Ted Cohen[7]

Abstract

Background: Congregate settings may serve as institutional amplifiers of tuberculosis (TB) and multidrug-resistant tuberculosis (MDR-TB). We analyze spatial, epidemiological, and pathogen genetic data prospectively collected from neighborhoods surrounding a prison in Lima, Peru, where inmates experience a high risk of MDR-TB, to investigate the risk of spillover into the surrounding community.

Methods: Using hierarchical Bayesian statistical modeling, we address three questions regarding the MDR-TB risk: (i) Does the excess risk observed among prisoners also extend outside the prison? (ii) If so, what is the magnitude, shape, and spatial range of this spillover effect? (iii) Is there evidence of additional transmission across the region?

Results: The region of spillover risk extends for 5.47 km outside of the prison (95% credible interval: 1.38, 9.63 km). Within this spillover region, we find that nine of the 467 non-inmate patients (35 with MDR-TB) have MDR-TB strains that are genetic matches to strains collected from current inmates with MDR-TB, compared to seven out of 1080 patients (89 with MDR-TB) outside the spillover region (p values: 0.022 and 0.008). We also identify eight spatially aggregated genetic clusters of MDR-TB, four within the spillover region, consistent with local transmission among individuals living close to the prison.

Conclusions: We demonstrate a clear prison spillover effect in this population, which suggests that interventions in the prison may have benefits that extend to the surrounding community.

Keywords: Antibiotic resistance, Bayesian statistics, Spatial analysis, Spillover analysis, Transmission

Background

In 2016, the latest year for which estimates are available, there were 490,000 incident cases of multidrug-resistant tuberculosis (MDR-TB) [1]. Individuals with MDR-TB have a disease that is resistant to at least isoniazid and rifampicin and they are at substantially elevated risk of treatment non-response, treatment-related side effects, and mortality, even if drug resistance is recognized and treatment with appropriate second-line drug regimens is available [2–4].

MDR-TB arises as a consequence of failed treatment or by direct transmission from an individual infectious with MDR-TB. Measures of the relative importance of failed treatment and direct transmission as drivers of MDR-TB are not easy to obtain in the setting of complex epidemics, where reports of treatment history and prior drug susceptibility results are often unreliable or unavailable. Nonetheless, an analysis based on programmatic data [5] and an inference based on fitting transmission dynamic models to data [6] reveal that direct transmission of MDR-TB is now the dominant mechanism driving incidence in most settings. Therefore, the success of interventions that aim to mitigate the rise of MDR-TB will depend critically on their ability to identify

* Correspondence: joshua.warren@yale.edu
[1]Department of Biostatistics, Yale University, New Haven, CT 06510, USA
Full list of author information is available at the end of the article

where transmission occurs and who is at the highest risk of infection.

It has been suggested that specific types of congregate settings, especially hospitals and prisons, can serve as institutional amplifiers of TB [7, 8], and in particular, MDR-TB [9–13]. This hypothesis suggests that the high incidence rates of TB and MDR-TB reported in congregate settings can lead to spillover risk in the community [14], especially in settings where there is a rapid turnover of members in the congregate setting or there are opportunities for interaction between community members and those in the congregate setting. Consistent with this hypothesis, a statistical analysis of country-level data from eastern Europe and central Asia found that rates of growth of the prison population were positively associated with increases in both TB incidence and the risk of MDR-TB [15]. Several studies have also documented the likely spillover of TB from prisons to communities [16] and an increased risk of MDR-TB in spatial proximity to prisons [12, 17] and in areas where former prisoners reside [18].

In this work, we develop hierarchical Bayesian statistical models to investigate the hypothesis that an elevated MDR-TB risk for prisoners (documented in an earlier study [19]) produces detectable spillover effects in the surrounding neighborhoods of Lima, Peru. In our analytic framework, we simultaneously test this hypothesis and estimate the magnitude, shape, and spatial range of the spillover effect. In addition, we further investigate the possibility of local transmission of MDR-TB within these neighborhoods through an analysis of the residual spatial correlation in risk among the patients and an exploration of genetic clusters of specific strains of *Mycobacterium tuberculosis*.

Methods
Data description
Between 2008 and 2010, sputum, as well as basic demographic and clinical data, were collected from all individuals with suspected TB living in two of the four large regions of metropolitan Lima (Callao and Lima Sur). The geographic region and study population are presented in Fig. 1 (jittered to protect confidentiality). These data were collected in the context of a population-wide implementation study of the Microscopic Observation Drug Susceptibility assay, a rapid test for TB and MDR-TB. Full details of the field methods are available in a previous publication [19]. All isolates included in this study have been tested for susceptibility to isoniazid and rifampin and have been genotyped by 15-loci MIRU-VNTR [20]. In total, approximately 71% of all culture-positive isolates had genotyping and geographic data and were included in this analysis [19].

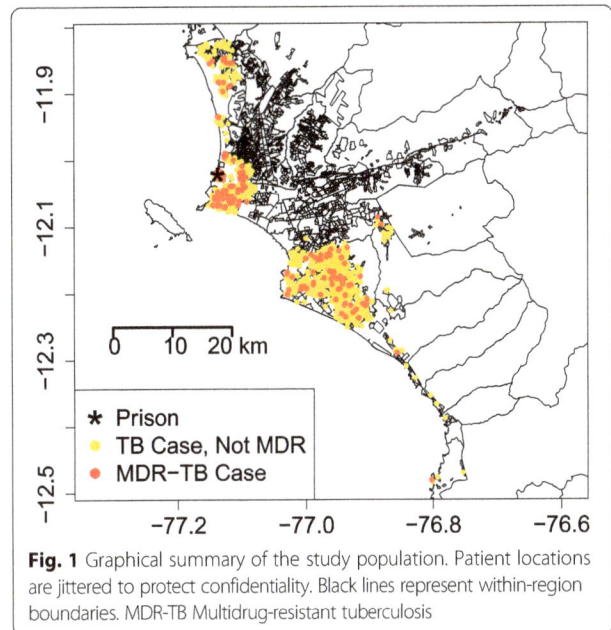

Fig. 1 Graphical summary of the study population. Patient locations are jittered to protect confidentiality. Black lines represent within-region boundaries. MDR-TB Multidrug-resistant tuberculosis

For this analysis, we used individual-level information about the patients including sex (male or female), sputum smear positivity indicator (yes or no), previous TB treatment status (yes or no), average socioeconomic status of their city block (lower, middle, and upper tertiles), population density of their city block (number of people per city block), age category (<25, 25–64, or 65+ years), prisoner status (yes or no), and longitude and latitude of residence at time of diagnosis. In total, our analysis includes 1587 TB patients after removing those with missing covariate information. Of these patients, 115 shared a residence with at least one other patient in the study. Table 1 displays the summary information for this population by MDR-TB status.

Spillover risk analysis
We develop hierarchical Bayesian statistical models that simultaneously account for the potential of elevated MDR-TB risk for an individual due to a number of sources including (i) individual-level risk factors, (ii) proximity to the prison (representing potential spillover), and (iii) spatial proximity to other MDR-TB cases (representing the possibility of local transmission). In our analyses, each TB patient is categorized as having MDR-TB or drug-susceptible TB (i.e., any phenotype that is not MDR-TB) and we model the probability that a patient has MDR-TB as a function of these different sources of risk.

Specifically, we define $Y_i(s_i) \mid p_i(s_i) \sim \text{Bernoulli}(p_i(s_i))$, $i = 1, ..., n$, where $Y_i(s_i)$ is equal to 1 if individual i residing at spatial location s_i has MDR-TB and is equal to 0 otherwise. $p_i(s_i)$ describes the individual's personal probability of being an MDR-TB patient and n is the number

Table 1 Study population characteristics

Characteristic	Tuberculosis type	
	Multidrug-resistant	Drug susceptible
Total	164	1423
Prisoner status (yes)	7 (0.04)	33 (0.02)
Sex (male)	102 (0.62)	897 (0.63)
Smear positive (yes)	147 (0.90)	1271 (0.89)
Previous treatment (yes)	79 (0.48)	346 (0.24)
Socioeconomic status category		
Upper tertile	9 (0.05)	73 (0.05)
Middle tertile	65 (0.40)	485 (0.34)
Lower tertile	90 (0.55)	865 (0.61)
Age category		
[18–25]	36 (0.22)	376 (0.26)
[25–65]	120 (0.73)	951 (0.67)
65+	8 (0.05)	96 (0.07)
Population density (per city block)	127.99 (57.84)	121.90 (57.38)
Distance to prison (kilometers)	15.07 (12.10)	18.36 (11.57)

Counts with proportions in parentheses are shown for categorical variables. Means with standard deviations in parentheses are shown for continuous variables

Table 2 Inference from the Gaussian spillover risk model

Parameter	Mean	SD	Quantile	
			0.025	0.975
Intercept	−2.23	0.71	−3.90	−1.20
Previous treatment: yes vs. no	0.81	0.24	0.44	1.35
Sex: female vs. male	0.11	0.16	−0.17	0.46
Smear positive: yes vs. no	0.11	0.22	−0.29	0.58
Socioeconomic status:				
Middle vs. upper	−0.19	0.30	−0.81	0.39
Lower vs. upper	−0.40	0.31	−1.10	0.15
Population density	0.01	0.09	−0.17	0.19
Age category				
[25–65] vs. [18–25]	−0.01	0.16	−0.33	0.31
65+ vs. [18–25]	−0.27	0.32	−1.00	0.30
Spillover magnitude (λ)	0.49	0.28	0.01	1.13
Spillover range (θ), kilometers	5.47	1.83	1.38	9.63
Regression parameter variance (σ_δ^2)	0.90	0.86	0.18	3.10
Spatial variance parameter (σ_w^2)	1.71	1.55	0.11	5.53

Posterior means, posterior SDs, and posterior quantiles are presented. Parameters whose 95% credible intervals do not include 0 are shown in bold, indicating an increased (positive effect) MDR-TB risk for a patient with the particular characteristic

MDR-TB multidrug-resistant tuberculosis, *SD* standard deviation

of individuals in the study. We note that multiple individuals can be located at the same residence, leading to identical spatial locations in the analysis. Therefore, we define the set of unique spatial locations as s_j^*. Each s_i maps to a particular s_j^* for $j = 1, ...m$, where m represents the total number of unique spatial locations and is less than the total number of patients, n.

Next, we introduce a model for an individual's personal probability of having MDR-TB that accounts for the patient's personal risk factors, distance to the prison, and spatial proximity to other individuals such that

$$\Phi^{-1}(p_i(s_i)) = \mathbf{x}_i^T \boldsymbol{\beta} + \lambda g(\|s_i - s_p\|; \theta) + w(s_i),$$

where $\Phi^{-1}(.)$ is the inverse cumulative distribution function of the standard normal distribution, resulting in a probit regression model. $\mathbf{x}_i$ is a vector of individual-level risk factors, which are displayed in Table 2. $\boldsymbol{\beta}$ is a vector of unknown regression parameters. The function $\lambda g(\|s_i - s_p\|; \theta)$ describes the impact of a patient's proximity to the prison on MDR-TB risk, where s_p is the longitude and latitude of the prison, $\|.\|$ is the Euclidean distance function, and λ, θ are unknown parameters that describe the magnitude of the spillover risk and the spatial range of the spillover effect, respectively. Finally, $w(s_i)$ is a spatially correlated random effect specific to the individual's location of residence that is useful in identifying residual MDR-TB risk based on spatial location alone, which is risk that is potentially due to local transmission.

We are primarily interested in determining if proximity to the prison has any impact on an individual's MDR-TB risk and formally test this hypothesis through the inclusion of $\lambda g(\|s_i - s_p\|; \theta)$. We test a number of competing options that each make a different assumption regarding the range and shape of the potential spillover effect, and formally compare the models using two Bayesian model selection techniques: the Watanabe–Akaike information criterion (WAIC) [21, 22] and D_k [23]. WAIC is used primarily when the model is intended for explanatory purposes while D_k, a posterior predictive loss metric, is used to compare the predictive capabilities of different models. Both metrics balance model fit and complexity with smaller values of each being preferred. Following [24], we set $k = 10^{10}$ and use the Bernoulli distribution deviance, with continuity correction, when calculating D_k. Our competing models are created by defining $g(\|s_i - s_p\|; \theta)$ as $1(\|s_i - s_p\| = 0)$ (prisoner indicator), $1(\|s_i - s_p\| \leq \theta)$ (constant spillover risk), $\exp\{-\|s_i - s_p\|\}1(\|s_i - s_p\| \leq \theta)$ (exponential spillover risk), and $\exp\{-\|s_i - s_p\|^2\}1(\|s_i - s_p\| \leq \theta)$ (Gaussian spillover risk), where $1(.)$ is an indicator function that is equal to 1 if the input statement is true and is equal to 0 otherwise.

The prison indicator model assumes that only those patients located at the prison have increased MDR-TB risk, indicating no spillover effect. The constant spillover risk model suggests that there is a spillover effect extending outside the prison that is constant in magnitude for all patients within the range of influence (controlled by the unknown parameter θ). The exponential spillover risk model suggests that the risk is highest at the prison and decays based on the function $\exp\{-\|s_i - s_p\|\}1(\|s_i - s_p\| \leq \theta)$ as distance from the prison increases. After a certain distance θ, the risk is, again, assumed to be zero. The Gaussian spillover risk model is similar to the exponential version, except that it replaces the exponential decay function with $\exp\{-\|s_i - s_p\|^2\}1(\|s_i - s_p\| \leq \theta)$.

We are also interested in understanding if there is additional residual risk associated with proximity to other MDR-TB cases. Therefore, we introduce random effects that aim to detect pockets of increased MDR-TB risk due to spatial location alone. The $w(s_i)$ parameters are spatially correlated random effects that account for any residual spatial variability in MDR-TB risk (after controlling for individual-level characteristics and proximity to the prison). The vector of spatially correlated random effects, $w = \{w(s_1^*), ..., w(s_m^*)\}^T$, is modeled using a Gaussian process prior distribution with spatially structured covariance matrix [25] such that $w \mid \phi \sim \text{MVN}(0, \sigma_w^2 \Sigma(\phi))$ where MVN(.,.) represents the multivariate normal distribution and $\sigma_w^2 \Sigma(\phi)$ describes the variance/covariance of the random effects. This specification allows us to determine if there are highly localized regions of MDR-TB risk, possibly due to transmission. Random effects associated with individuals who are separated by a short distance are assumed to be more similar a priori, leading to similar estimates of individual-level risk ($p_i(s_i)$). We allow the data to inform about the distance that this correlation extends from a particular location and what type of impact it has on MDR-TB risk in general. Specifically, we model the covariance between two of the random effects by defining $\sigma_w^2 \Sigma(\phi)_{ij}$ as

$$\text{Covariance}\left\{w\left(s_i^*\right), w\left(s_j^*\right)\right\} = \sigma_w^2 \rho\left(\left\|s_i^* - s_j^*\right\|; \phi\right),$$

where σ_w^2 represents the total variance of the random effect distribution, ϕ controls the range of spatial correlation (at what distance random effects are uncorrelated), and $\rho(.;.)$ is an isotropic spatial correlation function that describes the correlation between random effects as a function of the distance between spatial locations [25]. In our application of the model, we choose the spherical correlation structure because it provides us with an exact definition of the range of spatial correlation, $1/\phi$. The spherical correlation function is defined as

$$\rho(d; \phi) = \begin{cases} 1 - 1.5\phi d + 0.5(\phi d)^3, & \text{if } 0 \leq d \leq 1/\phi, \\ 0, & \text{if } d \geq 1/\phi, \end{cases}$$

where d is the distance between spatial locations.

Predicted probabilities of MDR-TB at new spatial locations are obtained through the posterior predictive distribution of individual-level probabilities, $f(p_i(s_i)\mid Y)$, where $Y = \{Y_1(s_1), ..., Y_n(s_n)\}^T$, using properties of the conditional multivariate normal distribution and composition sampling [25]. The mean and standard deviation of the posterior predictive distributions are plotted to assess the geographic risk of MDR-TB across the study region.

Molecular analysis

The spatially correlated random effects identify areas that have excess residual MDR-TB risk. To determine if this excess risk may be due to local transmission, we further interrogate these regions using 15-loci MIRU-VNTR genotypes [20]. If multiple genetically matched isolates are identified in a single high MDR-TB risk region, we deem local transmission to be probable. Specifically, we first identify estimated spatial random effects whose upper 95% credible intervals are larger than 0, indicating a statistically significant increased local risk of MDR-TB (i.e., $P(w(s_j^*) > 0\mid Y) \geq 0.95$). Next, based on the estimated spatial range of correlation for these random effects (posterior mean of $1/\phi$), we create buffers around these significant spatial random effects with a radius equal to this distance. We then look within these buffers to determine if there are at least two individuals with a statistically significant increased MDR-TB risk. For those buffers that meet these requirements, we examine whether the observed strains have identical MIRU-VNTR patterns.

We also examine the MDR-TB strains from individuals residing within the estimated range of the spillover effect from the prison (posterior mean of θ). These MDR-TB strains are then compared with MDR-TB strains from current inmates to investigate further the possible mechanism of the spillover effect identified through the spatial analysis.

Prior specification

To specify the model fully within the Bayesian framework, prior distributions must be selected for each of the unknown model parameters. When possible, we select weakly informative prior distributions for the data to drive the inference rather than our prior beliefs. The regression parameters are assumed to arise independently from a common Gaussian distribution such that $\beta_j, \lambda \sim N(0, \sigma_\delta^2)$ with $\sigma_\delta^2 \sim$ Inverse Gamma(0.01, 0.01). The spillover range parameter, θ, is assigned a Uniform(0, 10) kilometers prior based on the distribution of patients surrounding the prison and reasonable expectations regarding the distance of a spillover impact. The variance of the spatial random effect distribution, σ_w^2, is given an Inverse Gamma(0.01, 0.01) prior while a Gamma(0.10, 0.10) prior distribution is selected for the spherical correlation range parameter, ϕ. In addition, we assess the sensitivity of our results to the choice of prior distributions for the variance parameters by rerunning the final selected model while specifying σ_δ, $\sigma_w \sim$ Uniform$(0, 100)$.

Computing and model fitting

Each of the proposed models are fitted in the Bayesian setting using Markov chain Monte Carlo sampling techniques with R statistical software [26]. For each model, we collect 90,000 samples from the joint posterior distribution of the model parameters after a burn-in period of 10,000 iterations. To reduce the autocorrelation in the Markov chains and ease the computational burden of summarizing 90,000 posterior samples (particularly with respect to prediction), we thin the chains, resulting in a final set of 5000 posterior samples. Convergence was assessed through visual inspection of individual parameter trace plots and by monitoring the Geweke diagnostic measure [27]. Neither approach suggested any obvious signs of non-convergence.

Results

Data description

We have a total of $n = 1,587$ TB patients in $m = 1,509$ unique spatial locations. As shown in Table 1, 164 of the TB patients have MDR-TB (10.3%). The factor most closely associated with increased risk of MDR-TB is previous treatment for TB; 18.6% of previously treated individuals have MDR-TB compared to 7.3% of treatment naive individuals. We note that previous TB treatment status among those with MDR-TB is an imperfect proxy for transmitted MDR-TB. Individuals without previous treatment are assumed to have MDR-TB as a consequence of direct transmission, but those with previous treatment may have MDR-TB as a result of transmission or acquisition during their prior treatment. Current imprisonment is also associated with MDR-TB. Among the 40 inmates with TB, 17.5% have MDR-TB compared to 10.2% of individuals in the general population.

Spillover risk analysis

Additional file 1: Table S1 displays the model comparison results along with a measure of model complexity for each metric (p_{WAIC} for WAIC and P for D_k). The prisoner indicator model provides an improved fit over the constant spillover risk model, indicating that the assumption of constant risk in the area surrounding the prison may not accurately reflect the true nature of the spillover. However, a substantial improvement in model fit is observed when different shapes of spillover risk are considered. The exponential and Gaussian spillover risk models have an improved fit overall compared with the prisoner indicator model. This indicates that there may

be a spillover effect and that the resulting excess risk decreases as distance from the prison increases, before becoming 0.

The WAIC and D_k results between these two models are comparable overall, so we examine the inference for λ, the parameter controlling the magnitude of the spillover risk, to make our final model selection. While the posterior mean of λ is comparable between both models, the 95% credible interval of the parameter for the exponential spillover risk model is slightly below 0. The corresponding interval from the Gaussian spillover risk model excludes 0 (Table 2). Therefore, we further explore the results of the Gaussian spillover risk model in the remaining analyses but note that the results are generally comparable between both models.

In Table 2, we present the posterior inference for each of the parameters in the Gaussian spillover risk model. Parameters whose 95% credible intervals are strictly larger than 0 indicate an increased risk of MDR-TB for patients in those categories, with a similar interpretation for strictly negative results. As expected, patients who have been previously treated for TB are more likely to have MDR-TB than patients with no previous treatment history. No other individual-level risk factors are associated with increased or decreased risk of MDR-TB.

Inference for λ in Table 2 suggests that people living closer to the prison are at a higher risk of MDR-TB. The spatial range of the spillover effect, described by θ, is estimated to be 5.47 km, indicating that the increased risk extends beyond the prisoner population. The prior and posterior densities for λ and θ are shown in Additional file 1: Figures S1 and S2, respectively. Inside this spillover region, 14.8% of patients have MDR-TB while outside the spillover region the risk is only 8.2%. In Fig. 2, we display the predicted probability of MDR-TB across the region for a patient with previously treated TB while in Additional file 1: Figure S4, we display the predictions for a patient without previous TB treatment. We do not include the spatial random effects when calculating these probabilities to focus attention solely on the spillover risk. These figures clearly show the elevated MDR-TB risk surrounding the prison, the decay in risk as distance from the prison increases, and the large difference in risk between patients with and without a history of previous TB treatment. Posterior standard deviations for these plots are shown in Additional file 1: Figures S3 and S4.

Molecular analysis

Through incorporation of the MIRU-VNTR genotyping data, we also investigate the particular TB strains that are present within the estimated buffer of increased MDR-TB risk surrounding the prison. In total, there are 467 non-prisoner TB patients within 5.47 km (posterior

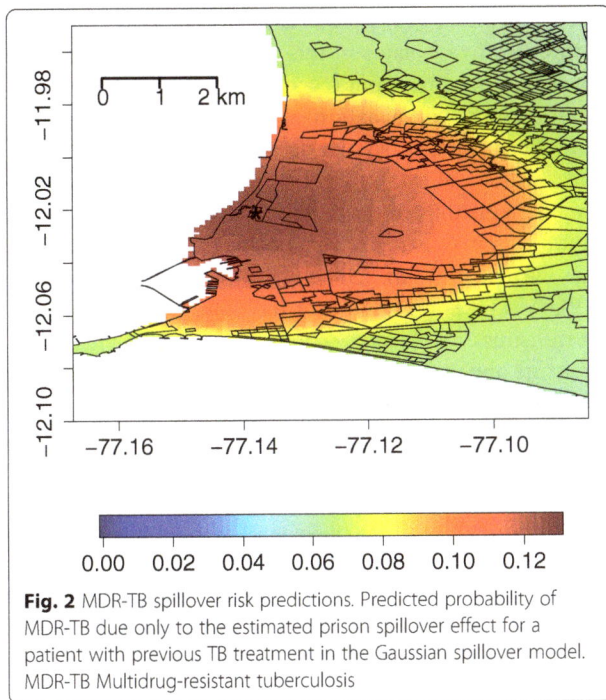

Fig. 2 MDR-TB spillover risk predictions. Predicted probability of MDR-TB due only to the estimated prison spillover effect for a patient with previous TB treatment in the Gaussian spillover model. MDR-TB Multidrug-resistant tuberculosis

mean of θ) of the prison. Of the TB strains observed in this spillover region, 249 (49%) do not have an exact MIRU-VNTR match. Nine MDR-TB patients outside the prison (but within the spillover buffer) share a common strain with an inmate with MDR-TB. In contrast, outside this prison spillover buffer, where there are over twice as many TB patients (1080), only seven MDR-TB patients share a common strain with inmates with MDR-TB (p = 0.022 from a two-sample test of proportions). When subsetting to only those patients with MDR-TB, we find nine out of the 35 MDR-TB patients within the prison spillover buffer share a common strain with an inmate compared to seven out of 89 MDR-TB patients outside the prison spillover buffer (p = 0.008). This provides further evidence to support the idea of potential MDR-TB spillover from the prison.

Estimation of the spherical correlation range parameter, ϕ, suggests that the residual spatial correlation has a highly localized impact (0.13 km, 95% credible interval: 0.04, 0.28 km). Individuals separated by distances greater than this are essentially independent of each other with respect to residual MDR-TB risk. Individuals living within this distance have a more similar risk of MDR-TB, based on their proximity to each other alone. In total, 18 out of the m = 1,509 unique spatial location random effects have an upper 95% credible interval larger than zero. From these significant random effects, we identified eight unique spatial clusters of at least two patients with increased residual MDR-TB risk, four of these clusters within

the prison buffer. Full information on each cluster is presented in Additional file 1: Table S2.

As an example of the role of residual spatial variability in local MDR-TB risk in this region, in Fig. 3 we display a cluster of four patients and the predicted risk of MDR-TB in the area assuming a patient had not been previously treated for TB (none of these patients had been previously treated). The posterior standard deviations are presented in Additional file 1: Figure S5. The elevated risk in this localized area, due to the inclusion of the spatial random effects, strongly suggests local transmission. In this cluster, where two of the patients were co-located, three of them share the same TB genotype. Interestingly, the two co-located patients do not match with respect to TB genotype, a phenomenon we have also seen in previous household studies of MDR-TB in Lima [28].

When investigating the robustness of our findings to the choice of prior distributions for the variance parameters, the sensitivity analysis results suggest that estimation of the spatial range of the spillover effect (5.29 vs. 5.47 km) and of the residual spatial correlation (0.11 vs. 0.13 km) were similar. Therefore, the estimated impact of the prison location and of potential local transmission on MDR-TB risk in the community remains consistent across the different sets of prior distributions.

Discussion

The availability of spatial and pathogen genetic data offers new opportunities to describe the transmission dynamics of pathogens across spatial scales [29], and these

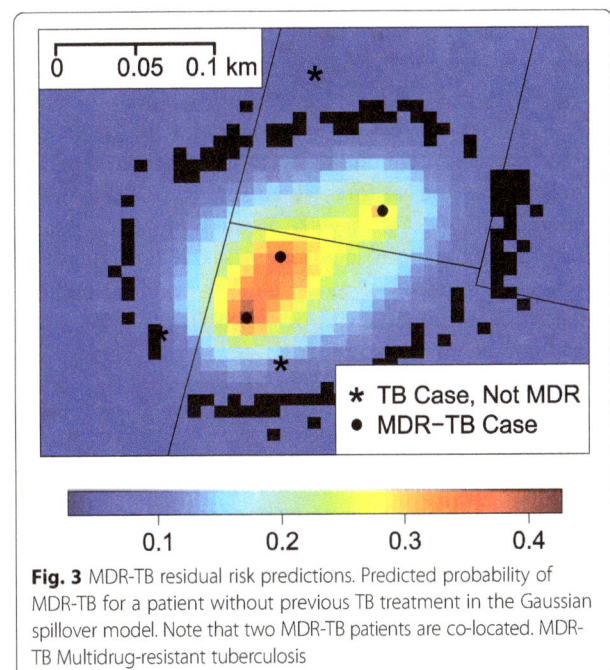

Fig. 3 MDR-TB residual risk predictions. Predicted probability of MDR-TB for a patient without previous TB treatment in the Gaussian spillover model. Note that two MDR-TB patients are co-located. MDR-TB Multidrug-resistant tuberculosis

types of data have been combined to gain a better understanding of how MDR-TB is transmitted within cities [30] and over larger geographic areas [18, 31], but the role of prisons in propagating epidemics of MDR-TB in the community has not previously been confirmed.

In this study, we found that the risk of MDR-TB was elevated among individuals diagnosed with TB in the area surrounding the prison in Lima. This spillover effect dissipated as distance from the prison increased, and the effect was non-significant at a distance of approximately 5 km. The individual covariate known to be most associated with MDR-TB (i.e., previous treatment for TB) remained a significant risk factor, but the distribution of cases reporting previous treatment did not explain the spatial concentration of MDR-TB around the prison location. As there is little reason to believe that risk of acquired resistance should be related to proximity to the prison, this spatial pattern suggests that the majority of MDR-TB cases among previously treated individuals in this area may be the result of transmitted resistance. Our approach allowed us to identify foci of residual risk of MDR-TB, for which interrogation of molecular epidemiological data revealed several probable hot spots of MDR-TB transmission with strains that are were also found within the prison. In summary, our analysis suggests that those living in the area closest to the prison experience a higher risk of MDR-TB spillover, and once such strains appear outside the prison, they can be transmitted further in the community. Demonstrating a clear prison spillover effect highlights the need to intervene in the prison to prevent both internal and external TB transmission. Figures from the Peruvian National Penitentiary Institute demonstrate that Sarita Colonia prison in Callao is overpopulated by 483%. The prison was designed to have a capacity of 573 inmates but in October 2016 it had a prison population of 3332 [32]. Daily mixing between the prison population and the surrounding community occurs because of the flux of prison staff and visitors, which includes conjugal and intimate visits, prisoners with permission to leave, and the continual intake of new inmates and the release of inmates. These types of movements provide a potential explanation for how the risk of MDR-TB can extend beyond the walls of the prison [33].

Our study has several notable limitations. First, we do not have data on whether individuals with TB in the community had previously been imprisoned or had known exposure to prisoners or ex-prisoners. This would have been useful in understanding the mechanism of increased risk experienced by those living closest to the prison. Second, our analysis is based solely on household location. As transmission of *Mycobacterium tuberculosis* may well occur outside the home, use of home location serves at best as a proxy of transmission risk.

Third, we had sufficient data to include 71% of culture-positive isolates in this analysis, and it is possible that selection bias could occur if individuals without bacteriological confirmation of TB or missing drug susceptibility testing or spatial data were at a systematically different risk of MDR-TB than those included in the analysis. Fourth, we have used MIRU-VNTR data to identify strains that are genetically clustered and thus, may be related in chains of transmission. While MIRU-VNTR is an important tool for identifying potential transmission clusters, whole-genome sequencing can break up apparent MIRU-VNTR clusters [34] and may have allowed us to infer transmission events better. [35] We are hopeful that future work, in which whole-genome sequencing is combined with spatial and epidemiological data to pin down the role of specific institutions in the propagation of TB epidemics, will inform the targeting of transmission-blocking interventions to settings where they can have the greatest effect. Finally, it is possible that ecological bias may be introduced by analyzing individual-level data using a combination of individual- and city block-level covariates. Associations could potentially differ if all covariates were measured on the same spatial scale.

Conclusions

We leveraged epidemiological, spatial, and pathogen genetic data to test the hypothesis that high rates of MDR-TB previously documented within a prison have led to a spillover risk in the surrounding community. Using Bayesian hierarchical spatial statistical modeling, we found strong evidence to support the hypothesis that the excess risk extends beyond the walls of the prison.

In combination with existing work, our results suggest that such institutions have potential to amplify epidemics and that efforts to control transmission within institutions can also have important indirect effects on reducing risk in the surrounding community.

Abbreviations
MDR-TB: Multidrug-resistant tuberculosis; SD: Standard deviation; TB: Tuberculosis; WAIC: Watanabe–Akaike information criterion

Funding
This work was supported by Clinical and Translational Science Awards (UL1 TR001863 and KL2 TR001862) from the National Center for Advancing Translational Science, the National Institutes of Health (grants R01 AI112438, R01 AI130058, and U54 GM088558), the National Institute for Health Research, the Academy of Medical Sciences, and the Wellcome Trust (grant 201470/Z/16/Z).

Authors' contributions

JLW, TC, LG, DAJM, JLZ, and JRA developed the primary question and overall plan for this study. LG, DAJM, AL, JC, and PS designed the original study and collected the data analyzed here. JLW and TC developed the analytic plan and JLW analyzed the data and contributed new analytic tools. JLW and TC wrote the first draft of the paper. LG, DAJM, JLZ, JRA, AL, JC, and PS provided feedback and key revisions to the initial draft. All authors read and approved the final manuscript.

Competing interests

The authors declare that they have no competing interests.

Author details

[1]Department of Biostatistics, Yale University, New Haven, CT 06510, USA. [2]Paediatric Infectious Diseases, Section of Paediatrics, Department of Medicine, Imperial College, London W2 1NY, UK. [3]Laboratorio de Investigacion y Desarrollo, Universidad Peruana Cayetano Heredia, San Martin de Porres, Lima, Peru. [4]TB Centre and Department of Clinical Research, London School of Hygiene and Tropical Medicine, London, UK. [5]Department of Epidemiology, University of Michigan, Ann Arbor, MI 48109, USA. [6]Department of Medicine, Stanford University, Stanford, CA 94305, USA. [7]Department of Epidemiology of Microbial Diseases, Yale University, New Haven, CT 06510, USA.

References

1. World Health Organization. Global tuberculosis report 2017. Licence: CC BY-NCSA 3.0 IGO. Geneva: WHO; 2017. http://www.who.int/tb/publications/global_report/en/.
2. Ahuja SD, Ashkin D, Avendano M, Banerjee R, Bauer M, Bayona JN, Becerra MC, Benedetti A, Burgos M, Centis R. Multidrug resistant pulmonary tuberculosis treatment regimens and patient outcomes: an individual patient data meta-analysis of 9,153 patients. PLoS Med. 2012;9(8):e1001300.
3. Dheda K, Limberis JD, Pietersen E, Phelan J, Esmail A, Lesosky M, Fennelly KP, te Riele J, Mastrapa B, Streicher EM. Outcomes, infectiousness, and transmission dynamics of patients with extensively drug-resistant tuberculosis and home-discharged patients with programmatically incurable tuberculosis: a prospective cohort study. Lancet Respir Med. 2017;5(4):269–81.
4. Gandhi NR, Nunn P, Dheda K, Schaaf HS, Zignol M, Van Soolingen D, Jensen P, Bayona J. Multidrug-resistant and extensively drug-resistant tuberculosis: a threat to global control of tuberculosis. Lancet. 2010; 375(9728):1830–43.
5. Cohen T, Jenkins HE, Lu C, McLaughlin M, Floyd K, Zignol M. On the spread and control of MDR-TB epidemics: an examination of trends in anti-tuberculosis drug resistance surveillance data. Drug Resist Updat. 2014;17(4): 105–23.
6. Kendall EA, Fofana MO, Dowdy DW. Burden of transmitted multidrug resistance in epidemics of tuberculosis: a transmission modelling analysis. Lancet Respir Med. 2015;3(12):963–72.
7. Basu S, Stuckler D, McKee M. Addressing institutional amplifiers in the dynamics and control of tuberculosis epidemics. Am J Trop Med Hyg. 2011; 84(1):30–7.
8. Yates T, Tanser F, Abubakar I. Plan Beta for tuberculosis: it's time to think seriously about poorly ventilated congregate settings. Int J Tuberc Lung Dis. 2016;20(1):5–10.
9. Biadglegne F, Rodloff A, Sack U. Review of the prevalence and drug resistance of tuberculosis in prisons: a hidden epidemic. Epidemiol Infect. 2015;143(5):887–900.
10. Nardell E, Dharmadhikari A. Turning off the spigot: reducing drug-resistant tuberculosis transmission in resource-limited settings. Int J Tuberc Lung Dis. 2010;14(10):1233–43.
11. Ruddy M, Balabanova Y, Graham C, Fedorin I, Malomanova N, Elisarova E, Kuznetznov S, Gusarova G, Zakharova S, Melentyev A. Rates of drug resistance and risk factor analysis in civilian and prison patients with tuberculosis in Samara Region, Russia. Thorax. 2005;60(2):130 5.
12. Shah L, Choi H, Berrang-Ford L, Henostroza G, Krapp F, Zamudio C, Heymann S, Kaufman J, Ciampi A, Seas C. Geographic predictors of primary multidrug-resistant tuberculosis cases in an endemic area of Lima, Peru. Int J Tuberc Lung Dis. 2014;18(11):1307–14.
13. Umubyeyi A, Shamputa IC, Rigouts L, Dediste A, Struelens M, Portaels F. Evidence of 'amplifier effect' in pulmonary multidrug-resistant tuberculosis: report of three cases. Int J Infect Dis. 2007;11(6):508–12.
14. Baussano I, Williams BG, Nunn P, Beggiato M, Fedeli U, Scano F. Tuberculosis incidence in prisons: a systematic review. PLoS Med. 2010;7(12): e1000381.
15. Stuckler D, Basu S, McKee M, King L. Mass incarceration can explain population increases in TB and multidrug-resistant TB in European and central Asian countries. Proc Natl Acad Sci. 2008;105(36):13280–5.
16. Sacchi FP, Praça RM, Tatara MB, Simonsen V, Ferrazoli L, Croda MG, Suffys PN, Ko AI, Andrews JR, Croda J. Prisons as reservoir for community transmission of tuberculosis, Brazil. Emerg Infect Dis. 2015;21(3):452–5.
17. Jones TF, Woodley CL, Fountain FF, Schaffner W. Increased incidence of the outbreak strain of Mycobacterium tuberculosis in the surrounding community after an outbreak in a jail. South Med J. 2003;96(2):155–7.
18. Jenkins HE, Plesca V, Ciobanu A, Crudu V, Galusca I, Soltan V, Serbulenco A, Zignol M, Dadu A, Dara M. Assessing spatial heterogeneity of multidrug-resistant tuberculosis in a high-burden country. Eur Respir J. 2013;42(5): 1291–301.
19. Grandjean L, Iwamoto T, Lithgow A, Gilman RH, Arikawa K, Nakanishi N, Martin L, Castillo E, Alarcon V, Coronel J. The association between Mycobacterium tuberculosis genotype and drug resistance in Peru. PLoS One. 2015;10(5):e0126271.
20. Supply P, Allix C, Lesjean S, Cardoso-Oelemann M, Rüsch-Gerdes S, Willery E, Savine E, de Haas P, van Deutekom H, Roring S. Proposal for standardization of optimized mycobacterial interspersed repetitive unit-variable-number tandem repeat typing of Mycobacterium tuberculosis. J Clin Microbiol. 2006; 44(12):4498–510.
21. Watanabe S. Asymptotic equivalence of Bayes cross validation and widely applicable information criterion in singular learning theory. J Mach Learn Res. 2010;11(Dec):3571–94.
22. Vehtari A, Gelman A, Gabry J. Practical Bayesian model evaluation using leave-one-out cross-validation and WAIC. Stat Comput. 2017;27(5):1413–32.
23. Gelfand AE, Ghosh SK. Model choice: a minimum posterior predictive loss approach. Biometrika. 1998;85(1):1–11.
24. Warren JL, Mwanza J-C, Tanna AP, Budenz DL. A statistical model to analyze clinician expert consensus on glaucoma progression using spatially correlated visual field data. Transl Vis Sci Technol. 2016;5(4):14.
25. Banerjee S, Carlin BP, Gelfand AE. Hierarchical modeling and analysis for spatial data. Boca Raton: CRC Press; 2014.
26. R Core Team. R: a language and environment for statistical computing. In: R Foundation for Statistical Computing; 2016.
27. Geweke J. Evaluating the accuracy of sampling-based approaches to the calculation of posterior moments, vol. 196. Minneapolis: Federal Reserve Bank of Minneapolis, Research Department; 1991.
28. Cohen T, Murray M, Abubakar I, Zhang Z, Sloutsky A, Arteaga F, Chalco K, Franke MF, Becerra MC. Multiple introductions of multidrug-resistant tuberculosis into households, Lima, Peru. Emerg Infect Dis. 2011;17(6):969–75.
29. Pybus OG, Suchard MA, Lemey P, Bernardin FJ, Rambaut A, Crawford FW, Gray RR, Arinaminpathy N, Stramer SL, Busch MP. Unifying the spatial epidemiology and molecular evolution of emerging epidemics. Proc Natl Acad Sci. 2012;109(37):15066–71.
30. Zelner JL, Murray MB, Becerra MC, Galea J, Lecca L, Calderon R, Yataco R, Contreras C, Zhang ZB, Manjourides J, et al. Identifying hotspots of multidrug-resistant tuberculosis transmission using spatial and molecular genetic data. J Infect Dis. 2016;213(2):287–94.
31. Shah NS, Auld SC, Brust JC, Mathema B, Ismail N, Moodley P, Mlisana K, Allana S, Campbell A, Mthiyane T. Transmission of extensively drug-resistant tuberculosis in South Africa. N Engl J Med. 2017;376(3):243–53.
32. Informe estad'istico penitenciario 2016 [https://www.inpe.gob.pe/documentos/estad%C3%ADstica/2016/90-octubre-2016/file.html]. Accessed 9 July 2018.
33. Manual de beneficios penitenciarios y de lineamientos del modelo procesal acusatorio [http://sistemas3.minjus.gob.pe/sites/default/files/documentos/

9

Cost-benefit analysis of vaccination: a comparative analysis of eight approaches for valuing changes to mortality and morbidity risks

Minah Park[1], Mark Jit[1,2,3†] and Joseph T. Wu[1*†]

Abstract

Background: There is increasing interest in estimating the broader benefits of public health interventions beyond those captured in traditional cost-utility analyses. Cost-benefit analysis (CBA) in principle offers a way to capture such benefits, but a wide variety of methods have been used to monetise benefits in CBAs.

Methods: To understand the implications of different CBA approaches for capturing and monetising benefits and their potential impact on public health decision-making, we conducted a CBA of human papillomavirus (HPV) vaccination in the United Kingdom using eight methods for monetising health and economic benefits, valuing productivity loss using either (1) the human capital or (2) the friction cost method, including the value of unpaid work in (3) human capital or (4) friction cost approaches, (5) adjusting for hard-to-fill vacancies in the labour market, (6) using the value of a statistical life, (7) monetising quality-adjusted life years and (8) including both productivity losses and monetised quality-adjusted life years. A previously described transmission dynamic model was used to project the impact of vaccination on cervical cancer outcomes. Probabilistic sensitivity analysis was conducted to capture uncertainty in epidemiologic and economic parameters.

Results: Total benefits of vaccination varied by more than 20-fold (£0.6–12.4 billion) across the approaches. The threshold vaccine cost (maximum vaccine cost at which HPV vaccination has a benefit-to-cost ratio above one) ranged from £69 (95% CI £56–£84) to £1417 (£1291–£1541).

Conclusions: Applying different approaches to monetise benefits in CBA can lead to widely varying outcomes on public health interventions such as vaccination. Use of CBA to inform priority setting in public health will require greater convergence around appropriate methodology to achieve consistency and comparability across different studies.

Keywords: Cost-benefit analysis, Economic evaluation, HPV, Vaccination

Background

Health economic evaluations are used to inform medical procurement and reimbursement decisions by public and private healthcare providers. The most popular form of health economic evaluation is cost-effectiveness analysis (CEA), which often presents the ratio of the incremental cost of an intervention (from the perspective of either the healthcare provider or society) to the incremental health benefits of an intervention. A review conducted for the Bill & Melinda Gates Foundation of health economic evaluations of interventions related to malaria, tuberculosis, HIV/AIDS and vaccination in low- and middle-income countries found that, of 204 studies published in 2000–2013, 202 (99%) were CEAs [1].

Economic evaluations of large public health interventions such as new vaccination programmes attract particularly

* Correspondence: joewu@hku.hk
†Mark Jit and Joseph T. Wu contributed equally to this work.
[1]WHO Collaborating Centre for Infectious Disease Epidemiology and Control, School of Public Health, Li Ka Shing Faculty of Medicine, The University of Hong Kong, G/F, Patrick Manson Building (North Wing), 7 Sassoon Road, Hong Kong SAR, People's Republic of China
Full list of author information is available at the end of the article

intense debates because of the high absolute costs (and potentially large benefits) involved [2]. A major focus of such debates has been about whether current economic evaluation techniques capture the full scope and value of these public health programmes. For instance, several reviews have found that vaccines may have broad, long-term societal consequences that are not always captured in CEAs [3, 4], although many of these benefits can, in principle, be monetised and included in CEA based on a broader societal perspective as recommended by the US Second Panel on Cost-Effectiveness in Health and Medicine [5, 6]. Such broader, non-health benefits of an intervention include effects on future productivity and consumption, social services, educational achievement and other societal impacts.

Several economists have instead proposed the use of cost-benefit analysis (CBA) [7, 8]. The term CBA is often informally used to refer to any analysis used in decision-making that compares the expected costs and benefits (both in monetary terms) of an investment. In principle, to be regarded as complete, a CBA should capture all benefits due to an intervention, valuing them either at their market value or at the level of consumption that individuals are willing to forego to obtain them. Hence, it has its conceptual roots in welfare economics, which quantifies social welfare in terms of individuals' willingness-to-pay (WTP) to increase welfare. By using a consistent, directly comparable metric to value all outcomes, CBA allows comparison with non-health interventions. A recent analysis estimated that the return on investment (a form of economic analysis that uses the same economic assumptions as CBA) for vaccines in low- and middle-income countries was comparable or superior to that for non-health interventions such as road safety [3].

The methodology for CEA has been well established, with the perspective or range of costs admissible in a CEA usually prescribed by 'reference cases' produced by particular health authorities. In CEAs, the perspective on costs can be narrow (costs and cost offsets falling to healthcare providers alone, as recommended by the National Institute for Health and Care Excellence (NICE) in the UK) [9] or broad (all costs and cost offsets falling on society, as recommended by the World Health Organization (WHO)) [10]. NICE's recommendation to take a narrow perspective when estimating costs is reasonable given that its evaluations are intended to promote the most efficient use of available resources allocated to the NHS (or publicly funded health sectors) in particular [11]. Conversely, the WHO Guide to Cost-Effectiveness Analysis [10] explicitly recommended all costs and health effects to be valued from the societal perspective, because there are always opportunity costs in every decision we make, such that all costs and resources used for a chosen health intervention (regardless

of who paid them) could have been used for other purposes in society, including non-health consumption. The guide further argued that the so-called 'decision-maker's approach' taking such a narrow perspective is not consistent with WHO's concern that governments should strive to maximise not only the overall health but also wellbeing of societies. The Second Panel on Cost-Effectiveness in Health and Medicine, composed of experts and leaders in the field of health economics, has also provided two reference cases for healthcare sector and societal perspectives, respectively, in their recent report. The Panel recommended that CEAs are undertaken based on both perspectives to improve the quality and comparability of CEAs [5].

Each of these approaches also affects the threshold by which an option with a particular cost-effectiveness ratio is deemed cost-effective. The CEA threshold is often determined based on one of the following: (1) the opportunity cost of new spending at the margin of a budget limit, (2) a multiple of GDP per capita, usually based on human capital arguments (although they have also been justified based on WTP) or (3) preference elicitation (based on WTP) [12]. Using a decision-maker's perspective and assuming that the decision-maker has control over a budget with the objective of maximising health, the threshold should arguably be set based on the opportunity cost of new spending at the margin of the decision-maker's budget. From a societal perspective, the threshold should arguably instead be set based on either the human capital value of improved health, or by preference elicitation (based on WTP) of societal willingness to improve health.

In contrast, there is less detail around CBA methodology in health. While there exists guidance on conducting CBAs for government policies [13–15], it generally is not as precise as 'reference cases' available for CEAs that specify the exact economic assumptions to be used in pharmacoeconomic evaluations. This is likely because CBA has not been used as extensively as CEA for informing decisions on specific healthcare resource allocation. While CBA is used to evaluate a broader range of public sector initiatives across multiple sectors, CEA guidelines are generally used in the health sector only.

Given the increasing interest in using CBA to evaluate the value of vaccinations and other major public health programmes (as in part evidenced by the Bill & Melinda Gates Foundation's recent efforts to develop a reference case for CBA), it is important to understand the implications of different approaches for capturing and monetising benefits. To this effect, we conducted a CBA of human papillomavirus (HPV) vaccination as a case study. HPV vaccination is a major public health investment that has been the topic of numerous CEAs with a total of more than 60 studies identified across a number of systematic reviews [16–18]. Indeed, vaccination in general has been subject to numerous studies assessing costs and benefits based on various monetisation methods [3, 19–22]. For the current study, we applied eight different approaches to monetise benefits of HPV vaccination and compared the results.

Methods

We conducted a CBA of HPV vaccination in the UK. HPV is the aetiological agent of a number of cancers and other diseases such as anogenital warts. Cervical cancer has the highest global burden among the HPV-related fraction of these cancers [23]. In particular, around 70% of cervical cancers are caused by HPV-16 and HPV-18. We have chosen this example as a large public health investment with a well-established model of HPV vaccine impact used for national decision-making, so that our focus in this study could be on the methodology of CBA rather than on the modelling of HPV epidemiology. For simplicity, we focus only on the value of vaccination in preventing cervical cancer due to HPV-16 and HPV-18.

The decision to introduce HPV vaccination in the UK was informed by a CEA that incorporated an epidemiological model of HPV transmission [24] to assess the impact of routine female adolescent two-dose vaccination on cervical cancer burden over a time horizon of 100 years. We adopted the same epidemiological model but used it as input for CBA. We assumed that (1) vaccination is given annually to 12-year-old girls at 80% coverage, with a catch-up campaign in the first year to age 16, and that (2) the vaccine provides lifelong protection against HPV-16 and HPV-18 without cross protection against other HPV types. Costs and benefits were discounted at 3.5% per annum. For the probability sensitivity analysis, we used Latin hypercube sampling to generate 1000 scenarios that encompass the uncertainties in epidemiologic and economic parameters.

The outcome in our CBA was threshold vaccine cost (TVC), which we defined as the maximum vaccine cost per person (including the administration cost) at which HPV vaccination has a benefit-to-cost ratio above one (i.e. the vaccination programme is cost-beneficial) (Additional file 1). The direct benefits of vaccination included all medical cost avoided due to reduced screening for and treatment of cervical cancer and pre-cancerous lesions (Additional file 2: Table S1).

We applied two conceptually different approaches to monetise benefits (lost production and WTP) to examine the impact of varying methods on the results. Estimates of WTP were derived from stated or revealed preference studies while lost production were measured using the human capital and friction cost methods as summarised in Table 1.

Lost production: Conventional production-based approaches

While conventional CBA generally assumes that individuals are the best judges of their own welfare (i.e. consumer sovereignty) and that monetary values should reflect individual willingness to exchange consumption for the outcomes of concern (e.g. [25], p. 30), lost production has also been commonly used in the CBA literature to value health [26–31]. Under these approaches, productivity loss averted due to reduction in morbidity and mortality were incorporated as indirect benefits of vaccination in terms of the wider economic effects of health as human capital (rather than its intrinsic value).

We considered the two most commonly used production-based approaches, namely the human capital (HC) and friction cost (FC) methods. From the perspective of affected individuals, the HC method assumes that production loss incurred by sick or deceased workers is irreplaceable. The duration of productivity loss for a sick worker was therefore assumed to be the same as the entire duration of disease treatment, whereas productivity loss due to premature death was estimated by assuming an average retirement age of 65. Specifically, production loss was measured with a cumulative sum of income lost over the duration of illness (morbidity) and the number of years lost due to premature death (mortality) using age-specific employment rates and mean personal incomes retrieved from the UK Office for National Statistics [32, 33].

In contrast, the FC method takes the employer perspective and assumes that there always exists some level of involuntary unemployment and hence a sick or deceased worker is replaceable by an otherwise unemployed worker [34]. As such, the FC method only accounts for productivity loss during the friction period, which is defined as the time between the first day of absence of a sick or deceased worker and the last day of training for a replaced worker. According to the 2015 UK Recruitment Trends Report [35] based on responses from major UK recruitment agencies, the average time to fill a vacancy (i.e. time between announcing a job and finding a successful applicant) ranged from 6 to 44 days in 2014. The average time in training for a new employee of 6.8 days was derived from the UK Employer Skills Survey 2015 [36]. As the friction period largely depends on the type of job (e.g. longer friction period for jobs requiring higher-level knowledge and skills) and economic or labour market conditions, it was difficult to find all the necessary data needed to estimate the friction period. We assumed that the sum of (1) the time period between the start of absence by a sick employee and the first day of job announcement and (2) the time period between the acceptance of job offer and the first day of training of a new employee to be approximately 3

Table 1 Overview of cost-benefit analysis (CBA) approaches to monetise benefits

Method	Rationale	Major limitations and uncertainties	How we accounted for methodological uncertainties
Human capital	• Individual perspective • Indirect benefits are productivity losses avoided by prevented or reduced morbidity and mortality • Productivity losses are valued by individual's cumulative income over the entire time absent from work	• Considers productivity loss incurred only by economically active individuals • Leads to biased decisions in favour of high-income earners and economically active individuals	• Sensitivity analysis was conducted to include homemakers in the calculation of productivity loss averted
Friction cost	• Employer perspective • Indirect benefits are productivity losses avoided by prevented or reduced morbidity and mortality • Productivity losses are valued by individual's gross earnings over the friction period • Assumes there always exists some level of involuntary unemployment • The sick/deceased worker is replaced by another worker who otherwise would have remained unemployed	• Disease- and job-specific data needed for estimating the friction period are often unavailable • Considers productivity loss incurred only by economically active individuals • Leads to biased decisions in favour of high-income earners and economically active individuals	• Sensitivity analysis was conducted to vary friction period – 55, 69 and 90 days – to account for uncertainties regarding the vacancy duration • Sensitivity analysis was conducted to include homemakers in the calculation of productivity loss averted
Value of a statistical life (VSL): Revealed Preference	• Individuals implicitly reveal how much they value mortality risk reduction in real markets (e.g. wage-risk trade-offs) • VSL is derived from observed behaviours	• Focus is mostly on job-related risks among working-age population, which largely result from injuries rather than illnesses	• A range of VSL estimates, including a VSL for cancer after adjusting for a 10-year latency period was used
VSL: Stated Preference	• Use contingent valuation with hypothetical scenario (i.e. surveys) to derive VSL	• Extra effort may be required to encourage survey participants for valid responses	• A range of VSL estimates, including one from a willingness-to-pay (WTP) study done in cervical cancer patients was used
Monetisation of quality adjusted life years (QALYs) (QM)	• QALY captures a broad range of health benefits • QALY can be monetised by multiplying the WTP with gains in QALYs	• Individuals cannot be expected to have a constant rate of substitution between QALYs and wealth	• Our QM approach with a £23,000/QALY WTP is analogous to NICE's cost-effectiveness reference case, which has a cost-effectiveness threshold of £20,000–£30,000/QALY [9]

to 5 weeks in total based on Koopmanschap's study [34]. The friction period in the UK was estimated to be approximately 34 to 86 days. In addition to productivity loss incurred over the friction period, we considered additional administrative costs related to hiring (£2610) [36] and training (£5433) [37] a new worker for all mortality and long-term morbidity cases (i.e. treatment time > friction period).

The conventional production-based approaches account for productivity loss from individuals with the paid jobs only and thus disregard homemakers who comprise a substantial proportion of cervical cancer cases (mean age 45, interquartile range 27–59) [38]. As indicated in one of WHO's guidelines on CBA, the economic value of unpaid work, such as homemaking and caring, is undervalued using this approach [39]. As such, we also considered modified versions of the conventional production-based methods (HC-M and FC-M) in which paid labour and homemakers within the same age group were assumed to have the same economic productivity. The assumption is in line with the UK's recent effort in recognising the value of unpaid work at home

and its contribution to the economy, by providing it with a monetary value equivalent to the average wages of those who are paid to do those tasks [40]. The proportion of homemakers in each age group was approximated based on the Office for National Statistics employment statistics [13].

Lost production: a new production-based approach

The conventional production-based approach has the advantage that it uses relatively objective and quantifiable measures (e.g. wage rates) compared to a WTP-based approach. However, the theoretical framework of neither the HC nor the FC method is completely sound, because (1) the HC method's underlying assumption of full employment is often considered unrealistic and (2) the friction period of the FC method largely varies across occupations, times and countries. In order to address both issues, we examined how easily job vacancies could actually be filled within the 'normal' friction period in the current UK labour market.

We considered a new approach for estimating productivity loss by interpolating between the HC and FC methods (HC/FC). Under this approach, productivity loss was a weighted average of that under the two methods where the weight for HC corresponded to the proportion of jobs that are unlikely to be filled within the friction period in the current labour market. We estimated this weight based on recent statistics on 'hard-to-fill vacancies' (HtFV) from the UK Commission's Employer Skills Survey 2015 (Additional file 3: Table S2) [36]. HtFV refer to vacancies that are difficult to fill due to skill-related (e.g. lack of qualified applicants) or non-skill-related reasons (e.g. low pay offered for the post). It was noted that there is a major gender difference in occupational employment in the UK [41], with women historically dominating employment in jobs such as leisure and caring while men dominating in construction industry, for example. To take into account the gender difference in occupational employment and largely varying proportions of HtFV by industry sector [36], we calculated the weighted proportion of HtFV for women to be used in the analysis. We compiled two recent UK employment statistics that provide (1) the distribution of female workforce [42] and (2) the proportion of HtFV in 13 industry sectors categorised according to the Standard Industrial Classification [36]. The distribution of females in the workforce largely varied by industry sector, ranging from 0.6% in agriculture to 22% in health and social work, while the proportion of HtFV (regardless of gender) ranged from 23% in education to 43% in construction.

WTP: the value of a statistical life (VSL) approach

Under this approach, the monetary values of both pecuniary (e.g. avoided medical expenses) and non-pecuniary (e.g. pain and suffering associated with the disease) benefits are presumed to be encapsulated by VSL estimates given that individuals' WTP takes into account the impact of mortality risk reductions on their wellbeing in every aspect. The VSL estimates are used to value mortality risk reductions and obtained via (1) revealed preferences (VSL-RP) based on labour-market or hedonic wage studies; or (2) stated preferences (VSL-SP) based on contingent valuation studies [8]. While the VSL generally does not address morbidity associated with non-fatal cases, it has been suggested that VSL-RP may as well include the value of the associated morbidity risk though it is likely to be minimal (6–25%) compared to the value of the fatality risk [43]. As for the VSL-SP, there has been mixed evidence regarding the morbidity premium (or cancer premium) to take into account the effects of morbidity associated with the fatality in the VSL estimate [44–46]. This highlights a key advantage of the VSL approach over the HC or FC methods that do not take into account the intrinsic value of health gains. We considered seven different VSL estimates derived from three individual studies (labelled as 'Lang', 'Viscusi'

and 'Gayer 1–2' in Fig. 1) and three normative national and international guidance ('UKHSE', 'USDoT' and 'OECD') (Additional file 4: Table S3). For VSL-RP, we selected (1) a VSL estimate currently in use by the US Department of Transportation ('USDoT') [47], which is very similar to that adopted by the US Department of Health and Human Services [14] and the US Environmental Protection Agency [15], as well as the estimated means from a meta-regression analysis, which adjusted for publication bias [48], and (2) a range of VSL for cancer risk reduction estimated based on hedonic housing prices in the US ('Gayer 1–2') [49]. For VSL-SP, we selected VSL estimates from (1) a WTP study conducted among cervical cancer patients in Taiwan ('Lang') [50], (2) a recent systematic review of VSL focusing on a 'cancer premium' ('Viscusi') [45], (3) recommendation of the UK Health and Safety Executive ('UKHSE') [13], and (4) OECD guidelines for EU-27 countries ('OECD') [44]. All VSL estimates were converted to the current UK currency based on the OECD guideline [44]. To convert VSL values varying across countries and over time to the UK 2015 value, we used the benefit transfer method with income adjustments. For example, to approximate VSL used by the US Department of Transportation, we used purchasing power parity (PPP)-adjusted GDP per capita in the following equation:

$$VSL_{UK,2015} = VSL_{US,2015}{}^{*}$$
$$\left(PPP\text{–}adjusted\ GDP\ per\ capita_{UK,2015} / PPP\text{–}adjusted\ per\ capita_{US,2015} \right).$$

Here, PPP-adjusted GDP per capita for both the UK and the US were extracted from the World Bank [51]. To convert the VSL (in USD) estimated from the above equation to the UK currency, we used PPP-adjusted exchange rates from OECD Statistics [52]. To update VSL values across different years (e.g. 2000 to 2015), we used the average Consumer Price Index and Real Income in the UK as follows:

$$VSL_{2015} = VSL_{2000}{}^{*}$$
$$\left(CPI_{2015} / CPI_{2000} \right)^{*} \left(Real\ Incomes_{2014/15} / Real\ Incomes_{1999/00} \right)$$

Data on Consumer Price Index and Real Incomes across different years were available at the UK Office for National Statistics website [53]. After the adjustment, the selected VSL estimates ranged from £1.1 million to £7.2 million. Each adjusted VSL estimate was then multiplied by the projected number of cervical cancer deaths prevented from vaccination.

WTP: the quality-adjusted life-year (QALY) monetisation (QM) approach

Under this approach, the health outcome in conventional cost-utility analyses, namely QALY, was monetised

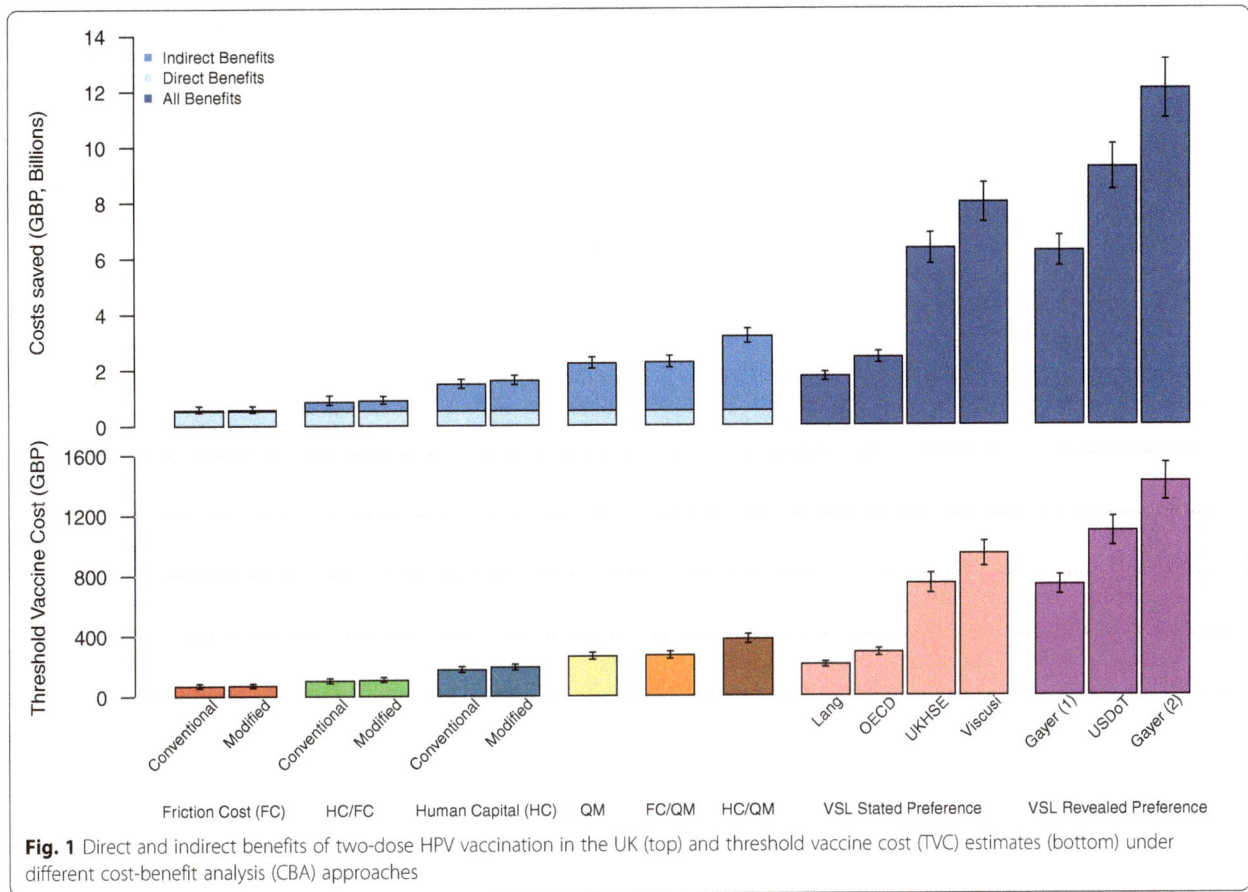

Fig. 1 Direct and indirect benefits of two-dose HPV vaccination in the UK (top) and threshold vaccine cost (TVC) estimates (bottom) under different cost-benefit analysis (CBA) approaches

using individual WTP for an additional QALY gained. Based on a study that assessed WTP for the respondent's own additional QALY gained (WTP$_{sel}$) in the UK [54], we applied £23,000 to the discounted QALY gained. Our QM approach with a £23,000/QALY WTP is analogous to NICE's cost-effectiveness reference case, which has a cost-effectiveness threshold of £20,000–£30,000/QALY [9], although our approach is based on individual rather than societal WTP arguments. Hence, it would be expected that the net present value of an intervention using our QM approach would correspond to its net monetary benefit evaluated using NICE's reference case.

Integration of production-based and QM approaches

Under these approaches, productivity loss from production-based approaches and monetised QALYs gained were both included when estimating the economic benefit of vaccination (e.g. HC/QM when HC is integrated with QM) to capture both the intrinsic and the instrumental value of better health. Such analyses are analogous to cost-utility analyses using a societal perspective.

Future deaths averted were discounted at 3.5% per annum back to the reference year, i.e. the year in which the vaccination programme is initiated. Subsequently,

the value attached to averted mortality was discounted further, depending on the method used. For production-based (HC and FC) and QM approaches, the productivity loss and QALYs lost for each year of life lost due to premature death was discounted back to the year of death. For the VSL-based approaches (VSL-RP and VSL-SP), the same value was ascribed to a prevented death regardless of the age of the woman or the number of life years averted, as has been standard practice for public policy analyses [55].

Results

Among all CBA methods considered, the WTP-based approach using the VSL yielded the highest TVC estimates. Specifically, the median TVC estimates ranged from £206 (interquartile range: £187–£223) to £939 (£855–£1021) under VSL-SP and £734 (£669–£798) to £1417 (£1291–£1541) under VSL-RP, which correspond to approximately 78.6% and 541% of the TVC estimated under the standard QM method (£262), respectively (Fig. 1). When the QM approach was integrated with the production-based approaches, the TVC estimates ranged from £268 (£244–£293) with FC/QM to £373 (£345–£407) with HC/QM and remained lower than that estimated under the VSL method.

Under the production-based approach, the direct benefit was £0.54 billion (£0.44 billion to £0.66 billion). The mean UK female employment rate used to measure the indirect benefits in terms of averted productivity loss was 36.9% for those aged 16–19 and 64.7–77.6% for those aged 20–64. The indirect benefits varied 9-fold across different monetisation methods utilising the production-based approach, at £33 million in FC, £37 million in FC-M, £946 million in HC, £1.1 billion in HC-M, and £324 million in HC/FC (Fig. 1). Consequently, the FC method resulted in the lowest TVC estimate of £69 (£56–£84), which is only 26% of the TVC estimated under the QM. When integrated with the QM method, the total indirect benefits increased by nearly 53-fold (£1.7 billion) and 2-fold (£2.6 billion) for the FC and HC methods, respectively. Similarly, with homemakers (around 8.9%–13.9% across the different age groups in 2015) included in the calculation of productivity loss under the modified production-based approaches, the TVC estimate increased by 1–2% (from £56–£84 to £57–£85) and 8–10% (from £157–£195 to £172–£211) under the FC and HC method, respectively (Additional file 5: Table S4).

Point estimates and error bars indicate medians and interquartile ranges across 1000 scenarios randomly generated. Benefits under the VSL approaches cannot be decomposed into direct and indirect components. VSL estimates used in Gayer–1 and –2 were derived from the same study using different level of cancer risk [49].

The proportion of HtFV varied by industry sector, ranging from 23% in education (in which 16% of women work) to 43% in construction (in which fewer than 2% of women work). Considering the gender difference and varying proportions of HtFV across different establishments, we estimated that the overall proportion of HtFV among the female workforce in the UK was 31% (Additional file 3: Table S2). That is, we estimated that 69% of all vacancies would be filled with a replaced worker within the friction period. The resulting TVC estimate was £101 (£88–£118) under HC/FC, which was 56% lower and 11% higher than that under HC and FC, respectively. Relative changes in TVC were similar when homemakers were included in the calculation of productivity loss.

We found that the economic benefits of vaccination against HPV-16 and HPV-18 in the UK could vary by as much as 20-fold depending on the method used to monetise benefits. In particular, two-dose HPV vaccination in the UK was found to be not cost-beneficial under the HC approach and all FC-related approaches except when integrated with QM.

Discussion

Our results suggest that using different approaches to monetise benefits can lead to divergent conclusions about the value of vaccination. Our TVC estimates for a vaccine against cervical cancer in the UK ranged over an order of magnitude (£69–£1417) depending on the method used to value the benefits of cervical cancer prevention. The TVC estimate was lowest (£69–£191) when benefits were valued in terms of productivity loss averted due to ill health and premature mortality, particularly if the friction cost method was used, and highest (£206–£1417) when VSL methodology was used. When an individual WTP for an additional QALY gained was used instead, the TVC estimates (£262–£373) were generally higher than that obtained by valuing productivity gains but lower than that obtained using VSL methods.

Our finding that measuring benefits based on WTP estimates (e.g. the VSL and QM approaches) yields larger benefit estimates than measuring benefits based on lost production (e.g. HC and FC) is unsurprising – this is likely because the former includes both financial (e.g. medical expenses and losses in future earnings) and non-financial (e.g. avoided pain and suffering) benefits of the intervention, whereas the latter solely focuses on lost production [56, 57]. The finding that the FC method yields much smaller benefit estimates than the HC method is likewise intuitive, because the FC method only takes into account temporary losses during the friction period while the HC method assumes lifetime losses during the entire period affected by morbidity and mortality.

Each of the methods used has advantages and limitations. Production-based approaches for valuing health gains have been criticised for not being consistent with the theoretical foundations of CBA in welfare economics, as they focus on changes in productivity rather than measuring overall welfare. Similarly, QALY-based approaches do not fit naturally within the conceptual framework of welfare economics, because they measure changes in health rather than overall welfare. The approach that most directly reflects the principles of welfare economics is to estimate the consumption that affected individuals are willing to trade-off to avoid morbidity or mortality [27, 58, 59].

Valuing benefits based on averted productivity loss has the advantage of being based on an easily measurable quantity (market income). However, for diseases such as cancer, which tend to cause long-term work absences, the difference in outcome between the production-based approaches can be large. In our study, productivity loss estimates under the HC approach were 29 times higher than that under the FC approach. Similarly, Oliva et al. [60] found that the annual productivity cost of mortality due to cervical cancer in Spain was €21.7 million based on HC and €0.39 million with FC (56-fold difference). Advocates of the FC method argue that there is always some level of involuntary unemployment, so the HC method overestimates the societal cost of long-term illness or death by measuring the 'potential' productivity loss over the entire period of absenteeism beyond the friction period [34]. The FC method purports to measure the 'actual' productivity loss to society from an employer's perspective by considering the time and related costs (e.g. hiring and training costs) needed to fully restore production levels with a replacement worker.

Both conventional production-based methods have been criticised for valuing life purely in terms of marketable productive capacity and not providing an explicit value for the health gains themselves (i.e. ignoring the additional value of avoided suffering, leisure time and unpaid labour) [61]. The concern is that this may lead to prioritising interventions that primarily benefit high-wage earners over low-wage earners and those doing unpaid labour (e.g. caregiving and housework). In our analysis, we have accounted for unpaid labour by employing the modified versions (namely HC-M and FC-M) and estimate that the TVC for HPV vaccination increases by 22% with the HC and 2% with the FC method if all females are included in productivity loss calculations (data not shown here), rather than those in the paid labour force only. It should be noted, however, that the market value approach that we used measures unpaid household work based on the population average wage, which differs from the conventional method of valuing household based on the average wage of a paid household worker or carer.

Measuring lost production by using wage rates raises a number of methodological questions, including (1) whether or not to assume full employment (we capture this uncertainty by showing results using both HC, which assumes full employment and competitive labour markets, and FC, which does not make these assumptions), (2) whether the economic value of lost productivity is best captured by the employer perspective (so measured in pre-tax wages including fringe benefits and indirect costs) or employee perspective (so measured in post-tax wages), and (3) how to capture labour market constraints on how much work an individual does, since there may be requirements to work a fixed number of hours [62]. For example, Bockstael et al. [63] found that individuals who are required to work a fixed number of hours valued the opportunity cost of time approximately 3.5-fold more than the wage rate, whereas those with flexible working hours valued it similarly to their wage rate.

We proposed an alternative production-based method that may be used instead of established methods, as it strikes a balance between the two approaches in terms of assumptions about unemployment. Weighting the outputs from the two methods according to the proportion of HtFV should theoretically give estimates closer to the actual productivity loss due to ill-health.

An alternative approach is the VSL method. The VSL reflects the marginal rate of substitution between money (or income) and mortality risk and infers the value of the consumption of market goods that individuals are willing to forgo to achieve a reduced risk of premature death [8]. Hence, VSL can be seen as a direct application of the welfarist principle of consumer sovereignty. Consistent with the conceptual framework for CBA, VSL estimates are highly context specific. In practice, however, researchers often rely on the averages across country populations (or even extrapolations from other countries), which can potentially cause under- or overestimations of the result. Furthermore, there are few VSL estimates from low- or middle-income countries. VSL estimates for cancer are particularly divergent, with debates around the existence and magnitude of a 'cancer premium' that inflates the VSL for a cancer death in comparison to a death from an acute fatality to incorporate the latency and morbidity period of cancer. For instance, Viscusi et al. [45] suggested the use of 1.21 for cancer premium, the US Environmental Protection Agency, the European Commission and several studies recommend a cancer premium of 1.5 [46, 64, 65], and the UK's Health and Safety Executive doubles the VSL (or the value of preventing a statistical fatality) estimates of accidental death to derive a VSL estimate for cancer [13]. We understand that there are concerns about transferring VSL between countries with different healthcare systems, income levels and cultural values that may affect mortality risk valuation. Nevertheless, we have used VSL estimates derived from other countries also for the following reasons: (1) there is disagreement and inconsistency with the use of a 'cancer premium' when applying a standard VSL to cancer studies and (2) there were few studies reporting cancer-specific VSLs at the time of the study, none of which was from the UK. To minimise such effects, we have adjusted for different income levels and costs between the countries using the 'unit transfer with income adjustments' method.

A third approach is to monetise individual WTP for an additional QALY gained. It offers policymakers the flexibility to incorporate additional units for the value of non-health outcomes not captured in measures such as QALYs, as well as to compare outcomes with non-health interventions. In practice, monetised QALYs has been used by government agencies such as the US Department of Health and Human Services [14] and US Food and Drug Administration for regulatory analyses [66]. However, there is still an on-going debate around the use of monetised QALYs in healthcare decision-making among health economists. During the meeting organised by the US National Institutes of Health in 2010, for example, it was argued that QALYs should not be monetised since this approach lacks theoretical and empirical support [67]. It should also be noted that adding productivity costs to monetised QALYs may lead to double counting, as there remains uncertainty about whether productivity loss has been fully captured in QALY measures [5, 6].

Hence, a key challenge to using CBA for priority setting around public health interventions is the great variety in the way benefits can be monetised and the relative lack of detail on normative guidance about the appropriate methodology to use.

Conclusions

In principle, CBA offers the opportunity to capture many benefits of public health interventions such as vaccination that may not naturally fit into a CEA framework. Other approaches, such as cost-consequences analysis and multiple criteria decision analysis, also admit a wider range of outcomes, but do not offer a straightforward way to synthesise multiple outcomes into a single measure. Wider use of CBA to evaluate public health interventions will require greater convergence around the appropriate methodology to use in order to achieve consistency and comparability across different studies. Ultimately, discussions around appropriate methodology for CBA could help us better understand what we actually value about health.

Abbreviations
CBA: cost-benefit analysis; CEA: cost-effectiveness analysis; FC: friction cost; FC-M: modified friction cost method; HC: human capital; HC-M: modified human capital method; HPV: human papillomavirus; HtFV: hard-to-fill vacancies; NICE: National Institute for Health and Care Excellence; PPP: purchasing power parity; QALY: quality-adjusted life-year; QM: monetisation of QALYs; TVC: threshold vaccine cost; VSL: value of a statistical life; VSL-RP: VSL based on revealed preference; VSL-SP: VSL based on stated preference; WHO: World Health Organization; WTP: willingness-to-pay

Funding
This study was supported by a commissioned grant (HSK-17-E15) from the Health and Medical Research Fund from the Government of the Hong Kong Special Administrative Region and Award Number U54GM088558 from the National Institute of General Medical Sciences. MJ was supported by the National Institute for Health Research Health Protection Research Units (NIHR HPRUs) in Immunisation at the London School of Hygiene and Tropical Medicine in partnership with Public Health England (PHE). The content is solely the responsibility of the authors and does not necessarily represent the official views of the National Institute of General Medical Sciences, the National Institutes of Health, the National Health Service, the NIHR, the Department of Health, or PHE.

Authors' contributions
MJ and JTW designed and conceived the study. MP collected and analysed the data. All authors contributed to interpreting the results and drafting the manuscript. All authors read and approved the final version before submission.

Competing interests
The authors declare that they have no competing interests.

Author details
[1]WHO Collaborating Centre for Infectious Disease Epidemiology and Control, School of Public Health, Li Ka Shing Faculty of Medicine, The University of Hong Kong, G/F, Patrick Manson Building (North Wing), 7 Sassoon Road, Hong Kong SAR, People's Republic of China. [2]Department of Infectious Disease Epidemiology, London School of Hygiene and Tropical Medicine, Keppel Street, London WC1E 7HT, UK. [3]Modelling and Economics Unit, Public Health England, 61 Colindale Avenue, London NW9 5EQ, UK.

References
1. Santatiwongchai B, Chantarastapornchit V, Wilkinson T, Thiboonboon K, Rattanavipapong W, Walker DG, et al. Methodological variation in economic evaluations conducted in low- and middle-income countries: information for reference case development. PLoS One. 2015;10(5):e0123853.
2. Christensen H, Hickman M, Edmunds WJ, Trotter CL. Introducing vaccination against serogroup B meningococcal disease: an economic and mathematical modelling study of potential impact. Vaccine. 2013;31(23):2638–46.
3. Ozawa S, Clark S, Portnoy A, Grewal S, Brenzel L, Walker DG. Return on investment from childhood immunization in low- and middle-income countries, 2011-20. Health Aff (Millwood). 2016;35(2):199–207.
4. Jit M, Hutubessy R, Png ME, Sundaram N, Audimulam J, Salim S, et al. The broader economic impact of vaccination: reviewing and appraising the strength of evidence. BMC Med. 2015;13:209.
5. Sanders GD, Neumann PJ, Basu A, Brock DW, Feeny D, Krahn M, et al. Recommendations for conduct, methodological practices, and reporting of cost-effectiveness analyses: second panel on cost-effectiveness in health and medicine. JAMA. 2016;316(10):1093–103.
6. Neumann PJ, Sanders GD, Russell LB, Siegel JE, Ganiats TG, editors. Cost-Effectiveness in Health and Medicine. 2nd ed. New York: Oxford University Press; 2017.
7. Bloom DE, Brenzel L, Cadarette D, Sullivan J. Moving beyond traditional valuation of vaccination: needs and opportunities. Vaccine. 2017;35(Suppl 1):A29–35.
8. Laxminarayan R, Jamison DT, Krupnick AJ, Norheim OF. Valuing vaccines using value of statistical life measures. Vaccine. 2014;32(39):5065–70.
9. National Institute for Health and Care Excellence (NICE). The Guidelines Manual: 7. Assessing Cost Effectiveness. 2012. https://www.nice.org.uk/process/pmg6/chapter/assessing-cost-effectiveness. Accessed 1 June 2017.
10. World Health Organization (WHO). Making Choices in Health: WHO Guide to Cost-Effectiveness Analysis. Geneva: WHO; 2003. p. 19–36.
11. National Institute for Health and Care Excellence (NICE). Guide to the Methods of Technology Appraisal 2013. https://www.nice.org.uk/process/pmg9/chapter/the-reference-case#framework-for-estimating-clinical-and-cost-effectiveness. Accessed 2 Mar 2017.
12. Shillcutt SD, Walker DG, Goodman CA, Mills AJ. Cost effectiveness in low- and middle-income countries: a review of the debates surrounding decision rules. Pharmacoeconomics. 2009;27(11):903–17.
13. HM Treasury. The Green Book: Central Government Guidance on Appraisal and Evaluation. 2018. https://assets.publishing.service.gov.uk/government/uploads/system/uploads/attachment_data/file/685903/The_Green_Book.pdf. Accessed 1 June 2018.
14. U.S. Department of Health and Human Services. Guidelines for Regulatory Impact Analysis 2016. https://aspe.hhs.gov/system/files/pdf/242926/HHS_RIAGuidance.pdf. Accessed 2 June 2018.
15. United States Environmental Protection Agency (EPA). Guidelines for Preparing Economic Analyses. 2010. https://www.epa.gov/environmental-economics/guidelines-preparing-economic-analyses. Accessed 3 June 2018.
16. Fesenfeld M, Hutubessy R, Jit M. Cost-effectiveness of human papillomavirus vaccination in low and middle income countries: a systematic review. Vaccine. 2013;31(37):3786–804.
17. Seto K, Marra F, Raymakers A, Marra CA. The cost effectiveness of human papillomavirus vaccines: a systematic review. Drugs. 2012;72(5):715–43.
18. Marra F, Cloutier K, Oteng B, Marra C, Ogilvie G. Effectiveness and cost effectiveness of human papillomavirus vaccine: a systematic review. PharmacoEconomics. 2009;27(2):127–47.
19. Ozawa S, Mirelman A, Stack ML, Walker DG, Levine OS. Cost-effectiveness and economic benefits of vaccines in low- and middle-income countries: a systematic review. Vaccine. 2012;31(1):96–108.

20. Zhou F, Shefer A, Wenger J, Messonnier M, Wang LY, Lopez A, et al. Economic evaluation of the routine childhood immunization program in the United States, 2009. Pediatrics. 2014;133(4):577–85.

21. Barnighausen T, Bloom DE, Canning D, Friedman A, Levine OS, O'Brien J, et al. Rethinking the benefits and costs of childhood vaccination: the example of the Haemophilus influenzae type b vaccine. Vaccine. 2011; 29(13):2371–80.

22. Sabot O, Cohen JM, Hsiang MS, Kahn JG, Basu S, Tang L, et al. Costs and financial feasibility of malaria elimination. Lancet. 2010;376(9752):1604–15.

23. Forman D, de Martel C, Lacey CJ, Soerjomataram I, Lortet-Tieulent J, Bruni L, et al. Global burden of human papillomavirus and related diseases. Vaccine. 2012;30(Suppl 5):F12–23.

24. Jit M, Brisson M, Laprise JF, Choi YH. Comparison of two dose and three dose human papillomavirus vaccine schedules: cost effectiveness analysis based on transmission model. BMJ. 2015;350:g7584.

25. Boardman AE, Greenberg DH, Vining AR, Weimer DL. Cost-Benefit Analysis. Concepts and Practice. 4th ed. Cambridge: Cambridge University Press; 2018.

26. Colombo GL, Ferro A, Vinci M, Zordan M, Serra G. Cost-benefit analysis of influenza vaccination in a public healthcare unit. Ther Clin Risk Manag. 2006; 2(2):219–26.

27. Drummond MF, Sculpher MJ, Torrance GW, O'Brien BJ, Stoddart GL. Methods for the Economic Evaluation of Health Care Programmes. Third ed. New York, NY: Oxford University Press; 2005.

28. Gasparini R, Lucioni C, Lai P, Maggioni P, Sticchi L, Durando P, et al. Cost-benefit evaluation of influenza vaccination in the elderly in the Italian region of Liguria. Vaccine. 2002;20(Suppl 5):B50–4.

29. Hayman DTS, Marshall JC, French NP, Carpenter TE, Roberts MG, Kiedrzynski T. Cost-benefit analyses of supplementary measles immunisation in the highly immunized population of New Zealand. Vaccine. 2017;35(37):4913–22.

30. Schoenbaum SC, Hyde JNJBL, Crampton K. Benefit-cost analysis of rubella vaccination policy. N Engl J Med. 1976;294(6):306–10.

31. Uzicanin A, Zhou F, Eggers R, Webb E, Strebel P. Economic analysis of the 1996-1997 mass measles immunization campaigns in South Africa. Vaccine. 2004;22(25–26):3419–26.

32. GOV.UK National Statistics: Personal Income by Tax Year Statistics. 2016. https://www.gov.uk/government/collections/personal-incomes-statistics. Accessed 28 July 2016.

33. Office for National Statistics (ONS). Annual Population Survey. 2016. https://www.nomisweb.co.uk/query/construct/summary.asp?mode=construct&version=0&dataset=17. Accessed 28 July 2016.

34. Koopmanschap MA, Rutten FF, van Ineveld BM, van Roijen L. The friction cost method for measuring indirect costs of disease. J Health Econ. 1995; 14(2):171–89.

35. Bullhorn. Growth and Impact: The 2015 UK Recruitment Trends Report 2015. https://www.bullhorn.com/uk/resources/2015-uk-recruitment-trends-report/?LS=Blog&LSD=UK_TrendsReport_2015. Accessed 3 Oct 2016.

36. UK Commission for Employment and Skills (UKCES). The UK Commission's Employer Skills Survey 2015: UK Results 2016. https://assets.publishing.service.gov.uk/government/uploads/system/uploads/attachment_data/file/704104/Employer_Skills_Survey_2015_UK_Results-Amended-2018.pdf. Accessed 3 Oct 2016.

37. Oxford Economics. The Cost of Brain Drain: Understanding the Financial Impact of Staff Turnover. 2014. http://www.oxfordeconomics.com/my-oxford/projects/264283. Accessed 4 Oct 2016.

38. Cancer Research UK. Cervical Cancer Incidence Statistics. 2014. http://www.cancerresearchuk.org/health-professional/cancer-statistics/statistics-by-cancer-type/cervical-cancer/incidence#heading-One. Accessed 5 Feb 2017.

39. World Health Organization (WHO). Guidelines for Conducting Cost–Benefit Analysis of Household Energy and Health Interventions. 2006. http://apps.who.int/iris/bitstream/handle/10665/43570/9789241594813_eng.pdf?sequence=1. Accessed 15 Oct 2016.

40. Office for National Statistics (ONS). Household Satellite Accounts: 2005 to 2014. 2016. https://www.ons.gov.uk/economy/nationalaccounts/satelliteaccounts/compendium/householdsatelliteaccounts/2005to2014. Accessed 30 May 2017.

41. Office for National Statistics (ONS). Women in the Labour Market: 2013. p. 2013. https://www.ons.gov.uk/employmentandlabourmarket/peopleinwork/employmentandemployeetypes/articles/womeninthelabourmarket/2013-09-25. Accessed 20 Feb 2017

42. Office for National Statistics (ONS). EMP04: Employment by Occupation. 2016. https://www.ons.gov.uk/employmentandlabourmarket/peopleinwork/employmentandemployeetypes/datasets/employmentbyoccupationemp04. Accessed 10 Jan 2017.

43. Gentry EP, Viscusi WK. The fatality and morbidity components of the value of statistical life. J Health Econ. 2016;46:90–9.

44. Organisation for Economic Co-operation and Development (OECD). Mortality Risk Valuation in Environment, Health and Transport Policies. 2012. http://www.oecd-ilibrary.org/environment/mortality-risk-valuation-in-environment-health-and-transport-policies_9789264130807-en. Accessed 3 Oct 2016.

45. Viscusi WK, Huber J, Bell J. Assessing whether there is a cancer premium for the value of a statistical life. Health Econ. 2014;23(4):384–96.

46. McDonald RL, Chilton SM, Jones-Lee MW, Metcalf HRT. Dread and latency impacts on a VSL for cancer risk reductions. J Risk Uncertainty. 2016;52(2):137–61.

47. U.S. Department of Transportation. Revised Departmental Guidance on Valuation of a Statistical Life in Economic Analysis. 2016. https://www.transportation.gov/sites/dot.gov/files/docs/2016%20Revised%20Value%20of%20a%20Statistical%20Life%20Guidance.pdf. Accessed 30 Oct 2016.

48. Viscusi WK. The role of publication selection Bias in estimates of the value of a statistical life. Am J Health Econ. 2015;1(1):27–52.

49. Gayer T, Hamilton JT, Viscusi WK. The market value of reducing cancer risk: hedonic housing prices with changing information. Southern Econ J. 2002; 69:266–89.

50. Lang HC, Chang K, Ying YH. Quality of life, treatments, and patients' willingness to pay for a complete remission of cervical cancer in Taiwan. Health Econ. 2012;21(10):1217–33.

51. The World Bank. International Comparison Program database. GDP, PPP (current international $). 2018. https://data.worldbank.org/indicator/NY.GDP.MKTP.PP.CD?end=2016&start=2005. Accessed 27 Mar 2017.

52. Organisation for Economic Co-operation and Development (OECD). OECD Stats: 4. PPPs and Exchange Rates. 2018. https://stats.oecd.org/Index.aspx?DataSetCode=SNA_TABLE4#. Accessed 20 Mar 2018.

53. Office for National Statistics (ONS). Inflation and Price Indices. 2018. https://www.ons.gov.uk/economy/inflationandpriceindices. Accessed 1 Apr 2017.

54. Shiroiwa T, Sung YK, Fukuda T, Lang HC, Bae SC, Tsutani K. International survey on willingness-to-pay (WTP) for one additional QALY gained: what is the threshold of cost effectiveness? Health Econ. 2010;19(4):422–37.

55. Robinson LA. Policy monitor: how US government agencies value mortality risk reductions. Rev Environ Econ Pol. 2007;1(2):283–99.

56. Landrigan PJ, Fuller R, Acosta NJR, Adeyi O, Arnold R, Basu NN, et al. The Lancet Commission on Pollution and Health. Lancet. 2018; 391(10119):462–512.

57. Narain U, Sall C. Methodology for Valuing the Health Impacts of Air Pollution: Discussion of Challenges and Proposed Solutions (English). 2016. http://documents.worldbank.org/curated/en/832141466999681767/Methodology-for-valuing-the-health-impacts-of-air-pollution-discussion-of-challenges-and-proposed-solutions.

58. Robinson LA, Hammitt JK. Valuing Nonfatal Health Risk Reductions in Global Benefit-cost Analysis. 2018. https://cdn2.sph.harvard.edu/wp-content/uploads/sites/94/2017/01/Robinson-Hammitt-Nonfatal-Risks.2018.03.121.pdf.

59. Robinson LA, Hammitt JK, O'Keeffe L. Valuing Mortality Risk Reductions in Global Benefit-Cost Analysis. 2018. https://cdn2.sph.harvard.edu/wp-content/uploads/sites/94/2017/01/Robinson-Hammitt-OKeeffe-VSL.2018.03.23.pdf.

60. Oliva J, Lobo F, Lopez-Bastida J, Zozaya N, Romay R. Indirect costs of cervical and breast cancers in Spain. Eur J Health Econ. 2005;6(4):309–13.

61. Sachs JD, World Health Organization. Macroeconomics and Health: Investing in Health for Economic Development: Report of the Commission on Macroeconomics and Health. Geneva: World Health Organization; 2001.

62. Baxter JR, Robinson LA, Hammitt JK. Valuing Time in U.S. Department of Health and Human Services Regulatory Impact Analyses: Conceptual Framework and Best Practices. 2017. https://aspe.hhs.gov/pdf-report/valuing-time-us-department-health-and-human-services-regulatory-impact-analyses-conceptual-framework-and-best-practices. Accessed 5 Jan 2018.

63. Bockstael NE, Strand IE, Hanemann WM. Time and the recreational demand model. Amer J Agr Econ. 1987;69:293–302.

10

Nordic diet, Mediterranean diet, and the risk of chronic diseases: the EPIC-Potsdam study

Cecilia Galbete[1,7], Janine Kröger[1], Franziska Jannasch[1], Khalid Iqbal[2,7], Lukas Schwingshackl[2,7], Carolina Schwedhelm[2,7], Cornelia Weikert[3,7], Heiner Boeing[2,7] and Matthias B. Schulze[1,4,5,6,7*]

Abstract

Background: The Mediterranean Diet (MedDiet) has been acknowledged as a healthy diet. However, its relation with risk of major chronic diseases in non-Mediterranean countries is inconclusive. The Nordic diet is proposed as an alternative across Northern Europe, although its associations with the risk of chronic diseases remain controversial. We aimed to investigate the association between the Nordic diet and the MedDiet with the risk of chronic disease (type 2 diabetes (T2D), myocardial infarction (MI), stroke, and cancer) in the EPIC-Potsdam cohort.

Methods: The EPIC-Potsdam cohort recruited 27,548 participants between 1994 and 1998. After exclusion of prevalent cases, we evaluated baseline adherence to a score reflecting the Nordic diet and two MedDiet scores (tMDS, reflecting the traditional MedDiet score, and the MedPyr score, reflecting the MedDiet Pyramid). Cox regression models were applied to examine the association between the diet scores and the incidence of major chronic diseases.

Results: During a follow-up of 10.6 years, 1376 cases of T2D, 312 of MI, 321 of stroke, and 1618 of cancer were identified. The Nordic diet showed a statistically non-significant inverse association with incidence of MI in the overall population and of stroke in men. Adherence to the MedDiet was associated with lower incidence of T2D (HR per 1 SD 0.93, 95% CI 0.88–0.98 for the tMDS score and 0.92, 0.87–0.97 for the MedPyr score). In women, the MedPyr score was also inversely associated with MI. No association was observed for any of the scores with cancer.

Conclusions: In the EPIC-Potsdam cohort, the Nordic diet showed a possible beneficial effect on MI in the overall population and for stroke in men, while both scores reflecting the MedDiet conferred lower risk of T2D in the overall population and of MI in women.

Keywords: Mediterranean diet, Nordic diet, regional diets, chronic diseases, diabetes, myocardial infarction, stroke, cancer, EPIC-Potsdam study, longitudinal analysis

Background

In the last years, the Nordic diet has emerged as a healthy regional eating option [1]. The Nordic diet tries to reflect the diet consumed in Nordic countries, particularly its healthier choices, including the intake of apples, pears and berries, root and cruciferous vegetables as well as cabbages, whole grain and rye bread as cereals, high intake of fish, low-fat dairy products, potatoes and vegetable fats, among others [1, 2]. To our knowledge, the long-term effects of the Nordic diet on major chronic diseases have only been investigated in prospective cohorts within Nordic countries (Denmark, Sweden, and Finland) [3–10] and the observed effects remain inconsistent.

Another regional diet, the Mediterranean diet (MedDiet), has been extensively evaluated in relation to chronic diseases. The MedDiet refers to the dietary habits in countries around the Mediterranean basin, based on the rural models. This diet postulates a high intake of fruits, nuts

---
* Correspondence: mschulze@dife.de
[1]Department of Molecular Epidemiology, German Institute of Human Nutrition Potsdam-Rehbruecke (DIfE), Nuthetal, Germany
[4]University of Potsdam, Institute of Nutritional Sciences, Nuthetal, Germany
Full list of author information is available at the end of the article

and seeds, vegetables, fish, legumes, cereals, low intake of meat and dairy products, moderate intake of alcohol, mainly from red wine, and extra virgin olive oil as a major fat source [11]. A large multicenter trial conducted in Spain, the PREDIMED (*Prevención con dieta mediterránea*) study, proved beneficial health effects of the MedDiet, primarily in the prevention of cardiovascular disease (CVD) [12], and similar effects have also been observed in prospective studies [13, 14]. The PREDIMED study also showed a reduction of the risk of type 2 diabetes (T2D) [15] and a reduction of incident breast cancer [16]. For T2D, this association was also confirmed in large prospective studies and meta-analyses [17–19]. Further, some beneficial effects have been also shown for certain types of cancer [20].

However, there is some controversy on the possible beneficial effects of the MedDiet outside of the Mediterranean region [21]. As stated by Hoffman and Gerber [21], certain factors, such as food availability, composition of foods available in the Mediterranean and non-Mediterranean countries, and culinary traditions, could complicate following a MedDiet. Similarly, the same could be stated for the application of the Nordic diet in a non-Nordic area. The EPIC-Potsdam (European Prospective Investigation into Cancer and Nutrition-Potsdam) cohort presents a suitable frame for the evaluation of the possible beneficial effects of these two regional diets on the onset of major chronic diseases in both non-Mediterranean and non-Nordic populations. Thus, we aimed to evaluate the association between the Nordic diet and the MedDiet with the risk of major chronic diseases (T2D, myocardial infarction (MI), stroke, and cancer) in the EPIC-Potsdam population.

Methods
Study population and design
The EPIC-Potsdam study is a prospective cohort based in Germany as part of the European-wide multicenter EPIC study. Briefly, it includes 27,548 men and women, aged mainly 35–65 years, recruited between 1994 and 1998. Participants were selected from the general population of Potsdam and surroundings and were invited to a baseline examination conducted by trained staff. At baseline, computer-guided interviews on lifestyle and medical history were also conducted. Every 2–3 years, participants received via mail a follow-up questionnaire in order to assess incident disease cases. The study was approved by the Ethical Committee of the Federal State of Brandenburg and written informed consent was obtained from all participants at the time of recruitment [22, 23].

Those participants who reported prevalent T2D, MI, stroke, or cancer were excluded, as well as those with missing follow-up time, those with missing information on diet, and those who reported implausibly high or low energy intake (< 800 or > 6000 kcal/day). Finally, the

analytical dataset included 9128 men and 14,357 women (*n* = 23,485). For the analysis on incident T2D, cases of other types of diabetes were excluded as well as those without verified T2D (final sample *n* = 23,411). In the case of the analysis for MI, stroke, and cancer, participants with non-verified positive self-reports were excluded, resulting in analytical samples of 23,409 for MI, 23,277 for stroke, and 23,152 for cancer.

Dietary assessment and diet scores
Habitual dietary intake was assessed at baseline by self-administered semiquantitative food-frequency questionnaires (FFQ). This consisted of 148 food items and inquired after the frequency of intake and portion sizes during the last 12 months. Questions about the fat content of the dairy products consumed as well as about the types of fats used for preparation and cooking were included. The reproducibility and validity of the FFQ have been previously reported [24, 25]. Briefly, a total of 104 men and women, aged 35–64 years, completed 12 monthly 24-h dietary recalls, and these were used as a reference method for the estimation of the relative validity of the FFQ. Spearman correlations between FFQ and the mean intake of the 24-h dietary recalls were calculated, ranging from 0.14 for legumes to 0.90 for alcoholic beverages. For bread, the correlation was 0.51, 0.42 for cereals, 0.50 for fruits, 0.34 for vegetables, 0.37 for potatoes, 0.18 for nuts and seeds, 0.56 for milk and milk products, 0.21 for fish, 0.53 for meat, and 0.57 for processed meat. Reproducibility was calculated by administering the FFQ at 6-month intervals in the same study sample. In this case, correlations of food group intake ranged from 0.49 for bread to 0.89 for alcoholic beverages (median = 0.70). For cereals, the calculated correlation was 0.73, 0.61 for fruits, 0.54 for vegetables, 0.70 for legumes, 0.71 for potatoes, 0.66 for nuts and seeds, 0.55 for milk and milk products, 0.77 for fish and for meat, and 0.73 for processed meat [24].

The construction of the Nordic diet score was based on previous publications [1, 5, 26–29], as well as on the data available in the FFQ. We created a score ranging from 0 to 18 points, incorporating 9 components (Table 1). After categorizing each food component into sex-specific tertiles of intake, the participants received a score of 0 to 2 points according to the first, second, and third tertile, respectively. Nine components were included, namely whole grain and rye bread, berries, apples and pears, fish, cabbage and cruciferous vegetables, root vegetables, low-fat dairy products, potatoes, and vegetable fats (excluding olive oil).

Two different scores for the MedDiet were calculated. The traditional MedDiet score (tMDS) was originally proposed by Trichopoulou et al. [30] and slightly modified for non-Mediterranean populations [21]. Our study

Table 1 Components and food items considered the score created to evaluate adherence to the Nordic diet

Food groups	Food items considered in each food group	Scoring criteria
Whole grain and rye bread	Whole grain bread, 'brown', rye, mix bread and grain flakes, grains, muesli	Sex-specific tertiles T1 = 0, T2 = 1, T3 = 2
Berries	Currants, blackberries, raspberries	Sex-specific tertiles T1 = 0, T2 = 1, T3 = 2
Apple and pear	Apple, pear	Sex-specific tertiles T1 = 0, T2 = 1, T3 = 2
Fish	Fish (preserved and smoked is also considered)	Sex-specific tertiles T1 = 0, T2 = 1, T3 = 2
Cabbage and cruciferous vegetables	Broccoli, red cabbage, cauliflower, white cabbage, sauerkraut, radish, coleslaw (*0.5)	Sex-specific tertiles T1 = 0, T2 = 1, T3 = 2
Root vegetables	Carrots, celery, salsify, radish, coleslaw (*0.5)	Sex-specific tertiles T1 = 0, T2 = 1, T3 = 2
Dairy products	Low-fat dairy products, high fat dairy products, low-fat cheese, high-fat cheese	Sex-specific tertiles T1 = 0, T2 = 1, T3 = 2
Potatoes	All kind of potatoes	Sex-specific tertiles T1 = 0, T2 = 1, T3 = 2
Fats	Overall vegetable fats (margarine + vegetable oil, olive oil not included)	Sex-specific tertiles T1 = 0, T2 = 1, T3 = 2

used a linear scale that incorporated nine key components, with a maximum of 18 points (Table 2). Each component was categorized into sex-specific tertiles of intake, except for alcohol and olive oil. For the five components presumed to reflect healthy components of the MedDiet (fruit, vegetables, legumes, fish, and cereals), 0 points were assigned to those participants in the lowest tertile of intake, 1 for those in the middle tertile, and 2 points to those in the highest tertile. This scoring was inverted for meat and

dairy products. Alcohol intake was considered optimal if consumed in moderation (2 points for consumption of 5–25 g/d for women and 10–50 g/d for men, 0 otherwise). In the case of olive oil, the scoring was adapted for the intake in non-Mediterranean countries as follows: 0 points were assigned to non-consumers and sex-specific medians were calculated within olive oil consumers. Two points were assigned to those with consumption over the median and 1 point to those below [17, 31].

Table 2 Components and food items considered in the score created to evaluate adherence to the Mediterranean diet score (tMDS) based on that established by Trichopoulou et al. [30]

Food groups	Food items considered in each food group	Scoring criteria
Cereals	Whole grain bread, other bread, grain flakes, grains, muesli, cornflakes, crisps, pasta, rice	Sex-specific tertiles T1 = 0, T2 = 1, T3 = 2
Fruits and nuts	Fresh fruit, nuts	Sex-specific tertiles T1 = 0, T2 = 1, T3 = 2
Vegetables	Raw vegetables, green salad, cruciferous vegetables, cooked vegetables, garlic, mushrooms	Sex-specific tertiles T1 = 0, T2 = 1, T3 = 2
Fish	Fish (preserved and smoked is also considered)	Sex-specific tertiles T1 = 0, T2 = 1, T3 = 2
Legumes	Legumes (green peas, green beans, lentil, peas, bean stew)	Sex-specific tertiles T1 = 0, T2 = 1, T3 = 2
Meat	Poultry, meat, meat products	Sex-specific tertiles T1 = 2, T2 = 1, T3 = 0
Dairy products	Butter, low-fat dairy products, high fat dairy products, low-fat cheese, high-fat cheese	Sex-specific tertiles T1 = 2, T2 = 1, T3 = 0
Alcohol	Beer, wine, spirits, other alcoholic beverages	5 to 25 g/day for women = 2 10–50 g/day for men = 2 Outside of the range = 0
Olive oil	Olive oil for salad dressing, preparation of vegetables, and preparation of meat	Non-consumers = 0 < sex-specific median = 1 ≥ sex-specific median = 2

The second score applied to assess the adherence to the MedDiet was based on the Mediterranean pyramid (MedPyr) recommendations [11], and calculated following the algorithm developed by Tong et al. [14]. This score categorizes 15 foods or food groups into those that should be consumed in high quantities, in moderation, or in low quantities. The pyramid also provides information on the number of servings recommended, per week or per day. Vegetables, legumes, and fish are food groups advised to be consumed in high quantities. Fruits, nuts, cereals, dairy products, white meat, egg, and alcohol are considered foods that should be consumed in moderation. Red meat, processed meat, potatoes, and sweets are recommended to be consumed in low quantities. Olive oil should represent the main fat source. Detailed information on the calculation of this score is provided in Table 3.

Outcome ascertainment

Information on incident chronic diseases (T2D, MI, stroke, and cancer) was obtained from self-reports during follow-up. These included self-reports on the respective condition, relevant medication, or reason for a reported change in diet. Further diagnoses were found by record linkages with the Common Cancer registry of the different Federal States [32]. Moreover, all potential incident cases were verified by contacting physicians, local cancer registries, and information of death certificates. Incident cases were coded based on the International Classification of Diseases (ICD-10 codes: I21 for myocardial infarction, I60, I61, I63, I64 for stroke, E11 for T2D, and C00–97 for cancer (except C44: non-melanoma skin cancer)). We considered data until the end of the fifth follow-up period (year 2009). Fatal cases due to MI or stroke were also included as incident cases.

Covariate assessment

General characteristics on sociodemographic, lifestyle, and health status were assessed at baseline using self-administered questionnaires. Educational attainment was categorized as (1) currently in training/no certificate or skill, (2) professional school (vocational training), and (3) college or higher education. Smoking status of the participants was categorized as never smoker, former smoker, current smoker, and smoking ≥ 20 cigarettes/day. Physical activity was defined as the mean time spent on leisure time physical activities and cycling (hours/week) during summer and winter, and further categorized (cycling: 0, > 0–2.5, > 2.5–5; > 5 h/week, and sports: 0, > 0–4; > 4 h/week). At baseline examination weight, height and waist circumference were measured

Table 3 Scoring criteria for the construction of the MedPyramid score (from Tong et al. [14])

Component	Recommended intake[a]	Score of 0[a]	Score of 1[a]
Vegetables[b]	≥ 6 /d	0 /d	≥ 6 /d
Legumes[b]	≥ 2 /wk	0 /wk	≥ 2 /wk
Fruits[c]	3–6 /d	0 /d	3–6 /d
Nuts[c]	1–2 /d	0 /d	1–2 /d
Cereals[c]	3–6 /d	0 /d	3–6 /d
Dairy[c]	2 /d	0 /d	1.5–2.5 /d
Fish[b]	≥ 2 /wk	0 /wk	≥ 2 /wk
Red meat[e]	‹ 2 /wk	≥ 4 /wk	‹ 2 /wk
Processed meat[e]	≤ 1 /wk	≥ 2 /wk	≤ 1 /wk
White meat[c]	2 /wk	0 /wk	1.5–2.5 /wk
Egg[c]	2–4 /wk	0 /wk	2–4 /wk
Potatoes[e]	≤ 3 /wk	≥ 6 /wk	≤ 3 /wk
Sweets[e]	≤ 2 /wk	≥ 4 /wk	≤ 2 /wk
Alcohol[d]	10–50 g/d for men, 5–25 g/d for women	> 50 g/d for men, > 25 g/d for women	10–50 g/d for men, 5–25 g/d for women
Olive oil[f]	Principal source of dietary lipids	Non-consumers	Consumers

[a]All recommendations are in number of servings per day or per week and we used continuous scoring for all components, except for olive oil and alcohol
[b]For those components for which a high consumption was recommended, continuous scores from 0 to 1 were assigned proportionally from no consumption to meeting the recommended level of consumption
[c]For components for which moderate consumption was recommended, we assigned a score of 1 for consumption within the recommended levels and 0 for no consumption, with consumption levels in between scored proportionately; overconsumption (double the mid-point value of the recommended intake) was penalized and received a maximum score of 0.5, with consumption between the recommended level and the penalty point scored proportionally
[d]For alcohol, we assigned a score of 1 for consumption levels within recommendation, non-consumption was scored 0.5 while overconsumption was scored 0
[e]For those components for which a low consumption was recommended, consumption below the recommended levels was assigned a score of 1 and double the recommended levels were assigned a score of 0; levels in between scored proportionally
[f]For olive oil, all non-consumers were scored 0 and all consumers 1

by trained staff. Prevalent hypertension diagnosis was based on blood pressure measured at baseline and self-report medication. Total energy intake (kcal/day) was calculated from the FFQ.

Statistical analysis

Cox proportional hazard regression models were used to investigate the association of the three different dietary pattern scores and the risk of incident chronic diseases (T2D, MI, stroke, and cancer, separately). Multivariable-adjusted hazard ratios (HRs) and 95% confidence intervals (CIs) were calculated across tertiles of dietary pattern scores, as well as considering the patterns as continuous variables (by 1 standard deviation (SD) and per 1 unit increment of the scores). The dependent time variable was defined as the time period between the age of recruitment and the age of exit (age of diagnoses or date of death or censoring). In order to be less sensitive to violations of the HR, the models were stratified by age in years. Two models were applied; the first adjusted for sex and the second additionally adjusted for body mass index (kg/m^2), waist circumference (cm) using the residual method adjusted for body mass index, total energy intake (kcal/day), education, smoking status, cycling, sports, and vitamin supplementation (yes/no). In addition, alcohol intake was considered in the analysis of the Nordic diet (0, > 0–6, > 6–12, > 12–24, > 24–60, > 60–96 g/d; plus one more category only for men, > 96 g/d). Prevalent hypertension status (yes/no) was also included in the analysis on T2D, MI, and stroke. Non-linear associations between the a priori defined scores and outcomes of interest were investigated using restricted cubic splines.

To determine the relative impact of the different components comprising the three dietary patterns on the observed associations, dietary scores were calculated alternately omitting each single component and adjusting Cox models for the excluded component.

Potential effect modification by sex was assessed by evaluating the cross-product term between sex and dietary pattern scores in the fully adjusted model. In case interactions were detected, stratified analyses by sex were applied.

Regression-based multiple imputation was conducted to impute missing information on covariates. Five imputed datasets were created. For the main analysis on the association of the patterns with the risk of onset of chronic diseases, missing covariates were observed in 2.5% of participants. Sensitivity analyses were performed by excluding participants with incident cases in the first 2 years of follow-up in the longitudinal analyses. In the analysis of the association of the dietary patterns with stroke, additional analyses were performed excluding incident hemorrhagic stroke cases.

Results

Cohort and dietary pattern characteristics

Sociodemographic lifestyle and anthropometric characteristics according to adherence to the three different diet scores are presented in Table 4. Participants with higher adherence to the Nordic diet where older than those with a low adherence, presented higher waist circumference, were more likely to be overweight and hypertensive, and less likely to be current or former smokers. They were also physically more active. Participants with higher scores for the tMDS diet were older, more likely to be men, higher educated, and physically more active than those with lower adherence. For the MedPyr score, participants with higher adherence were younger, less likely to be hypertensive, more likely with a higher education, and physically more active that those in the lowest tertile of adherence. All three diet scores were associated with each other, observing a stronger association between the two MedDiet scores and a lower one between the Nordic diet and the MedPyr scores (Additional file 1: Table S1). Apart from the differences directly related to the calculation of the scores, further differences were observed. Total energy and fiber intake were positively associated with the three scores, and somewhat more pronounced for the Nordic diet. Concerning macronutrient intake, higher intake of protein from plants was observed in participants with higher adherence to the Nordic diet than in those with a lower adherence; this was also observed for polyunsaturated fat intake. Participants with a higher score for the tMDS had lower intake of saturated fat. Concerning food intake, higher adherence to the Nordic diet was also associated with higher intake of legumes and higher intake of sweets. Higher scores for the tMDS and the MedPyr were also positively associated with sweets, whole grain cereals, and alcohol intake. Intake of potatoes was positively associated with the tMDS but inversely with the MedPyr score.

Dietary patterns and incidence of major chronic diseases

Table 5 shows the associations observed between the a priori defined diet scores and the four different outcomes considered (T2D, MI, stroke, and cancer). The cubic spline analysis did not show evidence for non-linearity for any of the diet score–chronic disease associations investigated. During 246,219 person-years of follow-up, 1376 participants reported a new diagnosis of T2D (mean follow-up of 10.5 years). Both MedDiet scores were associated with lower risk of T2D in the fully adjusted model. Participants in the highest tertile of adherence to the MedPyr presented 20% lower risk of T2D in comparison with those in the lowest tertile (HR$_{T3 \text{ vs. } T1}$ 0.80, 95% CI 0.70–0.92; HR$_{\text{per 1 SD}}$ 0.92, 95% CI 0.87–0.97). For the tMDS, participants with higher adherence

Table 4 General characteristics of the EPIC-Potsdam population according to the degree of adherence to diet scores

Variable	Total population (n = 23,485)	Nordic diet score		tMDS score		MedPyr score	
		Low adherence (n = 7686) 0–7 points	High adherence (n = 7637) 11–18 points	Low adherence (n = 7077) 0–7 points	High adherence (n = 6709) 11–18 points	Low adherence (n = 7828) < 6.2 points	High adherence (n = 7828) > 7.3 points
Sex (% of male)	38.9	39.0	39.3	35.8	41.1	38.8	38.1
Age at recruitment	49.8 (8.9)	48.5 (8.6)	50.8 (8.9)	49.1 (9.0)	50.1 (8.8)	50.7 (9.1)	48.9 (8.6)
BMI (kg/m^2)	26.1 (4.2)	25.8 (4.2)	26.3 (4.2)	26.1 (4.4)	26.0 (4.1)	26.2 (4.4)	26.0 (4.1)
% BMI ≥ 25 kg/m^2	55.9	53.1	58.1	55.4	54.8	56.6	55.0
Waist circumference (cm)	85.6 (12.8)	84.8 (12.9)	86.4 (12.5)	85.2 (13.0)	85.5 (12.7)	86.0 (12.9)	85.2 (12.8)
Prevalent hypertension (%)	46.1	43.4	48.9	44.6	46.9	47.5	44.9
Current or former smokers (%)	51.2	57.4	45.5	52.2	50.0	50.6	51.4
Education; university degree (%)	37.7	36.5	39.0	30.9	44.6	29.5	44.9
Total sport (h/week)[a]	2.0 (0.0–4.0)	1.5 (0.0–3.5)	2.0 (0.5–5.0)	1.5 (0.0–3.5)	2.0 (0.5–5.0)	1.5 (0.0–3.5)	2.0 (0.5–4.5)

Data are shown as mean (SD) unless otherwise stated
BMI body mass index, *MedPyr* Mediterranean diet score based on the Mediterranean Pyramid, *tMDS* Mediterranean diet score based on that established by Trichopoulou et al. [30]
[a]Data are shown as median (IQR)

presented 16% reduction of the risk (HR$_{T3 vs. T1}$ 0.84, 95% CI 0.73–0.97; HR$_{per 1SD}$ 0.93, 95% CI 0.88–0.98). No association was observed for the Nordic diet on the risk of incident T2D. In the analysis for MI, during 249,262 person-years, 312 participants developed MI (10.8 years follow-up on average). For the Nordic diet, a statistically not-significant inverse association with the onset of MI was observed (HR$_{T3 vs. T1}$ 0.88, 95% CI 0.64–1.20; HR$_{per 1 SD}$ 0.91, 95% CI 0.80–1.04). In the case of the MedDiet scores, an inverse but not-statistically significant association was observed for the MedPyr in the model corrected for sex and age. However, after the full adjustment for covariates, the association was attenuated, yet still suggesting a lower risk for higher adherence (HR$_{T3 vs. T1}$ 0.84, 95% CI 0.63–1.11; HR$_{per 1 SD}$ 0.92, 95% CI 0.82–1.04). For stroke, during 252,457 person-years follow-up, 321 new cases were identified (mean follow-up of 10.8 years), but no associations were observed. For cancer, from 244,339 person-years of follow-up, 1618 participants developed cancer (mean follow-up of 10.6 years). Similar to stroke, no associations were observed for overall cancer risk. Further sensitivity analysis excluding incident cases which occurred in the first 2 years of follow-up provided similar associations (Additional file 1: Table S2). For stroke, the exclusion of the hemorrhagic stroke cases did not show different associations (Additional file 1: Table S3). Stratified analyses were performed for sex when interaction between sex and the dietary patterns were detected in the fully adjusted model (Table 6). This was observed in the case of the Nordic diet on its association with stroke (p = 0.071). The stratified analyses revealed a decreased risk only in men (HR$_{T3 vs. T1}$ 0.85, 95% CI 0.56–1.29; HR$_{per 1 SD}$ 0.88, 95% CI 0.74–1.04). Possible interaction was also detected between sex and the MedPyr

score for the risk on MI (p = 0.070). After stratification, an inverse association was observed in women (HR$_{T3 vs. T1}$ 0.77, 95% CI 0.45–1.30; HR$_{per 1 SD}$ 0.81, 95% CI 0.65–1.00), but not in men. Sensitivity analyses omitting individual components in the calculation of the scores were performed to test the dependence of observed associations on these components (Table 7). These analyses revealed that, for T2D, the omission of alcohol in both MedDiet scores attenuated the associations from a HR$_{per 1 SD}$ of 0.93 (95% CI 0.88–0.98) to 0.95 (95% CI 0.90–1.01) in the case of the tMDS, and from 0.92 (95% CI 0.87–0.97) to 0.94 (95% CI 0.89–0.99) for the MedPyr score. The omission of alcohol in the calculation of the MedPyr score also led to the strongest attenuation of the association between this score and MI among women, from a HR$_{per 1 SD}$ of 0.81 (95% CI 0.65–1.00) to 0.88 (95% CI 0.71–1.08). Similar results were observed for the exclusion of potatoes and red meat. However, the opposite was observed for olive oil, where, when excluded, the inverse association with MI became stronger (HR$_{per 1 SD}$ 0.77, 95% CI 0.62–0.94).

Discussion
In this study, we have analyzed the association between the MedDiet and the Nordic diet with the incidence of major chronic disease in a German, middle aged, and apparently healthy population. With a mean of 10.6 years of follow-up, the two different MedDiet scores showed inverse associations with the risk of developing T2D. We also observed an inverse association of the MedPyr score and the risk of MI among women. The Nordic diet showed an inverse but not-statistically significant association with MI risk in the overall population, and with stroke in men. No association was observed for any of the scores with the incidence of cancer.

Table 5 Prospective associations between adherence to the diet scores and the incidence of major chronic diseases

	Low adherence	Moderate adherence		High adherence		p for trend	per 1 SD		per 1 unit	
	(Ref.)	HR	95% CI	HR	95% CI		HR	95% CI	HR	95% CI
DIABETES										
Nordic diet										
Cases, n/person-year	413/80,081	494/85,511		469/80,627						
Model 1	1.00	1.04	0.91–1.18	1.00	0.87–1.14	1.000	1.00	0.94–1.05	1.00	0.98–1.02
Model 2	1.00	1.02	0.89–1.17	1.01	0.87–1.18	0.827	1.00	0.94–1.07	1.00	0.98–1.02
tMDS										
Cases, n/person-year	445/73,939	578/101,702		353/70,578						
Model 1	1.00	0.87	0.77–0.99	0.75	0.65–0.87	< 0.001	0.89	0.84–0.94	0.96	0.94–0.98
Model 2	1.00	0.92	0.81–1.04	0.84	0.73–0.97	0.019	0.93	0.88–0.98	0.97	0.95–0.99
MedPyr										
Cases, n/person-year	549/81,156	448/82,176		379/82,887						
Model 1	1.00	0.84	0.74–0.96	0.75	0.65–0.84	< 0.001	0.88	0.84–0.93	0.90	0.87–0.94
Model 2	1.00	0.90	0.79–1.02	0.80	0.70–0.92	0.001	0.92	0.87–0.97	0.93	0.89–0.97
MYOCARDIAL INFARCTION										
Nordic diet										
Cases, n/person-year	94/81,983	123/87,572		95/82,706						
Model 1	1.00	1.11	0.85–1.45	0.85	0.64–1.14	0.272	0.91	0.81–1.02	0.97	0.94–1.01
Model 2	1.00	1.13	0.85–1.49	0.88	0.64–1.20	0.440	0.91	0.80–1.04	0.97	0.93–1.01
tMDS										
Cases, n/person-year	91/75,908	137/104,226		84/72,128						
Model 1	1.00	0.99	0.76–1.29	0.84	0.62–1.13	0.283	0.91	0.81–1.02	0.97	0.93–1.01
Model 2	1.00	1.06	0.81–1.39	0.95	0.70–1.28	0.816	0.95	0.85–1.07	0.98	0.94–1.03
MedPyr										
Cases, n/person-year	122/83,499	105/84,148		85/84,614						
Model 1	1.00	0.89	0.69–1.16	0.78	0.59–1.03	0.073	0.89	0.80–1.00	0.91	0.83–1.00
Model 2	1.00	0.91	0.70–1.19	0.84	0.63–1.11	0.224	0.92	0.82–1.04	0.94	0.85–1.03
STROKE										
Nordic diet										
Cases, n/person-year	108/81,956	100/87,741		113/82,760						
Model 1	1.00	0.78	0.59–1.02	0.87	0.66–1.13	0.297	0.92	0.82–1.03	0.97	0.94–1.01
Model 2	1.00	0.82	0.62–1.09	0.97	0.72–1.31	0.819	0.97	0.85–1.10	0.99	0.95–1.03
tMDS										
Cases, n/person-year	91/75,836	144/104,416		86/72,204						
Model 1	1.00	1.06	0.82–1.38	0.91	0.68–1.22	0.498	0.99	0.88–1.11	1.00	0.96–1.04
Model 2	1.00	1.10	0.85–1.44	0.98	0.72–1.32	0.832	1.02	0.91–1.14	1.01	0.96–1.05
MedPyr										
Cases, n/person-year	124/83,599	93/84,291		104/84,566						
Model 1	1.00	0.80	0.61–1.04	0.96	0.74–1.25	0.701	0.97	0.87–1.09	0.98	0.90–1.07
Model 2	1.00	0.83	0.63–1.09	1.03	0.79–1.35	0.870	1.01	0.90–1.13	1.01	0.92–1.10

Table 5 Prospective associations between adherence to the diet scores and the incidence of major chronic diseases *(Continued)*

	Low adherence	Moderate adherence		High adherence		*p* for trend	per 1 SD		per 1 unit	
	(Ref.)	HR	95% CI	HR	95% CI		HR	95% CI	HR	95% CI
CANCER										
Nordic diet										
Cases, n/person-year	503/79,442	559/85,025		556/79,872						
Model 1	1.00	0.93	0.83–1.05	0.94	0.83–1.06	0.243	0.97	0.92–1.01	0.99	0.97–1.00
Model 2	1.00	0.95	0.84–1.08	0.99	0.87–1.14	0.774	0.99	0.93–1.05	1.00	0.98–1.01
tMDS										
Cases, n/person-year	482/73,638	691/100,771		445/769,931						
Model 1	1.00	0.98	0.87–1.10	0.91	0.80–1.03	0.119	0.97	0.92–1.02	0.99	0.97–1.01
Model 2	1.00	1.00	0.89–1.12	0.95	0.83–1.08	0.345	0.99	0.94–1.04	0.99	0.98–1.01
MedPyr diet										
Cases, n/person-year	571/80,743	556/81,584		491/82,013						
Model 1	1.00	1.03	0.92–1.16	0.96	0.85–1.09	0.636	0.99	0.94–1.04	0.99	0.95–1.03
Model 2	1.00	1.04	0.93–1.17	1.00	0.88–1.13	0.979	1.01	0.96–1.06	1.00	0.96–1.05

Model 1: adjusted for age and sex
Model 2: Model 1 + smoking status, education, total energy (kcal/day), vitamin supplementation, body mass index (kg/m^2), waist circumference (cm), cycling, sports, prevalent hypertension (not in the analyses on cancer), alcohol intake (7 categories) (only for the Nordic diet analysis)
SD standard deviation, *HR* hazard ratio, *CI* confidence interval
tMDS Mediterranean diet score based on that established by Trichopoulou et al. [30], *MedPyr* Mediterranean diet score based on the Mediterranean Pyramid

To our knowledge, our analyses are the first to explore the associations between the Nordic diet and several different major chronic diseases in a prospective cohort outside of the Nordic region. Three large prospective cohorts have studied the effects of the Nordic diet on the onset of major chronic diseases. In the Diet, Cancer and Health study in Denmark, which included more than 55,000 men and women and followed them for more than 13 years, a higher adherence to the Nordic diet was associated with lower risk for total stroke, T2D, and colorectal cancer, the latter only among women [3, 5, 6]. The Swedish Women's Lifestyle and Health cohort included more than 44,000 women followed for over a median of

Table 6 Prospective associations between the diet scores and certain disease outcomes stratified by sex in the EPIC-Potsdam cohort

	Low adherence	Moderate adherence		High adherence		*p* for trend	per SD		per 1 unit		*p* for interaction
	(Ref.)	HR	95% CI	HR	95% CI		HR	95% CI	HR	95% CI	
Nordic diet score and stroke											0.071
Men											
Cases, n/person-year	63/31,471	60/33,485		52/32,401							
Fully adjusted model	1.00	0.95	0.65–1.37	0.85	0.56–1.29	0.406	0.88	0.74–1.04	0.96	0.91–1.01	
Women											
Cases, n/person-year	45/50,458	40/54,556		61/50,359							
Fully adjusted model	1.00	0.72	0.46–1.12	1.05	0.68–1.64	0.913	1.06	0.87–1.28	1.02	0.96–1.08	
Mediterranean pyramid score and myocardial infarction											0.070
Men											
Cases, n/person-year	82/31,889	75/32,219		61/32,325							
Fully adjusted model	1.00	0.97	0.71–1.34	0.87	0.62–1.22	0.397	0.98	0.86–1.13	0.99	0.88–1.10	
Women											
Cases, n/person-year	41/51,641	29/52,014		24/52,174							
Fully adjusted model	1.00	0.80	0.50–1.30	0.77	0.45–1.30	0.313	0.81	0.65–1.00	0.84	0.71–1.00	

Fully adjusted model: age, sex, smoking status, education, total energy (kcal/day), vitamin supplementation, body mass index (kg/m^2), waist circumference (cm), cycling, sports, prevalent hypertension, alcohol intake (7 categories) (only for the Nordic diet analysis)
SD standard deviation, *HR* Hazard ratio, *CI* confidence interval

Table 7 Prospective associations of the diet scores with type 2 diabetes mellitus and myocardial infarction, excluding single components

Diabetes						Myocardial infarction in women	
	tMDS		MedPyr			MedPyr	
	HR (per 1 SD)	95% CI		HR (per 1 SD)	95% CI	HR (per 1SD)	95% CI
Overall association	0.93	0.88–0.98	Overall association	0.92	0.87–0.97	0.81	0.65–1.00
Minus cereals	0.93	0.88–0.98	Minus cereals	0.91	0.87–0.96	0.81	0.66–1.00
Minus fruits and nuts	0.94	0.89–0.99	Minus fruits	0.92	0.87–0.97	0.81	0.66–1.00
			Minus nuts	0.92	0.87–0.97	0.82	0.67–1.02
Minus vegetables	0.94	0.89–1.00	Minus vegetables	0.92	0.87–0.97	0.81	0.65–1.00
Minus fish	0.92	0.87–0.98	Minus fish	0.91	0.86–0.96	0.82	0.67–1.02
Minus legumes	0.92	0.87–0.98	Minus legumes	0.91	0.86–0.96	0.80	0.65–0.99
Minus meat	0.94	0.89–1.00	Minus red meat	0.93	0.88–0.98	0.86	0.70–1.07
			Minus processed meat	0.92	0.88–0.98	0.80	0.65–0.99
			Minus white meat	0.91	0.87–0.97	0.81	0.65–1.00
			Minus egg	0.91	0.86–0.96	0.76	0.62–0.94
Minus dairy products	0.92	0.87–0.98	Minus dairy products	0.93	0.88–0.98	0.79	0.64–0.98
			Minus potatoes	0.93	0.88–0.98	0.86	0.69–1.06
Minus alcohol	0.95	0.90–1.01	Minus alcohol	0.94	0.89–0.99	0.88	0.71–1.08
			Minus sweets	0.91	0.86–0.96	0.83	0.67–1.02
Minus olive oil	0.95	0.89–1.00	Minus olive oil	0.91	0.87–0.97	0.77	0.62–0.94

Age, sex, smoking status, education, total energy (kcal/day), vitamin supplementation, body mass index (kg/m^2), waist circumference (cm), cycling, sports, prevalent hypertension, excluded component

CI confidence interval, *HR* hazard ratio, *SD* standard deviation

tMDS Mediterranean diet score based on that established by Trichopoulou et al. [30]]

MedPyr Mediterranean diet score based on the Mediterranean Pyramid

20 years [10]; however, no association between the Nordic diet and the risk of breast and colorectal cancer or CVD was observed [7, 9, 33]. In addition, in two Finnish prospective cohorts, the Helsinki Birth Cohort and the Health 2000 survey, no association between the Nordic diet and the risk of T2D was detected [4].

The construction of the Nordic diet score is probably the most important difference between previous studies and our present study. The Diet, Cancer and Health study [5] and the Swedish Women's Lifestyle and Health cohort [10] used a very similar index composed of six food groups, namely oatmeal, apples/pears, cabbages, root vegetables, fish, and rye bread in the Danish Diet, Cancer and Health cohort [5], but whole grain cereals in the Swedish Women's Lifestyles and Health study [10]. However, it would be too ambitious to hypothesize that this small disparity could lead to the different observations. The Helsinki Birth Cohort and the Health 2000 survey indicated no association between the Nordic diet and the risk of T2D, considering six components in line with the Nordic diet pyramid [4] (berries/apples/pears, vegetables, rye/oats/barley, fat-free milk/< 2% fat milk, salmon/freshwater fish, and polyunsaturated fatty acids/(saturated fatty acids + *trans*-fatty acids) ratio), two components that contradict

these (meat products and total fat (E%)), and alcohol, which should be consumed in moderation. Again, the composition of the pattern does not provide a possible explanation for this null association. Indeed, previous publications in the same cohorts already showed an inverse association of the Nordic diet with abdominal obesity [34] and low-grade inflammation [35]. Other items considered as part of the Nordic diet in other publications, like potatoes, low-fat dairy products and vegetable oils, were also included in our score [26, 36]. These discrepancies highlight the necessity to get into an agreement about the definition of Nordic diet.

Regarding the MedDiet, beneficial effects on the incidence of T2D have already been reported in a large randomized control trial, the PREDIMED study [15], as well as in large longitudinal cohorts, and summarized in several meta-analyses [17–19]. Moreover, we have shown that alcohol presented the highest contribution to the observed beneficial effect of both MedDiet scores. This observation is in line with EPIC-InterAct study, which also observed that high olive oil and low meat consumption, besides moderate alcohol consumption, are important components of the effect of the MedDiet on T2D. In line with these observations, a meta-analysis concluded that olive oil could have beneficial effects on the prevention and management of T2D [37]. Finally, another meta-analysis also determined that the intake of red and processed meat increased the risk. In our study, we also showed a marginal effect of these two components [38]. The association between MedDiet and the risk of CVD has been extensively explored [12–14, 39]. In our analysis, we observed a tendency of adherence to the MedPyr to lower the risk for incident MI, with a stronger effect in women than in men. Similarly to T2D, this association appeared to be at least in part attributable to alcohol intake. The protective effects of alcohol intake on cardiovascular risk have been a matter of substantial debate. A recent meta-analysis supported the idea that the health effects of alcohol intake depend on the amount as well as on the pattern of consumption [40]. Nevertheless, a recent study from Bell et al. [41] found heterogeneous associations for the level of alcohol consumption and different cardiovascular endpoints, encouraging for a more accurate and careful research and public health counseling.

In our study, we observed sex differences in the association of the a priori defined scores with CVD. Previous studies have already discussed the sex differences in response to diet, particularly fat-rich diets [42–44]. Grosso et al. [13] summarized prospective studies in a meta-analysis and observed an inverse association between adherence to the MedDiet and the occurrence of stroke. Recently, a work evaluated the associations of four different MedDiet scores with the risk of CVD in the EPIC-Norfolk prospective cohort [14]. An inverse association was observed for stroke with the MedPyr score but not for the three other scores assessed. The construction of the dietary scores (items included and cut-offs used) may directly affect the results. This is one of the major critic points and has been extensively discussed before [21, 45–47]. In this study, we decided to use one of the most frequently applied scores to represent the MedDiet in non-Mediterranean areas, the tMDS. For the calculation of this score, we used population-specific cut-off values for most component food groups, thus assigning score points based on relative ranking in the cohort rather than absolute food consumption levels. Another study conducted in the EPIC-Potsdam cohort evaluating the effects of the MedDiet on heart failure [48] suggested the use of observed medians in the EPIC-Greece cohort [30], arguing that, by using these, the calculated score better represents food consumption levels of the 'true' MedDiet. Apart from this, and following the suggestion from Tong et al. [14], we also used the MedPyr score, which is based on the Mediterranean pyramid proposed by the Mediterranean Diet Foundation [11]. This score has two major differences in comparison to the tMDS. First, the pyramid includes more food groups (15) – separating fruits and nuts, distinguishing between red, processed and white meat, and additionally including potatoes, eggs, and sweets. Second, score points are assigned to absolute food consumption levels rather than relative intake. For those food items included in both scores, the MedPyr score reflected somewhat smaller differences in absolute intake between those considered to have a high versus low score compared to tMDS (Additional file 1: Table S1). Both differences in the definition of components and in their intake levels are possible explanations for inconsistent associations observed for both scores in our cohort. The study of Tong et al. [14], in line with our observations, also showed the strongest associations with cardiovascular outcomes for the MedPyr score. However, they also conclude that the three scores used to assess adherence to the MedDiet (the MedPyr, the tMDs, and a third one based on the literature as proposed by Sofi et al. [49]) were useful in epidemiological settings [14]. Unfortunately, thus far, there are no data available regarding the utility and the use of different Nordic diet scores. On the other hand, for a better comparability among the created scores and with other previous publications, we decided to construct scores without adjusting components for total energy intake. We included total energy intake as a covariate in the regression models in order to achieve the equivalent of an isocaloric diet. This is in accordance with the methodology applied by Trichopoulou et al. [30, 50] when they first created and evaluated the MedDiet score and its implication on health. Still, the role of energy adjustment of components prior to dietary pattern score calculation remains a matter of scientific debate. First, heterogeneity exists across previous studies as to whether and what kind of energy adjustments were applied, which limits the comparability between studies. Secondly, few studies have been performed to evaluate the consequences of such methodological differences. For example, studies have found little difference in derived patterns if input variables were or not adjusted for energy. Additionally, expressing the input variables as contributions to energy intake might be less meaningful for food groups that might be important for health but contribute little to energy intake [51].

Some strengths and limitations of the present work should be mentioned. The EPIC-Potsdam study is a large follow-up study that includes a high number of apparently healthy participants at baseline. Together with the medical verification of the new incident cases, the validity of our observations was strengthened. On the other hand, the use of a FFQ as a tool for measuring habitual dietary intake is not exempt from limitations and there is much discussion on how well the FFQ captures habitual diet [52, 53]. For example, misreporting is a common problem, which could lead to measurement error and bias in the estimations. Moreover, diet and other lifestyle factors were only assessed at baseline, and possible changes have not been taken into account. Possible diet changes after the diagnosis of a chronic disease could have led to reverse causality and thus explain our observations. However, after the exclusion of prevalent cases of chronic disease and the further sensitivity analysis excluding incident cases within the first 2 years, we made an attempt to minimize this problem. We have also controlled our analysis for a large number of plausible confounders that could influence the association between the dietary patterns and risk of chronic diseases. Nevertheless, residual confounding is possible due to imperfect measurement or presence of unknown confounders. Due to possible limited power, we decided to combine overall cancer incidence as an outcome. However, this approach might complicate possible conclusions and interpretations of the null finding and, still, possible beneficial effects on specific cancer sites cannot be ruled out. The same problem on limited power could also apply to incident stroke and MI.

Conclusions

In summary, we have observed an inverse association of both MedDiet scores with the incidence of T2D, with alcohol being a relevant component within these. At the same time, we have observed that the MedPyr score was also associated with lower risk of MI in women, but not in men. However, we have not observed any other statistically significant association between the evaluated scores and the risk of stroke or overall cancer. Nevertheless, possible beneficial effects cannot be completely ruled out due to limited power to evaluate associations and the possibility of cancer site-specific effects. Thus, re-analysis of the associations in our cohort after extended follow-up would include a higher number of incident cases and provide further information.

Abbreviations

CI: confidence interval; CVD: cardiovascular disease; EPIC: European Prospective study into Cancer and Nutrition; FFQ: food frequency questionnaire; HR: hazard ratio; MedPyr: Mediterranean pyramid score; MI: myocardial infarction; PREDIMED: Prevención con dieta mediterránea; T2D: type 2 diabetes; tMED: traditional Mediterranean diet score

Acknowledgments

We thank Dr. Manuela Bergmann, who was responsible for the methodological and organizational work of data collection of exposures and outcomes, and Wolfgang Fleischhauer for his medical expertise, which was employed in case ascertainment and contacts with the physicians. We also want to thank Catarina Schiborn for the technical review.

Funding

This work was supported by NutriAct – Competence Cluster Nutrition Research Berlin-Potsdam funded by the German Federal Ministry of Education and Research (FKZ: 01EA1408A-G). The funders had no role in study design, data collection and analysis, decision to publish, or preparation of the manuscript.

Authors' contributions

Conceived and designed the analyses: CG, JK, FJ, MBS, HB. Performed the analyses: CG. Acquisition of the data: HB, MBS, CW. Interpretation of the data: CG, JK, FJ, KI, LS, CS, CW, HB, MBS. Wrote the first draft of the manuscript: CG. Contributed to the writing of the manuscript: CG, JK, FJ, KI, LS, CS, CW, MBS. Agree with the manuscript's results and conclusions: CG, JK, FJ, KI, LS, CS, CW, HB, MBS. All authors have read, and confirm that they meet, ICMJE criteria for authorship. All authors read and approved the final manuscript.

Competing interests

The authors declare that they have no competing interests.

Author details

[1]Department of Molecular Epidemiology, German Institute of Human Nutrition Potsdam-Rehbruecke (DIfE), Nuthetal, Germany. [2]Department of Epidemiology, German Institute of Human Nutrition Potsdam-Rehbruecke, Nuthetal, Germany. [3]Department of Food Safety, Federal Institute for Risk Assessment, Berlin, Germany. [4]University of Potsdam, Institute of Nutritional Sciences, Nuthetal, Germany. [5]German Center for Diabetes Research (DZD), München-Neuherberg, Germany. [6]DZHK (German Centre for Cardiovascular Research), partner site Berlin, Berlin, Germany. [7]NutriAct – Competence Cluster Nutrition Research Berlin-Potsdam, Nuthetal, Germany.

References

1. Mithril C, Dragsted LO, Meyer C, Blauert E, Holt MK, Astrup A. Guidelines for the new Nordic diet. Public Health Nutr. 2012;15(10):1941–7.
2. Adamsson V, Reumark A, Cederholm T, Vessby B, Riserus U, Johansson G. What is a healthy Nordic diet? Foods and nutrients in the NORDIET study. Food Nutr Res. 2012;56. https://doi.org/10.3402/fnr.v56i0.18189.
3. Hansen CP, Overvad K, Kyro C, Olsen A, Tjonneland A, Johnsen SP, et al. Adherence to a healthy Nordic diet and risk of stroke: a Danish cohort study. Stroke. 2017;48(2):259–64.
4. Kanerva N, Rissanen H, Knekt P, Havulinna AS, Eriksson JG, Mannisto S. The healthy Nordic diet and incidence of type 2 diabetes–10-year follow-up. Diabetes Res Clin Pract. 2014;106(2):e34–7.
5. Kyro C, Skeie G, Loft S, Overvad K, Christensen J, Tjonneland A, et al. Adherence to a healthy Nordic food index is associated with a lower incidence of colorectal cancer in women: the diet, Cancer and health cohort study. Br J Nutr. 2013;109(5):920–7.
6. Lacoppidan SA, Kyro C, Loft S, Helnaes A, Christensen J, Hansen CP, et al. Adherence to a healthy Nordic food index is associated with a lower risk of Type-2 diabetes–the Danish diet, Cancer and health cohort study. Nutrients. 2015;7(10):8633–44.
7. Li Y, Roswall N, Sandin S, Strom P, Adami HO, Weiderpass E. Adherence to a healthy Nordic food index and breast cancer risk: results from a Swedish cohort study. Cancer Causes Control. 2015;26(6):893–902.
8. Roswall N, Li Y, Kyro C, Sandin S, Lof M, Adami HO, et al. No association between adherence to a healthy Nordic food index and colorectal Cancer: results from a Swedish cohort study. Cancer Epidemiol Biomark Prev. 2015;24(4):755–7.
9. Roswall N, Sandin S, Lof M, Skeie G, Olsen A, Adami HO, et al. Adherence to the healthy Nordic food index and total and cause-specific mortality among Swedish women. Eur J Epidemiol. 2015;30(6):509–17.
10. Roswall N, Sandin S, Scragg R, Lof M, Skeie G, Olsen A, et al. No association between adherence to the healthy Nordic food index and cardiovascular disease amongst Swedish women: a cohort study. J Intern Med. 2015;278(5):531–41.

11. Bach-Faig A, Berry EM, Lairon D, Reguant J, Trichopoulou A, Dernini S, et al. Mediterranean diet pyramid today. Science and cultural updates. Public Health Nutr. 2011;14(12A):2274–84.

12. Estruch R, Ros E, Salas-Salvado J, Covas MI, Corella D, Aros F, et al. Primary prevention of cardiovascular disease with a Mediterranean diet. N Engl J Med. 2013;368(14):1279–90.

13. Grosso G, Marventano S, Yang J, Micek A, Pajak A, Scalfi L, et al. A comprehensive meta-analysis on evidence of Mediterranean diet and cardiovascular disease: are individual components equal? Crit Rev Food Sci Nutr. 2017;57(15):3218–32.

14. Tong TY, Wareham NJ, Khaw KT, Imamura F, Forouhi NG. Prospective association of the Mediterranean diet with cardiovascular disease incidence and mortality and its population impact in a non-Mediterranean population: the EPIC-Norfolk study. BMC Med. 2016;14:135.

15. Salas-Salvado J, Guasch-Ferre M, Lee CH, Estruch R, Clish CB, Ros E. Protective effects of the Mediterranean diet on type 2 diabetes and metabolic syndrome. J Nutr. 2016;146(4):920S–7S.

16. Toledo E, Salas-Salvado J, Donat-Vargas C, Buil-Cosiales P, Estruch R, Ros E, et al. Mediterranean diet and invasive breast Cancer risk among women at high cardiovascular risk in the PREDIMED trial: a randomized clinical trial. JAMA Intern Med. 2015;175(11):1752–60.

17. InterAct C, Romaguera D, Guevara M, Norat T, Langenberg C, Forouhi NG, et al. Mediterranean diet and type 2 diabetes risk in the European prospective investigation into Cancer and nutrition (EPIC) study: the InterAct project. Diabetes Care. 2011;34(9):1913–8.

18. Jannasch F, Kroger J, Schulze MB. Dietary patterns and type 2 diabetes: a systematic literature review and meta-analysis of prospective studies. J Nutr. 2017;147(6):1174–82.

19. Schwingshackl L, Missbach B, Konig J, Hoffmann G. Adherence to a Mediterranean diet and risk of diabetes: a systematic review and meta-analysis. Public Health Nutr. 2015;18(7):1292–9.

20. Schwingshackl L, Schwedhelm C, Galbete C, Hoffmann G. Adherence to Mediterranean diet and risk of Cancer: an updated systematic review and meta-analysis. Nutrients. 2017;9(10).

21. Hoffman R, Gerber M. Evaluating and adapting the Mediterranean diet for non-Mediterranean populations: a critical appraisal. Nutr Rev. 2013; 71(9):573–84.

22. Boeing H, Korfmann A, Bergmann MM. Recruitment procedures of EPIC-Germany. European investigation into Cancer and nutrition. Ann Nutr Metab. 1999;43(4):205–15.

23. Boeing H, Wahrendorf J, Becker N. EPIC-Germany–A source for studies into diet and risk of chronic diseases. European Investigation into Cancer and Nutrition. Ann Nutr Metab. 1999;43(4):195–204.

24. Bohlscheid-Thomas S, Hoting I, Boeing H, Wahrendorf J. Reproducibility and Relative validity of food group intake in a food frequency questionnaire developed for the German part of the EPIC project. European prospective investigation into Cancer and nutrition. Int J Epidemiol. 1997;26(Suppl 1):S59–70.

25. Kroke A, Klipstein-Grobusch K, Voss S, Moseneder J, Thielecke F, Noack R, et al. Validation of a self-administered food-frequency questionnaire administered in the European prospective investigation into Cancer and nutrition (EPIC) study: comparison of energy, protein, and macronutrient intakes estimated with the doubly labeled water, urinary nitrogen, and repeated 24-h dietary recall methods. Am J Clin Nutr. 1999;70(4):439–47.

26. Akesson A, Andersen LF, Kristjansdottir AG, Roos E, Trolle E, Voutilainen E, et al. Health effects associated with foods characteristic of the Nordic diet: a systematic literature review. Food Nutr Res. 2013;57. https://doi.org/10.3402/fnr.v57i0.22790.

27. Bere E, Brug J. Towards health-promoting and environmentally friendly regional diets - a Nordic example. Public Health Nutr. 2009;12(1):91–6.

28. Kanerva N, Kaartinen NE, Schwab U, Lahti-Koski M, Mannisto S. The Baltic Sea diet score: a tool for assessing healthy eating in Nordic countries. Public Health Nutr. 2014;17(8):1697–705.

29. Perala MM, von Bonsdorff M, Mannisto S, Salonen MK, Simonen M, Kanerva N, et al. A healthy Nordic diet and physical performance in old age: findings from the longitudinal Helsinki birth cohort study. Br J Nutr. 2016;115(5):878–86.

30. Trichopoulou A, Costacou T, Bamia C, Trichopoulos D. Adherence to a Mediterranean diet and survival in a Greek population. N Engl J Med. 2003; 348(26):2599–608.

31. Buckland G, Agudo A, Lujan L, Jakszyn P, Bueno-de-Mesquita HB, Palli D, et al. Adherence to a Mediterranean diet and risk of gastric adenocarcinoma within the European prospective investigation into Cancer and nutrition (EPIC) cohort study. Am J Clin Nutr. 2010;91(2):381–90.

32. Bergmann MM, Bussas U, Boeing H. Follow-up procedures in EPIC-Germany–data quality aspects. European prospective investigation into Cancer and nutrition. Ann Nutr Metab. 1999;43(4):225–34.

33. Roswall N, Eriksson U, Sandin S, Lof M, Olsen A, Skeie G, et al. Adherence to the healthy Nordic food index, dietary composition, and lifestyle among Swedish women. Food Nutr Res. 2015;59:26336.

34. Kanerva N, Kaartinen NE, Schwab U, Lahti-Koski M, Mannisto S. Adherence to the Baltic Sea diet consumed in the Nordic countries is associated with lower abdominal obesity. Br J Nutr. 2013;109(3):520–8.

35. Kanerva N, Loo BM, Eriksson JG, Leiviska J, Kaartinen NE, Jula A, et al. Associations of the Baltic Sea diet with obesity-related markers of inflammation. Ann Med. 2014;46(2):90–6.

36. Mithril C, Dragsted LO, Meyer C, Tetens I, Biltoft-Jensen A, Astrup A. Dietary composition and nutrient content of the new Nordic diet. Public Health Nutr. 2013;16(5):777–85.

37. Schwingshackl L, Lampousi AM, Portillo MP, Romaguera D, Hoffmann G, Boeing H. Olive oil in the prevention and management of type 2 diabetes mellitus: a systematic review and meta-analysis of cohort studies and intervention trials. Nutr Diabetes. 2017;7(4):e262.

38. Schwingshackl L, Hoffmann G, Lampousi AM, Knuppel S, Iqbal K, Schwedhelm C, et al. Food groups and risk of type 2 diabetes mellitus: a systematic review and meta-analysis of prospective studies. Eur J Epidemiol. 2017;32(5):363–75.

39. Widmer RJ, Flammer AJ, Lerman LO, Lerman A. The Mediterranean diet, its components, and cardiovascular disease. Am J Med. 2015; 128(3):229–38.

40. Mostofsky E, Chahal HS, Mukamal KJ, Rimm EB, Mittleman MA. Alcohol and immediate risk of cardiovascular events: a systematic review and dose-response meta-analysis. Circulation. 2016;133(10):979–87.

41. Bell S, Daskalopoulou M, Rapsomaniki E, George J, Britton A, Bobak M, et al. Association between clinically recorded alcohol consumption and initial presentation of 12 cardiovascular diseases: population based cohort study using linked health records. BMJ. 2017;356:j909.

42. Bedard A, Riverin M, Dodin S, Corneau L, Lemieux S. Sex differences in the impact of the Mediterranean diet on cardiovascular risk profile. Br J Nutr. 2012;108(8):1428–34.

43. Knopp RH, Paramsothy P, Retzlaff BM, Fish B, Walden C, Dowdy A, et al. Gender differences in lipoprotein metabolism and dietary response: basis in hormonal differences and implications for cardiovascular disease. Curr Atheroscler Rep. 2005;7(6):472–9.

44. Lapointe A, Balk EM, Lichtenstein AH. Gender differences in plasma lipid response to dietary fat. Nutr Rev. 2006;64(5 Pt 1):234–49.

45. Bach A, Serra-Majem L, Carrasco JL, Roman B, Ngo J, Bertomeu I, et al. The use of indexes evaluating the adherence to the Mediterranean diet in epidemiological studies: a review. Public Health Nutr. 2006;9(1A):132–46.

46. Davis C, Bryan J, Hodgson J, Murphy K. Definition of the Mediterranean diet; a literature review. Nutrients. 2015;7(11):9139–53.

47. Mila-Villarroel R, Bach-Faig A, Puig J, Puchal A, Farran A, Serra-Majem L, et al. Comparison and evaluation of the reliability of indexes of adherence to the Mediterranean diet. Public Health Nutr. 2011;14(12A):2338–45.

48. Wirth J, di Giuseppe R, Boeing H, Weikert C. A Mediterranean-style diet, its components and the risk of heart failure: a prospective population-based study in a non-Mediterranean country. Eur J Clin Nutr. 2016;70(9):1015–21.

49. Sofi F, Macchi C, Abbate R, Gensini GF, Casini A. Mediterranean diet and health status: an updated meta-analysis and a proposal for a literature-based adherence score. Public Health Nutr. 2014;17(12):2769–82.

50. Trichopoulou A, Kouris-Blazos A, Wahlqvist ML, Gnardellis C, Lagiou P, Polychronopoulos E, et al. Diet and overall survival in elderly people. BMJ. 1995;311(7018):1457–60.

51. Ocke MC. Evaluation of methodologies for assessing the overall diet: dietary quality scores and dietary pattern analysis. Proc Nutr Soc. 2013;72(2):191–9.

52. Kristal AR, Peters U, Potter JD. Is it time to abandon the food frequency questionnaire? Cancer Epidemiol Biomark Prev. 2005;14(12):2826–8.

53. Willett WC, Hu FB. Not the time to abandon the food frequency questionnaire: point. Cancer Epidemiol Biomark Prev. 2006;15(10):1757–8.

11

Medical end-of-life practices in Swiss cultural regions: a death certificate study

Samia A. Hurst[1] (ID), Ueli Zellweger[2], Georg Bosshard[3], Matthias Bopp[2*] and for the Swiss Medical End-of-Life Decisions Study Group

Abstract

Background: End-of-life decisions remain controversial. Switzerland, with three main languages shared with surrounding countries and legal suicide assistance, allows exploration of the effects of cultural differences on end-of-life practices within the same legal framework.

Methods: We conducted a death certificate study on a nationwide continuous random sample of Swiss residents. Using an internationally standardized tool, we sent 4998, 2965, and 1000 anonymous questionnaires to certifying physicians in the German-, French-, and Italian-speaking regions.

Results: The response rates were 63.5%, 51.9%, and 61.7% in the German-, French-, and Italian-speaking regions, respectively. Non-sudden, expected deaths were preceded by medical end-of-life decisions (MELDs) more frequently in the German- than in the French- or Italian-speaking region (82.3% vs. 75.0% and 74.0%, respectively), mainly due to forgoing life-prolonging treatment (70.0%, 59.8%, 57.4%). Prevalence of assisted suicide was similar in the German- and French-speaking regions (1.6%, 1.2%), with no cases reported in the Italian-speaking region. Patient involvement was smaller in the Italian- than in the French- and German-speaking regions (16.0%, 31.2%, 35.6%). Continuous deep sedation was more frequent in the Italian- than in the French- and German-speaking regions (34.4%, 26.9%, 24.5%), and was combined with MELDs in most cases.

Conclusion: We found differences in MELD prevalence similar to those found between European countries. On an international level, MELDs are comparably frequent in all regions of Switzerland, in line with the greater role given to patient autonomy. Our findings show how cultural contexts and legislation can interact in shaping the prevalence of MELDs.

Background

In many countries worldwide, there is persistent controversy surrounding end-of-life decisions, particularly in relation to assisted suicide and euthanasia. Debates regarding the legal status of such decisions assume that legislative differences [1] and care settings [2, 3] largely determine international variation in prevalence. Countries where these decisions are legal and where several cultures co-exist, such as Switzerland, Belgium, the US, and more recently Canada, thus present an important opportunity to explore the role of legal and cultural frameworks for variations of end-of-life decisions.

Switzerland allows suicide assistance if it is offered without selfish motive and even when it is practiced by non-physicians [4], without recognizing an entitlement to such assistance [5]. In contrast to the Netherlands, Belgium, and Luxemburg, but similarly to the US states allowing suicide assistance, euthanasia is not legal [6–8]. "Suicide tourism" toward Switzerland has influenced end-of-life debates in countries such as Germany, the UK, the US, and Canada, from which many assisted suicide candidates originate [9].

Switzerland has four official languages, German, French, Italian, and Romansh, within defined geographical areas. The language regions share many cultural features with the respective neighboring countries, offering an opportunity to explore the effects of cultural differences on end-of-life practices within the same legal context [10]. Reliable population-level data on this field has only been collected

---

* Correspondence: matthias.bopp@uzh.ch
[2]Epidemiology, Biostatistics and Prevention Institute, University of Zurich, Hirschengraben 84, CH-8001 Zürich, Switzerland
Full list of author information is available at the end of the article

once in Switzerland in 2001, within the EURELD study [11]. However, the Swiss sample was limited to the German-speaking region. Other studies suggest that French physicians' support for legalizing euthanasia could be greater [12], and German physicians' lesser [13], than their Swiss counterparts. The ETHICUS study showed an increase in frequency in withdrawal of life-sustaining treatment from South to North Europe [14]. In the EURELD study, however, Sweden and Denmark showed lower prevalence than Belgium and the Netherlands, and much lower prevalence than (German-speaking) Switzerland [15]. Further, data from Belgium suggests that cultural differences between regions affect euthanasia practices within a country [2]. In Switzerland, substantial variations were described in physicians' attitudes between language regions, the most striking being a reluctance of Italian-speaking doctors against any kind of end-of-life decisions – in close similarity to Italy [16].

In 2013, we performed a follow-up study of the Swiss part of the EURELD study using the same methodology and largely the same questionnaire [11], but including the French- and Italian-speaking regions. Comparative data related to the German-speaking region of Switzerland in 2001 and 2013 have been published recently [17, 18]. This paper presents cross-sectional data of the different language regions of Switzerland on medical end-of-life decisions (MELDs).

Methods

Participants

Study methods have been described in more detail elsewhere [17, 18]. A continuous random sample of death certificates of residents aged 1 year or older was selected on a weekly basis by the Swiss Federal Statistical Office. We differentiated between German- (71.6% of total population), French- (23.6%), and Italian-speaking (4.4%) areas. Since Romansh, the fourth national language, is only spoken by less than 1% of the national population and its geographical area is not contiguous, it was included into the German-speaking region. Taking into account the smaller population size, the French- and Italian-speaking regions were oversampled. The sample size was chosen in order to obtain reliable data from all three language regions while limiting the risk that some physicians in the smaller language regions received too many questionnaires. In total, 21.3%, 41.1%, and 62.9% of registered deaths were respectively sampled among residents of the German-, French-, and Italian-speaking regions of Switzerland, and certifying physicians were invited to participate. Between August 1, 2013, and January 31, 2014, we sent 4998, 2965, and 1000 questionnaires in weekly batches to the three respective language regions. The last completed questionnaire arrived on June 11, 2014.

Survey tool

If death was not sudden and unexpected, the case was considered eligible for questions regarding end-of-life decisions. In such cases, physicians were asked whether they had (1) withheld or withdrawn a probably life-prolonging medical treatment taking into account or explicitly intending to hasten the patient's death; (2) intensified the alleviation of pain and/or symptoms with drugs taking into account or partly intending to hasten the patient's death; or (3) prescribed or administered a drug with the explicit intention of ending the patient's life (physician-assisted death). For this study, we categorized cases as a physician-assisted death when a positive response was given to question (3), irrespective of answers to questions (1) and (2). Positive answers to question (3) were categorized as follows:

(3a) "assisted suicide", if patients self-administered the drug to end their life;

(3b) "euthanasia", if somebody else administered the drug and the question regarding explicit request of the patient was answered affirmatively;

(3c) "ending of life without the patient's explicit request", if the question regarding explicit request of the patient was not answered affirmatively.

To evaluate continuous deep sedation, physicians were asked if the patient received medicines to maintain them in a continuous deep sedation or coma until death.

The survey tool was translated into French and Italian, back translated for quality control, and checked by bilingual individuals. The final questionnaire (four pages) is available upon request.

Human participant protection

To guarantee anonymity, physicians were requested to return questionnaires to the Swiss Academy of Medical Sciences. Questionnaires were only forwarded to the investigators at the Epidemiology, Biostatistics, and Prevention Institute of the University of Zurich (then Institute of Social and Preventive Medicine) after confirmation that the code key had been deleted for this case. Questionnaire return was considered to imply consent to participate. The study was declared exempt from ethics review by the Zurich Cantonal Ethics Board (KEK-StV-Nr. 23/13).

Data analysis

Questionnaires were scanned and all data were weighted to adjust for region-, age-, and sex-specific differences in response rates. Weighted percentages and 95% confidence intervals for the comparison of the three language regions were calculated using STATA 13.1 survey tables for weighted data (StataCorp LP, College Station, TX, US).

Results

Sample

Of 8963 mailed questionnaires, 3173 (63.5%), 1538 (51.9%), and 617 (61.7%) were returned from the German-, French-, and Italian-speaking regions of Switzerland, respectively, which is comparable to other research using this method [6].

Medical end-of-life decisions (MELDs)

Non-sudden, expected deaths were preceded by at least one MELD in a majority of cases, more frequently (82.3%) in the German- than in the French- (75%) or Italian-speaking (74%) regions (Table 1). Focusing on the most explicit practice, forgoing life-prolonging treatment was the most frequent MELD in the German-speaking region and intensified alleviation of symptoms the most frequent in the French-speaking region (49.3% of non-sudden expected deaths and 39.8%, respectively), with both being similarly frequent in the Italian-speaking region (34.8% and 37.4%, respectively). Assisted suicide was reported in 1.6% and 1.2% of non-sudden expected deaths in the German- and French-speaking regions, with no cases reported in the Italian-speaking region in our sample.

MELDs were combined in approximately half of the cases (Table 2). When all cases including a decision to forgo life-prolonging treatment were considered, the intention to shorten life was more frequent than only taking this into account in the German-speaking region (44.2% vs. 25.8%), while there were no statistically significant differences in the other two regions. Intensified alleviation of symptoms was similarly prevalent in all language regions. There was no intention to shorten life in most cases of alleviation of pain and symptoms; however, in a minority of cases, shortening of life was partly intended (more often in the German- and Italian- than in the French-speaking region).

Continuous deep sedation (CDS)

Death was preceded by medication to bring about CDS in many non-sudden, expected deaths (Table 3). This was more frequent in the Italian-speaking region than in the German- and French-speaking regions (34.4% vs. 24.4% and 26.9%). CDS were combined with MELDs in most cases. Deaths preceded by CDS without a MELD were slightly, but statistically significantly more frequent in the Italian- than in the German-speaking region (with intermediate prevalence in the French-speaking region).

Table 1 Prevalence of medical end-of-life practices[a] in Switzerland 2013, by language region

Regions	German-speaking		French-speaking		Italian-speaking	
Number of non-sudden expected deaths (eligible for end-of-life decision)	N = 2256		N = 992		N = 430	
	%[b]	95% CI	%[b]	95% CI	%[b]	95% CI
No end-of-life practice	17.7%	(16.2–19.3)	25.0%	(22.4–27.9)	26.0%	(22.0–30.3)
Forgoing life-prolonging treatment	49.4%	(47.3–51.4)	31.6%	(28.8–34.6)	34.8%	(30.4–39.5)
- taking into account hastening of death[c]	6.4%	(5.4–7.5)	5.2%	(4.0–6.7)	4.7%	(3.0–7.1)
- intending hastening of death[d]	43.0%	(40.9–45.0)	26.5%	(23.8–29.3)	30.1%	(26–34.7)
Intensified alleviation of pain/symptoms	29.8%	(28.0–31.7)	39.8%	(36.8–42.9)	37.4%	(33.0–42.1)
- taking into account hastening of death[e]	26.9%	(25.1–28.8)	36.6%	(33.7–39.7)	33.8%	(29.5–38.4)
- partly intending hastening of death[f]	2.9%	(2.3–3.7)	3.2%	(2.3–4.5)	3.6%	(2.2–5.8)
Physician-assisted death	3.1%	(2.5–3.9)	3.5%	(2.5–4.8)	1.8%	(0.9–3.6)
- Assisted suicide[g]	1.6%	(1.1–2.2)	1.2%	(0.6–2.1)	–	
- Euthanasia[h]	0.5%	(0.3–0.9)	0.5%	(0.2–1.2)	0.5%	(0.1–1.8)
- Ending of life without the patient's explicit request[i]	1.1%	(0.8–1.6)	1.9%	(1.2–2.9)	1.4%	(0.6–3.0)

[a]If several practices were combined, the most explicit action was decisive; e.g., combinations of physician-assisted death with forgoing life-prolonging treatments or intensified alleviation of pain and symptoms were categorized under physician-assisted death

[b]100% = all non-sudden expected deaths; percentages weighted to region-sex-age-specific response rates

[c]Affirmative answer to the question, "Did you or another physician withhold or withdraw a medical treatment while taking into account the possible hastening of death?"

[d]Affirmative answer to the question, "Did you or another physician withhold or withdraw a medical treatment with the intention to hasten death?"

[e]Affirmative answer to the question, "Did you or another physician intensify the alleviation of pain and/or symptoms while taking into account the possible hastening of death?"

[f]Affirmative answer to the question, "Did you or another physician intensify the alleviation of pain and/or symptoms partly with the intention to hasten death?"

[g]Affirmative answer to the question, "Was death the consequence of the use of a drug that was prescribed or supplied by you or another physician with the explicit intention of enabling the patient to end his or her life?"

[h]Affirmative answer to the question, "Was death the consequence of the use of a drug that was prescribed or supplied by you or another physician with the explicit intention of hastening the patient's death?" AND affirmative answer to the question: "Was this decision made at the explicit request of the patient?"

[i]Affirmative answer to the question, "Was death the consequence of the use of a drug that was prescribed or supplied by you or another physician with the explicit intention of hastening the patient's death?" AND no affirmative answer to the question: "Was this decision made at the explicit request of the patient?"

Table 2 Forgoing life-prolonging treatment and intensified alleviation of pain and symptoms, Switzerland 2013, by language region

Regions	German-speaking		French-speaking		Italian-speaking	
Number of non-sudden expected deaths (eligible for end-of-life decision)	N = 2256		N = 992		N = 430	
	%[a]	95% CI	%[a]	95% CI	%[a]	95% CI
Forgoing life-prolonging treatment						
Total	70.0%	(68.1–71.9)	59.8%	(56.7–62.8)	57.4%	(52.7–62.0)
- taking into account hastening of death	25.8%	(24.0–27.6)	32.1%	(29.3–35.1)	25.7%	(21.8–30.1)
- intending hastening of death	44.2%	(42.2–46.3)	27.7%	(25.0–30.6)	31.7%	(27.5–36.3)
- not combined with other medical end-of-life practice (1)	17.3%	(15.8–18.9)	12.5%	(10.6–14.7)	10.2%	(7.7–13.5)
- combined with intensified alleviation of pain/symptoms only	51.2%	(49.1–53.2)	45.0%	(41.9–48.1)	45.4%	(40.7–50.1)
- ditto, only intended forgoing treatment (2)	32.0%	(30.1–34.0)	19.2%	(16.8–21.7)	24.6%	(20.7–28.9)
- combined with physician-assisted death	1.5%	(0.1–2.1)	2.3%	(1.5–3.5)	1.8%	(0.9–3.6)
Intensified alleviation of pain/symptoms						
Total	63.4%	(61.4–65.3)	61.4%	(58.3–64.4)	63.8%	(59.1–68.2)
- taking into account hastening of death	51.7%	(49.7–53.8)	53.8%	(50.7–56.9)	48.8%	(44.1–53.5)
- partly intending hastening of death	11.6%	(10.4–13.0)	7.6%	(6.1–9.4)	15.0%	(11.9–18.8)
- not combined with other medical end-of-life practice (3)	10.7%	(9.5–12.0)	14.0%	(12.0–16.4)	16.6%	(13.4–20.5)
- combined with forgoing life-prolonging treatment only	51.2%	(49.1–53.2)	45.0%	(41.9–48.1)	45.4%	(40.7–50.1)
- ditto, only non-intended forgoing treatment (4)	19.1%	(17.6–20.8)	25.8%	(23.2–28.7)	20.8%	(17.2–24.9)
- combined with physician-assisted death	1.5%	(0.1–2.1)	24.0%	(1.6–3.6)	1.8%	(0.9–3.6)

[a]100% = all non-sudden expected deaths; percentages weighted to region-sex-age-specific response rates
Data in this table include cases in which more than one end-of-life decision were taken
Forgoing life-prolonging treatment as most explicit end-of-life decision (cf. Table 1): (1) + (2)
Intensified alleviation of pain/symptoms as most explicit end-of-life decision (cf. Table 1): (3) + (4)

Place of death

As outlined in Table 4, non-sudden expected deaths were more likely to occur without MELDs at home (25.8%) than in hospitals (15.7%) or nursing homes (17.6%) in the German-speaking region (Table 4). Forgoing life-prolonging treatment was less frequent at home than in hospitals or long-term care homes in the German-speaking region, and less frequent at home than in hospitals in the French-speaking region. Intensified alleviation of symptoms showed similar prevalence in all places of death in the French- and Italian-speaking regions, but was more frequent in hospitals (68.8%) and less frequent for home (53.1%) deaths than in long-term care homes (62.7%) in the German-speaking region. Assisted suicide was more frequent at home in the German- (4.2%) and

French-speaking (9%) regions, and did not occur in our sample in the Italian-speaking region.

Shared decision-making

Most MELDs were discussed with the patient or relatives, or based on previously known patient wishes (Table 5), with only a minority being discussed with the patient at the time of the decision. Patient involvement was less frequent in the Italian-speaking region (16%), as compared to the French- (31.2%) and German-speaking (35.6%) regions. Even when patients were fully capable of decision-making, up to 40% of MELDs occurred without their involvement, and approximately 12% occurred even without involving their relatives and without knowledge of previously expressed patient wishes.

Table 3 Continuous deep sedation in Switzerland 2013, by language region

Regions	German-speaking		French-speaking		Italian-speaking	
Non-sudden expected deaths	N = 2256		N = 992		N = 430	
	%[a]	95% CI	%[a]	95% CI	%[a]	95% CI
Continuous deep sedation until death (CDS)	24.5%	(22.3–26.3)	26.9%	(24.2–29.7)	34.4%	(30.1–39.0)
- CDS without end-of-life decision	1.6%	(1.2–2.2)	3.2%	(2.2–4.5)	5.1%	(3.4–7.6)
- CDS combined with end-of-life decision	22.8%	(21.1–25.6)	23.7%	(21.2–26.5)	29.3%	(25.2–33.8)

[a]100% = all non-sudden expected deaths; percentages weighted to region-sex-age-specific response rates

Table 4 Prevalence of medical end-of-life practices, Switzerland 2013, by language region and place of death

Regions Number of non-sudden expected deaths (eligible for end-of-life decision)	German-speaking N = 2256		French-speaking N = 992		Italian-speaking N = 430	
	%[a]	95% CI	%[a]	95% CI	%[a]	95% CI
At home	N = 265		N = 96		N = 67	
	11.6%	*(10.4–13)*	*9.5%*	*(7.9–11.5)*	*15.6%*	*(12.4–19.3)*
No end-of-life practice	25.8	(20.9–31.4)	24.6	(17.0–34.2)	31.1	(21.1–43.2)
Forgoing treatment total	60.3	(54.2–66.0)	47.0	(37.2–57.1)	45.8	(34.2–57.8)
Alleviation of pain & symptoms total	53.1	(47.1–59.1)	60.2	(50.0–69.6)	63.1	(51.0–73.8)
vPhysician-assisted death total	5.7	(3.5–9.2)	15.4	(9.3–24.4)	1.6	(0.2–10.5)
- Assisted suicide	4.2	(2.3–7.5)	9.0	(4.6–17.0)	–	
In long-term care homes	N = 982		N = 371		N = 186	
	44.3%	*(42.3–46.4)*	*38.6%*	*(35.6–41.7)*	*43.1%*	*(38.5–47.8)*
No end-of-life practice	17.6	(15.3–20.1)	23.9	(19.8–28.5)	27.1	(21.2–34.0)
Forgoing treatment total	71.5	(68.6–74.3)	59.1	(53.9–64.0)	54.8	(47.6–61.8)
Alleviation of pain and symptoms total	62.7	(59.6–65.7)	63.2	(58.2–68.0)	63.1	(55.9–69.8)
Physician-assisted death total	1.2	(0.7–2.2)	3.0	(1.7–5.4)	3.1	(1.4–6.8)
- Assisted suicide	0.1	(0.0–0.8)	0.3	(0.0–2.0)	–	
In hospital	N = 973		N = 522		N = 174	
	42.5%	*(40.5–44.6)*	*51.5%*	*(48.4–54.7)*	*40.6%*	*(36.1–45.4)*
No end-of-life practice	15.7	(13.5–18.1)	26.0	(22.4–30.0)	22.7	(17.0–29.5)
Forgoing treatment total	73.6	(70.4–75.9)	62.6	(58.4–66.7)	64.5	(57.1–71.3)
Alleviation of pain and symptoms total	68.8	(65.8–71.6)	60.2	(55.9–64.4)	65.9	(58.6–72.6)
Physician-assisted death total	2.0	(1.3–3.1)	1.7	(0.9–3.2)	0.5	(0.1–3.8)
- Assisted suicide	–		0.4	(0.1–1.4)	–	

[a]100% = all non-sudden expected deaths; percentages weighted to region-sex-age-specific response rates
Data in this table include cases in which more than one end-of-life decision were taken

Table 5 Discussion of medical end-of-life decisions[a] in function of the patient's decision-making capacity, Switzerland 2013, by language region

Regions Deaths with end-of-life practice mentioned (eligible for involvement)	German-speaking N = 1856		French-speaking N = 744		Italian-speaking N = 318	
	%[b]	95% CI	%[b]	95% CI	%[b]	95% CI
Discussed with patient	35.6%	(33.4–37.5)	31.2%	(27.9–34.6)	16.0%	(12.4–20.4)
Patient fully capable	73.3%	(69.6–76.6)	71.2%	(65.3–76.5)	60.0%	(47.2–71.6)
Patient not fully capable	37.1%	(32.3–42.3)	30.3%	(22.9–38.8)	8.4%	(3.8–17.6)
Patient not capable at all	9.7%	(7.6–12.2)	5.8%	(3.4–9.6)	6.9%	(3.6–12.8)
Patient's capacity unknown	3.4%	(1.7–6.7)	–		–	
Discussed with patient and/or relatives and/or patient ever expressed wish	76.5%	(74.5–78.4)	73.8%	(70.5–76.9)	69.0%	(63.7–73.8)
Patient fully capable	87.8%	(85.0–90.2)	88.5%	(84.0–91.9)	87.4%	(76.5–93.6)
Patient not fully capable	85.3%	(81.2–88.6)	82.9%	(75.3–88.5)	75.6%	(64.4–84.1)
Patient not capable at all	79.8%	(76.5–82.7)	82.2%	(76.6–86.6)	82.8%	(75.3–88.4)
Patient's capacity unknown	22.1%	(17.2–28.0)	20.4%	(14.2–28.4)	13.1%	(6.6–24.2)

[a]CDS is not a MELD and is thus not included in this table
[b]100% = all deaths with reported end-of-life practice; percentages weighted to region-sex-age-specific response rates

Discussion

To our best knowledge, this is the first population-level death-certificate study allowing comparison of real practice MELDs other than euthanasia between different cultural regions within the same country. Our study shows that MELDs are more frequent overall in the German-speaking region, and the prevalence of the MELD deemed most explicit varies between the three language regions in Switzerland, supporting the view that cultural differences subsist under the same legal system [2]. The view of Switzerland as "Europe in miniature" [16] is at least partly corroborated by our results. International comparison nevertheless shows a generally high proportion of MELDs in all regions of Switzerland when compared to countries sharing a language, such as France [19] or Italy [11], with no data currently available on the practice of MELD in Germany or Austria. This is in line with other studies suggesting that Switzerland is among the European countries where patient autonomy is given a greater weight in MELDs [20, 21].

Previous studies have shown distinct national cultures of end-of-life care [22]. Cultural influence on physicians' views of MELDs within the same country have been reported in a former Swiss survey [16] as well as between Walloon and Flemish physicians in Belgium [2]. Differences in patients' and families' requests may have even more impact than physicians' attitudes [20]. Despite being limited to a single specialty, reports of practices by a Sentinel Network of General Practitioners in the Dutch- and French-speaking regions of Belgium had also shown that the prevalence of MELDs was higher in the Dutch- than in the French-speaking community [23].

Our data suggest greater reluctance in forgoing life-prolonging treatment in the French- and Italian-speaking regions than in the German-speaking region, with partial replacement through either intensified alleviation of symptoms or CDS in French- and Italian-speaking regions. This is consonant with data from Belgium, showing more negative attitudes towards euthanasia and lower rates of reporting from the French- as compared to the Dutch-speaking region [2], and higher prevalence of CDS among French- than among Dutch-speaking physicians in the Brussels area [24]. In contrast, variation of intensified alleviation of symptoms between regions was almost absent in our sample. It has been proposed that this could be due to a perception that this constitutes a more direct response to a clinical situation [20]. There were no significant differences in the practice of suicide assistance in the German- and French-speaking regions, yet our sample recorded no case of suicide assistance in the Italian-speaking region [25].

International comparisons show a generally high proportion of MELDs in all regions of Switzerland.

Although these data were collected at different times, overall prevalence for MELDs was somewhat lower in France than in the French-speaking region [19] and substantially lower in Italy than in the Italian-speaking region of Switzerland [11]. Further, forgoing life-prolonging treatment was somewhat less frequent, and intensified alleviation of symptoms somewhat more frequent, in France than in the French-speaking region of Switzerland [19]. No comparative data are available from Germany.

Greater reluctance to forgo life-prolonging treatment may not be due to identical factors in the French- and Italian-speaking regions. The observed greater prevalence of hospital deaths in the French-speaking region suggests a greater tendency to pursue treatment, a finding consonant with greater appreciation of curative, technological, and specialist medicine in the French-speaking than in the Dutch-speaking community in Belgium [23]. Additionally, it is also consistent with a health system focus on hospitals rather than nursing homes in the French-speaking region, and with data showing structural effects of health systems on place of death [26]. However, this cannot explain the greater reluctance in the Italian-speaking region, where more deaths occurred at home than in the French-speaking region.

That most assisted suicide found in our sample took place at home is consistent with many hospitals' reluctance to allow suicide assistance, but also with data suggesting that the key reasons for patients to choose their homes include a concern to avoid loss of control [25].

Patient involvement in decisions was less frequent in the Italian-speaking region. Although this was mostly the case for patients deemed "not fully capable", a similar trend was shown for fully capable patients and those allocated to this category represented an implausibly small proportion when compared to the other two language regions. These data suggest that Italian-speaking doctors may be loath to discuss MELD, possibly because they have remained ambivalent towards MELDs, as suggested by previous findings comparing attitudes [16]. This is also consistent with international data showing higher prevalence of treatment preference discussions with Belgian and Dutch than with Spanish and Italian patients [27]. We did not find differences in the involvement of patients in the German- and French-speaking regions. However, a comparison of patient involvement in the Flemish- and French-speaking regions of Belgium did not show significant differences in patient involvement either [23].

Although culture is being used as an "umbrella term" herein, encompassing many different elements, our findings are compatible with the view that, compared to the German-speaking region, a more family-oriented approach is prevalent in the Italian-speaking region and a more technology-oriented approach in the French-speaking region. End-of-life decisions are debated simultaneously within countries, within single-language transnational regions, and internationally. Although these differences require qualitative exploration in order to be better understood, our results may show how national and language-based discussions can interact.

Our study has several limitations. The optimal phrasing of the questionnaire for international comparison purposes remains controversial [28]; this, however, is unlikely to affect intra-national comparison. We cannot exclude the possibility of a non-response bias, especially since responding that death was sudden and unexpected offered an easy option to skip all potentially sensitive questions. This would not have affected the intra-national comparison, were it not for the fact that response rates were different in the three language regions. This effect is not likely to be large; indeed, response rates in our study were remarkably high, especially given the fact that our survey had no official monitoring mission. Even in the French-speaking region, where response rates were lowest, they were clearly higher than in France (40%) [19] and Italy (44%) [11]. We may nevertheless have underestimated the prevalence of MELDs. The observation unit was deaths and not physicians; several physicians filled in more than one questionnaire. Due to the anonymous nature of the survey, questionnaires stemming from the same physician could not be identified. Therefore, the results are not necessarily representative for Swiss physicians. Although our sample size was much larger than other similar studies [23], small differences in the prevalence of MELDs may nevertheless have escaped our sample size, especially in the smaller language regions. More importantly, this method only allows exploration of what physicians believe happened. Depending on respondents' technical knowledge regarding MELDs, their beliefs may sometimes have been mistaken [29]. Despite this, this kind of study is still widely accepted as the gold standard for assessing MELDs on a population level.

Conclusion

Differences within Switzerland partly reflect practices in countries with the same linguistic tradition, but international comparisons show a generally high proportion of MELDs in all areas of the country, in line with the greater role given to patient autonomy. Our findings show how cultural contexts and legislation can interact in shaping the prevalence of MELDs.

Acknowledgements
The authors wish to thank the Swiss National Science Foundation (grant 406740-139309, National Research Program 67 "End-of-Life") and the SwissLife Jubiläumsstiftung for funding and supporting this study, the Swiss Federal Statistical Office for the identification of certifying physicians, the Swiss Academy of Medical Sciences for the de-identification of participants, Sarah Ziegler and Yolanda Penders for very useful comments, as well as the members of the Swiss Medical End-of-Life Decisions Study Group Dr. Karin Faisst (St. Gallen), Prof. em. Dr. Felix Gutzwiller (Zürich), Dr. Christoph Junker (Neuchâtel), Prof. Dr. Milo Puhan (Zürich), and Dr. Margareta Schmid (Zürich).

Funding
This study and one of the coauthors (UZ) were supported by the Swiss National Science Foundation (grant 406740-139309, National Research Program 67 "End-of-Life") and by an unconditional grant of the SwissLife Jubiläumsstiftung. The funding organizations had no influence in study design, analysis, or interpretation of data.

Authors' contributions
SAH contributed to the study design, questionnaire adaptation, data collection, data interpretation, and wrote the first draft and revision of the manuscript. GB contributed to the study design, questionnaire adaptation, data collection, data interpretation, and revision of the manuscript. UZ contributed to the conduct of the study, data collection, entry and cleaning, data analysis, and revision of the manuscript. MB contributed to the data analysis and interpretation of results, and conception and revision of the manuscript. All authors approved the final version.

Competing interests
The authors declare that they have no competing interests.

Author details
[1]Institute for Ethics, History, and the Humanities, Geneva University Medical School, 1211 Genève, Switzerland. [2]Epidemiology, Biostatistics and Prevention Institute, University of Zurich, Hirschengraben 84, CH-8001 Zürich, Switzerland. [3]Clinic for Geriatric Medicine, Zurich University Hospital, and Center on Aging and Mobility, University of Zurich and City Hospital Waid, Rämistrasse 100, 8091 Zürich, Switzerland.

References
1. Battin MP, van der Heide A, Ganzini L, van der Wal G, Onwuteaka-Philipsen BD. Legal physician-assisted dying in Oregon and the Netherlands: evidence concerning the impact on patients in "vulnerable" groups. J Med Ethics. 2007;33(10):591–7.
2. Cohen J, Van Wesemael Y, Smets T, Bilsen J, Deliens L. Cultural differences affecting euthanasia practice in Belgium: One law but different attitudes and practices in Flanders and Wallonia. Soc Sci Med. 2012;75(5):845–53.
3. Cohen J, Bilsen J, Fischer S, Loefmark R, Norup M, van der Heide A, et al. End-of-life decision-making in Belgium, Denmark, Sweden and Switzerland: does place of death make a difference? J Epidemiol Commun H. 2007;61(12):1062–8.
4. Hurst SA, Mauron A. Assisted suicide and euthanasia in Switzerland: allowing a role for non-physicians. Brit Med J. 2003;326(7383):271–3.
5. Hurst SA, Mauron A. Assisted suicide in Switzerland: clarifying liberties and claims. Bioethics. 2017;31(3):199–208.

6. Chambaere K, Vander Stichele R, Mortier F, Cohen J, Deliens L. Recent trends in euthanasia and other end-of-life practices in Belgium. N Engl J Med. 2015;372(12):1179–81.

7. Onwuteaka-Philipsen BD, Brinkman-Stoppelenburg A, Penning C, de Jong-Krul GJF, van Delden JJM, van der Heide A. Trends in end-of-life practices before and after the enactment of the euthanasia law in the Netherlands from 1990 to 2010: a repeated cross-sectional survey. Lancet. 2012; 380(9845):908–15.

8. van der Heide A, van Delden JJM, Onwuteaka-Philipsen BD. End-of-life decisions in the Netherlands over 25 Years. N Engl J Med. 2017;377(5): 492–4.

9. Gauthier S, Mausbach J, Reisch T, Bartsch C. Suicide tourism: a pilot study on the Swiss phenomenon. J Med Ethics. 2015;41(8):611–7.

10. Faeh D, Minder C, Gutzwiller F, Bopp M. Swiss National Cohort Study G. Culture, risk factors and mortality: can Switzerland add missing pieces to the European puzzle? J Epidemiol Community Health. 2009;63(8):639–45.

11. van der Heide A, Deliens L, Faisst K, Nilstun T, Norup M, Paci E, et al. End-of-life decision-making in six European countries: descriptive study. Lancet. 2003;362(9381):345–50.

12. Peretti-Watel P, Bendiane MK, Pegliasco H, Lapiana JM, Favre R, Galinier A, et al. Doctors' opinions on euthanasia, end of life care, and doctor-patient communication: telephone survey in France. Brit Med J. 2003; 327(7415):595–6.

13. Maitra RT, Harfst A, Bjerre LM, Kochen MM, Becker A. Do German general practitioners support euthanasia? Results of a nation-wide questionnaire survey. Eur J Gen Pract. 2005;11(3–4):94–100.

14. Sprung CL, Cohen SL, Sjokvist P, Baras M, Bulow HH, Hovilehto S, et al. End-of-life practices in European intensive care units - The Ethicus study. JAMA. 2003;290(6):790–7.

15. Bosshard G, Nilstun T, Bilsen J, Norup M, Miccinesi G, van Delden JJM, et al. Forgoing treatment at the end of life in 6 European countries. Arch Intern Med. 2005;165(4):401–7.

16. Fischer S, Bosshard G, Faisst K, Tschopp A, Fisher J, Bar W, et al. Swiss doctors' attitudes towards end-of-life decisions and their determinants - A comparison of three language regions. Swiss Med Wkly. 2006;136(23–24): 370–6.

17. Bosshard G, Zellweger U, Bopp M, Schmid M, Hurst SA, Puhan MA, et al. Medical end-of-life practices in Switzerland: a comparison of 2001 and 2013. JAMA Intern Med. 2016;176(4):555–6.

18. Schmid M, Zellweger U, Bosshard G, Bopp M. Decisions SME-O-L. Medical end-of-life decisions in Switzerland 2001 and 2013: Who is involved and how does the decision-making capacity of the patient impact? Swiss Med Wkly. 2016;146:w14307.

19. Pennec S, Monnier A, Pontone S, Aubry R. End-of-life medical decisions in France: a death certificate follow-up survey 5 years after the 2005 act of parliament on patients' rights and end of life. BMC Palliat Care. 2012;11:25.

20. Onwuteaka-Philipsen BD, Fisher S, Cartwright C, Deliens L, Miccinesi G, Norup M, et al. End-of-life decision making in Europe and Australia: a physician survey. Arch Intern Med. 2006;166(8):921–9.

21. Miccinesi G, Fischer S, Paci E, Onwuteaka-Philipsen BD, Cartwright C, van der Heide A, et al. Physicians' attitudes towards end-of-life decisions: a comparison between seven countries. Soc Sci Med. 2005;60(9):1961–74.

22. Gysels M, Evans N, Menaca A, Andrew E, Toscani F, Finetti S, et al. Culture and end of life care: a scoping exercise in seven European countries. Plos One. 2012;7(4):e34188.

23. Van den Block L, Deschepper R, Bilsen J, Bossuyt N, Van Casteren V, Deliens L. Euthanasia and other end-of-life decisions: a mortality follow-back study in Belgium. BMC Public Health. 2009;9:79.

24. Chambaere K, Bilsen J, Cohen J, Raman E, Deliens L. Differences in performance of euthanasia and continuous deep sedation by French- and Dutch-speaking physicians in Brussels, Belgium. J Pain Symptom Manag. 2010;39(2):e5–7.

25. Gamondi C, Pott M, Payne S. Families' experiences with patients who died after assisted suicide: a retrospective interview study in southern Switzerland. Ann Oncol. 2013;24(6):1639–44.

26. Orlovic M, Marti J, Mossialos E. Analysis of end-of-life care, out-of-pocket spending, and place of death in 16 European countries and Israel. Health Aff (Millwood). 2017;36(7):1201–10.

27. Evans N, Pasman HR, Alonso TV, van den Block L, Miccinesi G, Van Casteren V, et al. End-of-life decisions: a cross-national study of treatment preference

discussions and surrogate decision-maker appointments. Plos One. 2013; 8(3):e57965.

28. van der Heide A, Onwuteaka-Philipsen B, Deliens L, van Delden JJM, van der Maas PJ. End-of-life decisions in the United Kingdom. Palliative Med. 2009; 23(6):565–6.

29. Smets T, Bilsen J, Cohen J, Rurup ML, Mortier F, Deliens L. Reporting of euthanasia in medical practice in Flanders, Belgium: cross sectional analysis of reported and unreported cases. BMJ. 2010;341:c5174.

12

Trauma and perceived social rejection among Yazidi women and girls who survived enslavement and genocide

Hawkar Ibrahim[1,2,3*], Verena Ertl[1,3], Claudia Catani[1,3], Azad Ali Ismail[2] and Frank Neuner[1,3]

Abstract

Background: In August 2014, the Islamic State of Iraq and Syria (ISIS), a terrorist organization, attacked the Yazidi's ancestral homeland in northwestern Iraq. Among other atrocities, they abducted thousands of women and girls and traded many of them into sexual slavery. The aim of this study is to determine the mental health of women and girl survivors of these events in relation to enslavement and experiences with genocide-related events, as well as perceived social rejection in their community.

Methods: Between February and July 2017, trained local assessors interviewed a sample of 416 Yazidi women and girls (65 of whom had survived sexual enslavement), aged between 17 and 75 years, and living in internally displaced person camps in the Kurdistan Region of Iraq. Post-traumatic stress disorder (PTSD) and depression symptoms were assessed using validated Kurdish versions of standard instruments. Scales for trauma exposure and perceived rejection were developed for the purpose of this study.

Results: Participants reported a high number of traumatic events. More than 80% of girls and women, and almost all participants who were formerly enslaved, met criteria for a probable DSM-5 PTSD diagnosis. Trauma exposure and enslavement predicted poor mental health. In addition, among formerly enslaved girls and women, perceived social rejection in their community mediated the relationship between traumatic enslavement events and depression symptoms.

Conclusions: In a context of maximum adversity, enslavement and war-related events contribute to high levels of PTSD and depression. Perceived social rejection seems to play a role in the relationship between trauma exposure and mental health among abducted genocide survivors. Providing psychosocial support and treatment for Yazidi people is essential and urgently required.

Keywords: Kurd, Yazidi, Genocide, Enslavement, PTSD, Depression, Perceived social rejection

Background

The Yazidis (*Êzidî*) are a Kurdish religious minority living in the north of Iraq, western Iran, eastern Turkey, and northern Syria [1]. They are followers of Yazidism, a non-Abrahamic, orally transmitted religion [2] that shares common characteristics with Christianity, Islam, and other monotheistic religions. Following the upheaval of the Arab Spring movement in the Middle East, an Islamic fundamentalist militant group, the so-called Islamic State of Iraq and Syria (ISIS), declared an Islamic Caliphate in Syria and Iraq. In June 2014, ISIS fighters captured the center of the Nineveh governorate in Iraq and announced a campaign to purify their Caliphate of non-Arab and non-Sunni Muslim communities, committing numerous atrocities against the civilian population. Due to their ethnicity and religion, Yazidis, as a Kurdish religious minority, were among the most severely affected communities [3]. In August 2014, ISIS attacked the Yazidi's ancestral homeland in northwestern Iraq, close to the Iraqi–Syrian border. During the attack, ISIS killed, kidnapped, and enslaved thousands of children, men, women, and girls, displacing the entire community to refugee camps in the

---

* Correspondence: hawkar@uni-bielefeld.de
[1]Department of Psychology, Clinical Psychology and Psychotherapy, Bielefeld University, Bielefeld, Germany
[2]Department of Clinical Psychology, Koya University, Koya, Kurdistan Region, Iraq
Full list of author information is available at the end of the article

process [4]. Based on survey data, Cetorelli et al. [5] estimated that 3100 Yazidis were killed and 6800 were kidnapped in this operation. The Independent International Commission of Inquiry on the Syrian Arab Republic by United Nations Human Rights Council investigated the violations committed against Yazidis and documented that the Yazidi people were subjected to mass killings, rape, sexual violence, enslavement, torture, and forcible transfer, leading the it to declare ISIS's crimes against the Yazidis as a genocide [6].

War and atrocities in the context of genocide have negative effects for the survivors at both the individual and collective levels. Multiple types of traumatic events during periods of genocide, including witnessing extreme violence, the disappearance and loss of family members, rape and sexual humiliation, torture, imprisonment, and kidnapping [7, 8], can have psychological consequences [9–11]. Research conducted in other conflict regions, including Rwanda [12] and Bosnia [13], has found that genocidal atrocities bring about long-lasting and severe effects for the survivors, with up to almost 70% of the survivors fulfilling criteria for trauma-related disorders. Studies among non-Yazidi Kurdish genocide survivors in the Middle East have shown that survivors still suffer from a wide range of mental health conditions years and even decades after the genocide campaigns [14–17]. A few recent studies with small- to medium-sized samples of forcibly displaced Yazidis have documented high rates of mental ill-health. Based on clinical interviews, Tekin et al. [18] found rates of 43% for PTSD and 40% for major depression among Yazidis displaced into Turkey. Similar levels were found for Yazidi children in Turkey [19, 20].

Sexual violence against women has commonly been systematically used during wars and genocide, with the aim of traumatizing the civilian population and the elimination of the targeted group through the desecration of individual group members [21]. Systematic rape and sexual violence have devastating effects on social, psychological, and physical health, including genital and non-genital injuries experienced by the survivors [22, 23]. Such violence contributes to a range of psychological disorders. Clinically significant psychological disorders have been documented in 69.4% of survivors of war-related sexual violence in northern Uganda. Sexual violence may occur over extended periods of time after the abduction of girls and women. Such extreme adversity hardly goes without long-term harm for the survivors, with almost 85% of the sample of abducted rape survivors from Bosnia and Congo presenting with trauma-related disorders [24]. A recent review of 20 studies of civilians who experienced war-related sexual violence from six countries across Africa and Europe concluded that the psychological sequelae of wartime sexual violence most often included extreme rates of PTSD, anxiety, and depression [25]. More

recently, Hoffman et al. [26] assessed the prevalence of PTSD as well as complex PTSD among 108 female Yazidi former ISIS captives and found that 50.9% of them had probable complex PTSD, while 20% had probable PTSD.

The negative impacts of rape and wartime sexual violence extend into the survivors' social lives. Victims of wartime sexual violence are commonly faced with rejection by their community and family members [27, 28]. Sexual violence has been associated with perceived levels of stigma and poor community relations among girls who were abducted by a rebel army in northern Uganda [29]. A recent study in the war region of eastern Congo [30] documented stigmatization, rejection, and abandonment among survivors of sexual violence. More than half of survivors of sexual violence had been told they should leave their home because they had been raped, and the same proportion perceived that their status in the community had decreased. More than two-thirds of survivors avoided attending church due to fear of being stigmatized as a survivor of sexual violence.

It is likely that the psychological and social consequences of sexual violence are more than independent outcomes that occur on different socioecological levels. Across different conceptual and theoretical frameworks, the association between social factors and psychological trauma has been well documented. Social support from the immediate environment has been identified as one of the most consistent predictor of psychological adaptation following a wide range of traumatic event types [31], including forced displacement [32, 33], although causality of this relationship remains unclear [34, 35]. Consistent with research on social support, the manner and extent to which people in the social community acknowledge the survivor's experiences of violence are associated with the survivor's well-being [36–39]. Conversely, social rejection seems to promote and maintain the symptoms of psychological disorders. A significant association between family rejection, PTSD, and depression symptoms has been documented among conflict-affected adult women in the eastern Congo [40]. A similar association between social discrimination and a range of mental health problems was also found in formerly abducted girls in northern Uganda [41].

While the negative psychosocial consequences of war-related mass sexual violence seem obvious given the background of current knowledge about trauma, there is a dearth of systematic research on individuals who experienced extreme levels of adversities during war, including enslavement. Herein, we compared two samples of Yazidi survivors of the ISIS atrocities in the Middle East, one with a history of enslavement and one without experiences of such. In this context, we aimed to determine predictors for poor mental health, specifically seeking to investigate whether enslavement has a unique contribution to PTSD and depression symptoms above and beyond other traumatic, war-related events. In addition, given the observation that some of the formerly abducted survivors reported rejection from their own communities, we aimed to test whether perceived social rejection contributed to the maintenance of poor mental health.

Methods

Participants

The participants consisted of 416 female Yazidi adult and youth survivors of the civil war in Syria and northern Iraq. A portion of them (15.6%) were survivors who had been abducted by ISIS and kept as slaves. Their periods of abduction and enslavement ranged from 1 day to 2.5 years (M = 9.01, SD = 9.21, in months). At the time of the interview, the age of participants ranged between 17 and 75 years (M = 31.68, SD = 12.63). The majority (78.4%) were currently married and more than half (54.3%) were illiterate. Only 10.4% of the married participants had no children, while the other married participants had between 1 and 12 children (M = 3.26, SD = 3.12). While a large majority of the participants (87.7%) had no regular monthly income, others had monthly incomes between 70,000 and 900,000 IQD (1390 IQD = 1 €, local rate). Only 18.5% of participants reported having received any type of psychosocial support (Table 1).

Procedures

Sampling

The sample was drawn from Yazidi women and girls residing in the Khanke and Arbat camps for internally displaced people (IDP), located in the Dohuk and Sulaymaniyah Governorates of the Kurdistan Region of Iraq (KRI). Of the 436 Yazidi women and girls invited to participate in this study, 22 refused. The most commonly reported reasons for refusing were "*I don't want to talk about this experience*" and "*I got tired of interviews*". The participants were selected based on a pragmatic sampling approach. The camps were subdivided into six to seven sections by the camp administrations, and tents were chosen based on a random selection of households by spinning a pen from the zone center. Trained interviewers visited the household that was in a straight line from the tip of the pen, identified the girls and women in the household and determined their eligibility for participation in the study. From each nuclear family, a maximum of two women or girls of at least 17 years of age were interviewed. All participants were interviewed individually by using a structured interview based on standardized questionnaires.

Protection and safety

All participants were informed about the availability of no-cost mental health services inside their IDP camps.

The address cards and contact details of relevant organizations were provided to educated participants. Before the start of data collection, we created a referral system in collaboration with local NGOs and camp administration for those participants who wished to receive psychological help and for those who were severely affected by displacement and enslavement events or by family issues. In Khanke camp, we referred our participants to the Rawshan center of People's Development Organization, supported by Norwegian People's Aid. Rawshan (*Rewşen*) is a People's Development Organization community center in Khanke camp that provides services to the majority of displaced people. Rawshan has a specific focus on women and young girls, especially to those who suffer from mental health problems, family, and gender-based violence. Rawshan center's mental health programs include psychiatric help provided by female psychiatrists, with psychotherapy and counseling provided by female psychologists trained at the BSc level.

In Arbat camp, we referred participants who needed support to the camp hospital to receive first aid psychiatric help or to NGOs that provided mental health rehabilitation programs. The location of the participants' tent and NGO's waiting list were taken into consideration when referring the individual to a specific NGO. In total, 32 participants (29 from Kahnke and 3 from Arbat camp) were referred for psychological/psychiatric help. Upon request of the participants, a 2-week follow-up was conducted by the first author, with the purpose of ensuring that the referred participants had received adequate support.

Interviewers

The interviews were conducted by 10 trained, local female BSc-level clinical psychologists who had experience with the displaced people living in KRI. As part of the training, intensive theoretical and practical training about the study instruments, mental health risk management, and diagnostic and ethical issues in mental health research studies were provided during a 7-day workshop. In addition, local interviewers also attended a 1-day tour to Arbat and Khanke camps to provide relevant information about the profile of the camps and to meet the administration staff and those local and international organizations who have psychosocial support programs based in the camps. The interviews took place in the participants' tents and lasted between 60 and 90 min.

The population in the camp, particularly the illiterate participants, expressed a strong distrust and skepticism of any official authority figures and were not willing to sign any document. Due to the skepticism of the population and to protect the participants, we relied on obtaining verbal rather than written informed consent through reading standardized written consent information sheets to the respondents. Each explicit verbal consent was

Table 1 Sociodemographic information and traumatic experiences

	Total sample (n = 416)	Non-slaves (n = 351)	Formerly enslaved (n = 65)
Age, mean (SD)[a]	31.68 (12.63)	30.48 (11.15)	38.16 (17.42)
Current marital status, n (%)			
Single	90 (21.6)	79 (22.5)	11 (16.9)
Married	326 (78.4)	272 (77.5)	54 (83.1)
Formal education, mean (SD)[a]	2.78 (3.69)	2.9 (3.74)	2.12 (3.40)
Place of growing up, n (%)			
Town	160 (38.5)	135 (38.5)	25 (38.5)
Village	256 (61.5)	216 (61.5)	40 (61.5)
Occupation, n (%)			
Currently working	26 (6.3)	18 (5.1)	8 (12.3)
Currently not working	390 (93.8)	333 (94.9)	57 (87.7)
Having regular income, n (%)			
No	365 (87.7)	311 (88.6)	54 (83.1)
Yes	51 (12.3)	40 (11.4)	11 (16.9)
Individual monthly income, mean (SD)[b]	27,824.51 (105,596.48)	25,470.08 (100,864.08)	40,538.46 (128,349.26)
Number of children, mean (SD)	3.26 (3.12)	3.19 (3.17)	3.60 (2.86)
Number of boys, mean (SD)	1.65 (1.83)	1.62 (1.84)	1.81 (1.75)
Number of girls, mean (SD)	1.59 (1.76)	1.56 (1.76)	1.78 (1.76)
Number of lifetime displacements, mean (SD)	1.10 (0.5)	1.11 (0.53)	1.06 (0.24)
Age during war, mean (SD)[a]	28.96 (12.68)	27.68 (11.17)	35.87 (17.40)
Location during war			
Town	161 (38.7)	137 (39)	24 (36.9)
Village	255 (61.3)	214 (61)	41 (63.1)
Number of family members directly affected by ISIS, mean (SD)[c]	6.16 (12.71)	4.20 (10.43)	16.73 (17.83)
Receiving psychosocial support			
No	339 (81.5)	294 (83.8)	45 (69.2)
Yes	77 (18.5)	57 (16.2)	20 (30.8)
Traumatic events, mean (SD)[d]	5.79 (3.02)	5.79 (3.02)	12.15 (4.30)
War-related events mean (SD)[e]	3.40 (2.05)	3.40 (2.05)	7.38 (2.19)
General life events[f]	2.76 (2.37)	2.39 (2.01)	4.76 (3.08)

[a] In years
[b] In Iraqi Dinar
[c] Score range: 0–140
[d] Score range: 0–25
[e] Score range: 0–10
[f] Score range: 0–15

documented by the interviewer and confirmed by her signature. The study and its procedure, including the reliance on verbal informed consents, were approved by the Ethical Committee of Bielefeld University in Germany as well as the Ethical Committee of Koya University in the KRI.

Instruments
Traumatic events
To examine general and war-related traumatic events experienced during the war, we developed the War and

Adversity Exposure Checklist as a combination of items that had been collected from various sources, including existing trauma instruments, such as the War Exposure Scale [42], Life Events Checklist for DSM-5 [43], and informal interviews with war survivors from the Syrian and Iraqi civil war. Both the War Exposure Scale and the Life Events Checklist for DSM-5 had been previously employed in the validation study among Kurdish and Arab displaced populations living in the KRI [42]. The trauma score was computed by summing the affirmative answers to the items on the instrument. The internal consistency of the War and Adversity Exposure Checklist, as measured by Cronbach's alpha, was acceptable ($\alpha = 0.77$).

Enslavement trauma scale

This checklist was specifically developed for this study to assess potentially traumatic events that occurred during enslavement. It was created on the basis of open discussions with ISIS slave survivors and key informants, including psychological staff in the camps. The 20-item events reflected Yazidi women's experiences of abuse by ISIS (e.g., forced religious conversion, being sold in ISIS sex slave markets, and witnessing people being beheaded or burnt to death, etc.). The checklist had a high internal consistency (Cronbach's alpha = 0.90).

Perceived social rejection

In order to examine the social experience of survivors within their family and social community post-enslavement, a short questionnaire of perceived social rejection was developed based on interviews with survivors who had previously been abducted by ISIS. The wording of existing stigma and social rejection scales were too complex to employ them with the population included in this study due to the high rates of illiteracy. The resulting questionnaire consisted of five questions ('Are you worried about not getting married or remaining married as result of what you have experienced?', 'Do you feel excluded by your family?', 'Do you feel excluded (or stigmatized) by members of your community?', 'Are you avoiding people or social situations (events) as a result of fear of being rejected or stigmatized?', and 'Are you worried about what other people think of what you have experienced?') with responses rated on a 4-point Likert scale. Response scores for each item ranged from 0 to 3 (Not at all = 0, A little = 1, Quite a bit = 2, Extremely = 3). The items of the perceived social rejection scale were factor analyzed using maximum likelihood factoring with oblique rotation. The Kaiser–Meyer–Olkin measure of sampling adequacy was 0.738, thus exceeding the recommended value of 0.6. Bartlett's test of sphericity was significant ($p < 0.0001$). The analysis produced one factor that explained 44.23% of the variance, and item loadings on this factor ranged between 0.753 and 0.559. This questionnaire had acceptable internal consistency (Cronbach's alpha = 0.79).

PTSD symptoms

We assessed PTSD symptoms with the Kurdish version of the PTSD Checklist for DSM-5 (PCL-5) [42]. The PCL-5 [44] is a self-report measure developed on the basis of the DSM-5 symptom criteria for PTSD, which contains 20 items, categorized into four symptom clusters and rated on a 5-point Likert scale, with scores ranging from 'Not at all' = 0 to 'Extremely' = 4. For the probable diagnosis of PTSD, the authors of the original version suggested a cut-off score of 33 [44], while a calibration study with the Kurdish version indicated a cut-off of 23 for the optimum fit with a diagnosis [42]. The internal consistency of the PCL-5 in the current study (Cronbach's alpha = 0.86) was quite close to the consistency in the validation study.

Depression symptoms

The second part of Hopkins Symptom Checklist-25 [45] was used to examine depression symptoms. This checklist had previously been used within Kurdish and Arab populations [42]. It consists of 15 items on a 4-point scale ('Not at all', 'A little', 'Quite a bit', and 'Extremely' rated 1 to 4, respectively). The mean scores range between 1 and 4, where higher scores indicate higher levels of symptoms. The internal consistency of Hopkins Symptom Checklist-25 in the current study was high (Cronbach's alpha = 0.89).

Data analysis

The collected data was analyzed using the Statistical Package for Social Sciences (SPSS-Mac version 25 and JMP 13). An exploratory data analysis was conducted to determine whether PTSD and depression scores were normally distributed, in addition to visual inspection of the histograms and a Q-Q plots. Results showed that the PTSD and depression scores were approximately normally distributed for non-enslaved, formerly enslaved, and across groups. The same exploratory data analysis was conducted for other variables and results showed that perceived social rejection and enslavement events were also normally distributed (Additional file 1: Table S1). T-tests were applied to determine group differences. Relationships between continuous variables were tested with bivariate Pearson correlations for normally distributed variables (PTSD, depression, enslavement events, and perceived social rejection), and with Spearman-rank correlations for continuous variables with non-normal distributions (age, education, number of children, income, number of lifetime displacement, and trauma score); the association between dichotomous variables and continuous variables were tested using point-biserial correlations. A mediation analysis was carried out based on a bootstrapping procedure using PROCESS macro version 3.0 [46] for SPSS to clarify the mediating role of perceived social rejection in the association between enslavement events and mental health. The bootstrap mediation analysis is a non-parametric method that can be applied to small and moderate sample sizes [47], regardless of the distribution of the sample. Direct and indirect effects of enslavement events on symptoms of depression and PTSD were estimated using a set of ordinary least squares regressions.

Standardized estimates of the resulting path coefficients, as well as tests of significance for each path were calculated using two regressions (one for the mediator as the outcome and one for the chosen measure of symptoms as the outcome). We used bootstrapping based on 5000 bootstrap samples to infer statistical significance (alpha level = 0.05). To determine the unique effect size and statistical significance of potential predictors of PTSD and depression symptoms we calculated linear models. Although the intracluster correlations were generally low (PTSD symptoms intracluster correlation coefficient = 0.0053; depression symptoms intracluster correlation coefficient = 0.0054), we accounted for cluster sampling using a mixed linear model calculated with JMP 13 (SAS Institute, Cary, NC, USA) that provides mixed models based on the SAS PROC MIXED procedure. Internal consistency was determined using Cronbach's alpha.

Results

Traumatic events

Participants reported experiencing between 0 and 20 traumatic events of different types ($M = 5.79$, $SD = 3.02$). Of all participants, 99% had experienced at least one traumatic event; 85.1% of participants reported that they had experienced food and water deprivation, 63.7% had direct exposure to armed- and combat-related events, and half of the participants were separated from their family members by force. Regarding general life events during the period of genocide, witnessing fire or explosion (43.5%), natural disaster (29.3%), and transportation accidents (26%) were among the most common traumatic life events. Formerly enslaved participants reported experiencing and/or witnessing a significantly higher number of traumatic events than did non-enslaved women and girls (non-enslaved: $M = 5.79$, $SD = 3.02$; formerly enslaved: $M = 12.15$, $SD = 4.30$; two-tailed t test (unequal variances): $t (76.07) = -11.38$, $p < .001$). Furthermore, formerly enslaved participants had also experienced a significantly higher number of general and war-related traumatic events (war related events: (non-enslaved: $M = 3.40$, $SD = 2.05$; formerly enslaved: $M = 7.38$, $SD = 2.19$; two-tailed t test (equal variances): $t (414) = -14.215$, $p < 0.001$); general life events: (non-enslaved: $M = 2.39$, $SD = 2.01$; formerly enslaved: $M = 4.76$, $SD = 3.08$; two-tailed t test (unequal variances): $t (74.4) = -7.94$, $p < 0.001$).

Enslavement events

As shown in Fig. 1, formerly enslaved participants experienced between 0 and 20 enslavement event types ($M = 7.96$, $SD = 5.21$). There was no statistically significant difference between women and girls in experiencing enslavement events (girls: $M = 8.09$, $SD = 6.93$; women: $M = 7.61$, $SD = 4.86$; two-tailed t test (equal variances): $t (63) = -0.276$, $p = 0.783$). There was no statistically significant relationship between enslavement events and age ($p > 0.05$).

Mental health symptomatology

Formerly enslaved subjects reported significantly higher levels of PTSD ($M = 61.5$ vs. 47.5) and depression ($M =$

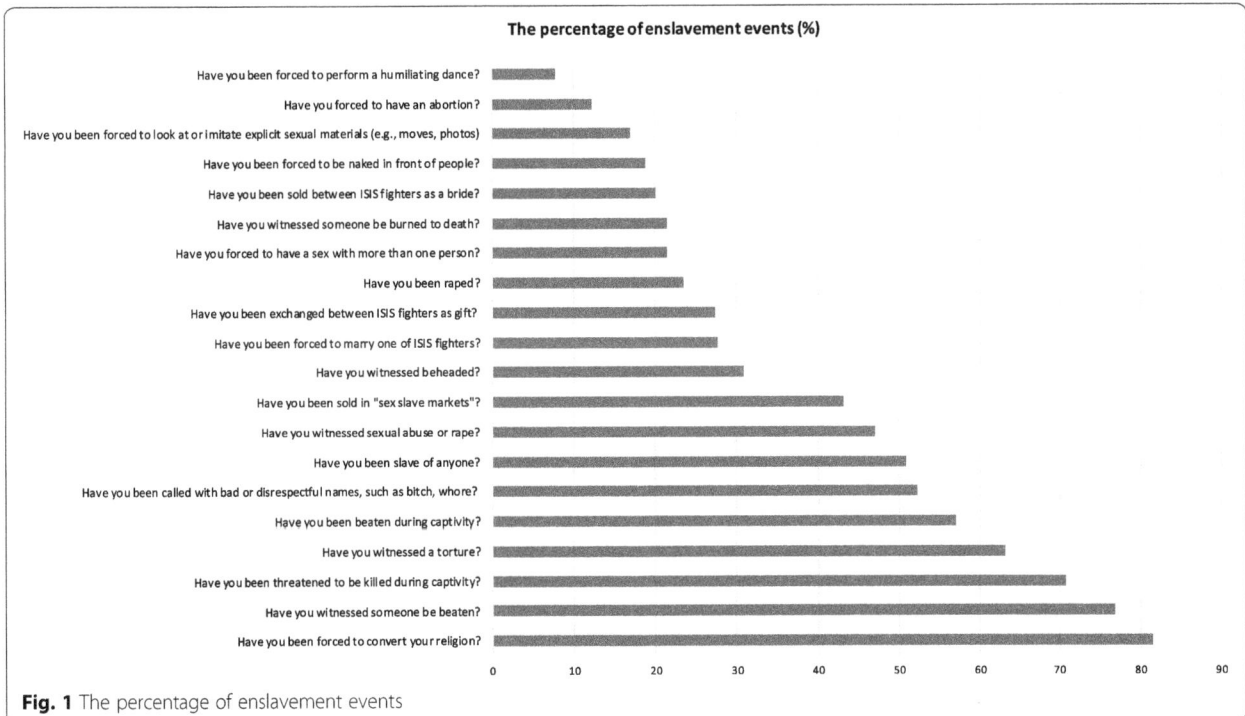

Fig. 1 The percentage of enslavement events

45.3 vs. 35.7) symptoms than did non-enslaved women and girls ($p < 0.001$). Using cut-off scores of 33 as a preliminary cut-point score suggested for the instrument [44], 88.9% of non-enslaved and 98.5% of formerly enslaved participants met DSM-5 symptom criteria for PTSD. When we used the culturally validated cut-off score of 23 [42], we found that all formerly enslaved and 97.2% of non-enslaved participants fulfilled the DSM-5 criteria for a PTSD diagnosis.

Perceived social rejection

Formally enslaved participants reported perceived social rejection ($M = 7.04$, $SD = 4.93$, range 0–15), with 32.3% being worried about not getting married or continuing in their marriage. The participants' feeling of exclusion by family and community members was high; 44.6% of formerly enslaved participants felt extremely excluded by community members. In addition, 49.2% reported extreme worry about what people thought of what they had experienced and 40% of them reported that they avoided people or social events as a result of fear of being rejected or stigmatized. The levels of perceived social rejection were not correlated with participants' level of education, age, or enslavement duration, but there was a significant positive relationship between perceived social rejection and the number of experienced enslavement events (Additional file 1: Table S2).

Associations of enslavement events, mental health, and perceived social rejection

As Fig. 2 illustrates, after controlling for the number of experienced traumatic events, the sum score of enslavement events was positively correlated with perceived social rejection ($\beta = 0.669$, $t = 4.49$, $p < 0.001$), PTSD ($\beta = 0.483$, $t = 3.59$, $p < 0.001$), and depression ($\beta = 0.678$, $t = 5.88$, $p < 0.001$). To examine the mediating role of perceived social rejection in this association we tested a simple mediation effect. After cntrolling for the mediating influence of perceived social rejection, the direct

effect of enslavement events on PTSD and depression was reduced but remained significant. The indirect effect was tested using a bootstrap estimation approach and results showed that the indirect effect reached significance for depression ($\beta = 0.194$, 95% CI 0.01 to 0.37) but not for PTSD ($\beta = 0.117$, 95% CI – 0.10 to 0.36).

Prediction of mental health symptomatology

Hierarchical linear model analyses were used to investigate potential predictors for PTSD and depression symptoms. The first model was created for the whole sample ($n = 416$). In this model, we entered age, years of formal education, marital status, individual monthly income, the number of family members who were directly affected by ISIS, trauma score, and enslavement as independent variables to predict PTSD and depression as dependent variables (Table 2). In addition, bivariate relationships were analyzed using zero-order correlations. The second model has been proposed to explain predictors of PTSD and depression among formerly enslaved participants ($n = 65$) (Table 3). The normality assumption of residuals for both models was checked using box plots and Q-Q plots, as well as Kolmogorov–Smirnov and Shapiro–Wilk tests. The results showed that standardized and unstandardized residuals of PTSD and depression scores in both models were normally distributed (Kolmogorov–Smirnov and Shapiro–Wilk $p > 0.05$).

Discussion

The current study demonstrated the psychosocial consequences of genocide and enslavement among Yazidi women and girls living in IDP camps in KRI. Findings suggest that high rates of mental health symptoms were mainly predicted by the intensity of trauma exposure. Enslavement predicted a worse outcome over and above the effect of traumatic event types. At the same time, our findings indicate that perceived social rejection plays a mediating role in the relationship between trauma and mental health.

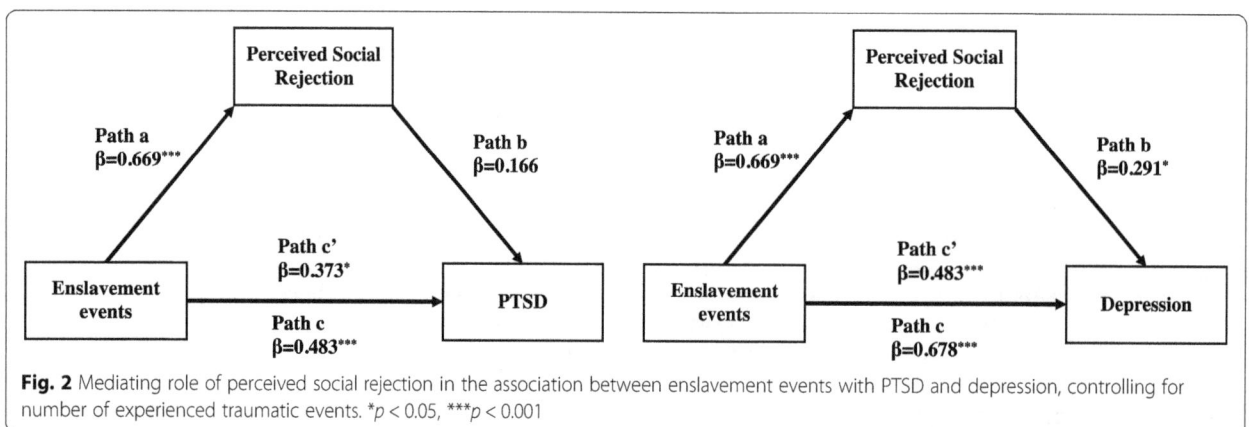

Fig. 2 Mediating role of perceived social rejection in the association between enslavement events with PTSD and depression, controlling for number of experienced traumatic events. *$p < 0.05$, ***$p < 0.001$

Table 2 Predictors of PTSD and depression symptoms among the total sample ($n = 416$)

Predictor	PTSD[a]		Depression[b]	
	Standardized ß-coefficient	Zero-order correlation	Standardized ß-coefficient	Zero-order correlation
Age	− 0.010	0.070	0.056	0.198**
Education	− 0.035	− 0.013	− 0.021	− 0.049
Marital status	− 0.013	0.020	0.082	0.139**
Income	0.089*	0.007	0.071	0.008
Number of family members directly affected by IS	0.195***	0.278***	0.213***	0.319***
Trauma score	0.182**	0.295***	0.196***	0.308***
Enslavement	0.171**	0.351***	0.127*	0.339***

[a] PTSD = (F (7,408) = 24.04, $p < 0.000$), with an R^2 of 0.19
[b] Depression = (F (7,408) = 15.62, $p < 0.001$), with an R^2 of 0.21
*$p = 0.05$, **$p < 0.01$, ***$p < 0.001$

Yazidi women who survived war atrocities represent a highly traumatized population. Rates of trauma exposure documented in our study are in line with numerous reports by international organizations about sexual and gender-based crimes against Yazidi women and girls [3, 6, 48]. It is also consistent with studies among female survivors of other genocides and armed conflicts [49–51]. The high exposure to adversities in this population is associated with very high rates of mental ill-health, which confirms previous reports of excessive rates of mental disorders in extremely traumatized war populations [52–54]. Yazidi women and girls who survived enslavement reported even more severe PTSD and depression symptoms. This effect remained stable after controlling for traumatic event types experienced by the survivors. While we are not aware of research on comparable populations reporting enslavement, studies with survivors of abduction, including victims of sex trafficking [55], child soldiers [56, 57], and formerly abducted people [58, 59], have confirmed the extraordinarily harmful effects of abduction. Even when considering the severity of trauma load

reported by the population, the prevalence rate of DSM-5 PTSD of approximately 90% found in this study is exceptionally high, especially when considering that a validated instrument was utilized. Such high prevalence of mental health disorders can be potentially attributed to the fact that all participants were females. Studies among genocide-affected populations showed that the prevalence rates of PTSD and depression are more than two times higher in women than in men [60, 61]. Moreover, subjects still lived in dependence and insecurity in refugee camps and less than one-quarter of the participants reported any type of professional psychosocial support. Furthermore, given that the Yazidis have a male-dominated and community-oriented culture, any intimate relationship outside of their social community is prohibited. Therefore, Yazidi women and girls who have a history of enslavement, rape, and sexual violence may find themselves isolated in the aftermath of enslavement, and this may contribute to severe mental health symptoms. Together, all these factors could be a potential explanation for the high

Table 3 Predictors of PTSD and depression among formerly enslaved women and girls ($n = 65$)

Predictor	PTSD[a]		Depression[b]	
	Standardized ß-Coefficient	Zero-order correlation	Standardized ß-Coefficient	Zero-order correlation
Age	− 0.119	− 0.189	0.059	− 0.042
Education	− 0.127	− 0.092	0.087	− 0.008
Marital status	0.026	− 0.005	0.183	0.152
Income	0.026	0.059	− 0.057	− 0.013
Number of family members who directly affected by ISIS	0.244*	0.415**	0.173	0.479***
Trauma score	0.019	0.212	− 0.040	0.315**
Enslavement events score	0.308*	0.509***	0.642***	0.669***

[a] PTSD = (F (7,57) = 3.14, $p < 0.05$), with an R^2 of 0.27
[b] Depression = (F (7,57) = 7.96, $p < 0.001$), with an R^2 of 0.49
*$p < 0.05$, **$p < 0.01$, ***$p < 0.001$

prevalence rates of mental health disorders in this study's sample.

Formerly enslaved women and girls perceived diverse levels of social rejection by their family and community members. The same phenomenon has been found among formerly abducted girls [62] and female victims of war-related sexual violence [27], who were likely to face or perceive stigma, discrimination, and social rejection. In line with research from Africa [41, 63], we found a significant relationship between mental health disorders and post-enslavement social stressors such as perceived stigma and social rejection. This finding is also consistent with results from meta-analytic studies that showed that, in general, perceived discrimination has negative outcomes on individual well-being [64, 65]. Furthermore, our findings indicate that the relationship between enslavement events and depression are partially mediated by perceived social rejection, while the mediation effect for PTSD did not reach significance. The nature of depression, associated with social conditions and life events, in contrast to PTSD, which may be conceptualized as a disorder of memory, could explain part of this finding.

This study has implications for the development of psychosocial and mental health programs. The high rates of mental health symptoms present should serve as a call to local and international organizations for urgent psychological intervention for Yazidi women and girls. Moreover, organizations could consider designing some social activity programs using the context of education for reintegrating formally enslaved females into their social community.

While our study is, to our knowledge, one of the first comprehensive studies to evaluate the mental health of Yazidi women and girls in the aftermath of genocide, several limitations should be noted. First, although we were careful to obtain an unbiased sample, it is impossible to evaluate to what extent the sample is representative of all female Yazidi survivors. Our sample consists only of those Yazidi women and girls who live in IDP camps in KRI, while some of the Yazidi survivors, especially those who were without male protection, live outside the camps. Further, although the majority of formally enslaved Yazidis were children and adolescents, we only interviewed those who were above the age of 17. Third, the results were also limited by the cross-sectional design, which prevents us from drawing temporal or even causal relationships in the interplay between traumatic events, social factors, and mental health outcomes. For example, it could be that PTSD and/or depressive symptoms mediate the effect on trauma exposure and perceived social rejection. Further longitudinal research could provide clarity to the links between these variables. Fourth, social rejection has been evaluated according to participants'

perception and, given that the majority of them are suffering from severe PTSD and depression symptoms, this may have an impact on the manner in which they perceive social reactions. Fifth, while participants had experienced repeated and multiple traumatic events, the current study only addressed PTSD, which is usually caused by a single traumatic event limited in duration. Complex PTSD, on the other hand, is a psychological syndrome following prolonged and multiple trauma.

Conclusion

Our results scientifically documented that Yazidi women and girls had experienced genocide and other instances of suppression and oppression by ISIS, with little action from the rest of the world to support them. The present study illustrates the devastating psychological consequences of genocide and enslavement. Our findings call for urgent psychosocial intervention for Yazidi survivors of genocide.

Abbreviations
IDP: internally displaced person; ISIS: Islamic State of Iraq and Syria; KRI: Kurdistan Region of Iraq; PCL-5: PTSD Checklist for DSM-5; PTSD: post-traumatic stress disorder

Acknowledgements
We are grateful to all study participants for their trust and generous involvement. We thank Ms. Bahar Munzir Osman, the general director of People's Development Organization, for her continued support. We are grateful to all mental health professionals from Rawshan community center, Arbat camp hospital, and other local and international NGOs who took care of our participants. Special thanks go to our local research team for their dedication and effort in this research project. We also thank camp managers, administration, and security staff for their facilitation.

Funding
This study was funded by Volkswagen Foundation. A part of this study was supported by a scholarship from the German Academic Exchange Service (DAAD) to the first author. The funders had no role in study design, data collection and analysis, decision to publish, or preparation of the manuscript.

Authors' contributions
HI and FN conceptualized and designed the study. HI is the co-principal investigator and project manager, carried out the informal interviews and focus group discussions with survivors, trained the local interviewers, supervised data acquisition, performed the statistical analysis as well as the interpretation of data, and wrote the manuscript. VE, CC, and AAI contributed to the statistical analysis and the interpretation of data. AAI is the co-principal investigator. FN is the chief investigator for this study, supervised data analyses, participated in the interpretation of the data, and critically revised the manuscript for important intellectual content. All authors read and approved the final manuscript.

Competing interests

The authors declare that they have no competing interests.

Author details

[1]Department of Psychology, Clinical Psychology and Psychotherapy, Bielefeld University, Bielefeld, Germany. [2]Department of Clinical Psychology, Koya University, Koya, Kurdistan Region, Iraq. [3]vivo International, Konstanz, Germany.

References

1. Allison C. The Yazidis. Oxford: Oxford University Press; 2017.
2. Açıkyıldız B. The Yezidis: the history of a community, culture and religion. London: I.B.Tauris & Co Ltd; 2010. https://www.hrw.org/sites/default/files/report_pdf/iraq1217web.pdf. Accessed 1 Mar 2018.
3. Human Rights Watch. Flawed Justice – Accountability for ISIS Crimes in Iraq. 2017.
4. Amnesty International. Escape from Hell: Torture and Sexual Slavery in Islamic State Captivity in Iraq. London: Amnesty International; 2014.
5. Cetorelli V, Sasson I, Shabila N, Burnham G. Mortality and kidnapping estimates for the Yazidi population in the area of Mount Sinjar, Iraq, in August 2014: A retrospective household survey. Plos Med. 2017;14: e1002297.
6. Independent International Commission of Inquiry on the Syrian Arab Republic. They Came to Destroy: ISIS Crimes Against the Yazidis. Geneva: Independent International Commission of Inquiry on the Syrian Arab Republic; 2016.
7. Rugema L, Mogren I, Ntaganira J, Gunilla K. Traumatic episodes experienced during the genocide period in Rwanda influence life circumstances in young men and women 17 years later. BMC Public Health. 2013;13:1235.
8. Roth M, Neuner F, Elbert T. Transgenerational consequences of PTSD: risk factors for the mental health of children whose mothers have been exposed to the Rwandan genocide. Int J Ment Health Syst. 2014;8:12.
9. Barel E, Van IJzendoorn MH, Sagi-Schwartz A, Bakermans-Kranenburg MJ. Surviving the holocaust: a meta-analysis of the long-term sequelae of a genocide. Psychol Bull. 2010;136:677–98.
10. Heim L, Schaal S. Rates and predictors of mental stress in Rwanda: investigating the impact of gender, persecution, readiness to reconcile and religiosity via a structural equation model. Int J Ment Health Syst. 2014;8:37.
11. Steel Z, Chey T, Silove D, Marnane C, Bryant RA, van Ommeren M. Association of torture and other potentially traumatic events with mental health outcomes among populations exposed to mass conflict and displacement. JAMA. 2009;302:537.
12. Schaal S, Elbert T. Ten years after the genocide: trauma confrontation and posttraumatic stress in Rwandan adolescents. J Trauma Stress. 2006; 19:95–105.
13. Weine SM, Becker DF, TH MG, Laub D, Lazrove S, Vojvoda D, Hyman L. Psychiatric consequences of 'ethnic cleansing': clinical assessments and trauma testimonies of newly resettled Bosnian refugees. Am J Psychiatry. 1995;152:536–42.
14. Dworkin J, Prescott M, Jamal R, Hardawan SA, Abdullah A, Galea S. The long-term psychosocial impact of a surprise chemical weapons attack on civilians in Halabja, Iraqi Kurdistan. J Nerv Ment Dis. 2008;196:772–5.
15. Bolton P, Michalopoulos L, Ahmed AMA, Murray LK, Bass J. The mental health and psychosocial problems of survivors of torture and genocide in Kurdistan, northern Iraq: a brief qualitative study. Torture. 2013;23:1–14.
16. Ahmad A, Sofi MA, Sundelin-Wahlsten V, Von Knorring AL. Posttraumatic stress disorder in children after the military operation 'Anfal' in Iraqi Kurdistan. Eur Child Adolesc Psychiatry. 2000;9:235–43.
17. Hall BJ, Bonanno GA, Bolton PA, Bass JK. A longitudinal investigation of changes to social resources associated with psychological distress among Kurdish torture survivors living in northern Iraq. J Trauma Stress. 2014;27:446–53.
18. Tekin A, Karadağ H, Süleymanoğlu M, Tekin M, Kayran Y, Alpak G, et al. Prevalence and gender differences in symptomatology of posttraumatic stress disorder and depression among Iraqi Yazidis displaced into Turkey. Eur J Psychotraumatol. 2016;7:28556.
19. Ceri V, Özlü-Erkilic Z, Özer Ü, Yalcin M, Popow C, Akkaya-Kalayci T. Psychiatric symptoms and disorders among Yazidi children and adolescents immediately after forced migration following ISIS attacks. Neuropsychiatrie. 2016;30:145–50.
20. Nasıroğlu S, Çeri V. Posttraumatic stress and depression in Yazidi refugees. Neuropsychiatr Dis Treat. 2016;12:2941–8.
21. Reid-Cunningham AR. Rape as a weapon of genocide. Genocide Stud Prev. 2008;3:279–96.
22. Longombe AO, Claude KM, Ruminjo J. Fistula and traumatic genital injury from sexual violence in a conflict setting in eastern Congo: case studies. Reprod Health Matters. 2008;16:132–41.
23. Tompkins TL. Prosecuting rape as a war crime: speaking the unspeakable. Notre Dame Law Rev. 1995;70:845–90.
24. Lončar M, Medved V, Jovanović N, Hotujac L. Psychological consequences of rape on women in 1991-1995 war in Croatia and Bosnia and Herzegovina. Croat Med J. 2006;47:67–75.
25. Ba I, Bhopal RS. Physical, mental and social consequences in civilians who have experienced war-related sexual violence: a systematic review (1981-2014). Public Health. 2017;142:121–35.
26. Hoffman YSG, Grossman ES, Shrira A, Kedar M, Ben-Ezra M, Dinnayi M, et al. Complex PTSD and its correlates amongst female Yazidi victims of sexual slavery living in post-ISIS camps. World Psychiatry. 2018;17:112–3.
27. Kelly JT, Betancourt TS, Mukwege D, Lipton R, VanRooyen MJ. Experiences of female survivors of sexual violence in eastern Democratic Republic of the Congo: a mixed-methods study. Confl Health. 2011;5:25.
28. Duroch F, McRae M, Grais RF. Description and consequences of sexual violence in Ituri province, Democratic Republic of Congo. BMC Int Health Hum Rights. 2011;11:5.
29. Amone-P'Olak K, Lekhutlile TM, Ovuga E, Abbott RA, Meiser-Stedman R, Stewart DG, et al. Sexual violence and general functioning among formerly abducted girls in northern Uganda: the mediating roles of stigma and community relations - the WAYS study. BMC Public Health. 2016;16:64.
30. Albutt K, Kelly J, Kabanga J, VanRooyen M. Stigmatisation and rejection of survivors of sexual violence in eastern Democratic Republic of the Congo. Disasters. 2017;41:211–27.
31. Brewin CR, Andrews B, Valentine JD. Meta-analysis of risk factors for posttraumatic stress disorder in trauma-exposed adults. J Consult Clin Psychol. 2000;68:748–66.
32. Siriwardhana C, Ali S, Roberts B, Stewart R. A systematic review of resilience and mental health outcomes of conflict-driven adult forced migrants. Confl Health. 2014;8:13.
33. Shishehgar S, Gholizadeh L, DiGiacomo M, Green A, Davidson PM. Health and socio-cultural experiences of refugee women: an integrative review. J Immigr Minor Heal. 2017;19:959–73.
34. King DW, Taft C, King LA, Hammond C, Stone ER. Directionality of the association between social support and posttraumatic stress disorder: a longitudinal Investigation. J Appl Soc Psychol. 2006;36:2980–92.
35. Barnes JB, Nickerson A, Adler AB, Litz BT. Perceived military organizational support and peacekeeper distress: A longitudinal investigation. Psychol Serv. 2013;10:177–85.
36. Wagner B, Keller V, Knaevelsrud C, Maercker A. Social acknowledgement as a predictor of post-traumatic stress and complicated grief after witnessing assisted suicide. Int J Soc Psychiatry. 2012;58:381–5.
37. Nietlisbach G, Maercker A. Social cognition and interpersonal impairments in trauma survivors with PTSD. J Aggress Maltreat Trauma. 2009;18:382–402.
38. Sommer J, Hinsberger M, Weierstall R, Holtzhausen L, Kaminer D, Seedat S, et al. Social acknowledgment of violent experiences and its role in PTSD and appetitive aggression among high-risk males in South Africa. Clin Psychol Sci. 2016;5:166–73.
39. Mueller J, Moergeli H, Maercker A. Disclosure and social acknowledgement as predictors of recovery from posttraumatic stress: a longitudinal study in crime victims. Can J Psychiatr. 2008;53:160–8.
40. Kohli A, Perrin NA, Mpanano RM, Mullany LC, Murhula CM, Binkurhorhwa AK, et al. Risk for family rejection and associated mental health outcomes among conflict-affected adult women living in rural eastern Democratic Republic of the Congo. Health Care Women Int. 2014;35:789–807.

41. Amone-P'Olak K, Ovuga E, Jones PB. The effects of sexual violence on psychosocial outcomes in formerly abducted girls in northern Uganda: the WAYS study. BMC Psychol. 2015;3:46.

42. Ibrahim H, Ertl V, Catani C, Ismail AA, Neuner F. Validation and calibration of the posttraumatic stress disorder checklist for DSM-5 (PCL-5) with Kurdish and Arab displaced populations living in the Kurdistan region of Iraq. BMC Psychiatry. 2018 (in press).

43. Weathers FW, Blake DD, Schnurr PP, Kaloupek DG, Marx BP, Keane T. The Life Events Checklist for DSM-5 (LEC-5). National Center for PTSD. 2013. National Center for PTSD. www.ptsd.va.gov. Accessed 9 Feb 2018.

44. Weathers FW, Litz BT, Keane TM, Palmieri PA, Marx BP, Schnurr PP. The PTSD Checklist for DSM-5 (PCL-5). National Center for PTSD. 2013. Instrument available from the National Center for PTSD at www.ptsd.va.gov

45. Hesbacher PT, Rickels K, Morris RJ, Newman H, Rosenfeld H. Psychiatric illness in family practice. J Clin Psychiatry. 1980;41:6–10.

46. Hayes AF. Introduction to Mediation, Moderation, and Conditional Process Analysis: A Regression-Based Approach. 2nd ed. New York: Guilford Press; 2018.

47. Shrout PE, Bolger N. Mediation in experimental and nonexperimental studies: new procedures and recommendations. Psychol Methods. 2002;7:422–45.

48. Global Justice Center. Human Rights Through Rule of Law. Genocide and Gender: Daesh's Crimes against Yazidi Women and Girls. 2016. http://globaljusticecenter.net/documents/Daesh's%20Crimes%20Against%20Yazidi%20Women%20and%20Girls.pdf. Accessed 1 Mar 2018.

49. Mlodoch K. Fragmented memory, competing narratives: the perspective of women survivors of the Anfal operations in Iraqi Kurdistan. In: Tejel J, Sluglett P, Bocco R, Bozarslan H, editors. Writing the Modern History of Iraq: World Scientific; 2012. p. 205–26. https://doi.org/10.1142/9789814390576_0014.

50. Suarez EB. The association between post-traumatic stress-related symptoms, resilience, current stress and past exposure to violence: a cross sectional study of the survival of Quechua women in the aftermath of the Peruvian armed conflict. Confl Health. 2013;7:21.

51. Johnson K, Scott J, Rughita B, et al. Association of sexual violence and human rights violations with physical and mental health in territories of the eastern Democratic Republic of the Congo. JAMA. 2010;304:553–62.

52. Stevanović A, Frančišković T, Vermetten E. Relationship of early-life trauma, war-related trauma, personality traits, and PTSD symptom severity: a retrospective study on female civilian victims of war. Eur J Psychotraumatol. 2016;7:30964.

53. Rieder H, Elbert T. The relationship between organized violence, family violence and mental health: findings from a community-based survey in Muhanga, southern Rwanda. Eur J Psychotraumatol. 2013;4 https://doi.org/10.3402/ejpt.v4i0.21329.

54. Ibrahim H, Hassan CQ. Post-traumatic stress disorder symptoms resulting from torture and other traumatic events among Syrian Kurdish refugees in Kurdistan region, Iraq. Front Psychol. 2017;8:241.

55. Muftić LR, Finn MA. Health outcomes among women trafficked for sex in the United States: a closer look. J Interpers Violence. 2013;28:1859–85.

56. Ovuga E, Oyok TO, Moro EB. Post traumatic stress disorder among former child soldiers attending a rehabilitative service and primary school education in northern Uganda. Afr Health Sci. 2008;8:136–41.

57. Betancourt TS, Brennan RT, Rubin-Smith J, Fitzmaurice GM, Gilman SE. Sierra Leone's former child soldiers: a longitudinal study of risk, protective factors, and mental health. J Am Acad Child Adolesc Psychiatry. 2010;49:606–15.

58. Pfeiffer A, Elbert T. PTSD, depression and anxiety among former abductees in northern Uganda. Confl Health. 2011;5:14.

59. Winkler N, Ruf-Leuschner M, Ertl V, Pfeiffer A, Schalinski I, Ovuga E, et al. From war to classroom: PTSD and depression in formerly abducted youth in Uganda. Front Psychiatry. 2015;6:2.

60. Umubyeyi A, Mogren I, Ntaganira J, Krantz G. Intimate partner violence and its contribution to mental disorders in men and women in the post genocide Rwanda: findings from a population based study. BMC Psychiatry. 2014;14:315.

61. Rugema L, Mogren I, Ntaganira J, Krantz G. Traumatic episodes and mental health effects in young men and women in Rwanda, 17 years after the genocide. BMJ Open. 2015;5:e006778.

62. Amone-P'Olak K, Lekhutlile TM, Ovuga E, Abbott RA, Meiser-Stedman R, Stewart DG, et al. Sexual violence and general functioning among formerly abducted girls in northern Uganda: the mediating roles of stigma and community relations--the WAYS study. BMC Public Health. 2016;16:64.

63. Amone-P'Olak K, Elklit A, Dokkedahl SB. PTSD, mental illness, and care among survivors of sexual violence in northern Uganda: findings from the WAYS study. Psychol Trauma. 2018;10(3):282–9.

64. Schmitt MT, Branscombe NR, Postmes T, Garcia A. The consequences of perceived discrimination for psychological well-being: a meta-analytic review. Psychol Bull. 2014;140:921–48.

65. Pascoe EA, Smart Richman L. Perceived discrimination and health: a meta-analytic review. Psychol Bull. 2009;135:531–54.

13

Real-world data reveal a diagnostic gap in non-alcoholic fatty liver disease

Myriam Alexander[1], A. Katrina Loomis[2], Jolyon Fairburn-Beech[1], Johan van der Lei[3], Talita Duarte-Salles[4], Daniel Prieto-Alhambra[5], David Ansell[6], Alessandro Pasqua[7], Francesco Lapi[7], Peter Rijnbeek[3], Mees Mosseveld[3], Paul Avillach[8], Peter Egger[1], Stuart Kendrick[1], Dawn M. Waterworth[1], Naveed Sattar[9†] and William Alazawi[10*†] ⓘD

Abstract

Background: Non-alcoholic fatty liver disease (NAFLD) is the most common cause of liver disease worldwide. It affects an estimated 20% of the general population, based on cohort studies of varying size and heterogeneous selection. However, the prevalence and incidence of recorded NAFLD diagnoses in unselected real-world health-care records is unknown. We harmonised health records from four major European territories and assessed age- and sex-specific point prevalence and incidence of NAFLD over the past decade.

Methods: Data were extracted from The Health Improvement Network (UK), Health Search Database (Italy), Information System for Research in Primary Care (Spain) and Integrated Primary Care Information (Netherlands). Each database uses a different coding system. Prevalence and incidence estimates were pooled across databases by random-effects meta-analysis after a log-transformation.

Results: Data were available for 17,669,973 adults, of which 176,114 had a recorded diagnosis of NAFLD. Pooled prevalence trebled from 0.60% in 2007 (95% confidence interval: 0.41–0.79) to 1.85% (0.91–2.79) in 2014. Incidence doubled from 1.32 (0.83–1.82) to 2.35 (1.29–3.40) per 1000 person-years. The FIB-4 non-invasive estimate of liver fibrosis could be calculated in 40.6% of patients, of whom 29.6–35.7% had indeterminate or high-risk scores.

Conclusions: In the largest primary-care record study of its kind to date, rates of recorded NAFLD are much lower than expected suggesting under-diagnosis and under-recording. Despite this, we have identified rising incidence and prevalence of the diagnosis. Improved recognition of NAFLD may identify people who will benefit from risk factor modification or emerging therapies to prevent progression to cardiometabolic and hepatic complications.

Keywords: Epidemiology, Population, NAFLD, NASH

Background

Non-alcoholic fatty liver disease (NAFLD) is rapidly becoming the most common cause of chronic liver disease worldwide [1]. NAFLD is a spectrum of diseases that encompasses uncomplicated steatosis, non-alcoholic steatohepatitis (NASH) and fibrosis, which in a small proportion can lead to complications including cirrhosis, liver failure and hepatocellular carcinoma [2]. NAFLD is a multisystem disease with a multidirectional relationship with the metabolic syndrome [3–5]. NAFLD is associated with increased risk of cardiovascular disease [5–7] and cancer [8]. Among other high-risk groups [9], people with diabetes and NAFLD are at increased risk of micro- and macrovascular complications [10, 11] and these patients have a twofold increased risk of all-cause mortality [12].

The estimated point prevalence of NAFLD in the general Western population is 20–30%, largely based on cohort studies with heterogeneous inclusion criteria and research methods [13]. The prevalence of NAFLD rises to 40–70% among patients with type 2 diabetes and up to 90% among patients with morbid obesity [14–16]. Moreover, as the rates of diabetes and obesity rise worldwide, it is expected that NAFLD will become even more

* Correspondence: w.alazawi@qmul.ac.uk
†Naveed Sattar and William Alazawi contributed equally to this work.
[10]Barts Liver Centre, Blizard Institute, Queen Mary, University of London, London, UK
Full list of author information is available at the end of the article

common. NAFLD-related cirrhosis is currently the third most common indication and is anticipated to become the leading indication for liver transplantation in the USA within the next one to two decades [17].

There is much debate about whether screening programmes in the general population or in at-risk groups, such as people with diabetes [9], should be implemented [18, 19]. This debate is based on our current understanding of the epidemiology and natural history of NAFLD, which, in turn, derives from cohort or cross-sectional studies [13]. These are often highly selected studies of individuals with metabolic risk factors, or they involve extensive phenotyping that would be unrealistic in routine practice.

A pragmatic approach is to focus on real-world patients for whom the diagnosis of NAFLD has been made during routine clinical care. A diagnosis of NAFLD is often made following abnormal imaging of the liver or elevated serum liver enzymes (so-called liver function tests) and involves exclusion of other causes of liver injury, such as excess alcohol consumption and viral hepatitis. Although routinely collected data can represent only the visible part of the clinical iceberg, there is a growing body of literature that has used well-curated electronic health records (EHRs) to study disease characteristics and epidemiology in large numbers of people [20–22].

In many European countries where health care is largely state funded and there are low or absent primary-care co-payments, the population has unrestricted access to health care with primary-care physicians acting as gatekeepers (including referral to secondary care) [23]. Healthy people register with primary-care centres when they move to an area to access health care when it is be needed and so primary-care EHR represent data that are as close to a general population as possible, with near universal coverage of the population in the region where the data is collected. Recording of a diagnosis in European primary-care databases is not driven by reimbursement and the patient population is relatively stable compared to other types of EHRs, such as US claims databases. Primary-care databases hold comprehensive medical records, which include diagnoses, prescriptions, laboratory values, lifestyle and health measures, and demographic information for a large and representative sample of patients. Concerns around the degree of data completeness are now largely historic as the vast majority of practices are paper-free and therefore, these data represent the only clinical record for care, administration and re-imbursement. Thus, within the areas that utilise these databases, coverage is near universal. If a practice joins the database, all the patients of that practice are registered in the database. Although there is an option for individual patients to opt out, this is minimal (<1%).

In this study, we harmonised health-care records for 17.7 million adults from four large European primary-health-care databases to estimate the prevalence and incidence of recorded diagnoses of NAFLD and, where available, NASH, in patients in primary care and to compare these with estimates from cohort studies. We sought to ascertain the changes in prevalence and incidence of recorded diagnoses of NAFLD from 2007 to 2015, and the effect of age and sex. We compared the characteristics of patients with an NAFLD diagnosis in the different databases and reported, where possible, the proportion of patients with markers of advanced disease in the diagnosed population.

Methods
Databases
Ethical approval was obtained by data custodians of each primary-care database according to local institutional review board requirements. Anonymised data were extracted from the Health Search Database (HSD) in Italy [24], the Integrated Primary Care Information (IPCI) in the Netherlands [25], The Health Improvement Network (THIN) in the UK [26] and the Information System for Research in Primary Care (SIDIAP) in the Catalonia region of Spain [27] (Additional file 1: Table S1).

THIN, HSD and IPCI had all reached high levels of patient registration from January 2004 onwards. SIDIAP started data collection in 2005 and has high quality data from 2006. Data entered between 1 January 2004 (SIDIAP from 1 January 2007) and up to 31 December 2015 were included in incidence estimates. Individuals were excluded if they had less than 1 year of follow-up post registration into the database. Individuals with a diagnosis of NAFLD were not included in the analyses if they also had a recorded history of alcohol abuse. To maximise data completeness, we included only patients whose NAFLD diagnosis occurred within ±6 months of a general practitioner (GP) visit when describing patients' characteristics (Table 1 and Additional file 1: Table S3).

Patient involvement
All eligible patients were included in the study. Routine health-care records were collected from patients at each encounter with a health-care practitioner. Following local regulations, patients who did not wish to share their data were able to withdraw from the databases.

Semantic harmonisation and case ascertainment
The four databases each use different coding systems (Additional file 1: Table S1). As a result, the capture of NAFLD and NASH diagnoses differed across databases. In HSD and IPCI, NAFLD and NASH were captured in a single code as 'NAFLD or NASH'. In SIDIAP and THIN, NAFLD and NASH were coded separately,

Table 1 Flow chart of identification of NAFLD patients

Flow chart	HSD (Italy)	IPCI (Netherlands)	SIDIAP (Spain)	THIN (UK)	Total
Total number of individuals ever enrolled by December 2015	1,571,651	2,225,925	5,488,397	12,695,046	21,981,019
Number of individuals with ≥1 year of registration in adulthood	1,544,573	1,780,500	5,259,575	9,085,325	17,669,973
Number of NAFLD patients	NAFLD: 27,002	NAFLD: 48,036 (19,048 were incident post IPCI starting date)	NAFLD: 77,547 NASH only: 1887	NAFLD: 23,529 NASH only: 1133	NAFLD: 176,114

The descriptive tables (Table 2 and Additional file 1: Table S3) include only patients with an incident diagnosis made within the study period and with a record of a GP visit within ±6 months of diagnosis. Numbers for NAFLD/NASH were as follows: HSD 24,027, IPCI 18,865, SIDIAP 77,107 and THIN: 12,385 individuals. Note in HSD and IPCI, 'NAFLD' is likely to include patients with NASH since no separate term for NASH exists in these databases. The number in the 'Total' column includes patients within SIDIAP and THIN who have NASH

GP general practitioner, HSD Health Search Database, IPCI Integrated Primary Care Information, NAFLD non-alcoholic fatty liver disease, NASH non-alcoholic steatohepatitis, SIDIAP Information System for Research in Primary Care, THIN The Health Improvement Network

branching out of a 'NAFLD or NASH' code. In this study, we extracted all 'NAFLD or NASH' diagnoses as well as 'NASH only diagnoses' where available. For simplicity, we labelled 'NAFLD or NASH' as 'NAFLD' and 'NASH only' as 'NASH'. Code lists were generated for the four terminologies (ICD9CM, Read Codes, SNOMEDCTUS and ICD10) that mapped to the same Unified Medical Language System (UMLS) concepts [28] (Additional file 1: Table S2).

Clinical diagnoses were defined with these code lists using the same process of harmonisation (code lists available on request). In SIDIAP, we used a combination of clinical codes and answers to questionnaires on alcohol consumption to identify alcohol abuse.

Given the absence of a code for NAFLD in the IPCI terminology, we additionally used text-mining in this database. The algorithm to identify NAFLD in IPCI is detailed in Additional file 1: Figure S1. Patients with records for the following search terms were extracted: 'NASH', 'NAFLD', 'steatohepatitis' or 'fatty liver disease' as distinct words preceded by a space and followed by a space, or at the beginning or end of a sentence. Patients with relevant search terms preceded by a negation term (e.g. 'no' or 'not') were excluded. To validate the text-mining, 100 individuals identified using free-text were randomly sampled. Their complete medical charts were manually reviewed to confirm that the clinical data support the text-mining-derived diagnosis.

Use of historical data

Governance rules differed between the different databases. In HSD and SIDIAP, there were no records available prior to a primary-care practice joining the database. In THIN, data from patients who had already left the practice were available, so NAFLD/NASH diagnoses made prior to the patient's primary-care practice joining THIN were counted in both incidence and prevalence estimates. However, in IPCI, records that predated their primary-care practice joining the database were available only for patients who remained in the practice (since leavers did not have the opportunity to refuse to participate). Therefore,

historic diagnoses could be included in the point prevalence. However, given that both the number of new diagnoses made as well as the total number of patients at risk in a given period were unknown, we could not include diagnoses made before the patient joined a practice in incidence estimates in IPCI.

Other data extraction

Demographic information, lifestyle and medical history of relevant morbidities were also extracted for all NAFLD and NASH patients identified in the four databases. Medical records for type 2 diabetes and hypertension at any time prior to NAFLD or NASH diagnosis were extracted. Code lists for those diagnoses were harmonised across the databases using the semantic harmonisation described in 'Methods', which aligns all terms for the same list of UMLS concepts (code lists available on request).

Laboratory values for aspartate transaminase (AST), alanine transaminase (ALT) and platelet count were extracted. We used the values closest to the time of NAFLD diagnosis (up to 2 years prior to diagnosis or less than 6 months after). Body mass index (BMI) was calculated for all NAFLD patients with weight recorded between 2 years prior to and 6 months after diagnosis, and with height recorded anytime in adulthood. We excluded values that were likely to be implausible: BMI below 15 kg/m^2, laboratory values greater than the mean in the database plus 3 times the standard deviation, AST and ALT less than 5 IU/L, and platelet counts below 5×10^9 L^{-1}.

The FIB-4 index was calculated to provide an estimate of the severity of fibrosis in patients at the time of their NAFLD diagnosis. The formula for FIB-4 is: Age [years] × AST [U/L] / (platelet [10^9] × $\sqrt{}$ALT [U/L]) [29]. The cut-offs for FIB-4 scoring for NAFLD are <1.30 for a low risk of advanced fibrosis or cirrhosis, between 1.30 and 2.67 for an indeterminate score and 2.67 for a high risk of advanced fibrosis or cirrhosis [30].

Statistical methods

Quantitative variables were reported as mean and 95% confidence interval (CI) of the mean assuming a normal distribution, and qualitative variables as percentages. Differences in patients' characteristics between the four databases were tested by an ANOVA test for quantitative characteristics and a chi-square test for categorical characteristics.

Incidence in the adult population aged ≥18 years old was estimated by dividing the number of individuals with a diagnosis of NAFLD (or NASH where relevant) by the total number of person-years at risk. Incidence was reported by predefined age categories, gender and calendar year.

Point prevalence was estimated for 1 January of each calendar year available in the data, by gender and by predefined age categories. Point prevalence was defined as the total number of individuals with a recorded NAFLD diagnosis at or prior to 1 January of a calendar year and who were still active in the database, divided by the total number of active patients in the database on that date.

In addition, the 1-year period prevalence was estimated in a sensitivity analysis to account for potential differences in length of follow-up across databases, and over time within databases. The 1-year period prevalence was defined for each calendar year available as the number of new individuals with a recorded diagnosis of NAFLD in a calendar year divided by the average number of active patients in that year (defined as the number on 1 January plus the number on 31 December divided by 2).

Age was computed at the end of the year for period prevalence (31 December of the year of interest). For point prevalnce, age was computed on 1 January of the year of interest. Within each database, incidence estimates were compared by calendar year (assuming a linear relationship), sex (males are the reference group) and age group (age 60–69 is the reference group) by fitting Poisson distributions. Prevalence estimates were compared by fitting logistic regressions and performing chi-square tests. $P < 0.001$ was considered as significant, although note that with such large datasets, a high level of significance can be achieved even for minimal absolute differences in prevalence and incidence levels.

Incidence and prevalence estimates were pooled for each calendar year across the four databases using a random effects meta-analysis after natural log-transformation (weighting by the inverse of the variance). We reported the I^2 statistic, which gives the percentage of variation among databases attributable to heterogeneity, and the p values of heterogeneity (p-het), tested using Q statistics. To investigate sources of heterogeneity, we tested for a linear association between incidence and point prevalence with calendar year by fitting a meta-regression.

Data were extracted and analysed using the European Medical Information Framework (EMIF) with a distributed network approach that allows data custodians to maintain control over their protected data [31]. Each data custodian extracted data from their database into four common files: prescriptions, measurements, events and patients. These files were transformed locally by the data transformation tool Jerboa Reloaded, which produces analytical datasets that can be shared with data analysts in a central remote research environment for further post-processing. The analytical datasets contained characteristics for each patient with a NAFLD diagnosis, as well as aggregated results on incidence and prevalence by age, gender and calendar year. Quality controls were run on each database and the research team communicated with data custodians to confirm results. Statistics and graphics were generated in the remote research environment using the statistical software Stata/SE 14.1.

Results

Semantic harmonisation to identify the European NAFLD cohort

In total, the four European databases held data on 21,981,019 patients, of whom 17,699,973 adults had been registered for at least 1 year in adulthood (Table 1). Using semantic harmonisation, we identified 176,114 patients who had a recorded diagnosis of NAFLD (including NASH). This represents 1.0% of the total population, ranging from 0.3% in the UK (THIN) to 2.7% in the Netherlands (IPCI). The largest number of NAFLD patients was in the Spanish cohort (SIDIAP, $n = 77,547$, Table 1). Recording of NASH diagnoses was possible only in Spain (SIDIAP, $n = 1887$) and in the UK (THIN, $n = 1133$), as the other two databases did not have specific codes distinguishing NAFLD from NASH. Given the small numbers overall, we did not pursue an analysis of NASH incidence and prevalence further and we included these patients within the total number of patients with a recorded diagnosis of NAFLD.

In the Dutch database (IPCI), the majority of patients were identified via free-text mining with seed words 'NAFLD', 'NASH', 'fatty liver' or 'steatosis', and a minority from diagnostic codes only (see Additional file 1: Figure S1). The code for 'liver steatosis' (D97.05) identified 1282 patients. The code for 'cirrhosis/other liver disease' (D97.00) identified 4228 patients when combined with a free-text search on the code label and 1214 additional patients when combined with a free-text search anywhere in the medical records. Searching for the search terms in free text in the absence of a relevant code identified 44,442 additional patients. Of these, 19,048 patients had an incident NAFLD diagnosis (recorded at a time when the patient's general practice was contributing to IPCI). In the sample of 100 cases that were manually reviewed, the positive predictive value for a text-mined diagnosis of NAFLD was 98%.

We identified only a small proportion of patients with a recorded diagnosis of NAFLD who also drank alcohol in excess of recommended limits: 3130 (7.0%) NAFLD patients in IPCI, 921 in HSD (3.3%), 12,461 in SIDIAP (14.1%) and 925 in THIN (3.8%). These patients were excluded from the statistical analysis.

The characteristics of the populations of patients with an incident diagnosis of NAFLD made during the study period, after exclusions, are shown in Table 2 for the individual databases. There were minor differences in the mean age, proportion of patients with impaired fasting glucose or diabetes, and platelet count in each of the four databases. However, we observed that HSD had statistically significantly higher proportions of males and patients with hypertension than other databases. There was considerable variation in recorded BMI (29.7 kg/m^2 in HSD to 32.4 kg/m^2 in THIN), alanine transaminase (ALT) levels (median 28 IU/L in HSD to 39 IU/L in THIN) and aspartate transaminase (AST) levels (median 24 IU/L in HSD to 32 IU/L in THIN). Moreover, we observed variation in clinical practice with higher rates of BMI being recorded and ALT requests in THIN and SIDIAP compared to IPCI and HSD (Table 2 and Additional file 1: Table S3).

Non-invasive scores that estimate the degree of liver fibrosis can be calculated from clinical parameters and are used to risk-stratify patients with NAFLD. Although both ALT and AST are required to calculate the majority of such non-invasive scores, ALT was more frequently available than AST in all four databases (Additional file 1: Table S3). An AST result was available for 21% (THIN) to 68% (HSD) and an ALT result for 67% (IPCI) to 86% (SIDIAP). This is reflected in the proportion of patients in whom a FIB-4 non-invasive assessment of liver fibrosis could be calculated, ranging from 11% in THIN to 54% in SIDIAP. Despite having the smallest number (and percentage) of patients in whom we could calculate FIB-4, the THIN database had the highest proportion of patients with high-risk scores indicative of advanced fibrosis or even cirrhosis (10.0% vs 2.9–4.3%, $p < 0.001$). In practice, patients with indeterminate or high-risk scores are often managed with further assessment leading to a liver biopsy. The proportion of patients with intermediate/high-risk scores was lower in IPCI (29.8%) compared to the other databases (35.0–35.7%); albeit the number of people for whom we could calculate FIB-4 was variable.

The rising prevalence of NAFLD diagnosis

The overall (pooled) prevalence of NAFLD diagnosis was low at 1.85% (95% CI: 0.91–2.79) (I^2 = 99.99%, p-het < 0.001) on 1 January 2015, but it had trebled from 0.60% (0.41–0.79) (I^2 = 99.97%, p-het < 0.001) on 1 January 2007 (Fig. 1 and Additional file 1: Table S4).

The prevalence of recorded NAFLD diagnosis rose over time in all databases, albeit levels and rates of rise

Table 2 Descriptive characteristics of patients with an incident diagnosis of NAFLD in four European primary-care databases

Characteristics	HSD (N = 24,027)	IPCI (N = 18,865)	SIDIAP (N = 77,107)	THIN (N = 23,385)	Test of difference p value
	% / Mean (SD) / median (IQR)	% / Mean (SD) / median (IQR)	% / Mean (SD) / median (IQR)	% / Mean (SD) / median (IQR)	
Age in years	56.2 (14.3)	56.8 (13.9)	56.0 (13.4)	53.7 (13.4)	<0.0001
Gender (males)	57.3%	49.3%	52.7%	51.5%	<0.0001
Body mass index in kg/m^2	29.7 (5.0)	30.8 (5.4)	31.3 (5.1)	32.4 (5.9)	<0.0001
History of diabetes or impaired fasting glucose	18.0%	20.5%	20.0%	21.0%	<0.0001
History of hypertension	47.5%	36.0%	42.8%	40.5%	<0.0001
Aspartate transaminase (IU/L)	24 (19–33)	29 (22–40)	29 (22–40)	32 (24–47)	<0.0001
Alanine transaminase (IU/L)	30 (20–48)	37 (25–56)	34 (22–53)	45 (28–68)	<0.0001
Platelet counts (10^9/L)	238 (65)	262 (68.6)	244 (61.2)	250 (75.3)	<0.0001
AST to ALT ratio	0.87 (0.34)	0.80 (0.36)	0.83 (0.38)	0.82 (0.38)	<0.0001
FIB-4 score					<0.0001
Low risk (FIB-4 < 1.30)	64.3%	70.4%	65.5%	65.0%	
Indeterminate risk (FIB-4: 1.30–2.67)	31.4%	26.7%	30.3%	25.0%	
High risk (FIB-4 > 2.67)	4.3%	2.9%	4.2%	10.0%	

Arithmetic means were reported for age, BMI, platelet counts and AST to ALT ratio; median (IQR) were reported for albumin, AST and ALT. P values are from ANOVA test of difference between means for continuous variables (for log-transformed AST and ALT), and Chi-2 test of difference for categorical variables. Number of patients with data available on each of these variables is provided in Additional file 1: Table S3

ALT alanine transaminase, ANOVA analysis of variance, AST aspartate transaminase, BMI body mass index, HSD Health Search Database, IPCI Integrated Primary Care Information, IQR interquartile range, SD standard deviation, SIDIAP Information System for Research in Primary Care, THIN The Health Improvement Network

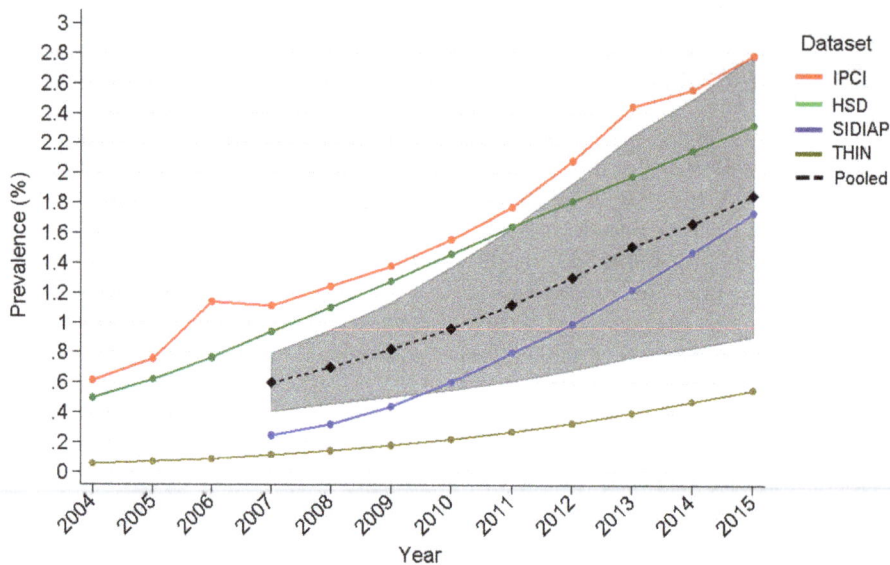

Fig. 1 Point prevalence of NAFLD (per 100 persons) by calendar year. Results are shown for each database and pooled across databases by meta-analysis. The pooled estimate is provided from 2007 only as data from SIDIAP were available only from that year onward. The pooled estimate confidence interval is shaded grey. HSD Health Search Database, IPCI Integrated Primary Care Information, NAFLD non-alcoholic fatty liver disease, SIDIAP Information System for Research in Primary Care, THIN The Health Improvement Network

differed between databases, being highest in the Netherlands (IPCI) and lowest in the UK (THIN). To confirm that those trends were not due to more complete medical records being available in more recent years, we also estimated 1-year period prevalence and observed rising trends for the four databases (Additional file 1: Table S5).

There were no significant differences in prevalence between sexes in any database, but prevalence did vary by age. Peak prevalence was in patients aged 60–79 in whom it was >20 times higher than in 18–29 years old in IPCI (4.89% versus 0.24%) and 10–14 times higher in the other databases (Fig. 2 and Additional file 1: Table S6).

Incidence of NAFLD has doubled since 2007

The overall (pooled) incidence of recorded NAFLD diagnoses was 2.35 (1.29–3.40; I^2 = 99.92%, p-het < 0.001) per 1000 person-years in 2015, having approximately doubled since 2007 (1.32; 0.83–1.82)) (see Fig. 3 and Additional file 1: Table S7).

We observed heterogeneity between databases. In IPCI and SIDIAP, there was a clear and consistent rise in incidence with a 2.7-fold increase from 2004 to 2015 to 4.09 per 1000 person-years in IPCI and 3.2-fold increase from 2007 to 2015 to 2.61 per 1000 person-years in SIDIAP. In HSD, there was no statistically significant change in incidence between 2005 and 2015 (Additional file 1: Table S6). Although the rate of rise in THIN was comparable to IPCI and SIDIAP, the very low starting rate meant that despite a fivefold increase, the absolute increase was still modest and the incidence in 2014 was 1.08 per 1000 person-years.

There was a significant difference between sexes in HSD and SIDIAP ($p < 0.05$) but not in IPCI and THIN. In HSD, IPCI and SIDIAP, peak incidence was in 60–69 year olds, and in 50–59 year olds in THIN (but the estimate was not significantly different from that in 60–69 year olds) and then decreased in older age groups (Fig. 4, Additional file 1: Table S8).

Discussion

In the largest real-world study of its kind to date, we report the incidence and prevalence of recorded NAFLD diagnoses among 17.7 million adults in four different European countries.

The databases used have been validated, are broadly representative of the population of the country and have been extensively used for pharmaco-epidemiology research [17, 20] (Additional file 1: Table S1). Despite a rise in incidence, our study found a large shortfall in Europe between the expected number of patients with NAFLD and NASH and the number with recorded diagnoses. Although others have suggested that this might be the case at a local level or in small questionnaire-based exercises [32], this study has identified the scale of that diagnostic gap across four European territories. Under-recording of NAFLD in primary care may reflect (i) missed opportunities to make the diagnosis by investigating abnormal liver enzyme values or imaging findings, (ii) a lack of confidence to make the diagnosis even if liver enzymes are in the reference range or (iii) under-recognition of the diagnosis in secondary care. Furthermore, many patients who do have the diagnosis

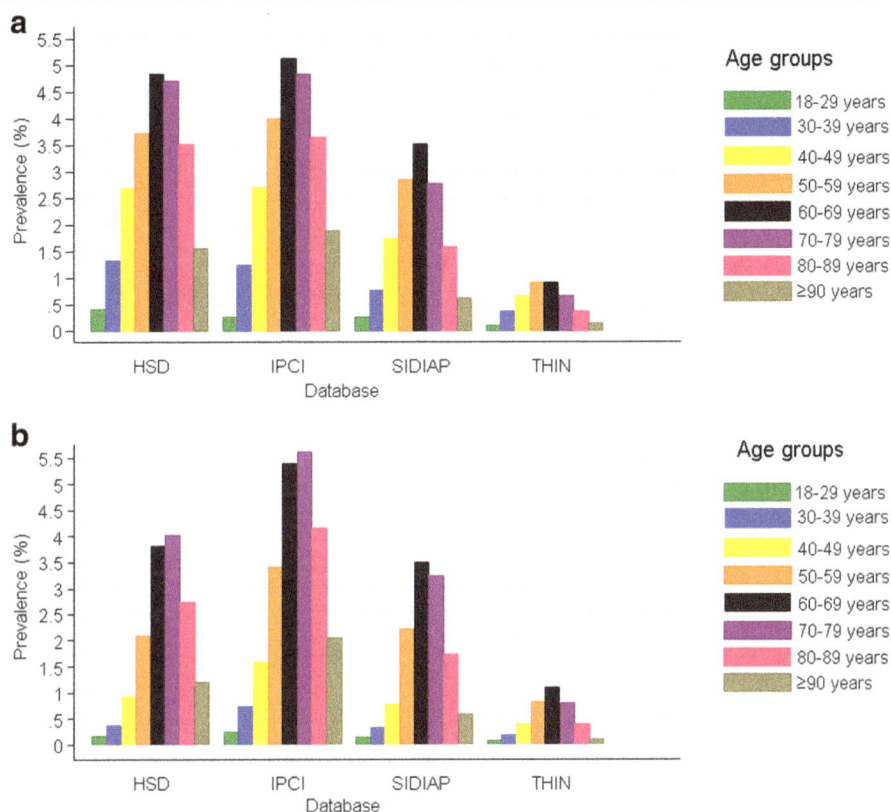

Fig. 2 Point prevalence of NAFLD (per 100 persons) by age group on 1 January 2015 in **a** males and **b** females. HSD Health Search Database, IPCI Integrated Primary Care Information, NAFLD non-alcoholic fatty liver disease, SIDIAP Information System for Research in Primary Care, THIN The Health Improvement Network

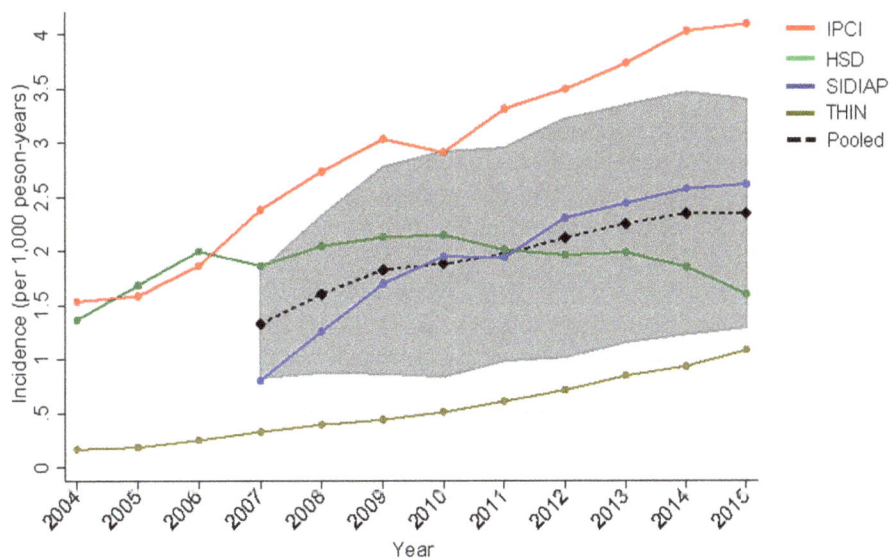

Fig. 3 Incidence of NAFLD (per 1000 person-years) by calendar year in four primary-care databases, and pooled across databases by a random effects meta-analysis. The pooled estimate is provided from 2007 only as data from SIDIAP were available only from that year onward. The pooled estimate confidence interval is shaded grey. HSD Health Search Database, IPCI Integrated Primary Care Information, NAFLD non-alcoholic fatty liver disease, SIDIAP Information System for Research in Primary Care, THIN The Health Improvement Network

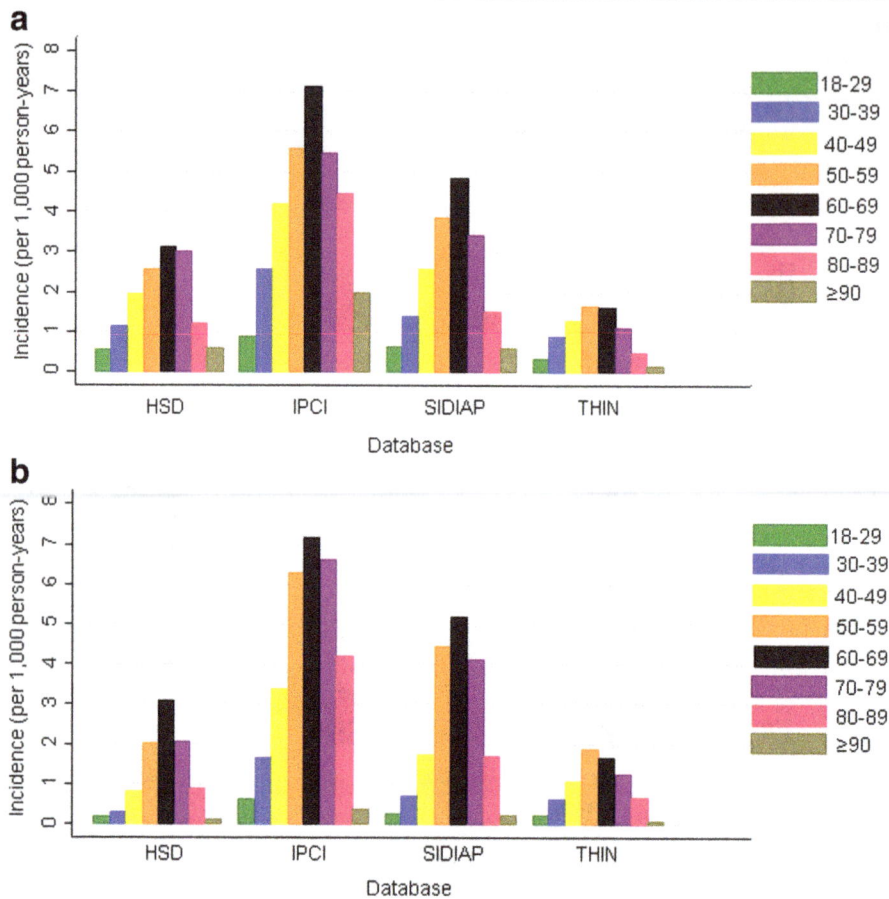

Fig. 4 Incidence of NAFLD (per 1000 person-years) by age group for the four primary care databases for 2015 in **a** males and **b** females. HSD Health Search Database, IPCI Integrated Primary Care Information, NAFLD non-alcoholic fatty liver disease, SIDIAP Information System for Research in Primary Care, THIN The Health Improvement Network

have not had the investigations required for appropriate risk-stratification and therefore, specialist care may not be offered to those at greatest need. The current study represents a departure from existing population-level study designs of NAFLD. Notwithstanding the limitations discussed below, by using real-world data, we have gained insight into current practice and attitudes to NAFLD and into the changing face of NAFLD in primary care.

We used UMLS semantic harmonisation to extract primary-care EHR data and identify 176,114 patients with a recorded diagnosis of NAFLD. Despite variations in coding systems, in the characteristics of the populations and in the health-care systems in each country, the results from all four territories are broadly consistent. They show rising incidence and prevalence of NAFLD; however, the levels of recorded NAFLD in EHR primary-care databases is many-fold lower than those anticipated based on prior observation studies, which estimated the prevalence of NAFLD in the general European population to be 20–30% [33]. The characteristics

of patients in that study were comparable with those with NAFLD in a recent systematic review of the literature and meta-analysis that included 101 studies [13]. That study reported the European prevalence of NAFLD diagnosed by imaging to be 24% (95% CI: 16–34%) and diagnosed by blood tests to be 13% (95% CI: 4–33%). Thus, our pooled prevalence in European EHR databases of 1.9% is at best ~1/6 and more likely only ~1/12 of the estimates based on cohort data. Our estimates of incidence in 2015 ranged from 1.1 to 4.1 per 1000 and are approximately 10 times lower than expected based on cohort studies: 28 (95% CI: 19–41) per 1000 person-years in Israel and 52 (95% CI: 28–97) per 1000 in Asia [13].

The prevalence of NAFLD diagnosis has trebled and incidence has doubled over the period of this study. The rising rates of co-morbid conditions such as diabetes and obesity may be responsible for this. Other probable factors include increased awareness among primary-care and non-liver physicians, improved communication of the diagnosis from secondary to primary care, and the increased use of blood tests and imaging to investigate common complaints such as abdominal pain or monitoring long-term conditions. Our data do not allow us to test these hypotheses further; however, studies from other groups also suggest that the total number of people developing NAFLD is rising, as is the number of people with NAFLD who develop life-threatening complications [13].

Despite the consistency in overall findings, the differences between the databases are indicative of differing practices. SIDIAP had a relatively large proportion of patients with a history of alcohol abuse (14.1%), although all databases included at least some NAFLD patients with recorded alcohol abuse. This reflects uncertainty in the community as to whether an individual can have fatty liver disease associated with metabolic syndrome even if they drink alcohol in excess of recommended limits, or indeed have any other cause of chronic liver injury such as viral hepatitis. While clinical trials make very precise distinctions between alcoholic and non-alcoholic fatty liver disease, the reality is that an obese, diabetic and hypertensive patient can consume alcohol in excess of recommended limits and have liver injury. There is no way to distinguish which aetiology is the dominant cause, and so clinicians are quite comfortable with co-existing diagnoses. Indeed, some authors now refer to BAFLD – both alcoholic and fatty liver disease. An alternative explanation may be that specialists making the diagnosis of fatty liver are unaware of the high alcohol use, either because of under-reporting by patients or poor communication from GP practices.

In HSD, prevalence increased over time whereas incidence has decreased in recent years. This can be explained by a relatively stable population in which nearly all patients were enrolled in 2000, see Additional file 1: Figure S3, and remained in the database until December 2015.

Text-mining in IPCI increased the number of NAFLD diagnoses by over eightfold. This suggests that while the diagnosis of NAFLD is being made, GPs are not recording it, despite there being a code for liver steatosis in IPCI. IPCI had the lowest level of ALT recording. A recent survey of Dutch GPs explored attitudes to the importance of NAFLD [34]. Only 47% of doctors used liver tests in patients with NAFLD and non-invasive scores were never used by 73% of respondents (we were able to calculate FIB-4 scores in only 27% in IPCI).

The UK THIN database appears to outlie from the others in several ways. The prevalence of recorded NAFLD in THIN (0.2%) is much lower than the other databases and markedly lower than that found in a study of almost 700,000 adults in a primary-care EHR study in London, UK (0.9%) [35]. Higher rates of alcohol recording in the UK alone are unlikely to account for all this difference. The median ALT was highest in THIN. This

may suggest that the diagnosis of NAFLD is more likely to be made in the UK by investigating abnormal liver enzymes than in other territories. However, the data required to calculate FIB-4 were available in only 11% of patients in THIN (Additional file 1: Table S3). NAFLD patients in THIN had the highest mean BMI. Moreover, THIN had the highest proportion of NAFLD patients with diabetes or impaired fasting glucose and the highest proportion of NAFLD patients with high-risk FIB-4 scores. Large-scale liver-biopsy-based cross-sectional studies or replication of the current study in cohorts with systematic ascertainment of the component of FIB-4 would be needed to confirm that patients are diagnosed with NAFLD at more advanced stages in the UK compared to other European countries.

Limitations of the study

When interpreting the data, it is important to consider the following issues. In IPCI, a diagnostic code for NAFLD was not available, therefore we devised an algorithm based on the diagnostic code 'liver steatosis' and excluding excess alcohol consumption. We did not do this for all databases because the IPCI terminology contains only 1073 clinical terms and therefore, general practitioners often utilise the free text to record information with greater precision, whereas the other coding systems contain many more such concepts: ICD9CM contains 40,855 terms, ICD10 contains 13,505 terms and Read Codes contains 347,568 terms [36].

The number of cases of recorded NASH is too small to make meaningful estimates of incidence and prevalence: 2–4% of patients with NAFLD in THIN and SIDIAP in which NASH was coded. This is far short of the 12.2% estimated from a US biopsy-based study [37]. This shortfall between coded NASH and the true burden of disease is probably due to the same factors that result in under-recording of NAFLD diagnosis: recognition, referral and coding in primary care, and under-diagnosis or poor communication in secondary care.

It is not possible to verify the accuracy or origin of recorded diagnoses, although the characteristics of the patients derived from the four databases are in keeping with the population one would expect with a NAFLD diagnosis. Some individuals not in this study may have undiagnosed NAFLD. Therefore, our results do not represent the true disease burden in the epidemiological sense, rather they tell us what is actually happening with people who currently have a diagnosis of NAFLD and they can inform the arguments for or against greater action in this area. While we cannot exclude the possibility (however unlikely) that all the other millions of expected NAFLD patients exist in other databases, we do not make any conclusions about people outside this dataset. Although primary-care data contain a large body of information, this does not diminish the value of well-phenotyped cohort studies in which NAFLD can be ascertained systematically using standardised screening methods (e.g. measuring liver enzymes or performing ultrasound in all patients). That said, the databases included in this study have been extensively used for research and have been validated for diagnoses other than NAFLD [24, 27, 38].

Conclusions

Clinical practice is evolving in this emerging field and as yet there are no recommendations to screen formally for NAFLD, even in high risk groups [39, 40]. One school of thought is that if the only available intervention for NAFLD or NASH is lifestyle change, then doctors are already giving such advice to their patients, although the extent to which patients take up such advice varies. However, hepatic steatosis is an independent predictor of diabetes [41, 42] and could, therefore, identify patients who stand to benefit from lifestyle changes to prevent diabetes and hepatic complications. Furthermore, the emerging data suggesting hepatic steatosis is an independent cardiovascular risk factor may be an additional incentive for physicians to increase their awareness of the early stages of NAFLD. At the more severe end of the scale, novel therapies targeted at NASH and fibrosis are already in phase III clinical trials and are expected to be available in the next few years. These may change the treatment paradigm. Therefore, the scale of the health-care challenge posed by NAFLD and its sequelae cannot simply be side-stepped by dismissing NAFLD as pre-disease. Further research is required to quantify the associations of NAFLD with outcomes and to determine whether Wilson's criteria for effective screening can be fulfilled [43], thereby informing the screening debate.

Additional file

Additional file 1: Table S1. Characteristics of the primary-care databases included in the study. **Figure S1.** Identification of NAFLD patients in the IPCI database. **Table S2.** List of codes for the identification of NAFLD and description in ICD9CM, ICD10, Read Codes and SNOMEDCT US terminologies. **Table S3.** Number and proportion of patients with individual patient characteristic data available. **Table S4.** Point prevalence (95% CI) of NAFLD and NASH (per 100 persons) on 1 January of each calendar year in four primary-care databases, and pooled across databases. **Table S5.** One-year period prevalence (95% CI) of NAFLD (per 100 persons) on 1 January of each calendar year in four primary-care databases. **Table S6.** Point prevalence (95% CI) of NAFLD (per 1000 persons) by age categories and gender on 1 January 2015 in four primary-care databases. **Table S7.** Incidence estimates (95% CI) of NAFLD (per 1000 person-years) by calendar year in four primary-care databases, and pooled estimates across databases. **Table S8.** Incidence estimates (95% CI) of NAFLD (per 1000 person-years) in 2015 by age categories and gender in four primary-care databases. **Figure S2.** Pooled **a** prevalence (per 100 persons) and **b** incidence (per 1000 person-years) regressed over calendar year by meta-regression. **Figure S3.** Distribution of entry date for patients in the four databases. (DOCX 203 kb)

Abbreviations

ALT: Alanine transaminase; ANOVA: Analysis of variance; AST: Aspartate transaminase; BMI: Body mass index; CI: Confidence interval; EHR: Electronic health record; EMIF: European Medical Information Framework; ERC: European Research Council; GP: General practitioner; HSD: Health Search Database; IPCI: Integrated Primary Care Information; NAFLD : Non-alcoholic fatty liver disease; NASH: Non-alcoholic steatohepatitis; NIHR: National Institute for Health Research; SIDIAP: Information System for Research in Primary Care; THIN: The Health Improvement Network; UK: United Kingdom; UMLS: Unified Medical Language System; US: United States

Acknowledgements

EMIF is a collaboration between industry and academic partners that aims to develop common technical and governance solutions to facilitate access to diverse electronic medical and research data sources. These analyses were supported by the Innovative Medicines Initiative Joint Undertaking under EMIF grant agreement 115372, whose resources include financial contributions from the European Union's Seventh Framework Programme (FP7/2007-2013) and in-kind contributions from European Federation of Pharmaceutical Industries and Associations companies. The authors would like to acknowledge Nicholas Galwey for his advice on the statistical methods, Alba Jene for her administrative support and support during submission to ethical review boards, and Derek Nunez for support during the early protocol design stage.

Funding

Funding was received from FP7 Ideas under European Research Council (ERC) award 115372. ERC had no role in the design of the study, the collection, analysis, and interpretation of data, or in writing the manuscript. DPA is funded by a National Institute for Health Research (NIHR) Clinician Scientist award (CS-2013-13-012). This article presents independent research funded by the NIHR. The views expressed are those of the authors and not necessarily those of the National Health Service in the UK, the NIHR or the Department of Health. This work was partially supported by the NIHR Biomedical Research Centre, Oxford. WA is in receipt of a Medical Research Council New Investigator Award.

Authors' contributions

MA, AKL, PE, SK, DW, NS and WA designed the study. TDS and PA undertook the semantic harmonisation. PR was responsible for the data transformation and federated data analysis. MA and JFB analysed the data. MA, NS and WA wrote the manuscript. All authors interpreted the results, edited the manuscript and gave approval for submission.

Competing interests

MA was contracted to work at, and JFB, PE, SK and DW are employees of, GlaxoSmithKline, which has conducted clinical research including trials of therapeutic agents in NAFLD. AKL is an employee of Pfizer, which is conducting clinical research including trials of therapeutic agents in NAFLD. DPA has received unrestricted research grants from UCB, Amgen and Servier, and consultancy fees (paid to his department or research group) from UCB Pharma. DA has provided consultancy and advice to many pharmaceutical companies on undertaking outcome studies using real-world evidence. FL has provided consultancy for AlfaSigma, Bayer and Abbvie. PE and SK are employees and stockholders of GlaxoSmithKline. NS has consulted for Boehringer Ingelheim, Eli Lilly, Novo Nordisk and Janssen, and has received grants from Astrazeneca and BI. WA is a consultant and has delivered sponsored lectures to UCB Pharma, Gilead, Intercept and Medimmune. TDS has no conflicts of interest to declare.

Author details

[1]GlaxoSmithKline, London, UK. [2]Worldwide Research and Development, Pfizer, Connecticut, USA. [3]Erasmus Universitair Medisch Centrum, Rotterdam, The Netherlands. [4]Fundació Institut Universitari per a la Recerca a l'Atenció Primària de Salut Jordi Gol i Gurina, Barcelona, Spain. [5]Centre for Statistics in Medicine, NDORMS, University of Oxford, Oxford, UK. [6]Quintile IMS, London, UK. [7]Health Search, Italian College of General Practitioners and Primary Care, Florence, Italy. [8]Harvard Medical School, Harvard, Boston, MA, USA. [9]University of Glasgow, BHF Glasgow Cardiovascular Research Centre, Glasgow, UK. [10]Barts Liver Centre, Blizard Institute, Queen Mary, University of London, London, UK.

References

1. Sattar N, Forrest E, Preiss D. Non-alcoholic fatty liver disease. BMJ. 2014;349:g4596.
2. Tai FW, Syn WK, Alazawi W. Practical approach to non-alcoholic fatty liver disease in patients with diabetes. Diabet Med. 2015;32(9):1121–33.
3. Mantovani A, et al. Nonalcoholic fatty liver disease and risk of incident type 2 diabetes: a meta-analysis. Diabetes Care. 2018;41(2):372–82.
4. Mantovani A, et al. Nonalcoholic fatty liver disease increases risk of incident chronic kidney disease: a systematic review and meta-analysis. Metabolism. 2018;79:64–76.
5. Targher G, et al. Non-alcoholic fatty liver disease and risk of incident cardiovascular disease: a meta-analysis. J Hepatol. 2016;65(3):589–600.
6. Ekstedt M, et al. Fibrosis stage is the strongest predictor for disease-specific mortality in NAFLD after up to 33 years of follow-up. Hepatology. 2015; 61(5):1547–54.
7. Söderberg C, et al. Decreased survival of subjects with elevated liver function tests during a 28-year follow-up. Hepatology. 2010;51(2):595–602.
8. Sanna C, et al. Non-alcoholic fatty liver disease and extra-hepatic cancers. Int J Mol Sci. 2016;17(5):171.
9. Lonardo A, et al. Epidemiological modifiers of non-alcoholic fatty liver disease: focus on high-risk groups. Dig Liver Dis. 2015;47(12):997–1006.
10. Targher G, Day CP, Bonora E. Risk of cardiovascular disease in patients with nonalcoholic fatty liver disease. N Engl J Med. 2010;363(14):1341–50.
11. Targher G, Lonardo A, Byrne CD. Nonalcoholic fatty liver disease and chronic vascular complications of diabetes mellitus. Nat Rev Endocrinol. 2018;14(2):99–114.
12. Allen AM, et al. Nonalcoholic fatty liver disease incidence and impact on metabolic burden and death: a 20 year-community study. Hepatology. 2016;64(6):2165–72.
13. Younossi ZM, et al. Global epidemiology of nonalcoholic fatty liver disease-meta-analytic assessment of prevalence, incidence, and outcomes. Hepatology. 2016;64(1):73–84.
14. Williamson RM, et al. Prevalence of and risk factors for hepatic steatosis and nonalcoholic fatty liver disease in people with type 2 diabetes: the Edinburgh type 2 diabetes study. Diabetes Care. 2011;34(5):1139–44.
15. Vernon G, Baranova A, Younossi ZM. Systematic review: the epidemiology and natural history of non-alcoholic fatty liver disease and non-alcoholic steatohepatitis in adults. Aliment Pharmacol Ther. 2011;34(3):274–85.
16. Bedossa P, et al. Systematic review of bariatric surgery liver biopsies clarifies the natural history of liver disease in patients with severe obesity. Gut. 2017; 66(9):1688–96.
17. Zezos P, Renner EL. Liver transplantation and non-alcoholic fatty liver disease. World J Gastroenterol. 2014;20(42):15532–8.
18. Rinella ME. Screening for nonalcoholic fatty liver disease in patients with atherosclerotic coronary disease?–in principle yes, in practice not yet. Hepatology. 2016;63(3):688–90.
19. Wong VW, Chalasani N. Not routine screening, but vigilance for chronic liver disease in patients with type 2 diabetes. J Hepatol. 2016;64(6):1211–3.
20. Booth H, et al. Incidence of type 2 diabetes after bariatric surgery: population-based matched cohort study. Lancet Diabetes Endocrinol. 2014;2(12):963–8.
21. Farmer RD, et al. Population-based study of risk of venous thromboembolism associated with various oral contraceptives. Lancet. 1997; 349(9045):83–8.
22. Hobbs FDR, et al. Clinical workload in UK primary care: a retrospective analysis of 100 million consultations in England, 2007-14. Lancet. 2016; 387(10035):2323–30.
23. Kringos D, et al. The strength of primary care in Europe: an international comparative study. Br J Gen Pract. 2013;63(616):e742–50.
24. Gini R, et al. Chronic disease prevalence from Italian administrative databases in the VALORE project: a validation through comparison of population estimates with general practice databases and national survey. BMC Public Health. 2013;13:15.
25. Vlug AE, et al. Postmarketing surveillance based on electronic patient records: the IPCI project. Methods Inf Med. 1999;38(4–5):339–44.
26. Blak BT, et al. Generalisability of the health improvement network (THIN) database: demographics, chronic disease prevalence and mortality rates. Inform Prim Care. 2011;19(4):251–5.
27. Garcia-Gil Mdel M, et al. Construction and validation of a scoring system for the selection of high-quality data in a Spanish population primary care database (SIDIAP). Inform Prim Care. 2011;19(3):135–45.
28. Avillach P, et al. Harmonization process for the identification of medical events in eight European healthcare databases: the experience from the EU-ADR project. J Am Med Inform Assoc. 2013;20(1):184–92.
29. Sterling RK, et al. Development of a simple noninvasive index to predict significant fibrosis in patients with HIV/HCV coinfection. Hepatology. 2006; 43(6):1317–25.
30. Shah AG, et al. Comparison of noninvasive markers of fibrosis in patients with nonalcoholic fatty liver disease. Clin Gastroenterol Hepatol. 2009;7(10): 1104–12.
31. Coloma PM, et al. Combining electronic healthcare databases in Europe to allow for large-scale drug safety monitoring: the EU-ADR project. Pharmacoepidemiol Drug Saf. 2011;20(1):1–11.
32. Nascimbeni F, et al. From NAFLD in clinical practice to answers from guidelines. J Hepatol. 2013;59(4):859–71.
33. Loomba R, Sanyal AJ. The global NAFLD epidemic. Nat Rev Gastroenterol Hepatol. 2013;10(11):686–90.
34. van Asten M, et al. The increasing burden of NAFLD fibrosis in the general population: time to bridge the gap between hepatologists and primary care. Hepatology. 2017;65(3):1078.
35. Alazawi W, et al. Ethnicity and the diagnosis gap in liver disease: a population-based study. Br J Gen Pract. 2014;64(628):e694–702.
36. Medicine, N.L.o. Unified Medical Language System. 2017; Available from: https://www.nlm.nih.gov/research/umls/sourcereleasedocs/mrsabfields.html.
37. Williams CD, et al. Prevalence of nonalcoholic fatty liver disease and nonalcoholic steatohepatitis among a largely middle-aged population utilizing ultrasound and liver biopsy: a prospective study. Gastroenterology. 2011;140(1):124–31.
38. Coloma PM, et al. Identification of acute myocardial infarction from electronic healthcare records using different disease coding systems: a validation study in three European countries. BMJ Open. 2013;3(6):e002862.
39. Chalasani N, et al. The diagnosis and management of nonalcoholic fatty liver disease: practice guidance from the American Association for the Study of Liver Diseases. Hepatology. 2018;67(1):328–57.
40. European Association for the Study of the, L., D. European Association for the Study of, and O. European Association for the Study of. EASL-EASD-EASO clinical practice guidelines for the management of non-alcoholic fatty liver disease. J Hepatol. 2016;64(6):1388–402.
41. Sung KC, Kim SH. Interrelationship between fatty liver and insulin resistance in the development of type 2 diabetes. J Clin Endocrinol Metab. 2011;96(4):1093–7.
42. Zelber-Sagi S, et al. Non-alcoholic fatty liver disease independently predicts prediabetes during a 7-year prospective follow-up. Liver Int. 2013;33(9):1406–12.
43. Wilson JMG, Jungner Gja. Principles and practice of screening for disease [by] J. M. G. Wilson [and] G. Jungner. Geneva: World Health Organization; 1968.

14

Migration and tuberculosis transmission in a middle-income country

Julia Moreira Pescarini[1,3*], Vera Simonsen[2], Lucilaine Ferrazoli[2], Laura C. Rodrigues[3], Rosangela S. Oliveira[2], Eliseu Alves Waldman[1†] and Rein Houben[3,4†]

Abstract

Background: Little is known about the impact of growing migration on the pattern of tuberculosis (TB) transmission in middle-income countries. We estimated TB recent transmission and its associated factors and investigated the presence of cross-transmission between South American migrants and Brazilians.

Methods: We studied a convenient sample of cases of people with pulmonary TB in a central area of São Paulo, Brazil, diagnosed between 2013 and 2014. Cases with similar restriction fragment length polymorphism (IS*6110*-RFLP) patterns of their *Mycobacterium tuberculosis* complex isolates were grouped in clusters (recent transmission). Clusters with both Brazilian and South American migrants were considered mixed (cross-transmission). Risk factors for recent transmission were studied using logistic regression.

Results: Isolates from 347 cases were included, 76.7% from Brazilians and 23.3% from South American migrants. Fifty clusters were identified, which included 43% South American migrants and 60.2% Brazilians (odds ratio = 0.50, 95% confidence interval = 0.30–0.83). Twelve cross-transmission clusters were identified, involving 24.6% of all clustered cases and 13.8% of all genotyped cases, with migrants accounting for either an equal part or fewer cases in 11/12 mixed clusters.

Conclusions: Our results suggest that TB disease following recent transmission is more common among Brazilians, especially among those belonging to high-risk groups, such as drug users. Cross-transmission between migrants and Brazilians was present, but we found limited contributions from migrants to Brazilians in central areas of São Paulo and vice versa.

Keywords: Tuberculosis, Molecular epidemiology, Transmission, Migration, Middle-income; disease control

Background

Tuberculosis (TB) in high-income countries is often driven by migration from countries with a higher TB burden, which can account for up to 80% of the total TB burden [1]. As a result, migrants tend to be seen as a potential source of transmission to the local-born population [2, 3]. However, molecular research from high-income countries has shown that transmission from migrants to the local-born population is often limited [4]. As former high burden countries in the Global South grow economically and make progress in TB control, they are facing a similar challenge through increasing South-South migration [5].

Molecular epidemiology studies can estimate the number of TB cases due to recent transmission between local-born and migrant populations (cross-transmission) [6]. Results from high-income countries suggest that cross-transmission is bidirectional, limited and has wide variation among study settings [7–9]. There is little evidence available from middle-income countries [10, 11], where *Mycobacterium tuberculosis* complex (*Mtbc*) transmission between migrants and local-born people, in the South-South migration context,

* Correspondence: juliapescarini@gmail.com
†Equal contributors
[1]Faculdade de Saúde Pública, Universidade de São Paulo, São Paulo, Brazil
[3]Department of Infectious Disease Epidemiology, Faculty of Epidemiology and Public Health, London School of Hygiene and Tropical Medicine, London, UK
Full list of author information is available at the end of the article

might be more pronounced because of increased mixing through cultural proximity and social integration [12].

Regional migration has increased significantly in South America over the past 15 years, with a predominance of young, healthy and more feminized populations involved in labour migration towards large urban centres in Argentina, Brazil and Chile [13]. While regional migration in South America can contribute to more social integration, the vulnerability of migrants can be enhanced by the already poor social context found in metropolitan areas of South America [14–16]. The vulnerability of the local-born population and the contexts in which migrants find themselves might contribute to more TB cross-transmission than what is evidenced in high-income countries [4, 12, 13].

While the World Health Organization (WHO) End TB Strategy recognizes migrants as one of the vulnerable populations who must be targeted [17], many middle-income countries do not have specific TB policies for internal or external migrants [18–20]. For this to change, evidence is needed to establish whether migration is contributing to the TB burden in middle-income countries and to ongoing transmission among the local population. Here, we estimated recent transmission of TB and its associated factors and investigated the presence of cross-transmission between South American migrants and Brazilians in central districts of the city of São Paulo.

Methods
Study design, area and population
We conducted a cross-sectional study in the municipality of São Paulo, Brazil. The Brazilian Health System (SUS) guarantees access to free and universal healthcare services, irrespective of country of origin [19], which is important for TB treatment completion and cure among migrants [21]. Migration flows in SP are predominantly from other parts of Brazil and other South American countries. The number of TB notifications among South American migrants has increased in the last ten years [21]. Migrants coming from Bolivia accounted for almost half of the notified cases in some city districts [21], and this probably reflects the three times higher yearly incidence of TB in Bolivia than in Brazil (117/100,00 inhabitants/year and 41 inhabitants/year in 2015) [22].

Our study focused on the central area of São Paulo, where vulnerable populations including a significant number of recently arrived migrants live. We selected four Administrative Regions (administrative division of the municipality based on grouped districts) with the highest absolute number of cases of TB among South American migrants (study area). Almost 2 million individuals live in this densely populated study area (11,934 residents/km^2), where the proportion of *near poor*[1] reached more than 30% in some regions in 2010 (see Fig. 1) [23]. Many live in

a combination of squatting and informal dwellings, including migrants under precarious work conditions living in the workplace [24]. The mean pulmonary TB (PTB) incidence rate for 2013/2014 ranged from 13 to 131/100,000 inhabitants/year in the districts, and the proportion of new PTB cases among individuals of South American origin in 2013 and 2014 ranged from 14% to 30% in each of the Administrative Regions studied. In this context, TB transmission is favourable in areas of overcrowding, poverty and inequality [17].

The Brazilian TB Control Programme recommends further confirmation by both culture and drug susceptibility test for TB cases in high-risk groups for TB. This includes people living with HIV (PLHIV), drug users, people in contact with drug-resistant TB cases, smear-positive cases after 2 months on TB treatment, retreatment TB cases and other members of the 'vulnerable population' including migrants from South American countries [19, 25].

Our reference population was all PTB cases among residents in the study area, and the study population included only patients with TB for whom there was a culture available, without age or sex restrictions. All *Mtbc* culture-positive PTB cases among Brazilians and migrants, available at the State Reference Laboratory for TB (Instituto Adolfo Lutz-São Paulo (IAL-SP)) between 1 January 2013 and 31 December 2014, were eligible for the study. We included only the first available respiratory sample with culture (including sputum and bronchoalveolar lavage) from all the individuals and excluded migrants from outside South America.

Data collection
Socio-demographic, clinical and epidemiological data were obtained from the São Paulo Tuberculosis Control Program database (SINAN-TBWEB) and laboratory information from the IAL-SP database (SIGH).

Molecular characterization
We performed the molecular characterization of *Mtbc* isolates by restriction fragment length polymorphism (IS*6110*-RFLP) at the IAL-SP [26]. Analysis of the *Mtbc* pattern was conducted in Bionumerics v.7.2 (Applied Maths, Kortrijk, Belgium). We excluded similar patterns with less than five bands.

Data analysis and definitions
Cases with a unique IS*6110*-RFLP pattern were identified and considered to result from reactivation, not in a transmission chain in the sample. Two or more cases with identical patterns or with one band difference were defined as a cluster (i.e. part of the same recent transmission chain). Clusters consisting of either all Brazilian or all South American migrant cases were defined as simple clusters, and those with at least one Brazilian and

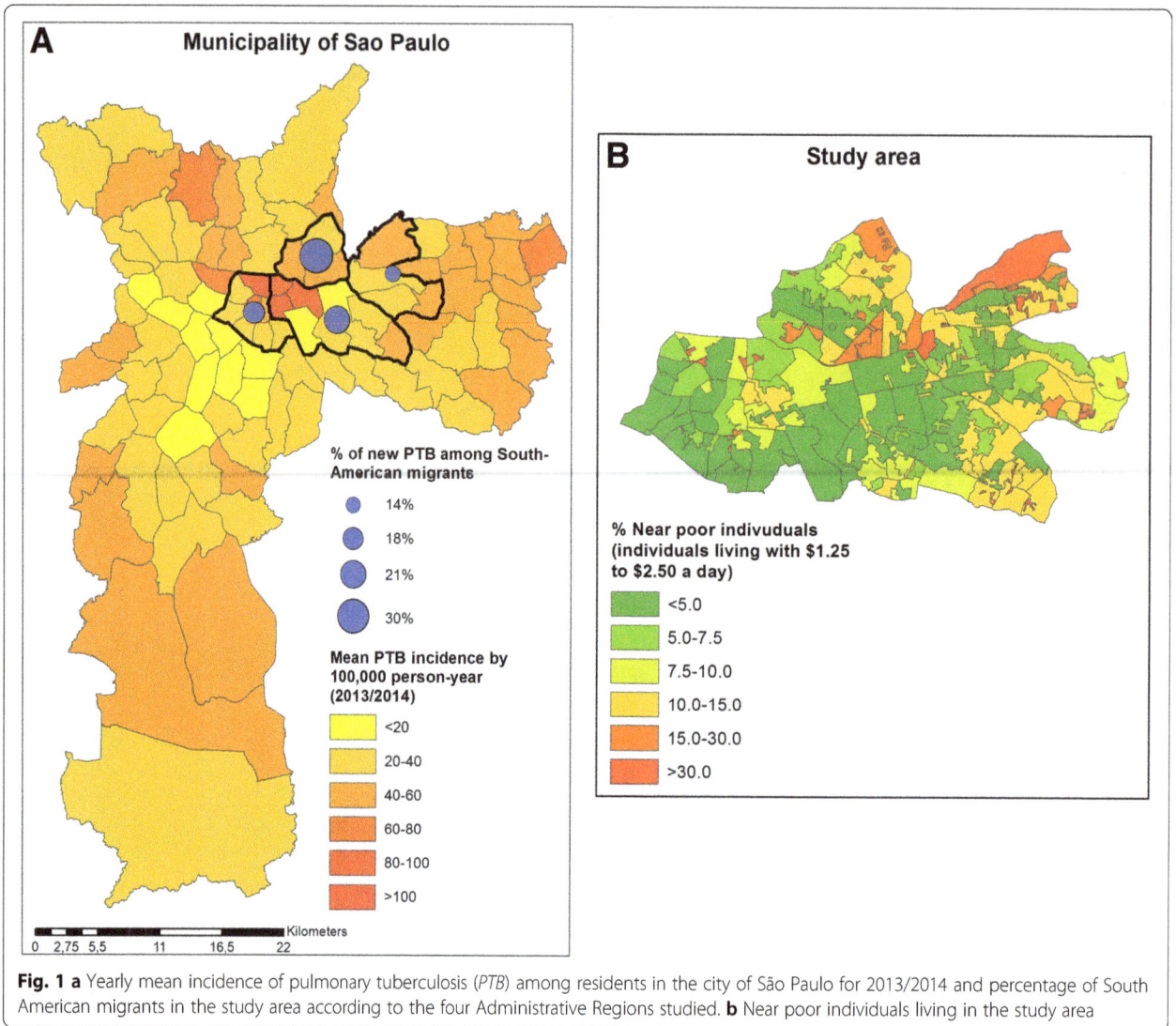

Fig. 1 a Yearly mean incidence of pulmonary tuberculosis (*PTB*) among residents in the city of São Paulo for 2013/2014 and percentage of South American migrants in the study area according to the four Administrative Regions studied. **b** Near poor individuals living in the study area

one South American migrant were defined as mixed clusters. Statistical analyses were conducted in Stata 14. 1. Specific analyses included the following:

1. *Descriptive analysis of the population.* We described the socio-demographic and epidemiological characteristics of all the TB cases in the studied area (reference population) and in the studied sample, stratified by origin (Brazilians or other South American migrants), in order to characterize Brazilians and migrants with PTB in our sample and to identify potential selection bias resulting from over-representation of potential high-risk populations for recent transmission within the sample (drug users, alcohol abusers and PLHIV).

2. *Clustering analysis.* The '*n*' method was used to estimate the proportion of cases involved in recent transmission in the central area of São Paulo. The

alternative, the '*n* − 1' method, which discounts one case from each cluster that may have occurred by disease reactivation, is vulnerable to strong underestimation of ongoing transmission when the sampling proportion is small, as was likely in our study [6, 27]. We described the simple and mixed clusters in our sample, emphasizing the proportion of clustering in Brazilians and South American migrants. We investigated the associated factors of belonging to a cluster compared to unique profiles for the studied individuals estimating the odds ratio (OR) and its 95% confidence interval (95% CI) using univariate and multiple logistic regression.

3. *Sensitivity analyses.* We estimated the proportion of clusters that would be found under a more restrictive cluster definition and considered only identical isolates as part of a cluster. A second sensitivity analysis explored the bias introduced by

overrepresentation of high-risk groups. We removed all PLHIV, drug users and alcohol abusers from the second analysis to estimate the proportion of overall clusters and mixed clusters.

Results

Descriptive analysis of the population

During 2013 and 2014, 1764 cases of people with PTB were reported in the study area. Approximately 79% were Brazilians, and 19% were from other South American countries. The remaining 2% (36 cases) were migrants from other regions and were excluded from this analysis. We genotyped *Mtbc* isolates of 347 cases from 631 (55%) which were culture-positive. Our sample was set by isolates from 19.7% of all cases, 266 (19.1%) Brazilian cases and 81 (24.2%) South American cases which occurred in the study area in both years (see Fig. 2).

Table 1 shows the socio-demographic and epidemiologic characteristics of the sampled PTB cases, stratified by origin. Compared to overall cases that occurred in the studied area (Additional file 1: Table S1), our sample had a higher frequency of retreatments or relapses (22.7% vs 16.7%), sputum smear-positive diagnosis (79.

1% vs 72.9%) and a greater proportion of PLHIV (25.6% vs 18.4%) and drug users (16.7% vs 11.5%). We observed this trend among sampled Brazilians but not among sampled South American migrants, who shared similar characteristics with cases among South Americans in the studied area.

Overall, our sample was predominantly male (72.1%), almost half of the sample attended school for 8 to 11 years (46.1%) and more than 77% were workers. The TB diagnosis was performed by active case finding for 6.4% cases; nearly 30% of all persons had five or more household contacts, and 61 of 135 individuals (30.4%) reported 12 or more weeks between disease onset and the start of drug therapy. South Americans were younger than Brazilians (mean age 27.0 vs 38.0, $p < 0.001$), and a higher proportion of them were females (34.6% vs 25.9%, $p = 0.191$). There was a lower proportion of retreatment and relapses (6.2% vs 27.8%, $p < 0.001$) and a similar cure proportion (77.8 vs 70.1%, $p = 0.318$). Among South American migrants smaller numbers of PLHIV (2.8% vs 32.5%, $p < 0.001$), alcohol abusers (3.7% vs 17.7%, $p = 0.002$) and drug users (2.5% vs 21.1%, $p < 0.001$) were observed.

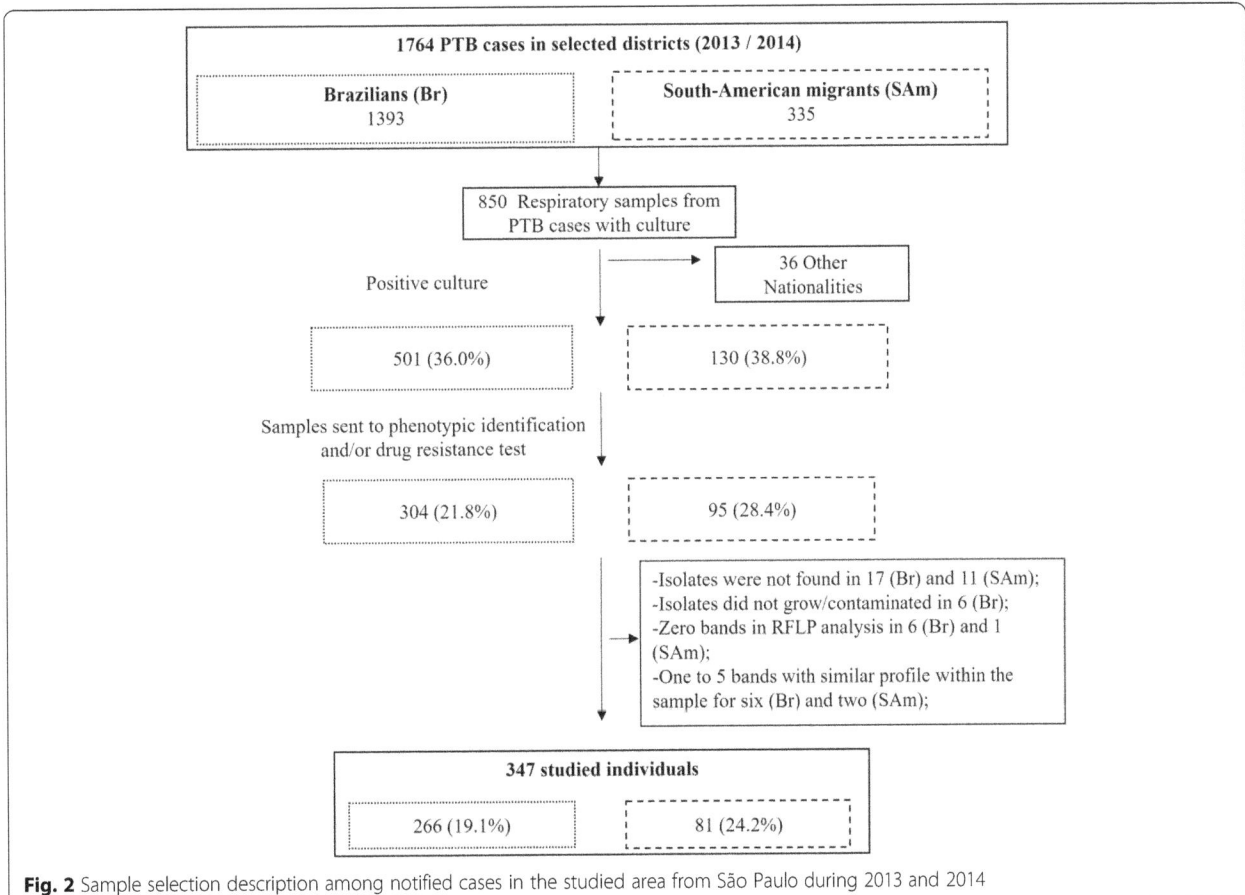

Fig. 2 Sample selection description among notified cases in the studied area from São Paulo during 2013 and 2014

Table 1 Characteristics of PTB cases identified in the study area and in the sample, stratified by Brazilian or other South American nationalities

	Brazilians (n = 266)	South American migrants (n = 81)	Total (n = 347)	
	N (%)	N (%)	N (%)	p value*
Mean age in years (SD)	38.0 (13.6)	27.0 (8.9)	35.4 (13.5)	< 0.001
Sex				0.130
Male	197 (74.1)	53 (65.4)	250 (72.1)	
Female	69 (25.9)	28 (34.6)	97 (27.9)	
School attendance				0.191
0–3	17 (7.62)	3 (4.9)	20 (7.0)	
4–7	74 (33.2)	14 (22.9)	88 (31.0)	
8–11	101 (45.3)	30 (49.2)	131 (46.1)	
12+	31 (13.9)	14 (23.0)	284 (15.9)	
Case				< 0.001
New	187 (72.2)	75 (93.8)	262 (77.3)	
Retreatment/relapse	72 (27.8)	5 (6.2)	77 (22.7)	
Treatment outcome				0.318
Cure	178 (70.1)	56 (77.8)	234 (71.8)	
Loss of follow-up	60 (23.6)	11 (15.3)	71 (21.8)	
Death/failure	16 (6.3)	5 (2.8)	21 (6.4)	
Sputum smear				0.160
Negative	50 (19.2)	21 (26.6)	71 (20.9)	
Positive	210 (80.8)	58 (73.4)	268 (79.1)	
Drug resistance[a]				0.596
No	210 (87.5)	70 (89.7)	280 (88.1)	
Yes	30 (12.5)	8 (10.3)	38 (11.9)	
HIV test				< 0.001
Negative	162 (67.5)	70 (97.2)	232 (74.4)	
Positive	78 (32.5)	2 (2.8)	80 (25.6)	
Diabetes				–
No	251 (94.4)	81 (100)	332 (95.7)	
Yes	15 (5.6)	0 (0)	15 (4.3)	
Alcohol abuse				0.002
No	219 (82.3)	78 (96.3)	297 (85.6)	
Yes	47 (17.7)	3 (3.7)	50 (14.4)	
Drug user				< 0.001
No	210 (78.9)	79 (97.5)	289 (83.3)	
Yes	56 (21.1)	2 (2.5)	58 (16.7)	

The percentage in brackets is calculated based on non-missing data. The difference between the total number of Brazilians, South American migrants or Total and each variable category corresponds to missing data
*Two tailed t test used for mean age comparison and Pearson chi-square for categorical variables
[a]Resistant to at least one drug

Clustering analysis

From the 347 individuals with typed *Mtbc* isolates, 152 (43.8%) had unique profiles and 195 (56.2%) were grouped in 58 clusters, of which 46 were simple and 12 were mixed. In the simple clusters, 40 contained only Brazilians and 6 only South American migrants. Simple clusters ranged from 2 to 18 individuals in Brazilians and from two to three in migrants. Forty-eight individuals were grouped in 12 mixed clusters, representing 13.8% of all genotyped cases or 24.6% of clustered cases. Figure 3 illustrates all the mixed clusters

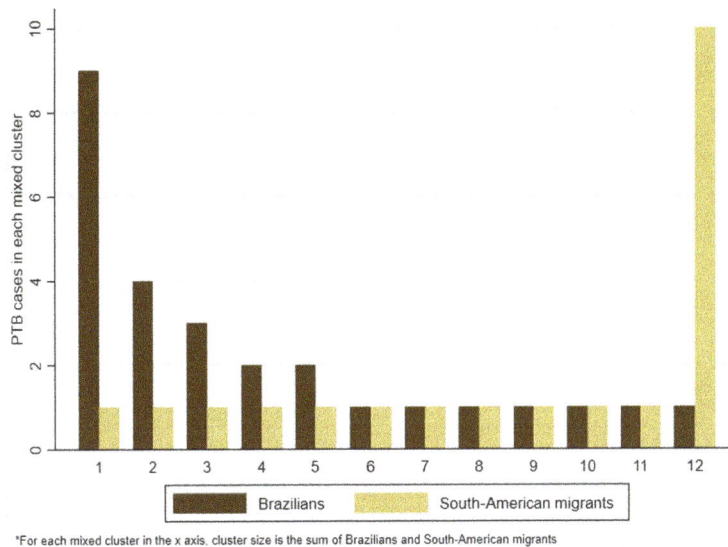

Fig. 3 Number of individuals involved in mixed clusters. For each mixed cluster on the x axis, *brown* represents the number of Brazilians and *beige* the number of South American migrants

and their distribution according to their origin. Of the 12 mixed clusters, six had only two individuals — one Brazilian and one South American — five had more Brazilians than South American migrants and one had more migrants than Brazilians.

In Table 2 we compare clusters with unique patterns according to their social, demographic and clinical characteristics. South American migrants made up 23.3% (81/347) of the sample. The cluster proportion was 43.2% (35/81) among South American migrants and 60.2% (160/266) among Brazilians (OR = 0.50, 95% CI = 0.30–0.83). Overall, drug users were more likely to be part of a cluster (OR = 2.11, 95% CI = 01.15–3.89), while the proportion of HIV/TB individuals in clusters did not differ between clusters and non-clustered cases (OR = 1.56, 95% CI = 0.92–2.65). After adjustment for age, sex, case type and TB/HIV co-infection, drug users (OR adj = 1.77, 95% CI = 0.85–3.68) and being South American (OR adj = 0.66, 95% CI = 0.35–1.27) were no longer strongly linked with clustering.

Sensitivity analysis

When we considered only identical patterns as clustered, we found a lower proportion clustered in both populations, but the OR for belonging to a cluster in South American migrants vs Brazilians remained consistent with the main analysis (OR = 0.56, 95% CI 0.33–0.94; Table 3, rows for Clusters). The proportion of mixed clusters decreased to 12.3% of all recent transmitted cases and to 6.3% of all the cases sampled.

After removing TB cases from high-risk groups for TB (PLHIV, drug users and alcohol abusers), 119 Brazilians and 68 South American migrants remained in our sample.

The proportion of clusters decreased from 60.2% to 42.9% among Brazilians and from 43.2% to 33.8% among South American migrants (OR = 0.68, 95% CI 0.37–1.27) (see Table 3, rows for Clusters). Six mixed clusters remained. The proportion of recent transmission involved in mixed clusters increased from 24.6% to 25.7% (19/74), which corresponded to 10.2% of overall cases in our sample.

Discussion

Our results suggest that TB disease following recent transmission in central areas from São Paulo is more common among Brazilians. Also, we suggest that cross-transmission between migrants and Brazilians is present; however, it is limited in both directions, i.e. from migrants to Brazilians and vice versa. These areas of São Paulo concentrate vulnerable populations for TB infection including a significant number of recently arrived migrants [21, 25].

In our study, 56.2% of cases of people with TB were possibly involved in clusters suggesting recent transmission. The proportion of clusters was smaller among South American migrants compared to Brazilians and higher among drug users. One out of four cases involved in recent transmission contained both Brazilians and South American migrants (mixed clusters). In most mixed clusters there was a predominance of Brazilians, with only one cluster with more South American migrants than nationals. In both our sample and in the study area, Brazilians and South American migrants differ in sociological, demographic and clinical characteristics: South American migrants tend to be younger, have higher levels of education, tend to be female and do not use drugs or carry HIV, reflecting the characteristics of healthy labour migration in the context of South America [13, 21].

Table 2 Distribution of cases clustered and non-clustered in our sample according to potential associated factors

Characteristics (N)	Clusters (n = 195)	Unique profiles (n = 152)	Univariate logistic regression	
	N (%)	N (%)	Crude OR (95% CI)	p value
Mean Age in years (SD)	35.3 (13.5)	35.6 (13.5)	1.00 (0.98–1.02)	0.868
Sex				
Male	140 (71.8)	110 (72.4)	1.00	
Female	55 (28.2)	42 (27.6)	1.03 (0.64–1.65)	0.906
Nationality				
Brazilian	160 (82.1)	106 (69.7)	1.00	
South American migrant	35 (17.9)	46 (30.3)	0.50 (0.30–0.83)	0.008
Education in years				
0–3	8 (4.9)	12 (10.0)	1.00	
4–7	52 (31.7)	36 (30.0)	2.17 (0.80–5.83)	0.126
8–11	81 (49.4)	50 (41.7)	2.43 (0.93–6.36)	0.070
12+	23 (14.0)	22 (18.3)	1.57 (0.54–4.56)	0.409
Worker				
Yes	140 (77.3)	109 (77.3)	1.00	
Retired/housewife	12 (6.6)	11 (7.8)	0.85 (0.36–2.00)	0.708
Unemployed	24 (13.3)	19 (13.5)	0.98 (0.51–1.89)	0.960
Prisoners	5 (2.8)	2 (1.4)	1.95 (0.37–10.22)	0.431
PTB incidence[a] in district of residence				
< 40	64 (32.8)	47 (30.9)	1.00	
40–80	74 (38.0)	55 (36.2)	0.99 (0.59–1.65)	0.963
> 80	57 (29.2)	50 (32)	0.84 (0.49–1.43)	0.515
Case type				
New	145 (75.1)	117 (80.1)	1.00	
Retreatment/relapse	48 (24.9)	29 (19.9)	1.33 (0.73–2.25)	0.277
Sputum smear				
Negative	46 (24.3)	25 (16.7)	1.00	
Positive	143 (75.7)	125 (82.3)	0.62 (0.36–1.07)	0.086
Diagnosis	184 (94.4)	140 (92.7)	1.00	
Passive	11 (5.6)	11 (7.3)	0.76 (0.32–1.81)	0.535
Active case finding				
Drug resistance				
No	158 (89.8)	122 (85.9)	1.00	
Yes	18 (10.2)	20 (14.1)	0.69 (0.35–1.37)	0.294
Treatment outcome				
Cure	128 (70.7)	106 (73.1)	1.00	
Loss of follow-up	41 (22.7)	30 (20.7)	1.13 (0.66–1.94)	0.651
Death/failure	12 (6.6)	9 (6.2)	1.10 (0.45–2.72)	0.829
Household contacts				
0	16 (14.7)	11 (11.5)	1.00	
1–2	41 (37.6)	33 (34.4)	0.85 (0.35–2.09)	0.730
3–4	19 (17.4)	24 (25.0)	0.54 (0.20–1.44)	0.222
5+	33 (30.3)	28 (29.2)	0.81 (0.32–2.03)	0.653

Table 2 Distribution of cases clustered and non-clustered in our sample according to potential associated factors *(Continued)*

Characteristics (N)	Clusters (n = 195)	Unique profiles (n = 152)	Univariate logistic regression	
	N (%)	N (%)	Crude OR (95% CI)	p value
Treatment delay in weeks				
0–2	12 (16.0)	14 (23.7)	1.00	
3–4	24 (32.0)	11 (18.6)	2.55 (0.89–7.27)	0.081
5–11	15 (20.0)	17 (28.8)	1.03 (0.36–2.91)	0.956
12 or more	24 (32.0)	17 (28.8)	1.65 (0.62–4.43)	0.323
Alcohol abuse				
No	166 (85.1)	131 (86.2)	1.00	
Yes	30 (14.9)	21 (13.8)	1.09 (0.59–2.00)	0.781
Drug use				
No	154 (79.0)	135 (88.8)	1.00	
Yes	41 (21.0)	17 (11.2)	2.11 (1.15–3.89)	0.016
TB/HIV co-infection				
No	126 (70.8)	106 (79.1)	1.00	
Yes	52 (29.2)	28 (20.9)	1.56 (0.92–2.65)	0.097
Diabetes				
No	189 (96.9)	143 (94,1)	1.00	
Yes	6 (3.1)	9 (5.9)	0.50 (0.18–1.45)	0.204

The percentage in brackets is calculated based on non-missing data. The difference between the total number of Brazilians, South American migrants or Total and each variable category corresponds to missing data

[a]Incidence per 100,000 person years

The overall clustering proportion found in our study was similar to that found in high-income countries [4, 28, 29], but lower than in middle- and low-income countries with a high TB burden [30, 31]. Other studies carried out in Brazil found less than 34% of cases due to recent transmission [32]. In our sample, South American migrants were less likely to belong to a cluster than Brazilians. These results differ from those in Iran with relapse cases [11] and agree with studies conducted in high-income settings, where in general there are higher proportions of clustering among the local-born population [4]. Nevertheless, being Brazilian or being a drug user was not independently associated with clustering. This is a likely reflection of the differences between South American migrants and Brazilians regarding social and demographic characteristics and the lower proportion of comorbidities among migrants.

The incidence ratio between migrants and the local born population are generally higher in South-North migration than in South-South. Studies in high- and middle-income countries have found similar proportions of cross-transmission to those in our study, around 30–40% [4, 11], suggesting a limited impact of cross-transmission on TB burden. When we removed all individuals belonging to high-risk groups for TB resistance (drug users, PLHIV and alcohol abusers), which were predominantly Brazilians, the proportion of recently transmitted cases among South American migrants and Brazilians became similar. On the other hand, the mixed clustering proportion was unchanged. Our results add to growing evidence from low- and middle-income countries (LMICs) that belonging to these high-risk groups might still be an important factor for recent TB transmission among Brazilians [30, 33, 34].

Table 3 Distribution of individuals by origin in clusters: sensitivity analysis with clusters restricted to those with identical patterns and excluding TB high-risk groups

Cluster proportion		South American migrants	Brazilians	Overall		
		N (%)	N (%)	N (%)	OR (95% CI)	p value
Identical patterns	Clusters	26 (32.1)	122 (45.9)	148 (42.7)	0.56 (0.33–0.94)	0.029
	Unique profiles	55 (67.9)	144 (54.1)	199 (57.3)		
Similar patterns, excluding HIV, drug users and alcohol abusers	Clusters	23 (33.18)	51 (42.9)	74 (39.6)	0.68 (0.37–1.27)	0.225
	Unique profiles	45 (66.18)	68 (57.1)	113 (60.4)		

The key limitations of our study are the short study duration and limited sampling frame. Combined with insufficient epidemiological information on contact tracing, this prevents us from assigning a likely source case. However, in larger clusters, for example where only one out of nine or more cases is from a different origin group, transmission was most likely to this individual, rather than in the opposite direction. This could suggest that cross-transmission from Brazilians to migrants is more likely than that from migrants to Brazilians, which would be in line with other studies where a majority rule is used to designate the origin of the 'primary' case in that cluster [7, 12]. Furthermore, variables such as country of origin and time since arrival in Brazil (for migrants), which could add more information to TB incidence in the country of origin and to the risk of clustering, were not available in the Brazilian notification system when this study was conducted. More studies are needed to estimate the most likely direction of TB transmission, in order to study the characteristics and measure the impact of migration in our setting.

The short duration and low sampling proportion are also likely to lead to an underestimation of the clustering in both populations [6, 27] in potentially equal measure. However, due to the oversampling of Brazilian drug users and PLHIV, who are more likely to be part of a cluster, clustering is probably overestimated in Brazilians. As migrants are considered a priority group for sputum culture in the study area, our sample provided a more accurate estimate of transmission in migrants. We therefore suspect that underestimation of clustering among South American migrants is more likely than among Brazilians, which could mean that the contribution of mixed clusters to ongoing transmission in the study area is higher than found here [6]. Cross-contamination must always be considered in a unique cluster of migrants with only one Brazilian, although we observed strict protocols during the collection of molecular characterization data.

Because of these sampling biases, we should consider this study exploratory, and it reflects the challenges of conducting molecular epidemiological studies in low- and middle-income settings. Another possible limitation of the study is the use of RFLP instead of whole genome sequencing (WGS). This could have provided lower estimates of recent transmission, especially if strain variability in countries of origin were low [35], although it is unlikely that RFLP overestimated cross-transmission. Also WGS would have provided more information on the most likely direction of transmission. Nevertheless, the existence of mixed clusters provides strong evidence for the existence of cross-transmission and the need to explore the direction and more precise estimates of the contribution of migration to the transmission of TB in LMICs.

Conclusions

This study contributes to our understanding of the influence of South-South migration on TB recent transmission and cross-transmission in the central area of São Paulo. Marked social inequalities in middle-income countries and in the context of regional migration must be considered to reach the End TB Strategy targets. TB care and prevention policies should contemplate the characteristics of migration and the living conditions in host countries, as has been done in high-income countries [36], and target those groups, both migrants and local-born populations, in which recent transmission is more evident.

Endnote

[1]The population considered near poor in a monetary sense has an equivalent income of more than $1.25 a day but less than $2.50 a day [23].

Abbreviations

IAL-SP: Instituto Adolfo Lutz-São Paulo; *Mtbc: Mycobacterium tuberculosis* complex; PLHIV: People living with HIV; PTB: Pulmonary tuberculosis; RFLP: Restriction fragment length polymorphism; SINAN-TBWEB: São Paulo Tuberculosis Control Program database; TB: Tuberculosis; WHO: World Health Organization

Acknowledgements

We would like to thank all the staff of the 'Coordenacao de Vigilancia em Saude' of São Paulo Municipal Department of Health for giving us access to their data and for providing inputs for the study.

Funding

This work was supported by National Council for Scientific and Technological Development (CNPq) from Brazil (141998/2013-0, 202310/2015-9 to JMP and 309647/2015-0 to EAW).

Authors' contributions

JMP and EAW designed the original study. VS, LF, RH and LCR made substantial contributions to the study design. JMP, VS, RSO and LF conducted the molecular typing and analysed the molecular data. JMP, RH, EAW and LCR interpreted the epidemiological and molecular data. JMP and RH wrote the manuscript. All the authors contributed substantially to the data interpretation, literature search and the manuscript writing, and they approved its final version. EAW and RH are joint senior authors. All authors read and approved the final manuscript.

Competing interests

The authors declare that they have no competing interests.

Author details
[1]Faculdade de Saúde Pública, Universidade de São Paulo, São Paulo, Brazil.
[2]Instituto Adolfo Lutz, São Paulo, Brazil. [3]Department of Infectious Disease Epidemiology, Faculty of Epidemiology and Public Health, London School of Hygiene and Tropical Medicine, London, UK. [4]TB Modelling Group, TB Centre, London School of Hygiene and Tropical Medicine, London, UK.

References

1. Alvarez GG, Gushulak B, Abu Rumman K, et al. A comparative examination of tuberculosis immigration medical screening programs from selected countries with high immigration and low tuberculosis incidence rates. BMC Infect Dis. 2011;11:3.
2. Borgdorff M, Nagelkerke N, van Soolingen D, de Haas P, Veen J, van Embden J. Analysis of tuberculosis transmission between nationalities in the Netherlands in the period 1993-1995 using DNA fingerprinting. Am J Epidemiol. 1998;147(2):187–95.
3. Bandera A, Gori A, Catozzi L, et al. Molecular epidemiology study of exogenous reinfection in an area with a low incidence of tuberculosis. J Clin Microbiol. 2001;39(6):2213–8.
4. Sandgren A, Schepisi MS, Sotgiu G, et al. Tuberculosis transmission between foreign- and native-born populations in the EU/EEA: a systematic review. Eur Respir J. 2014;43(4):1159–71.
5. Van Rie A, Victor TC, Richardson M, et al. Reinfection and mixed infection cause changing Mycobacterium tuberculosis drug-resistance patterns. Am J Respir Crit Care Med. 2005;172(5):636–42.
6. Murray M, Alland D. Methodological problems in the molecular epidemiology of tuberculosis. Am J Epidemiol. 2002;155(6):565–71.
7. Kamper-Jorgensen Z, Andersen AB, Kok-Jensen A, et al. Migrant tuberculosis: the extent of transmission in a low burden country. BMC Infect Dis. 2012;12:60.
8. Goldblatt D, Rorman E, Chemtob D, et al. Molecular epidemiology and mapping of tuberculosis in Israel: do migrants transmit the disease to locals? Int J Tuberc Lung Dis. 2014;18(9):1085–91.
9. Borrell S, Espanol M, Orcau A, et al. Tuberculosis transmission patterns among Spanish-born and foreign-born populations in the city of Barcelona. Clin Microbiol Infect. 2010;16(6):568–74.
10. Liang QF, Pang Y, Chen QY, et al. Genetic profile of tuberculosis among the migrant population in Fujian Province. China Int J Tuberc Lung Dis. 2013; 17(5):655–61.
11. Parissa-Farnia MMR, Varahram M, Mirsaeidi M, Ahmadi M, Khazampour M, et al. The recent-transmission of Mycobacterium tuberculosis strains among Iranian and Afghan relapse cases: a DNA-fingerprinting using RFLP and spoligotyping. BMC Infect Dis. 2008;8:109.
12. Barniol J, Niemann S, Louis VR, et al. Transmission dynamics of pulmonary tuberculosis between autochthonous and immigrant sub-populations. BMC Infect Dis. 2009;9:197.
13. IOM. South America: The regional migration context. International Organization of Migration: Regional Office for South America; 2016. https://www.iom.int/south-america. Accessed 1 Apr 2017
14. Pescarini JM, Rodrigues LC, Gomes MG, Waldman EA. Migration to middle-income countries and tuberculosis-global policies for global economies. Glob Health. 2017;13(1):15.
15. Goldberg A. Contextos de vulnerabilidad social y situaciones de riesgo para la salud: tuberculosis en inmigrantes bolivianos que trabajan y viven en talleres textiles clandestinos de Buenos Aires. Cuadernos de Antropología Social. 2014;39:91–114.
16. Barreto ML, Teixeira MG, Bastos FI, Ximenes RAA, Barata RB, Rodrigues LC. Successes and failures in the control of infectious diseases in Brazil: social and environmental context, policies, interventions, and research needs. Lancet. 2011;377(9780):1877–89.
17. WHO. Draft global strategy and targets for tuberculosis prevention, care and control after 2015 — Report by the Secretariat. Geneva: World Health Organization; 2014.
18. del VA Y. Tuberculosis en inmigrantes: situación Chile-Perú. Rev chil enferm respir. 2010;26(3):161–4.
19. Brasil. Ministério da Saúde. Secretaria de Vigilância em Saúde. Departamento de Vigilância Epidemiológica. Manual de recomendações para o controle da tuberculose no Brasil. Brasilia: Ministério da Saúde; 2011.
20. Zhou C, Chu J, Geng H, Wang X, Xu L. Pulmonary tuberculosis among migrants in Shandong, China: factors associated with treatment delay. BMJ Open. 2014;4(12):e005805.
21. Martinez VN, Komatsu NK, De Figueredo SM, Waldman EA. Equity in health: tuberculosis in the Bolivian immigrant community of Sao Paulo, Brazil. Tropical Med Int Health. 2012;17(11):1417–24.
22. WHO. Global tuberculosis report 2016. Geneva: World Health Organization; 2016.
23. UNDP. Atlas of Human Development in Brazil. 2018. http://www.atlasbrasil.org.br/2013/en/. Accessed 15 Feb 2018.
24. Silveira C, Carneiro Junior N, Ribeiro MC, Barata Rde C. Living conditions and access to health services by Bolivian immigrants in the city of São Paulo, Brazil. Cad Saude Publica. 2013;29(10):2017–27.
25. SES-SP, CCD, CVE, Tuberculose Dd. Boletim TB 2011. Sao Paulo: Secretaria Estadual de Saude de SP. Centro de Controle de Doenças. Coordenadoria de Vigilancia em Saude. Divisão de Tuberculose. 2011.
26. Embden V. Strain Identification of Mycobacterium tuberculosis by DNA Fingerprinting: Recommendations for a standardized methodology. J Clin Microbiol. 1993;31(2):406–9.
27. Glynn JR, Bauer J, Boer AS, et al. Interpreting DNA fingerprint clusters of Mycobacterium tuberculosis. Int J Tuberc Lung Dis. 1999;3(12):1055–60.
28. Houben RM, Glynn JR. A systematic review and meta-analysis of molecular epidemiological studies of tuberculosis: development of a new tool to aid interpretation. Tropical Med Int Health. 2009;14(8):892–909.
29. Nava-Aguilera E, Andersson N, Harris E, Mitchell S, Hamel C, Shea B, et al. Risk factors associated with recent transmission of tuberculosis: systematic review and meta-analysis. Int J Tuberc Lung Dis. 2009;13(1):17–26.
30. Asiimwe BB, Joloba ML, Ghebremichael S, Koivula T, Kateete DP, Katabazi FA, et al. DNA restriction fragment length polymorphism analysis of Mycobacterium tuberculosis isolates from HIV-seropositive and HIV-seronegative patients in Kampala, Uganda. BMC Infect Dis. 2009;9:12.
31. Verver S, Warren RM, Munch Z, Vynnycky E, van Helden PD, Richardson M, et al. Transmission of tuberculosis in a high incidence urban community in South Africa. Int J Epidemiol. 2004;33(2):351–7.
32. Ribeiro FK, Pan W, Bertolde A, Vinhas SA, Peres RL, Riley L, et al. Genotypic and spatial analysis of Mycobacterium tuberculosis transmission in a high-incidence urban setting. Clin Infect Dis. 2015;61(5):758–66.
33. Godfrey-Faussett P, Sonnenberg P, Shearer SC, Bruce MC, Mee C, Morris L, et al. Tuberculosis control and molecular epidemiology in a South African gold-mining community. Lancet. 2000;356(9235):1066–71.
34. Fok A, Numata Y, Schulzer M, FitzGerald MJ. Risk factors for clustering of tuberculosis cases: a systematic review of population-based molecular epidemiology studies. Int J Tuberc Lung Dis. 2008;12(5):480–92.
35. Stucki D, Ballif M, Egger M, et al. Standard genotyping overestimates transmission of Mycobacterium tuberculosis among immigrants in a low-incidence country. J Clin Microbiol. 2016;54(7):1862–70.
36. Pareek M, Greenaway C, Noori T, Munoz J, Zenner D. The impact of migration on tuberculosis epidemiology and control in high-income countries: a review. BMC Med. 2016;14(1):48.

15

Quantifying where human acquisition of antibiotic resistance occurs: a mathematical modelling study

Gwenan M. Knight[1]*[iD], Céire Costelloe[1], Sarah R. Deeny[2], Luke S. P. Moore[1,3], Susan Hopkins[1,4,5,6], Alan P. Johnson[1,6], Julie V. Robotham[1,4,7] and Alison H. Holmes[1,3]

Abstract

Background: Antibiotic-resistant bacteria (ARB) are selected by the use of antibiotics. The rational design of interventions to reduce levels of antibiotic resistance requires a greater understanding of how and where ARB are acquired. Our aim was to determine whether acquisition of ARB occurs more often in the community or hospital setting.

Methods: We used a mathematical model of the natural history of ARB to estimate how many ARB were acquired in each of these two environments, as well as to determine key parameters for further investigation. To do this, we explored a range of realistic parameter combinations and considered a case study of parameters for an important subset of resistant strains in England.

Results: If we consider all people with ARB in the total population (community and hospital), the majority, under most clinically derived parameter combinations, acquired their resistance in the community, despite higher levels of antibiotic use and transmission of ARB in the hospital. However, if we focus on just the hospital population, under most parameter combinations a greater proportion of this population acquired ARB in the hospital.

Conclusions: It is likely that the majority of ARB are being acquired in the community, suggesting that efforts to reduce overall ARB carriage should focus on reducing antibiotic usage and transmission in the community setting. However, our framework highlights the need for better pathogen-specific data on antibiotic exposure, ARB clearance and transmission parameters, as well as the link between carriage of ARB and health impact. This is important to determine whether interventions should target total ARB carriage or hospital-acquired ARB carriage, as the latter often dominated in hospital populations.

Keywords: Antibiotic resistance, Mathematical modelling, Community, Hospital, Resistance acquisition, Intervention design

Background

Infections due to antibiotic-resistant bacteria (ARB) are associated with higher morbidity and mortality levels [1]. Globally, numbers of infections with ARB are increasing [2]. To tackle ARB, we need to develop interventions that optimise treatment outcomes whilst slowing the dissemination of antibiotic resistance. In order to develop these interventions we need to quantify the important transmission routes of ARB [3] and determine how much each setting contributes to the overall ARB burden. Without this information, we are potentially wasting resources on poorly targeted interventions [3, 4], resulting in delays in clinical care improvement and the continued spread of ARB to potentially irreversible levels [5].

ARB encountered in clinical situations may originate from any setting in which bacteria are exposed to antibiotics [6]. Such settings include hospitals, nursing homes, soil and wastewater from pharmaceutical plants [7, 8]. Although we know that antibiotics exist in many environments, we do not know what proportion of infections

* Correspondence: gwen.knight@lshtm.ac.uk
[1]National Institute of Health Research Health Protection Research Unit in Healthcare Associated Infections and Antimicrobial Resistance, Department of Infectious Diseases, Imperial College London, London W12 0NN, UK
Full list of author information is available at the end of the article

caused by ARB is due to the antibiotic exposure in each environment. For example, although a significant proportion of antibiotics is used in agriculture [9], there is an on-going debate about how much this usage selects for ARB that are ultimately transmitted to humans [10]. We therefore cannot currently predict the likely human health impact of reducing agricultural antibiotic use, although recent modelling work suggests that reducing transmission from livestock may be more important [11].

In this work we focus on two broad settings: the community and hospitals, as both are important for human ARB acquisition [12]. We define the "community" to be the population of individuals not in a healthcare setting. We did not include any settings with indirect pathways to human carriage of ARB, as the estimates are currently highly uncertain due to a lack of data (e.g. for agriculture [10]).

Although the vast majority (~ 80%) of healthcare antibiotics prescribed in England in 2013 were for patients in the community [13], the per capita exposure is greater and more infections with ARB occurred in hospitals [14]. This is worrying, as the hospital population suffer more serious consequences. What is unknown is whether, under a broad range of realistic parameters, ARB are commonly being acquired within the hospital setting or in the community and repeatedly introduced into hospitals within which they then spread. The former hypothesis suggests that antibiotic control in the community will do little to reduce the burden of serious ARB infections in hospitals, whilst the latter suggests that it may be key.

To address this unknown, we present a dynamic transmission mathematical model that tracks the acquisition of ARB by humans in each setting for a range of scenarios. The model structure is similar to previous modelling work exploring ARB movement between community and hospital settings (e.g. [12, 15–17]), but it is novel in that it generalises to multiple pathogen/antibiotic combinations to ask: Are there broad trends for acquisition that can be found, and under what parameter conditions are most ARB acquired in the community? Previous modelling work has focused on invasion of community strains into the hospital setting (e.g. [15, 18]) or mechanisms which drive maintenance of resistance in hospitals (e.g. [16, 19]). There is also a large body of work quantifying the different relative contribution of various colonisation or transmission routes of ARB in hospital wards [3, 4, 20–22]. This work expands on this quantification in the hospital, to explore the contribution of the hospital vs. community setting to acquisition of ARB under a large set of parameter combinations.

With this quantification we can explore whether broad trends exist using multiple scenarios, such as whether we would expect *most* ARB to be selected in the community or in the hospital and where interventions for

ARB should be targeted. This adds to existing clinical data, which usually only report where the patient was when ARB carriage (asymptomatic or an infection) was detected but cannot differentiate where or how resistance was acquired: e.g. did a patient with a bloodstream infection in a hospital ward acquire that ARB in the hospital, or before, in the community? To link to a specific example, we considered the set of parameters for a case study of *Escherichia coli* resistant to third-generation cephalosporins in England, which are an increasing problem [23].

Our long-term aim is to quantify the sources of ARB [24]. With this study, we explore the relative contributions of two important environments and provide the basic structure to be expanded upon in future quantification work. This first step demonstrates what can and should be done for ARB research and also highlights the gaps in our existing understanding.

Methods

To determine where humans acquire ARB, we split a population of 100,000 people into subpopulations based on their setting (community or hospital) and bacterial status (with no bacteria or susceptible bacteria, or with ARB acquired within the hospital or community) (Fig. 1). Here "with bacteria" incorporates both carriage and infection. The community setting was taken to be broadly representative of the general population.

Within the population, people moved from the community (C_X) into the hospital (H_X) at the hospitalisation rate per day (α) and exited at a rate (l). Assuming that all hospitals are full [16], we initially set a constant percentage of 0.25% of the total population to be in hospital (but varied this in sensitivity analyses). People were grouped by their bacterial carriage status: carrying no bacteria or susceptible bacteria (C_s, H_s), carrying ARB acquired in the hospital (C_{Rh}, H_{Rh}) or carrying ARB acquired in the community (C_{Rc}, H_{Rc}). We did not differentiate people by age, gender, co-morbidity or colonisation/infection status. We assumed that infected and colonised people have the same infectivity [16, 25, 26], but that those "with" bacteria who become infected had a higher mortality rate [27].

ARB was acquired either by transmission at a rate ($\beta_c\omega_c/N_c$, $\beta_h\omega_h/N_h$) from an exogenous source or by de novo emergence ($\epsilon\omega_c$, $\epsilon\omega_h$) (Fig. 1). Here, β_c, β_h are the transmission rates, ω_c, ω_h the antibiotic exposure rates and N_c, N_h the population sizes in the hospital and community respectively. ϵ is the proportion of people who acquire resistance during each antibiotic treatment. We chose a frequency-dependent transmission formulation to reflect likely transmission by the hands of healthcare workers in the hospital setting, where the likelihood of colonisation of the healthcare worker will depend on the

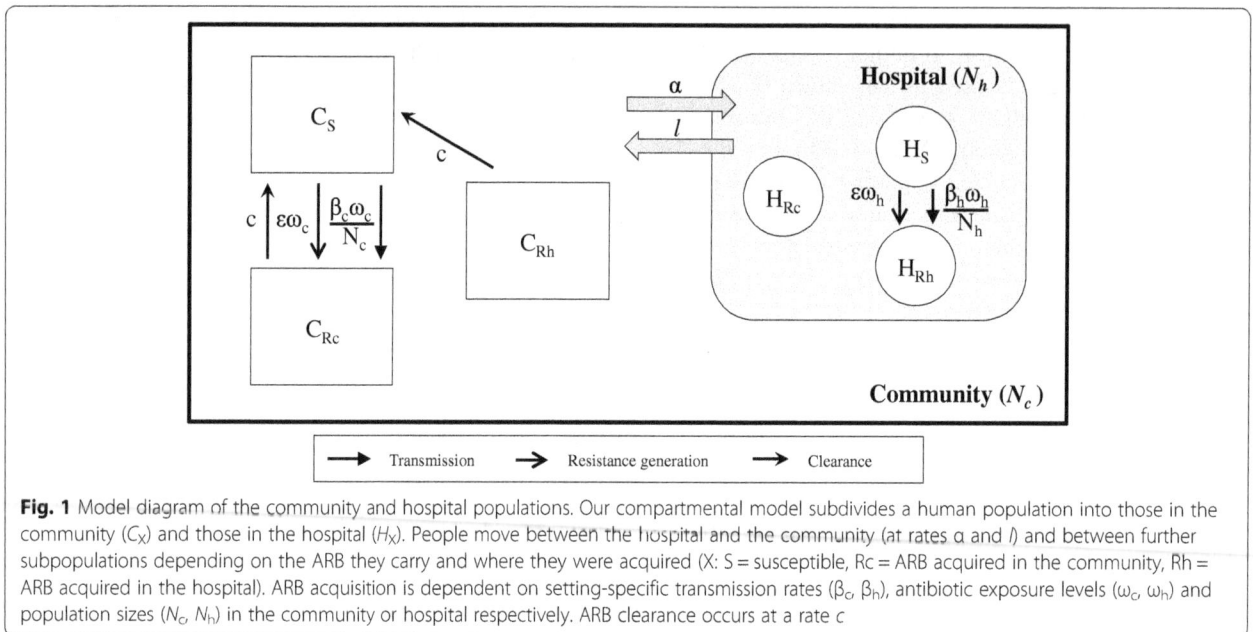

Fig. 1 Model diagram of the community and hospital populations. Our compartmental model subdivides a human population into those in the community (C_X) and those in the hospital (H_X). People move between the hospital and the community (at rates a and l) and between further subpopulations depending on the ARB they carry and where they were acquired (X: S = susceptible, Rc = ARB acquired in the community, Rh = ARB acquired in the hospital). ARB acquisition is dependent on setting-specific transmission rates (β_c, β_h), antibiotic exposure levels (ω_c, ω_h) and population sizes (N_c, N_h) in the community or hospital respectively. ARB clearance occurs at a rate c

proportion of patients carrying ARB, rather than the density. We used the same assumption in the community for consistency. Both acquisition rates (via transmission and de novo emergence) were dependent on exposure to antibiotics, as antibiotic use clears sensitive bacterial carriage, predisposing a host to colonisation with the (new) ARB. Linking transmission directly to antibiotic exposure captures this impact of selection on both the source of transmission (antibiotic exposure increases the ARB load) and the receiver (antibiotic exposure increases the chance of successful ARB transmission).

A higher transmission rate was (usually) assumed in the hospital (some models assume all transmission occurs only in hospitals, e.g. [16]). This is due to patient proximity, increased bacterial load and a high prevalence of immunocompromised patients in hospitals. The total number of contacts is likely to be greater in the community, due to the likely higher relative mobility of people in the community; however, each contact is likely to have a lower chance of successful bacterial transfer.

"Acquired" was defined by where the ARB were acquired, regardless of from whom they were transmitted. This is important in the public health context, as many infections with ARB are endogenous [28, 29], and hence knowledge of the original source of ARB acquisition is highly important for targeting interventions to reduce infections with ARB. The rate of transmission was taken to be a mass action assumption with random mixing in the hospital and community separately.

Those carrying bacteria can become infected (i_c, i_h) and die (μ_c, μ_h) at a higher rate than the background mortality rate. Due to potential fitness costs to resistant strains, it was assumed that resistant strains are equally or less likely to cause an infection than susceptible strains (by a factor r_{inf}) [30]. People do not remain persistently colonised with ARB in the community, but instead carriage is lost at a rate c. Due to the short duration of stay and the likely higher transmission rates in hospital, it was assumed that resistant bacterial carriage is not lost in the hospital setting.

These bacterial and patient dynamics (Fig. 1) were captured using a compartmental, deterministic model (see Additional file 1). All parameter values are listed in Table 1. Our results, as they are proportions, remain the same for any large population size. Detailed explanations of methods to determine the ranges for each parameter are given in Additional file 1.

Case study

To give a specific parameter combination, we considered a case study of *E. coli* in England, focusing on phenotypic resistance to third-generation cephalosporins, which is commonly, but not exclusively, mediated by production of extended-spectrum β-lactamases (ESBLs). We chose this due to the frequent use of β-lactams in both community and hospital settings, the existence of mandatory surveillance data for *E. coli* bacteraemia and due to the increasing problem of resistance (see Additional file 1) [23].

Total population analysis

Our primary outcome measure was the proportion of the total population with resistance who had acquired it in the hospital (Eq. (1)).

Table 1 Parameter values with description and range of parameters explored as well as the values used in the case study. For all details on calculations see Additional file 1

Symbol	Parameter description	Range	Case study	Notes and references
N	Total population size	100,000	100,000	Fixed
N_h	Size of the total population in hospital	(0.02% to 3%)N	0.25%	Fixed in baseline [37], explored in sensitivity analysis
N_c	Size of the total population in the community	$(1 - [0.02\% \text{ to } 3\%])N$	1–0.25%	Depends on N_h
a	Rate at which those in the community enter the hospital	2×10^{-4} to 2×10^{-3} per day	8×10^{-4} per day	Linked to number of admissions per day [38]
l	Rate at which those hospitalised return to the community	0.05 to 1 per day	0.32 per day	Varied to fit N_h
b	Background death rate	Fixed	1/(81*365)	Inverse of life expectancy [39]
ε	Proportion that acquire resistance during each antibiotic treatment	0.0008 to 0.13	0.0135 per treatment	Estimates taken from a range of studies (see Additional file 1)
ω_c	Rate of antibiotic exposure in community	(1 to 15)/1000 per day	8.6/1000 per day	Using total consumption in England in 2014 [23] and point prevalence surveillance data [40]
ω_h	Rate of antibiotic exposure in hospital	(0.5 to 1.00)ω_c	0.22 per day	
β_h	Transmission rate in the hospital	0.1 to 10 per day	1.8 per day	Case study value calibrated [14, 41]. Assumed to be the same or lower in the community
β_c	Transmission rate in the community	$\beta_h/25$ to $2\beta_h$	β_h	
c	Rate of clearance of resistant bacteria in community	1/730 to 1/42 per day	1/127 per day	Estimates taken from a range of studies (see Additional file 1)
i_c	Rate of infection in the community	$(1.4 \text{ to } 2.8) \times 10^{-6}$	1.75×10^{-6}	[42]
i_h	Rate of infection in the hospital	(5 to 500)i_c	100i_c	Assumed to be higher in hospitals due to patient co-morbidities.
r_{inf}	Decreased rate of infection by resistant organisms	0.5 to 1	0.8	Most ARB have reduced fitness, which can be ameliorated. (see Additional file 1)
μ_r	Proportion of infections with resistant bacteria that result in death	0.4 to 0.9	0.6	Case study value based on bacteraemia data [27]
μ_c	Proportion of infections with susceptible bacteria that result in death	0.1 to 0.5	0.2	

Proportion of resistance in total population acquired in hospital

$$= \frac{H_{Rh} + C_{Rh}}{H_{Rc} + H_{Rh} + C_{Rc} + C_{Rh}}$$

$$(1)$$

Due to the high levels of parameter uncertainty, our results are presented across many parameter combinations to encompass many possible resistance types. Firstly, we performed bivariate parameter analysis, with all other parameters held at the values in the case study. Secondly, in order to further explore multivariate effects, we used Latin hypercube sampling (LHS) (a method by which a well-distributed set of parameters is generated from a multidimensional distribution) to generate 10,000 parameter sets from our parameter ranges (Table 1). These 10,000 parameter sets allowed us to explore, within reasonable bounds, many possible combinations of values for each of the clinical variables in the model,

for example, high antibiotic usage in hospitals with low lengths of patient stay and vice versa. Extreme parameter combinations resulted in negative population sizes, which arose due to our use of a discrete-time simulation. We removed these values, to leave our final valid parameter set. With the variation in exit and entry rates, the size of our "hospital" population varied from 0 to 4% of the total population. This could reflect a larger hospital population than is currently the case for England, or our "hospital" setting representing a hospital population plus other populations with similar characteristics (e.g. high antibiotic exposure) such as nursing homes, where approximately 0.5% of the English population resides [31].

Using the valid LHS parameter samples we performed a sensitivity analysis to consider which parameters drive relative acquisition and hence should be targeted for both interventions and further data collection. This was done using a partial rank correlation coefficient analysis (PRCC) [32].

Hospital population analysis

The preceding multivariate analysis was repeated for the hospital subpopulation with a similar outcome measure: what proportion of those with ARB in hospital had acquired it in the hospital setting (Eq. (2)). This allowed us to explore whether those in the hospital setting have a different place of ARB acquisition than the total population.

$$= \frac{H_{Rh}}{H_{Rc} + H_{Rh}}$$

Proportion of resistance in hospital population acquired in hospital

$$(2)$$

A sensitivity analysis was also performed for this outcome (Eq. (2)) and for the prevalence of resistance in the population.

Results

Analysis of the total population

The minority of human ARB acquisition in our case study of *E. coli* resistant to third-generation cephalosporins occurs in the hospital (5%) (targets in Fig. 2).

Under most of our parameter combinations (bivariate and multivariate) the majority of the ARB in the total population was acquired in the community (Fig. 2). Only under certain scenarios was more resistance acquired in the hospital (Fig. 2, green to blue shaded areas above the 50% cut-off dashed line). Importantly, if the rate of transmission in the hospital is increased (*y* axis, Fig. 2a), then acquisition in the hospital is greater when the level of transmission in the community is lower by a factor of six or more (we explored up to a factor of 25 times lower). At extremely low transmission levels, more resistance is acquired in the community setting, due to a reversal to de novo resistance generation (instead of transmission) domination in the larger community population.

Even when antibiotic exposure is much higher in the hospital than in the community setting, acquisition in the hospital does not dominate in our model (Fig. 2b). Similarly, even when the exit rate from hospital is extremely low (i.e. there are long lengths of stay in hospital) or the rates of clearance of resistance in the community are high, acquisition in the hospital does not dominate (Fig. 2c–d). Varying the infection or mortality rates had little impact on these results (see Additional file 1).

More of the total ARB burden was acquired in the community under the majority (76%) of the valid (6562) LHS parameter sets (Fig. 2e). The proportion of acquisition in the community varied by parameter set, with a mean of 69% of ARB acquired in the community (see Additional file 1). Similar results were seen across different hospital population sizes (see Additional file 1).

Our sensitivity analysis showed that the most influential parameters on the proportion of ARB acquired in the hospital are those of relative antibiotic exposure, exit/entry rates and transmission in the hospital (Fig. 3).

Analysis of the hospital population

In the hospital population, the minority of human ARB acquisition in our case study of *E. coli* resistant to third-generation cephalosporins also occurs in the hospital (35%) (targets in Fig. 4). This was an exception to the majority of parameter scenarios, where most patients with ARB in hospital had acquired this resistance whilst in the hospital setting (Fig. 4). The exceptions were when transmission in the hospital was high, and similar in the community (Fig. 4a); when there was high antibiotic use in the community or similar levels in both settings (Fig. 4b); and when the rate of clearance in the community was low (Fig. 4d). Varying the exit and entry rates from those assumed in our case study (Fig. 4c) also generated no scenarios where most ARB in the hospital setting were acquired in the hospital setting.

When considering only those with ARB in the hospital, more had acquired them in the hospital under the majority (78%) of the valid LHS parameter samples (Fig. 4e). The proportion acquired in hospital varied across parameter sets, with a mean of 71% of ARB acquired in hospitals (see Additional file 1).

Our sensitivity analysis showed that the most influential parameters on the proportion of ARB acquired in the hospital for those patients in hospital are those of antibiotic exposure, rate of clearance of resistance in the community and length of stay (hospital exit rate) (see Additional file 1). For overall prevalence of resistance (see Additional file 1), the rate at which resistance is cleared and antibiotic exposure in the community, as well as the proportion that acquire resistance during antibiotic exposure are the most important parameters.

Discussion

Our work suggests that most ARB in the total population are acquired in the community setting. If instead we consider the small hospital subpopulation, under the majority of parameters considered, those patients in hospital with ARB had acquired them in the hospital. Quantitative assessment frameworks such as this can be used to make much sought-after predictions regarding the spread of ARB and the impact of interventions [7]. For example, this output forms part of the evidence base required for the recommended interventions, such as where to prioritise vaccine or diagnostic roll-out, in the recent UK O'Neill Report on "tackling drug-resistant infections globally" [33]. Such information is urgently needed, as ARB is already a major societal issue globally [2, 10].

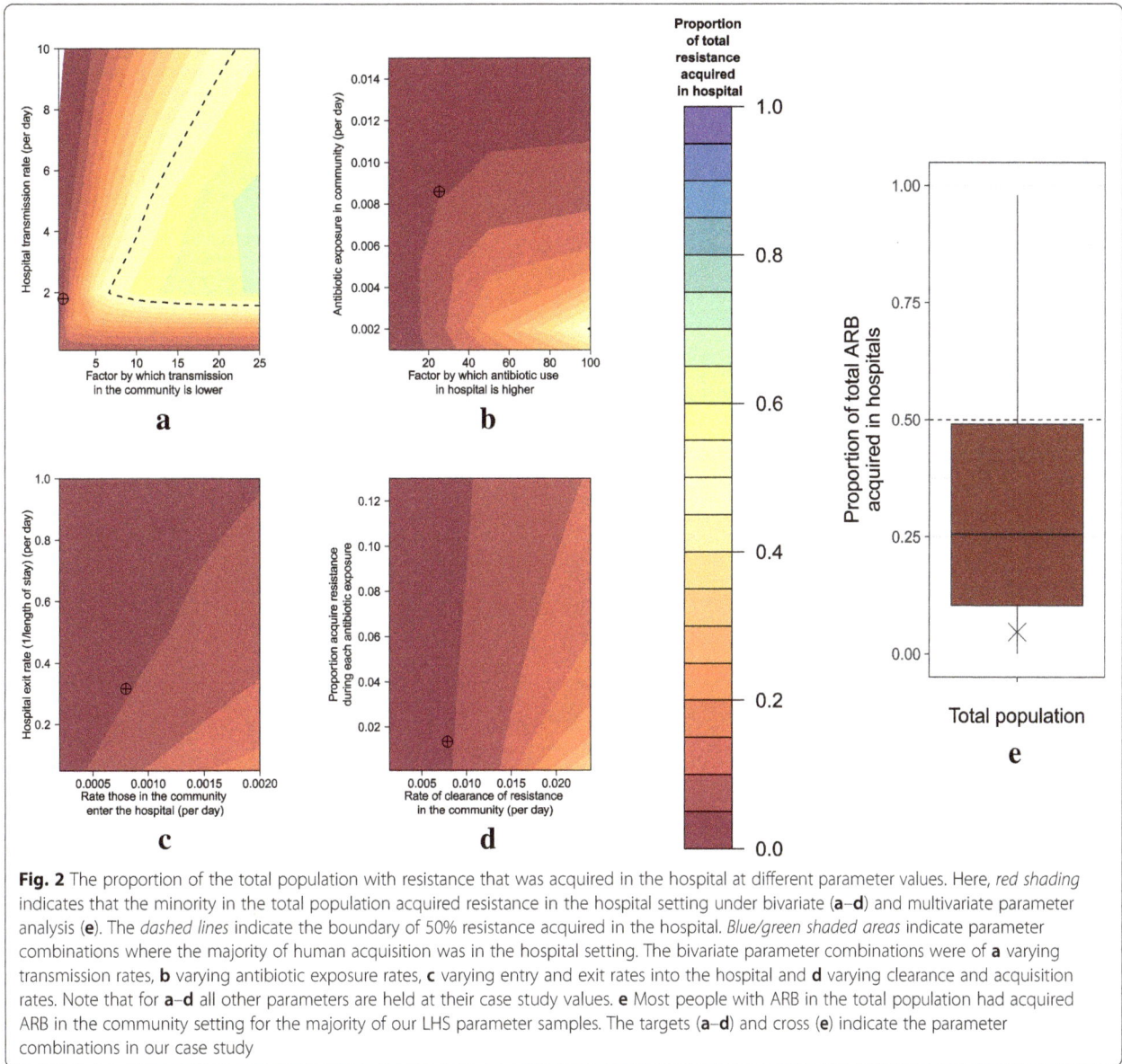

Fig. 2 The proportion of the total population with resistance that was acquired in the hospital at different parameter values. Here, *red shading* indicates that the minority in the total population acquired resistance in the hospital setting under bivariate (**a–d**) and multivariate parameter analysis (**e**). The *dashed lines* indicate the boundary of 50% resistance acquired in the hospital. *Blue/green shaded areas* indicate parameter combinations where the majority of human acquisition was in the hospital setting. The bivariate parameter combinations were of **a** varying transmission rates, **b** varying antibiotic exposure rates, **c** varying entry and exit rates into the hospital and **d** varying clearance and acquisition rates. Note that for **a–d** all other parameters are held at their case study values. **e** Most people with ARB in the total population had acquired ARB in the community setting for the majority of our LHS parameter samples. The targets (**a–d**) and cross (**e**) indicate the parameter combinations in our case study

The key parameters that alter where resistance is acquired are antibiotic use, length of hospital stay and the rate of transmission of ARB. Only under scenarios of much greater levels of transmission (Fig. 2a, upper right-hand corner) or antibiotic use in hospitals (Fig. 2b, lower right-hand side) is human ARB acquisition in the total population driven by hospitals. The predominance of human acquisition of ARB in the community is linked to the substantially higher numbers of people in the community (~ 98% of our population). If we increase the percentage of the population in our "hospital" setting, then the proportion acquired in hospitals increases, as seen by Kouyos et al. when exploring hospital size and ARB [17]. It is then crucial for intervention design and our understanding of ARB that we know the details of the heterogeneous settings in our populations and their interrelationships.

If reducing the total acquisition of ARB is our goal, then this model suggests interventions should target antibiotic exposure in the community setting. There are many ways that this could be done, for example by using educational interventions [34] or by targeting the symptoms most likely to be inappropriately prescribed antibiotics, such as sore throat [35]. Within the hospital setting, this model suggests that to reduce acquisition of ARB here, interventions should target transmission (for example by improved hand hygiene) and reduced antibiotic exposure. More acquisition also occurs in the hospital setting if clearance rates are higher in the community, suggesting that post-discharge decolonisation regimes, whilst aiding in driving down resistance prevalence, may shift the majority of ARB acquisition from occurring in the community to the hospital setting.

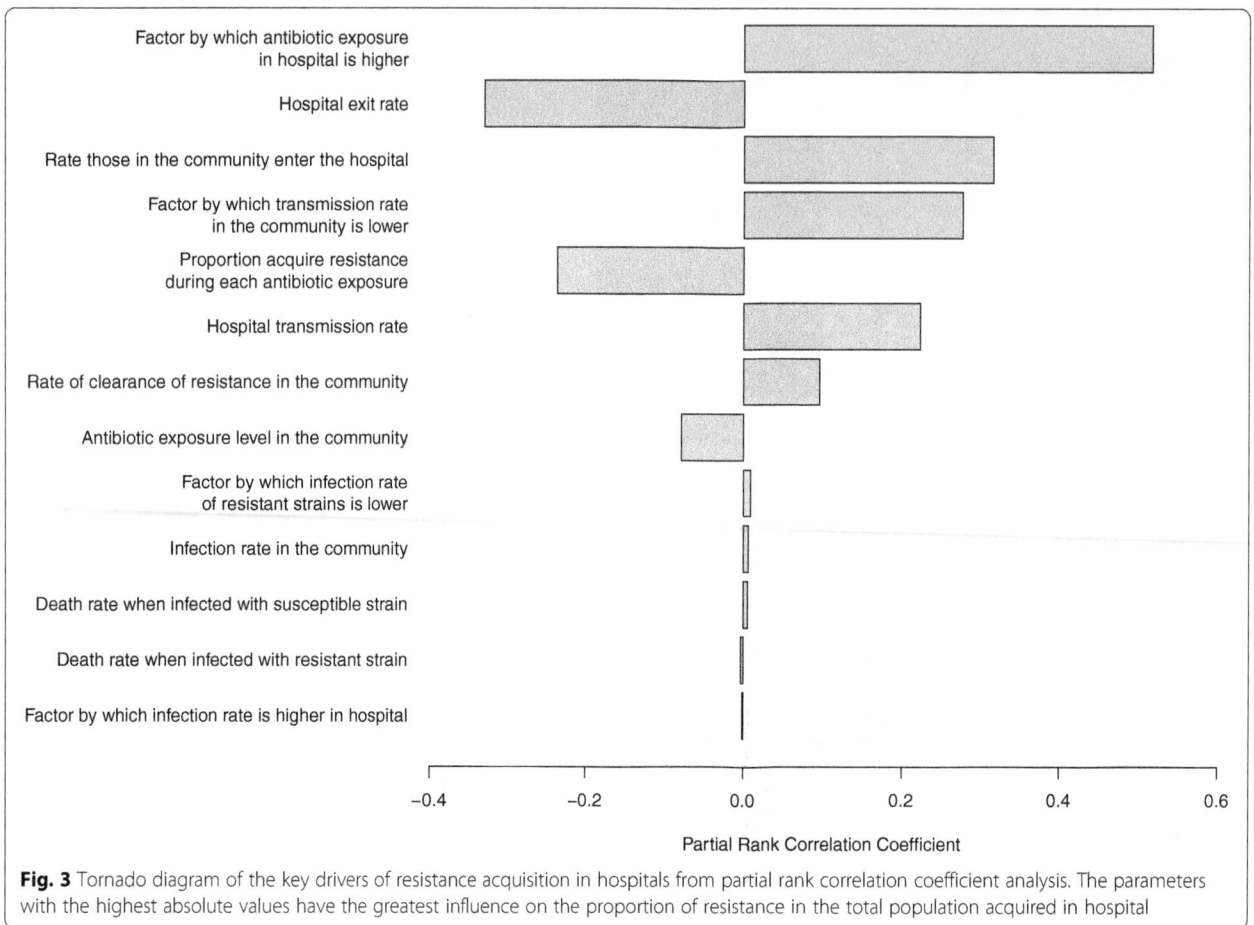

Fig. 3 Tornado diagram of the key drivers of resistance acquisition in hospitals from partial rank correlation coefficient analysis. The parameters with the highest absolute values have the greatest influence on the proportion of resistance in the total population acquired in hospital

Length of stay was also an important driver of where acquisition occurs, which could be targeted by tackling fundamental infrastructure (e.g. improved outpatient care).

To understand the clinical implications of this work we also need to consider the following question: does a reduction in human acquisition of ARB, which we model here, directly lead to a decrease in their associated health burden? We found that to reduce total ARB carriage requires interventions against acquisition of ARB in the community. However, the majority of those with ARB in hospitals had acquired them in the hospital. Although the hospital population is very small (< 4% of the total population), it is the one in which infection with ARB is potentially far more serious due to the higher proportion of people with immunocompromised status. Hence, it could be argued that reducing ARB burden in hospitals would have a bigger health impact. Targeting ARB in hospitals may also have a knock-on effect if those in hospital are the key sources of on-going transmission due to their immunocompromised status and increased bacterial load. Thus, the link between ARB acquisition and impact on health burden needs to be determined. Similarly, the routes to successful acquisition need to be established. For example, in exploring antibiotic use in

agriculture, what proportion of those who eat meat contaminated with ARB subsequently become infected?

Our case study highlights that our choice of where we target interventions should be tailored by the type of resistance and pathogen under consideration. Here, for *E. coli* resistant to third-generation cephalosporins, this work suggests that interventions should be focused on the community setting, as the majority of ARB acquisition (even in the hospital population) was always in the community (crosses in Figs. 2e and 4e). This reflects the parameters of this case study, where we assumed that transmission rates were the same in the hospital and community, that acquisition rates per treatment were low and, importantly, that high levels of cephalosporins are used in the community. For other ARB with high levels of antibiotic exposure in the community (such as other β-lactams) it may be that most acquisition is always in the community setting. However, for the majority of our parameter combinations, and hence other ARB, the picture is more complex, and the levels of use of the specific antibiotic in each setting will be critically important in determining where acquisition occurs. This can be seen through the dependence of our results on antibiotic exposure in the sensitivity analysis (Fig. 3).

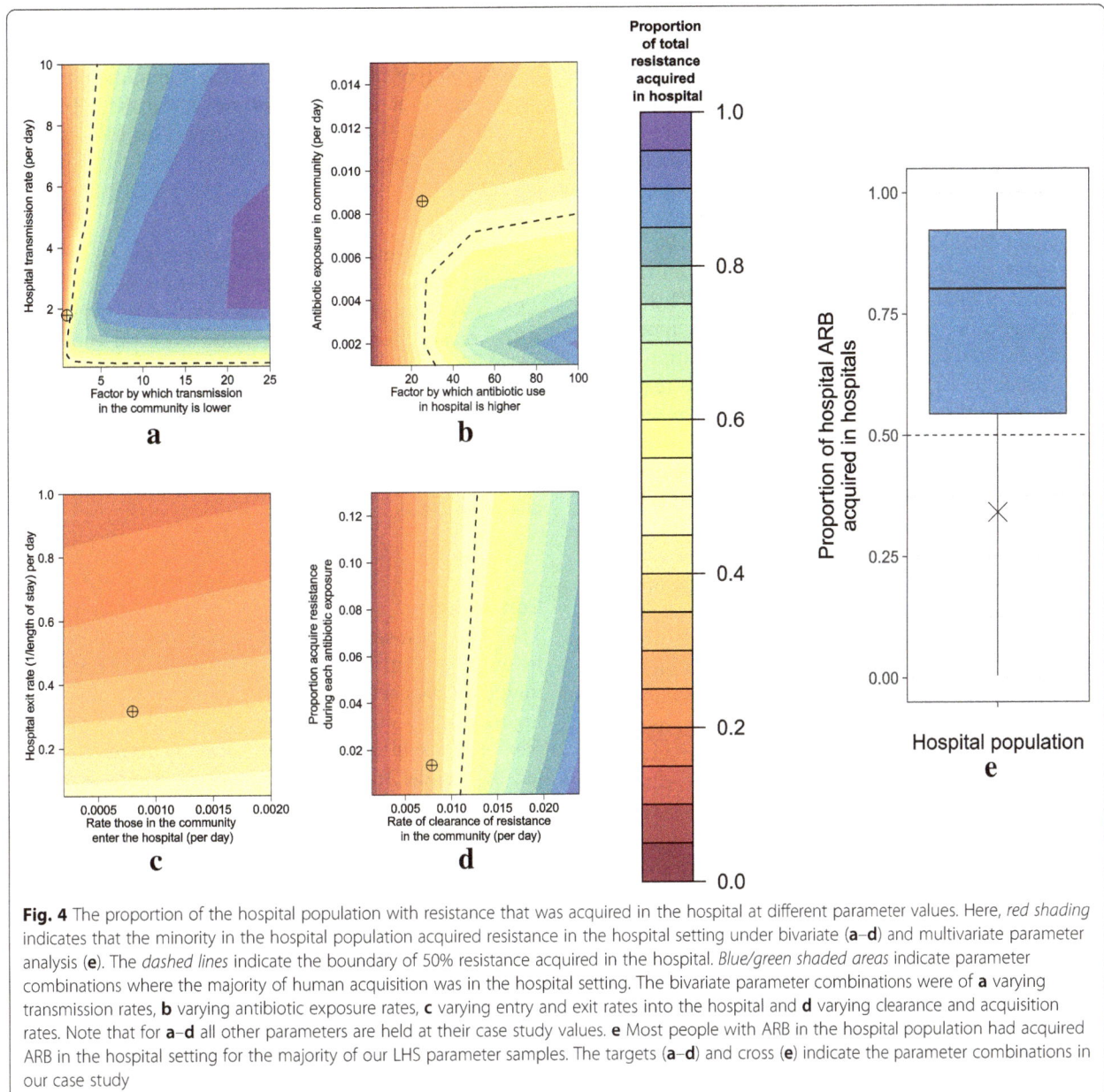

Fig. 4 The proportion of the hospital population with resistance that was acquired in the hospital at different parameter values. Here, *red shading* indicates that the minority in the hospital population acquired resistance in the hospital setting under bivariate (**a–d**) and multivariate parameter analysis (**e**). The *dashed lines* indicate the boundary of 50% resistance acquired in the hospital. *Blue/green shaded areas* indicate parameter combinations where the majority of human acquisition was in the hospital setting. The bivariate parameter combinations were of **a** varying transmission rates, **b** varying antibiotic exposure rates, **c** varying entry and exit rates into the hospital and **d** varying clearance and acquisition rates. Note that for **a–d** all other parameters are held at their case study values. **e** Most people with ARB in the hospital population had acquired ARB in the hospital setting for the majority of our LHS parameter samples. The targets (**a–d**) and cross (**e**) indicate the parameter combinations in our case study

The strengths of our study are that it uses a transparent quantitative framework to explore a broad parameter range that encompasses a wide set of potential scenarios for ARB acquisition. As there are few good estimates for many of these parameters (e.g. transmission rates), this allows for only broad conclusions to be drawn. Moreover, this model captures only a subset of the dynamics — both important human population and environmental stratifications are missing. Including missing human population stratifications (e.g. age, colonisation and infection status, and co-morbidities) would alter the movements between settings, requiring lengths of stay and contact pattern distributions, antibiotic exposure rates, as well as mortality rates. In particular, it is known that

resistance prevalence is highest in those with longer lengths of hospital stay. Environmental stratifications could include agricultural and waste water contact.

In comparison to previous work, our analysis is novel in that it considers acquisition of ARB from a broader, more general quantitative perspective, namely: how much ARB is acquired in which setting? This differs from previous mathematical models of ARB spread in the community and hospital [12, 16, 17, 25] which consider the importance of community reservoirs and the contribution of incoming carriage rates to their primary focus of the hospital.

The parameter sensitivity analysis suggests that future work should focus on determining better estimates for levels of transmission, antibiotic exposure and the rate at which ARB are cleared. Their correlation with the proportion of resistance acquired in the hospital suggests that these parameters are also key targets for interventions.

The next steps for this model would be to include the additional structural complexities that can be parameterised. Specifically, the entry and exit rates for the population should be stratified, potentially by age, as these rates were found to be key influences on the proportion of resistance acquired in hospitals. This lack of heterogeneity is the main limitation of this model. Including further human population stratification would likely result in acquisition differences by age (e.g. more acquisition in the community in certain age groups than others). The model could also be tailored to suit different pathogens and resistance types, as the quantitative contributions of different environments are likely to vary. One assumption to be varied is the 100% carriage rate, which is not true for pathogens such as *Staphylococcus aureus* and its important resistant subpopulation (methicillin-resistant *S. aureus*, MRSA). Complexity here would need to be added in the form of assumptions around the protective effect of prior colonisation.

Strikingly, most antibiotic resistance modelling studies tackle only populations in the community, hospitals, families and schools [36]. Extending our framework, for example to build on previous work showing the likely contribution of livestock antibiotic usage [11], could be used to test hypotheses, evaluate trends in resistance development over time and test the relative impact of new interventions. Furthermore, if we could extend our model to quantify how much ARB acquisition takes place in different hospital settings, such as wards, then we could potentially design better treatment options (e.g. if little ARB acquisition occurs in intensive care units, then last line antibiotics could be used there for critically ill patients).

To test our model results would require new data to be collected; for example, there could be a large prospective longitudinal study, tracking where and how people acquire ARB. This could be done by routinely sampling an individual's microbiome and that of his/her environment, to determine when (if at all) and where (community or hospital) acquisition of ARB occurs. The study would have to be large and long (~years) to be powered to detect hospital vs. community differences due to the low rate of hospitalisation and low prevalence of ARB. In the absence of such a large trial, efforts to determine differences in parameters, such as average antibiotic exposure levels in community and hospital settings, could be used to improve our parameter estimates. This would narrow the range of parameters explored within this model and allow us to be more confident as to where acquisition

is occurring. Our model predictions of relative levels of acquisition at these new estimates could then be tested by targeting interventions either at the community or hospital (whichever the model deems to be the setting of most acquisition) and comparing impact on ARB carriage and infection levels.

This study provides a new framework for ARB source quantification. We need now to not focus solely on where ARB infections are detected but on the settings where ARB are acquired. With this knowledge we can target ARB acquisition at its source, rather than fire fight at the clinical endpoint. More research is crucially needed on ARB prevalence across healthcare and environmental settings, transmission routes for ARB that result in human health burden and the levels and acquisition effects of antibiotic usage.

Conclusions

This is the first step to building a quantitative framework to test the relative contributions of all of the complex multidimensional drivers of ARB acquisition and hence improve intervention design. Here, we highlight the complex relationships that are likely to be uncovered by showing that, under the majority of our resistance scenarios, although the majority of ARB acquisition occurs in the community, most people with ARB in the hospital have acquired it in the hospital setting. Future work needs to develop this model to capture the full spectrum of ARB sources and to capture data on acquisition and transmission across these source environments.

Abbreviations

ARB : Antibiotic-resistant bacteria; ESBL: Extended-spectrum β-lactamase; LHS: Latin hypercube sampling; MRSA: Methicillin-resistant *Staphylococcus aureus*; PRCC: Partial rank correlation coefficient analysis

Acknowledgements

The authors also wish to acknowledge support from the National Institute for Health Research (NIHR) Imperial Biomedical Research Centre provided to LSPM and AHH.

Funding

The work was supported by the NIHR Health Protection Research Unit (HPRU) in Healthcare Associated Infections and Antimicrobial Resistance at Imperial College London in partnership with Public Health England (PHE). The views expressed are those of the author(s) and not necessarily those of the National Health Service (NHS), the NIHR, the Department of Health or PHE.

Authors' contributions
The concept was designed through discussions between GMK, AHH, CC and LSPM. The modelling was performed by GMK with technical support from SD and JVR. Results analyses and interpretation were performed by all authors. GMK wrote the first draft. All authors read, commented on and then approved the final manuscript.

Competing interests
AHH has received an Honorarium for presenting at a conference entitled South African Antibiotic Stewardship Programme Annual Workshop, sponsored by Merck (MSD Hoddesdon) from Medical Services, MSD Hoddesdon. LSPM consulted for bioMerieux in 2014 and for DNA Electronics in 2015, held an unrelated research grant from Leo Pharma in 2016 and received travel/meeting/accommodation expenses from Eumedica in 2016.

Author details
[1]National Institute of Health Research Health Protection Research Unit in Healthcare Associated Infections and Antimicrobial Resistance, Department of Infectious Diseases, Imperial College London, London W12 0NN, UK. [2]Data Analytics, The Health Foundation, London, UK. [3]Imperial College Healthcare NHS Trust, London, UK. [4]Antimicrobial Resistance Programme, Public Health England, London, UK. [5]Royal Free London NHS Foundation Trust Healthcare, London, UK. [6]Division of Healthcare-Associated Infection & Antimicrobial Resistance, National Infection Service, Public Health England, London, UK. [7]Modelling and Economics Unit, National Infection Service, Public Health England and Health Protection Research Unit in Modelling Methodology, London, UK.

References
1. Friedman ND, Temkin E, Carmeli Y. The negative impact of antibiotic resistance. Clin Microbiol Infect. 2016;22(5):416–25.
2. WHO: Antimicrobial resistance: global report on surveillance. 2014.
3. Pelupessy I, Bonten MJ, Diekmann O. How to assess the relative importance of different colonization routes of pathogens within hospital settings. Proc Natl Acad Sci U S A. 2002;99(8):5601–5.
4. Mikolajczyk RT, Sagel U, Bornemann R, Kramer A, Kretzschmar M. A statistical method for estimating the proportion of cases resulting from cross-transmission of multi-resistant pathogens in an intensive care unit. J Hosp Infect. 2007;65(2):149–55.
5. Global Antimicrobial Resistance Surveillance System (GLASS) report: early implementation 2016–17. Geneva: World Health Organization; 2017. http://apps.who.int/iris/bitstream/10665/259744/1/9789241513449-eng.pdf?ua=1. Accessed July 2018.
6. Department of Health UK. Antimicrobial resistance (AMR) systems map. 2014. https://www.gov.uk/government/publications/antimicrobial-resistance-amr-systems-map. Accessed July 2018.
7. Berendonk TU, Manaia CM, Merlin C, Fatta-Kassinos D, Cytryn E, Walsh F, et al. Tackling antibiotic resistance: the environmental framework. Nat Rev Microbiol. 2015;13(5):310–7.
8. Tello A, Austin B, Telfer TC. Selective pressure of antibiotic pollution on bacteria of importance to public health. Environ Health Perspect. 2012;120(8):1100–6.
9. UK one health report: joint report on human and animal antibiotic use, sales and resistance. 2015. https://www.gov.uk/government/publications/uk-one-health-report-antibiotics-use-in-humans-and-animals. Accessed July 2018.
10. Review on Antimicrobial Resistance. Tackling drug-resistant infections globally: An overview of our work. https://amr-review.org/Publications.html. Accessed July 2018.
11. van Bunnik BAD, Woolhouse MEJ. Modelling the impact of curtailing antibiotic usage in food animals on antibiotic resistance in humans. R Soc Open Sci. 2017;4:161067. https://doi.org/10.1098/rsos.161067.
12. Austin DJ, Anderson RM. Studies of antibiotic resistance within the patient, hospitals and the community using simple mathematical models. Philos Trans R Soc Lond Ser B Biol Sci. 1999;354(1384):721–38.
13. Ashiru-Oredope D, Hopkins S, English Surveillance Programme for Antimicrobial Utilization and Resistance Oversight Group. Antimicrobial stewardship: English Surveillance Programme for Antimicrobial Utilization and Resistance (ESPAUR). J Antimicrob Chemother. 2013;68(11):2421–3.
14. Moore LS, Freeman R, Gilchrist MJ, Gharbi M, Brannigan ET, Donaldson H, Livermore DM, Holmes AH. Homogeneity of antimicrobial policy, yet heterogeneity of antimicrobial resistance: antimicrobial non-susceptibility among 108,717 clinical isolates from primary, secondary and tertiary care patients in London. J Antimicrob Chemother. 2014;69(12):3409–22.
15. D'Agata EM, Webb GF, Horn MA, Moellering RC Jr, Ruan S. Modeling the invasion of community-acquired methicillin-resistant Staphylococcus aureus into hospitals. Clin Infect Dis. 2009;48(3):274–84.
16. Cooper BS, Medley GF, Stone SP, Kibbler CC, Cookson BD, Roberts JA, Duckworth G, Lai R, Ebrahim S. Methicillin-resistant Staphylococcus aureus in hospitals and the community: stealth dynamics and control catastrophes. Proc Natl Acad Sci U S A. 2004;101(27):10223–8.
17. Kouyos RD, Abel Zur Wiesch P, Bonhoeffer S. On being the right size: the impact of population size and stochastic effects on the evolution of drug resistance in hospitals and the community. PLoS Pathog. 2011;7(4):e1001334.
18. Hetem DJ, Westh H, Boye K, Jarlov JO, Bonten MJ, Bootsma MC. Nosocomial transmission of community-associated methicillin-resistant Staphylococcus aureus in Danish hospitals. J Antimicrob Chemother. 2012;67(7):1775–80.
19. van Kleef E, Luangasanatip N, Bonten MJ, Cooper BS. Why sensitive bacteria are resistant to hospital infection control. Wellcome Open Res. 2017;2:16.
20. Bootsma MC, Bonten MJ, Nijssen S, Fluit AC, Diekmann O. An algorithm to estimate the importance of bacterial acquisition routes in hospital settings. Am J Epidemiol. 2007;166(7):841–51.
21. Forrester M, Pettitt AN. Use of stochastic epidemic modeling to quantify transmission rates of colonization with methicillin-resistant Staphylococcus aureus in an intensive care unit. Infect Control Hosp Epidemiol. 2005;26(7):598–606.
22. McBryde ES, Pettitt AN, Cooper BS, DL ME. Characterizing an outbreak of vancomycin-resistant enterococci using hidden Markov models. J R Soc Interface. 2007;4(15):745–54.
23. English Surveillance Programme for Antimicrobial Utilisation and Resistance (ESPAUR) 2010 to 2014: report 2015. 2015. https://www.gov.uk/government/publications/english-surveillance-programme-antimicrobial-utilisation-and-resistance-espaur-report. Accessed July 2018.
24. Knight GM, Costelloe C, Murray KA, Robotham JV, Atun R, Holmes AH. Addressing the unknowns of antimicrobial resistance: quantifying and mapping the drivers of burden. Clin Infect Dis. 2018;66(4):612–6.
25. Kardas-Sloma L, Boelle PY, Opatowski L, Brun-Buisson C, Guillemot D, Temime L. Impact of antibiotic exposure patterns on selection of community-associated methicillin-resistant Staphylococcus aureus in hospital settings. Antimicrob Agents Chemother. 2011;55(10):4888–95.
26. Austin DJ, Kristinsson KG, Anderson RM. The relationship between the volume of antimicrobial consumption in human communities and the frequency of resistance. Proc Natl Acad Sci U S A. 1999;96(3):1152–6.
27. Melzer M, Petersen I. Mortality following bacteraemic infection caused by extended spectrum beta-lactamase (ESBL) producing E. Coli compared to non-ESBL producing E. Coli. J Infect. 2007;55(3):254–9.
28. Robinson TP, Bu DP, Carrique-Mas J, Fevre EM, Gilbert M, Grace D, Hay SI, Jiwakanon J, Kakkar M, Kariuki S, et al. Antibiotic resistance is the quintessential one health issue. Trans R Soc Trop Med Hyg. 2016;110(7):377–80.
29. Health matters: preventing infections and reducing antimicrobial resistance. 2017. https://www.gov.uk/government/publications/health-matters-preventing-infections-and-reducing-amr/health-matters-preventing-infections-and-reducing-antimicrobial-resistance. Accessed July 2018.
30. Andersson DI, Hughes D. Antibiotic resistance and its cost: is it possible to reverse resistance? Nat Rev Microbiol. 2010;8(4):260–71.
31. Changes in the older resident care home population between 2001 and 2011. London: Office for National Statistics; 2014. http://webarchive.

nationalarchives.gov.uk/20160105160709/http://www.ons.gov.uk/ons/
dcp171776_373040.pdf. Accessed July 2018.

32. Iman RL, Helton JC, Campbell JE. An approach to sensitivity analysis of
    computer models. Part 2. Ranking of input variables, response-surface
    validation, distribution effect and technique synopsis. J Qual Technol. 1981;
    13(4):232–40.

33. Review on Antimicrobial Resistance. Tackling drug-resistant infections
    globally. Final report and recommendations. 2016. http://amr-review.org/.
    Accessed July 2018.

34. Roque F, Herdeiro MT, Soares S, Teixeira Rodrigues A, Breitenfeld L, Figueiras
    A. Educational interventions to improve prescription and dispensing of
    antibiotics: a systematic review. BMC Public Health. 2014;14:1276.

35. Smieszek T, Pouwels KB, Dolk FCK, Smith DRM, Hopkins S, Sharland M, Hay
    AD, Moore MV, Robotham JV. Potential for reducing inappropriate antibiotic
    prescribing in English primary care. J Antimicrob Chemother. 2018;
    73(suppl_2):ii36–43.

36. Opatowski L, Guillemot D, Boelle PY, Temime L. Contribution of
    mathematical modeling to the fight against bacterial antibiotic resistance.
    Curr Opin Infect Dis. 2011;24(3):279–87.

37. Average number of available and occupied beds open overnight by sector.
    https://www.england.nhs.uk/statistics/statistical-work-areas/bedavailability-
    and-occupancy/bed-data-overnight/. Accessed July 2018.

38. Hospital Episode Statistics: Admitted Patient Care, England - 2013-2014.
    http://www.hscic.gov.uk/catalogue/PUB16719 . Accessed July 2018.

39. World Development Indicators. http://data.worldbank.org/country/united-
    kingdom. Accessed July 2018.

40. English National Point Prevalence Survey on Healthcare-associated
    Infections and Antimicrobial Use, 2011. London: Health Protection Agency;
    2012.

41. Wickramasinghe NH, Xu L, Eustace A, Shabir S, Saluja T, Hawkey PM. High
    community faecal carriage rates of CTX-M ESBL-producing Escherichia coli
    in a specific population group in Birmingham, UK. J Antimicrob Chemother.
    2012;67(5):1108–13.

42. Public Health England. Annual epidemiological commentary: mandatory
    MRSA, MSSA and E. coli bacteraemia and C. difficile infection data, 2013/14.
    https://www.gov.uk/government/statistics/mrsa-mssa-and-e-coli-
    bacteraemia-and-c-difficile-infection-annual-epidemiological-commentary.
    Accessed July 2018.

16

A cut-off of daily sedentary time and all-cause mortality in adults: a meta-regression analysis involving more than 1 million participants

Po-Wen Ku[1], Andrew Steptoe[2], Yung Liao[3], Ming-Chun Hsueh[4*] and Li-Jung Chen[5*]

Abstract

Background: The appropriate limit to the amount of daily sedentary time (ST) required to minimize mortality is uncertain. This meta-analysis aimed to quantify the dose-response association between daily ST and all-cause mortality and to explore the cut-off point above which health is impaired in adults aged 18–64 years old. We also examined whether there are differences between studies using self-report ST and those with device-based ST.

Methods: Prospective cohort studies providing effect estimates of daily ST (exposure) on all-cause mortality (outcome) were identified via MEDLINE, PubMed, Scopus, Web of Science, and Google Scholar databases until January 2018. Dose-response relationships between daily ST and all-cause mortality were examined using random-effects meta-regression models.

Results: Based on the pooled data for more than 1 million participants from 19 studies, the results showed a log-linear dose-response association between daily ST and all-cause mortality. Overall, more time spent in sedentary behaviors is associated with increased mortality risks. However, the method of measuring ST moderated the association between daily ST and mortality risk ($p < 0.05$). The cut-off of daily ST in studies with self-report ST was 7 h/day in comparison with 9 h/day for those with device-based ST.

Conclusions: Higher amounts of daily ST are log-linearly associated with increased risk of all-cause mortality in adults. On the basis of a limited number of studies using device-based measures, the findings suggest that it may be appropriate to encourage adults to engage in less sedentary behaviors, with fewer than 9 h a day being relevant for all-cause mortality.

Keywords: Sedentary behavior, Sitting, Inactivity, Review, Cut-point, Recommendation

Background

A sedentary lifestyle is prevalent among adults in the present era. A recent multi-country study based on 12 sites in 10 countries including the USA, Brazil, the UK, Denmark, the Czech Republic, and China (Hong Kong) of adults aged 18–66 using accelerometry found that the average sedentary time (ST) per day was 8.65 h (standard deviation [SD] = 1.8) [1]. ST was estimated to be responsible for 3.8% of all-cause mortality in adults according to a meta-analysis pooling data across 54 countries [2]. Prolonged ST has been increasingly recognized as a serious issue in public health [3], and recommendations have begun to appear in public health guidelines [4], suggesting that all adults should minimize the amount of ST [5, 6]. To conduct screening and surveillance of the health hazards of a sedentary lifestyle and develop feasible intervention strategies and evidence-based recommendations, it is crucial to identify a cut-off or limit on the amount of ST per day, above which health is impaired.

* Correspondence: boxeo@ntnu.edu.tw; ljchen@gm.ntupes.edu.tw
[4]Department of Physical Education, National Taiwan Normal University, NO.162, He-ping East Road, Section 1, Taipei 106, Taiwan
[5]Department of Exercise Health Science, National Taiwan University of Sport, No. 16, Section 1, Shuang-Shih Rd., Taichung 404, Taiwan
Full list of author information is available at the end of the article

The Australian government has proposed that that the cut-off point for risk is approximately 7 or 8 h a day [7], but the current evidence is inconsistent. Based on six studies (five using self-reported measures vs. one using a device-based measure), a meta-analysis examining the relationships between daily ST and all-cause mortality revealed that more than 7 h per day is associated with increased mortality risk [8]. In contrast, another recent meta-analysis based on 13 studies (all based on self-reported measures) found an increased risk of all-cause mortality among adults spending 4 or more hours per day in sedentary behaviors [9], which could be attenuated by the levels of moderate-to-vigorous physical activity (MVPA) as a moderator. Although the evident discrepancy may be due to heterogeneity across studies, one of the major limitations is that almost all the studies included in these two meta-analyses were based on self-report ST. Compared with devices, subjective measures such as questionnaires tend to be less accurate due to recall bias [10, 11]. Currently, there is insufficient evidence on which to provide specific public health recommendations regarding the appropriate limit to the amount of daily ST required to minimize mortality, especially using device-based assessments.

To address these shortfalls, our study involved meta-regression analyses to quantify the dose-response association between daily ST and all-cause mortality in adults aged 18–64 years old and to explore the cut-off duration associated with elevating the risk of all-cause mortality through reviewing evidence based on subjective measurements and recent studies using device-based ST [12–15]. We also examined whether there are distinct differences between studies involving self-report ST and those using device-based measures of ST.

Methods
Search strategy and selection criteria
Five databases, MEDLINE, PubMed, Scopus, Web of Science, and Google Scholar, were searched up to January 31, 2018 to identify potential studies examining relationships of sedentary behaviors with all-cause mortality in adults (aged 18–64 years). The following search strings were used: (("sitting time" OR "sedentary behavior" OR "sedentary behavior") AND (mortality OR mortalities OR death OR fatal)) AND (risk OR Cox OR hazard OR survival analysis OR odds). Additional studies were identified by manually checking the reference lists of included papers.

Article eligibility for inclusion was based on the following criteria: (1) original articles published in English before January 31, 2018; (2) articles involving a prospective cohort design; (3) involvement of participants in the age range of 18 to 64 years or the mean age in this range at baseline; (4) daily total ST or overall sitting time used as an exposure variable and all-cause mortality as an outcome variable; and (5) reported effect estimates of relative risk (RR) or odds ratios (ORs) or hazard ratios (HRs) with 95% confidence intervals (CIs) for all-cause mortality.

The exclusion criteria were applied to articles that: (1) focused on clinical populations such as patients with cardiovascular diseases, type 2 diabetes, or cancer etc.; (2) did not provide cut-off durations of total sedentary or sitting time; or (3) did not adjust for physical activity, since physical activity may be a confounding factor for the relationships of death with prolonged ST [12, 13].

Data extraction and quality assessment
The following data were extracted from the retrieved articles: author(s), year of publication, country, study population (sample size/death, age at baseline, and gender), follow-up time, total ST measure, covariates that were adjusted for in the analysis, and the HR estimates with corresponding 95% CIs for the models. Two authors independently extracted the data from each study and compared them for consistency. Any discrepancies between the two reviewers were settled through discussion, and a third reviewer's help was sought for resolving disagreements.

The study appraisal criteria and characteristics for each study are presented in Additional file 1: Table S1. Using the study quality checklist proposed by Kmet, Lee, and Cook [16], two authors (MH and YL) independently assessed the studies, and any disagreements were resolved by consensus. Studies were scored (0 for no, 1 for partial, 2 for yes) on 14 criteria by the following questions: Question/objective sufficiently described? and Study design evident and appropriate? [16], and the score of each study is presented in Additional file 2: Table S2. The sum of all scores was then divided by the highest possible score, giving quality scores ranging from 0 (worst) to 1 (best). A score ≥ 0.85 was defined as being of high quality [9].

Statistical analysis
Categorization of ST was based on the data available from each study. The maximally adjusted HR estimates from multivariable proportional hazards models were utilized to reduce the confounding effect in each study. To identify the cut-off of ST duration for increasing the risk of all-cause mortality, "dose of ST" was assigned, using the median or mean level of ST in each category, to the corresponding relative risk for each study. When ST was reported by ranges of time, the midpoint of the range was estimated. When the highest category was open ended, the length of the open-ended interval was assumed to be the same as that of the adjacent interval.

When the lowest category was open ended, the lower boundary was set to zero [17, 18]. Measures of association (HRs) and the corresponding CIs were transformed into the natural logarithm of the HRs and their variances. The statistical heterogeneity among studies was evaluated using I^2 (i.e., the proportion of total variation contributed by between-study variance) [19].

To assess the shape of the associations of ST with log-transformed risk of all-cause mortality using pooled data extracted from the 19 prospective cohort studies, random-effects meta-regression models were used. Linear, quadratic, and cubic models were fitted to determine the model of best fit for the pooled dose-response data first [20]. Additionally, to explore a range of possible functions such as U-shaped and J-shaped patterns, second-order fractional polynomial models, including the quadratic model, were also comprehensively evaluated: $(\log HR \mid X) = \beta_1 X^{P1} + \beta_2 X^{P2}$. In this equation, P1 and P2 were chosen from a predefined set $P = [-2, -1, -0.5, 0, 0.5, 1, 2]$ [21]. The results of goodness-of-fit tests among these models (including the linear model, the second-order fractional polynomial models, and the cubic model) are shown in Additional file 3: Table S3. The model selection was based on two criteria: (1) more variance between studies were explained by the model (i.e., R^2 analog) [22]; (2) the coefficients of each regression model were significantly different from zero. Among them, the linear model was chosen. Therefore, a random-effects meta-regression model based on linear dose-response relationships with restricted maximum likelihood estimations was utilized in the following analyses. To estimate the dispersion across studies and provide more accurate estimates, the Knapp-Hartung method was applied in the random-effects meta-regression analyses; this method additionally uses a refined estimator of between-studies variance of the effect estimator via a Student's t distribution instead of a Z distribution [23, 24]. This method has the effect of expanding the width of the CIs and yields a more conservative inference.

Several random-effects meta-regression models were used as follows. First, the linear dose-response relationship between ST and all-cause mortality was examined based on all studies (Model 1). Second, the independent effects of ST and measurement of ST (device-based [1] vs. subjective [0]) on the heterogeneity of mortality risks were assessed in Model 2. Third, to assess whether measurement of ST moderates the association of ST with subsequent mortality risks across studies, Model 2 was rerun by further including an interaction term (ST × measurement of ST). Finally, given the statistically significant interaction effect ($p < 0.05$), two separate meta-regression models were conducted for studies using subjective measures and those with device-based instruments (Models 3 and 4).

Sensitivity analyses were performed to address potential confounding effects. The study-level variables, which may account for the heterogeneity of mortality risks, were scrutinized in a simple meta-regression model. In addition to measurement of ST (subjective vs. device-based), gender, mean age, year of publication, and mean length of follow-up were assessed. Among them, only mean length of follow-up reached significance ($p < 0.05$). Because of potential confounding due to the differences in length of study follow-up, the time for follow-up was further included in Model 2 (Model 5). Model 5 was also repeated by further including in it an interaction term (ST × measurement of ST).

To visualize the association of ST and mortality risk and identify the potential cut-off of ST, scatter plots with regression lines and 95% CIs (Model 2: total studies, Model 3: studies with self-reported ST, and Model 4: studies with device-based ST) were obtained using meta-regression models. The follow-up time of each study as a continuous variable was further included in the three models for adjustment.

Publication bias was evaluated by a visual investigation of funnel plots for potential asymmetry and assessed with Egger's test [25] and Duval and Tweedie's "trim and fill" test [26].

All analyses were performed with Comprehensive Meta-Analysis Version 3.3.070 (Biostat, Englewood, NJ, USA) [22]. All p values were two-sided and were considered significant at $p < 0.05$.

Results

Study characteristics

A total of 254 articles were identified through five different database searches ($n = 238$) and reference list searches ($n = 16$) (see the Preferred Reporting Items for Systematic Reviews and Meta-Analyses [PRISMA] flow-chart in Fig. 1) [27]. Subsequently, after duplicates were removed, a total of 240 articles were retrieved to endnote. When the abstracts were screened, a total of 28 full-text articles were obtained for further review. We removed 9 of these based on the following exclusion criteria after contacting the authors of the original studies when missing information was not available in their articles: (1) mean age of the study population was ≥ 65 ($n = 4$) [28–31]; (2) the study sample was based on participants in clinical trials on hormone therapy ($n = 1$) [32]; (3) the cut-off point of the total sitting time was not provided ($n = 2$) [33, 34]; (4) there was no adjustment for physical activity in the multivariable model ($n = 1$) [35]; (5) devices were used to estimate ST without excluding sleep time ($n = 1$) [36]. Finally, 19 studies were included for meta-analysis, and the quality scores were high in all studies (average = 0.96; ≥ 0.85 was defined as high quality) [9] (see Additional file 2: Table S2).

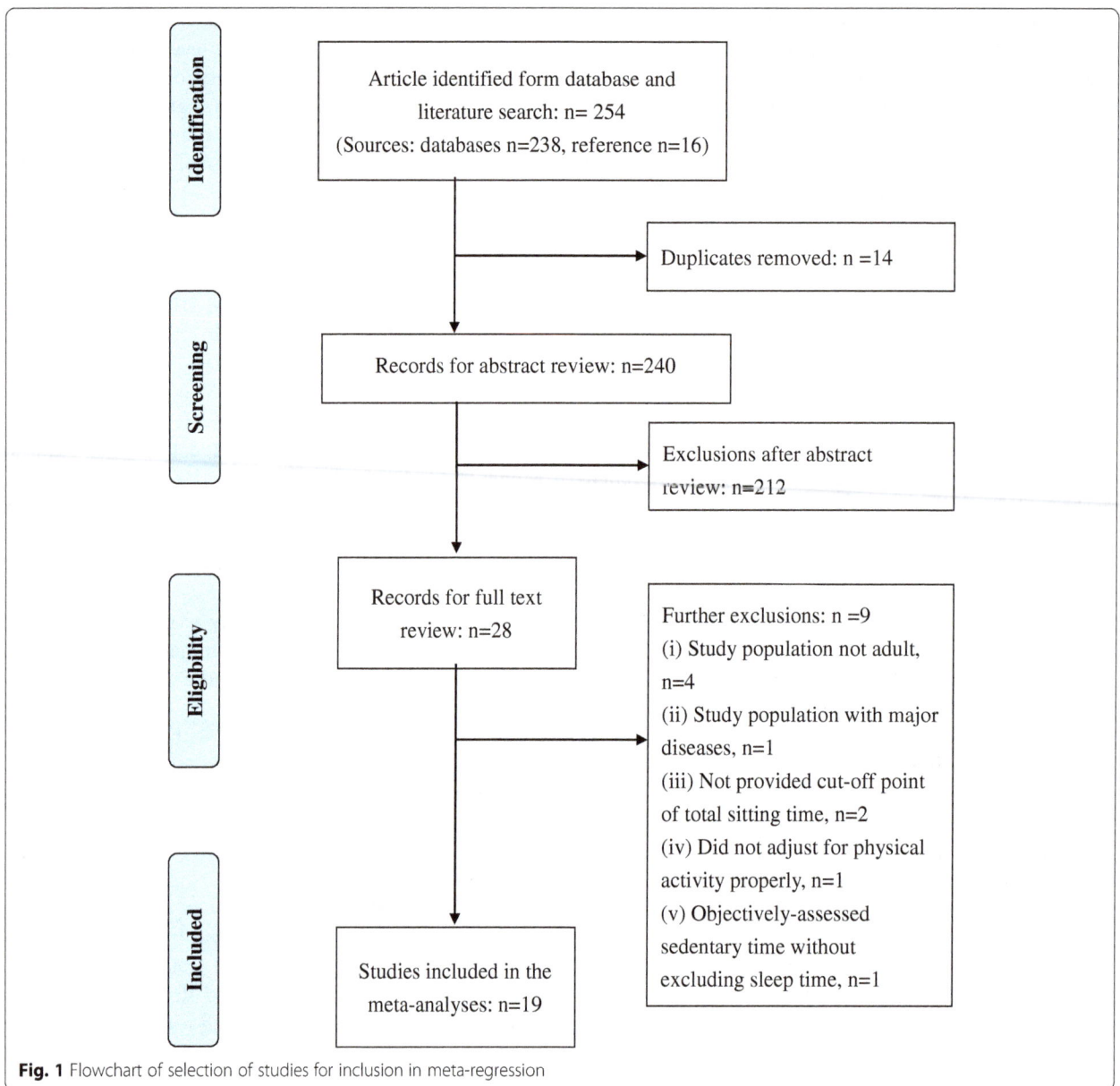

Fig. 1 Flowchart of selection of studies for inclusion in meta-regression

Data from all studies were extracted and are summarized in Additional file 1: Table S1. The 19 studies in the meta-analysis included 1,259,482 individuals who were followed up for 2.8–15.7 (mean time = 7.8) years, among whom 86,671 (6.9%) died [12–15, 37–47]. The mean age of participants in these studies ranged from 39.7 to 63.8 years old. Twelve studies assessed data by self-report ST [37–48] in comparison with seven studies with device-based ST [12–15, 49–51]. The measures of self-report ST among the 12 studies were brief. Seven studies utilized a single item [37–40, 42, 47, 48], three studies used two items [41, 45, 46], one used three items [44], and another one used five items [43]. The cut-off points for the categories were not consistent across the studies (see Additional file 1: Table S1). All studies adjusted for multiple potential confounding factors including at least gender, age, and physical activity, while 16 out of 19 studies also adjusted for education and smoking, 14 studies for body mass index (BMI), and 12 studies for alcohol consumption. Other covariates used for adjustment in the studies in this meta-analysis comprised race, marital status, urbanization, occupation, income, and comorbidity (see Additional file 1: Table S1).

The heterogeneity of effect estimates among studies based on I^2 was 85.64%, suggesting a relatively high inconsistency across the findings in the included studies [52].

Sedentary time and mortality: dose-response meta-regression

The meta-regression based on all included studies indicated a linear dose-response relationship between daily ST and log-transformed risk of all-cause mortality (Model 1 in Table 1). The Model 2 analyses demonstrated that both daily ST and measurement of ST (device-based vs. subjective) independently account for the heterogeneity in mortality risks. Model 2 was rerun after further inclusion of an interaction term, revealing a statistically significant interaction effect ($p = 0.02$).

Two separate meta-regression models were then conducted for studies using subjective measures and those with device-based instruments (Models 3 and 4). ST was significantly associated with all-cause mortality in both models. However, the magnitude of associations was stronger in studies using devices (regression coefficient = 0.09) than in those based on subjective instruments (regression coefficient = 0.03).

In sensitivity analyses, we explored several study-level variables, such as gender, mean age, year of publication, and mean length of follow-up, which may account for the heterogeneity of mortality risks and possess potential confounding effects. Among them, only mean length of follow-up reached significance ($p < 0.05$), which was further included in Model 2 (Model 5). The results showed that studies with longer follow-up periods tended to have weaker associations between daily ST and mortality risks (see Table 1). The moderation effect of ST measurement was further examined in Model 5,

indicating that the interaction effect remained similar ($p = 0.01$).

Visual assessment of dose-response relationships

The scatter plot of Model 1 illustrates the association of log-transformed mortality risk and doses of sitting time per day treated as a continuous variable (Fig. 2). The regression line and the upper and lower lines for 95% CI showed that increased hazards of death from all causes became significant when total ST exceeded approximately 7.5 h/day.

The scatter plot of Model 3 (Fig. 3a) revealed that mortality risk significantly increased when daily ST exceeded 7 h/day in studies with subjective measurement. In contrast, the potential cut-off time duration for those with device-based assessment was close to 9 h (Fig. 3b).

Assessment of publication bias

No evidence of funnel plot asymmetry was observed (Additional file 4: Figure S1). There was no indication of publication bias with Egger's test, $p = 0.46$ or with the "trim and fill" adjustment. The observed point estimate in log units was 0.11 (95% CI 0.07–0.15), which is similar to the adjusted estimate after imputing two studies: 0.10 (95% CI 0.06–0.14).

Discussion

The present meta-regression analyses based on pooled data for more than 1 million participants from 19 well-designed

Table 1 Dose-response relationships of sedentary time with all-cause mortality assessed using random-effects meta-regression models

Models	Number of ES	Coefficients (SE)	t	p value
Model 1	57			
Sedentary time		0.03 (0.01)	4.92	< 0.001
Model 2	57			
Sedentary time		0.03 (0.01)	5.08	< 0.001
Measurement (device-based = 1)		0.11 (0.05)	2.39	0.03
Model 3 (subjective measures)	36			
Sedentary time		0.03 (0.01)	5.09	< 0.001
Model 4 (device-based measures)	21			
Sedentary time		0.09 (0.03)	3.04	0.001
Model 5 (sensitivity analysis)	57			
Sedentary time		0.03 (0.005)	6.21	< 0.001
Measurement (device-based = 1)		0.09 (0.04)	2.19	0.03
Follow-up (5–9 vs. < 5 years)		−0.09 (0.04)	−2.16	0.04
Follow-up (10+ vs. < 5 years)		−0.16 (0.04)	−3.88	< 0.001

ES effect size, SE standard error

To test for moderation effects, the interaction term (sedentary time × measurement [device-based vs. subjective measure]) was further added into Model 2 ($p = 0.02$) and Model 5 ($p = 0.01$)

t Knapp-Hartung method

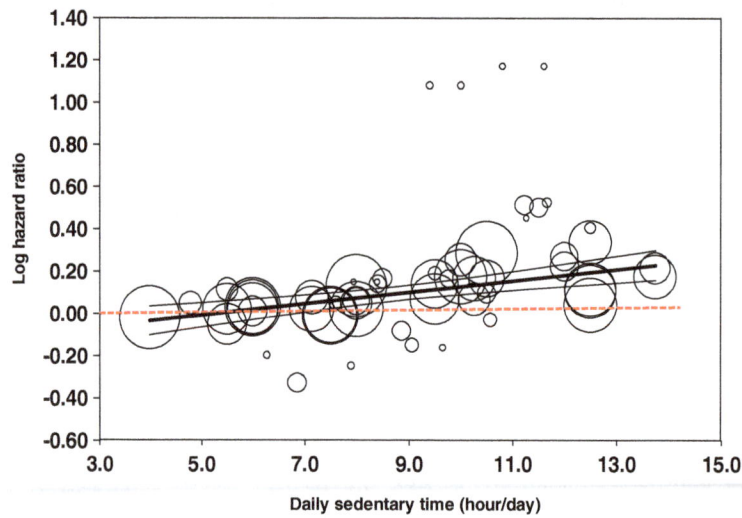

Fig. 2 Meta-regression of all-cause mortality risk on daily sedentary time (including all studies). Each study is represented by a *circle*. The *size* of each circle is proportional to that study's weight. The *center line* and the *upper and lower lines* show the predicted values and their 95% confidence intervals. Note: The meta-regression model was adjusted for follow-up time of each study

prospective cohort studies revealed a significant log-linear association between daily ST and all-cause mortality (i.e., HR) in adults. Overall, more time spent in sedentary behaviors is prospectively associated with increased mortality risks. Interestingly, there is a role for the method of measurement of ST in modulating the effect of daily ST on subsequent mortality risks across studies. The cut-off duration of daily ST in studies with subjective measures was more than 7 h. In contrast, the cut-off point for those with device-based measures was close to 9 h. These findings were supported by the meta-regression analyses adjusting for follow-up periods of each study. All of the pooled estimates were derived from large-scale prospective cohort studies with high-quality design and adjusted for multiple underlying confounding factors, including MVPA. Collectively, they provide additional evidence for ST recommendation.

The current meta-analysis study based on 19 prospective cohort studies (12 self-reported vs. 7 device-based) found that the optimal amount of daily ST in adults should be less than 7.5 h. This is close to a previous meta-analysis of cohort studies (5 self-reported vs. 1 device-based) [8], suggesting a cut-off time interval of 7 h, and is somewhat higher than the cut-off of 5 h (the midpoint of the category 4–6 h/day) revealed by another recent meta-analysis of cohort studies (13 studies all based on self-report measures) [9]. This inconsistency may be partly due to variation in the studies included in each review, which comprised studies based on different measures of ST.

This review using meta-regression found that the measurement method may moderate the associations between ST and all-cause mortality across studies. The magnitude of associations was stronger in studies using

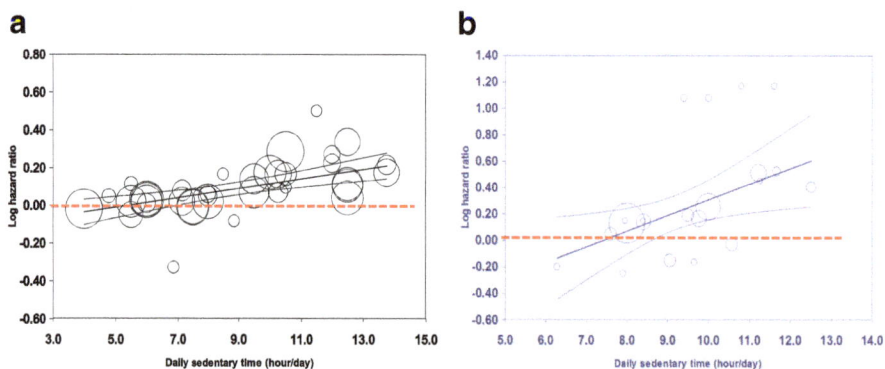

Fig. 3 Meta-regression of all-cause mortality risk on daily sedentary time based on studies with different measures (**a** subjective vs. **b** device-based). Each study is represented by a *circle*. The *size* of each circle is proportional to that study's weight. The *center line* and the *upper and lower lines* show the predicted values and their 95% confidence intervals. Note: The meta-regression models were adjusted for follow-up time of each study

device-based devices than in those with self-report ST. Previous evidence suggests that questionnaires involving multiple contexts for assessing daily ST are more likely to overestimate total ST in comparison with accelerometer-based devices [53]. In contrast, daily ST assessed using a single item such as the International Physical Activity Questionnaire (IPAQ) leads to an underestimate of total daily ST ranging from 2 to 3.5 h [54, 55]. In the present review, 10 out of the 12 studies based on self-report ST employed only one or two items to assess daily ST. It is possible that a questionnaire with one or two items is not able to capture the variability of sedentary behaviors that occurs in different contexts. This may partially explain why the cut-off in studies with subjective measurement was 7 h/day in comparison with 9 h/day in those with device-based assessment, and why the magnitude of relationships was greater in studies using device-based measures. Therefore, the appropriate cut-off duration for daily ST in adults may be around 9 h, although this finding is based on a small number of studies with device-based measures. It is worth noting that the relationships of mortality risk (i.e., HR) with ST are log-linear. Participants spending more than 9 h/day had a significant increased risk of mortality (HR = 1.22), with a rapid escalation from 10 h/day (HR = 1.35), 12 h/day (HR = 1.63), to 14 h/day (HR = 1.96) (based on Model 1 in Table 1, data not shown).

The moderating effect of type of measurement on the relationships of ST with mortality risks was further supported by the sensitivity analysis that took the length of follow-up into account. Studies with longer follow-up periods were more likely to have weaker associations between daily ST and mortality risks. This issue has not been documented in previous relevant meta-analyses [8, 9], and there is no clear explanation for the result. But it is possible that sedentary behaviors change over time, attenuating the associations between baseline estimates and all-cause mortality. Although the studies with a shortened period of follow-up may increase the possibility of reverse causality, several studies included in this review have demonstrated that similar results remained after excluding those dying in the first year [15, 40, 47] or in the first 3 years [42].

There are several strengths in this meta-analysis. First, it is the first meta-regression based on 19 high-quality cohort studies that has examined the moderating effect of type of ST measurement on the dose-response relationships with mortality risk. Second, the large-scale pooled data for more than 1 million participants allowed the dose-response analyses to yield more precise effect estimates than previously obtained. Finally, mortality ascertainment was based on official death registry records, which is more likely to be accurate than other methods of assessment.

The main limitation of this meta-analysis is the small number of high-quality studies, especially those with device-based ST [8]. Furthermore, although the pooled estimates were based on large-scale prospective cohort studies with high-quality design and adjusted for multiple underlying confounding factors including moderate-to-vigorous physical activity (MVPA), there remains the possibility of reverse causality or unmeasured confounding [8]. The mean age of participants in the studies analyzed ranged from 39.7 to 63.8 years old, which may limit the generalizability of the findings to the wider adult population. Additionally, the studies using device-based measures in the current review provide more accuracy of ST estimation, but they could not detect the difference between standing and sitting, which is a limitation of monitoring daily sedentary time. Finally, the current analyses were based on all-cause mortality as the outcome, and other thresholds for ST duration may be relevant to different outcomes, such as non-fatal illness or adiposity.

An international study involving 10 countries using accelerometry found that average sedentary time (ST) per day was 8.65 h among adults [1], which is close to the cut-off (9 h) of daily ST in adults observed in the current study. This means that nearly half of adults are at risk of increased mortality, and immediate action is needed to address the rise of sedentary lifestyle as a global trend. A previous meta-analysis demonstrated that MVPA potentially moderates the association of ST with mortality. Those who were active for about 60–75 min of MVPA every day did not have an increased risk of mortality even if they sat for more than 8 h per day [9]. Notably, those findings indicated distinct sitting-mortality effects at different levels of MVPA, revealing that the cut-off of ST may be different among adults with different levels of MVPA. However, those meta-analyses were all based on studies using self-reported measures of ST, which should be further verified using studies with device-based ST, especially with a large sample size.

Conclusions

This meta-analysis suggests that there is a log-linear dose-response association between daily ST and all-cause mortality in adults. The method of measurement could moderate the relationships of daily ST with subsequent mortality risks. This review suggests that it is appropriate to encourage adults to engage in less sedentary behaviors, with fewer than 9 h a day being relevant for all-cause mortality. There is a pressing need for more longitudinal studies involving device-based measures of ST and examining other thresholds for ST duration for all-cause mortality and other different outcomes such as non-fatal illness or adiposity.

Abbreviations

BMI: Body mass index; CI: Confidence interval; HR: Hazard ratio; M: Mean; MVPA: Moderate to vigorous physical activity; OR: Odds ratio; PA: Physical activity; RR: Relative risk; SE: Standard error; ST: Sedentary time

Funding

This study was funded by the Taiwan Ministry of Science and Technology (MOST 105–2628-H-018-001-MY2). The funders had no role in the study design, data collection, data analysis and interpretation, or the content of the final manuscript.

Authors' contributions

PK, AS, and LC conceived and designed the study. YL and MH acquired the data, checked data extractions, and conducted the assessment of study quality. PK obtained funding and carried out the statistical analysis. AS interpreted the data, advised on the structure of the manuscript, and revised the draft of the paper. PK and LC drafted the manuscript, and all authors critically revised the manuscript. All authors have read and approved the final manuscript. PK and MH had full access to all the data and take responsibility for the integrity of the data and the accuracy of the data analysis.

Competing interests

The authors declare that they have no competing interests.

Author details

[1]Graduate Institute of Sports and Health, National Changhua University of Education, Changhua City, Taiwan. [2]Department of Behavioural Science and Health, University College London, London, UK. [3]Department of Health Promotion and Health Education, National Taiwan Normal University, Taipei, Taiwan. [4]Department of Physical Education, National Taiwan Normal University, NO.162, He-ping East Road, Section 1, Taipei 106, Taiwan. [5]Department of Exercise Health Science, National Taiwan University of Sport, No. 16, Section 1, Shuang-Shih Rd., Taichung 404, Taiwan.

References

1. van Dyck D, Cerin E, De Bourdeaudhuij I, Hinckson E, Reis RS, Davey R, Sarmiento OL, Mitas J, Troelsen J, MacFarlane D. International study of objectively-measured physical activity and sedentary time with body mass index and obesity: IPEN adult study. Int J Obesity. 2015;39(2):199–207.

2. de Rezende LF, Sá TH, Mielke GI, Viscondi JYK, Rey-López JP, Garcia LMT. All-cause mortality attributable to sitting time: analysis of 54 countries worldwide. Am J Prev Med. 2016;51(2):253–63.

3. Biddle SJH, Bennie JA, Bauman AE, Chau JY, Dunstan D, Owen N, Stamatakis E, van Uffelen JGZ. Too much sitting and all-cause mortality: is there a causal link? BMC Public Health. 2016;16(1):635.

4. Young D, Hivert M-F, Alhassan S, Camhi S, Ferguson J, Katzmarzyk P, Lewis C, Owen N, Perry C, Siddique J, et al. Sedentary behavior and cardiovascular morbidity and mortality: a science advisory from the American Heart Association. Circulation. 2016;134:e262–79.

5. UK Department of Health. Physical activity guidelines for adults (19–64 years). London: Department of Health; 2011.

6. Australian Department of Health. Australia's Physical Activity and Sedentary Behaviour Guidelines for Adults (18–64 years). Canberra: Department of Health; 2014.

7. Australian National Preventive Health Agency. Obesity: Sedentary behaviours and health. Sydney: Australian National Preventive Health Agency; 2014.

8. Chau JY, Grunseit AC, Chey T, Stamatakis E, Brown WJ, Matthews CE, Bauman AE, van der Ploeg HP. Daily sitting time and all-cause mortality: a meta-analysis. PLoS One. 2013;8(11):e80000.

9. Ekelund U, Steene-Johannessen J, Brown WJ, Fagerland MW, Owen N, Powell KE, Bauman A, Lee IM. Does physical activity attenuate, or even eliminate, the detrimental association of sitting time with mortality? A harmonised meta-analysis of data from more than 1 million men and women. Lancet. 2016;388(10051):1302–10.

10. Kang M, Rowe DA. Issues and challenges in sedentary behavior measurement. Meas Phys Educ Exerc Sci. 2015;19(3):105–15.

11. Clark B, Sugiyama T, Healy G, Salmon J, Dunstan D, Owen N. Validity and reliability of measures of television viewing time and other non-occupational sedentary behaviour of adults: a review. Obesity Review. 2009; 10(1):7–16.

12. Koolhaas CM, Dhana K, van Rooij FJ, Kocevska D, Hofman A, Franco OH, Tiemeier H. Sedentary time assessed by actigraphy and mortality: The Rotterdam Study. Prev Med. 2017;95:59–65.

13. Matthews CE, Keadle SK, Troiano RP, Kahle L, Koster A, Brychta R, Van Domelen D, Caserotti P, Chen KY, Harris TB. Accelerometer-measured dose-response for physical activity, sedentary time, and mortality in US adults. Am J Clin Nutr. 2016;104(5):1424–32.

14. Edwards MK, Loprinzi PD. All-cause mortality risk as a function of sedentary behavior, moderate-to-vigorous physical activity and cardiorespiratory fitness. Phys Sportsmed. 2016;44(3):223–30.

15. Koster A, Caserotti P, Patel KV, Matthews CE, Berrigan D, Domelen DR, Brychta RJ, Chen KY, Harris TB. Association of sedentary time with mortality independent of moderate to vigorous physical activity. PLoS One. 2012;7:e37696.

16. Kmet LM, Lee RC, Cook LS: Standard quality assessment criteria for evaluating primary research papers from a variety of fields, vol. 22. Edmonton: Alberta Heritage Foundation for Medical Research; 2004.

17. Aune D, Chan DS, Lau R, Vieira R, Greenwood DC, Kampman E, Norat T. Dietary fibre, whole grains, and risk of colorectal cancer: systematic review and dose-response meta-analysis of prospective studies. BMJ. 2011;343:d6617.

18. Grosso G, Micek A, Godos J, Pajak A, Sciacca S, Galvano F, Giovannucci EL. Dietary flavonoid and lignan intake and mortality in prospective cohort studies: Systematic review and dose-response meta-analysis. Am J Epidemiol. 2017;185(12):1304–16.

19. Higgins J, Thompson SG. Quantifying heterogeneity in a meta-analysis. Stat Med. 2002;21(11):1539–58.

20. Burgers AMG, Biermasz NR, Schoones JW, Pereira AM, Renehan AG, Zwahlen M, Egger M, Dekkers OM. Meta-analysis and dose-response metaregression: circulating insulin-like growth factor I (IGF-I) and mortality. J Clin Endocrinol Metabol. 2011;96(9):2912–20.

21. Bagnardi V, Zambon A, Quatto P, Corrao G. Flexible meta-regression functions for modeling aggregate dose-response data, with an application to alcohol and mortality. Am J Epidemiol. 2004;159(11):1077–86.

22. Borenstein M, Hedges L, Higgins J, Rothstein H. Comprehensive Meta-Analysis Version 3. Englewood: Biostat; 2014.

23. Knapp G, Hartung J. Improved tests for a random effects meta-regression with a single covariate. Stat Med. 2003;22(17):2693–710.

24. Borenstein M, Hedges LV, Higgins J, Rothstein HR. Introduction to meta-analysis. Chichester: Wiley Online Library; 2009.

25. Egger M, Smith GD, Schneider M, Minder C. Bias in meta-analysis detected by a simple, graphical test. BMJ. 1997;315(7109):629–34.

26. Duval S, Tweedie R. A nonparametric "trim and fill" method of accounting for publication bias in meta-analysis. J Am Stat Assoc. 2000;95(449):89–98.

27. Moher D, Liberati A, Tetzlaff J, Altman DG, Group P. Preferred reporting items for systematic reviews and meta-analyses: The PRISMA statement. PLoS Med. 2009;6:e1000097.

28. Matthews CE, Moore SC, Sampson J, Blair A, Xiao Q, Keadle SK, Hollenbeck A, Park Y. Mortality benefits for replacing sitting time with different physical activities. Med Sci Sports Exerc. 2015;47(9):1833.

29. Dohrn M, Sjöström M, Kwak L, Oja P, Hagströmer M. Accelerometer-measured sedentary time and physical activity—a 15 year follow-up of mortality in a Swedish population-based cohort. J Sci Med Sport. 2017; https://doi.org/10/1016/j.jsams.2017.10.035

30. Diaz KM, Howard VJ, Hutto B, Colabianchi N, Vena JE, Safford MM, Blair SN, Hooker SP. Patterns of sedentary behavior and mortality in US middle-aged and older adults: a national cohort study. Ann Intern Med. 2017;167(7):465–75.

31. Schmid D, Ricci C, Leitzmann MF. Associations of objectively assessed physical activity and sedentary time with all-cause mortality in US adults: the NHANES study. PLoS One. 2015;10(3):e0119591.

32. Wang A, Qin F, Hedlin H, Desai M, Chlebowski R, Gomez S, Eaton CB, Johnson KC, Qi L, Wactawski-Wende J. Physical activity and sedentary behavior in relation to lung cancer incidence and mortality in older women: The Women's Health Initiative. Int J Cancer. 2016;139(10):2178–92.

33. Stamatakis E, Rogers K, Ding D, Berrigan D, Chau J, Hamer M, Bauman A. All-cause mortality effects of replacing sedentary time with physical activity and sleeping using an isotemporal substitution model: a prospective study of

A cut-off of daily sedentary time and all-cause mortality in adults: a meta-regression analysis involving...

175

201,129 mid-aged and older adults. Int J Behav Nutr Phys Act. 2015;12:121.

34. Katzmarzyk PT, Church TS, Craig CL, Bouchard C. Sitting time and mortality from all causes, cardiovascular disease, and cancer. Med Sci Sports Exerc. 2009;41:998–1005.

35. Krokstad S, Ding D, Grunseit AC, Sund ER, Holmen TL, Rangul V, Bauman A. Multiple lifestyle behaviours and mortality, findings from a large population-based Norwegian cohort study—the HUNT Study. BMC Public Health. 2017; 17(1):58.

36. Schmid D, Ricci C, Baumeister SE, Leitzmann MF. Replacing sedentary time with physical activity in relation to mortality. Med Sci Sports Exerc. 2016; 48(7):1312–9.

37. Inoue M, Iso H, Yamamoto S, Kurahashi N, Sasazuki S, Tsugane S. Daily total physical activity level and premature death in men and women: results from a large-scale population-based cohort study in Japan (JPHC Study). Ann Epidemiol. 2008;18:522–30.

38. Matthews CE, Cohen SS, Fowke JH, Han X, Xiao Q, Buchowski MS, Hargreaves MK, Signorello LB, Blot WJ. Physical activity, sedentary behavior, and cause-specific mortality in black and white adults in the Southern Community Cohort Study. Am J Epidemiol. 2014;180(4):394–405.

39. Matthews CE, George S, Moore S, Bowles H, Blair A, Park Y, Troiano R, Hollenbeck A, Schatzkin A. Amount of time spent in sedentary behaviors and cause-specific mortality in US adults. Am J Clin Nutr. 2012;95:437–45.

40. van der Ploeg HP, Chey T, Korda RJ, Banks E, Bauman A. Sitting time and all-cause mortality risk in 222,497 Australian adults. Arch Intern Med. 2012; 172(6):494–500.

41. Petersen CB, Bauman A, Grønbæk M, Helge JW, Thygesen LC, Tolstrup JS. Total sitting time and risk of myocardial infarction, coronary heart disease and all-cause mortality in a prospective cohort of Danish adults. Int J Behav Nutr Phys Act. 2014;11(1):13.

42. Grunseit AC, Chau JY, Rangul V, Holmen TL, Bauman A. Patterns of sitting and mortality in the Nord-Trøndelag health study (HUNT). Int J Behav Nutr Phys Act. 2017;14(1):8.

43. Kim Y, Wilkens LR, Park S-Y, Goodman MT, Monroe KR, Kolonel LN. Association between various sedentary behaviours and all-cause, cardiovascular disease and cancer mortality: the Multiethnic Cohort Study. Int J Epidemiol. 2013;42:1040–56.

44. Pulsford RM, Stamatakis E, Britton AR, Brunner EJ, Hillsdon M. Associations of sitting behaviours with all-cause mortality over a 16-year follow-up: the Whitehall II study. Int J Epidemiol. 2015;44(6):1909–16.

45. Seguin R, Buchner DM, Liu J, Allison M, Manini T, Wang C-Y, Manson JE, Messina CR, Patel MJ, Moreland L. Sedentary behavior and mortality in older women: the Women's Health Initiative. Am J Prev Med. 2014;46(2):122–35.

46. Hagger-Johnson G, Gow AJ, Burley V, Greenwood D, Cade JE. Sitting time, fidgeting, and all-cause mortality in the UK Women's Cohort Study. Am J Prev Med. 2016;50(2):154–60.

47. Chau JY, Grunseit A, Midthjell K, Holmen J, Holmen TL, Bauman AE, Ploeg HP. Sedentary behaviour and risk of mortality from all causes and cardiometabolic diseases in adults: evidence from the HUNT3 population cohort. Br J Sports Med. 2015;49:737–42.

48. Ding D, Rogers K, van der Ploeg H, Stamatakis E, Bauman AE. Traditional and emerging lifestyle risk behaviors and all-cause mortality in middle-aged and older adults: evidence from a large population-based Australian cohort. PLoS Med. 2015;12(12):e1001917.

49. Evenson KR, Herring AH, Wen F. Accelerometry-assessed latent class patterns of physical activity and sedentary behavior with mortality. Am J Prev Med. 2017;52(2):135–43.

50. Evenson KR, Wen F, Herring AH. Associations of accelerometry-assessed and self-reported physical activity and sedentary behavior with all-cause and cardiovascular mortality among US adults. Am J Epidemiol. 2016;184(9):621–32.

51. Lee PH. Examining non-linear associations between accelerometer-measured physical activity, sedentary behavior, and all-cause mortality using segmented Cox regression. Front Physiol. 2016;7:272.

52. Higgins J, Thompson SG, Deeks JJ, Altman DG. Measuring inconsistency in meta-analyses. BMJ. 2003;327(7414):557–60.

53. Busschaert C, De Bourdeaudhuij I, Van Holle V, Chastin SF, Cardon G, De Cocker K. Reliability and validity of three questionnaires measuring context-specific sedentary behaviour and associated correlates in adolescents, adults and older adults. Int J Behav Nutr Phys Act. 2015;12(1):117.

54. Gupta N, Christiansen CS, Hanisch C, Bay H, Burr H, Holtermann A. Is questionnaire-based sitting time inaccurate and can it be improved? A cross-sectional investigation using accelerometer-based sitting time. BMJ Open. 2017;7(1):e013251.

55. Chastin S, Culhane B, Dall P. Comparison of self-reported measure of sitting time (IPAQ) with objective measurement (activPAL). Physiol Meas. 2014; 35(11):2319.

17

Do hotspots fuel malaria transmission: a village-scale spatio-temporal analysis of a 2-year cohort study

Gillian H. Stresman[1*†], Julia Mwesigwa[2,3†], Jane Achan[2,3], Emanuele Giorgi[4], Archibald Worwui[2,3], Musa Jawara[2,3], Gian Luca Di Tanna[5], Teun Bousema[6], Jean-Pierre Van Geertruyden[3], Chris Drakeley[1] and Umberto D'Alessandro[1,2,3]

Abstract

Background: Despite the biological plausibility of hotspots fueling malaria transmission, the evidence to support this concept has been mixed. If transmission spreads from high burden to low burden households in a consistent manner, then this could have important implications for control and elimination program development.

Methods: Data from a longitudinal cohort in The Gambia was analyzed. All consenting individuals residing in 12 villages across the country were sampled monthly from June (dry season) to December 2013 (wet season), in April 2014 (mid dry season), and monthly from June to December 2014. A study nurse stationed within each village recorded passively detected malaria episodes between visits. *Plasmodium falciparum* infections were determined by polymerase chain reaction and analyzed using a geostatistical model.

Results: Household-level observed monthly incidence ranged from 0 to 0.50 infection per person (interquartile range = 0.02–0.10) across the sampling months, and high burden households exist across all study villages. There was limited evidence of a spatio-temporal pattern at the monthly timescale irrespective of transmission intensity. Within-household transmission was the most plausible hypothesis examined to explain the observed heterogeneity in infections.

Conclusions: Within-village malaria transmission patterns are concentrated in a small proportion of high burden households, but patterns are stochastic regardless of endemicity. Our findings support the notion of transmission occurring at the household and village scales but not the use of a targeted approach to interrupt spreading of infections from high to low burden areas within villages in this setting.

Keywords: Hotspot, Foci, Geostatistics, Cohort, Spatial epidemiology

Background

Within populations, heterogeneity in exposure to malaria has been widely documented; it is generally estimated that 20% of the population experience 80% of the disease burden [1–3]. The skewed distribution of exposure has been observed at every spatial scale, in different transmission landscapes, and is expected to be more pronounced when transmission is low [4]. Several

studies have documented both spatial and spatio-temporal high burden areas of malaria, typically referred to as hotspots but here defined as clusters, and have fueled the notion of spatially targeting interventions for control and elimination [5–7].

The consistent presence of spatial clusters of high malaria burden within populations contributed to the hypothesis that there may be hotspots, or certain households, or subsets of households within foci (spatially discrete areas with sustained transmission) that fuel transmission [8]. The number and size of clusters within foci and the delineation of a foci itself will likely depend on the specific setting. For example, on the coast

* Correspondence: Gillian.Stresman@lshtm.ac.uk
†Gillian H. Stresman and Julia Mwesigwa contributed equally to this work.
[1]Department of Immunology and Infection, London School of Hygiene and Tropical Medicine, London, UK
Full list of author information is available at the end of the article

of Kenya, multiple clusters were identified per foci [2], whereas a single cluster was observed in a highland setting [6]. If such clusters are in fact hotspots, meaning they are drivers of malaria transmission, and they could be easily identified and targeted with interventions, then resources could be used more effectively and their impact on transmission intensity may be greater than that of a uniform approach [8, 9]. For a hotspot-driven approach at the sub-village level to be viable, it is critical to determine whether the observed heterogeneity at the village scale is a feature of malaria transmission and supports the notion of "hotspots" fueling transmission or whether it follows a more stochastic pattern [10].

The notion of hotspots as intrinsic drivers of malaria transmission being an inherent part of the transmission landscape is plausible with risk being driven by macroscale and microscale characteristics [11, 12]. For example, the observed seasonality in transmission is associated with climate, specifically the rainfall patterns and temperature [13, 14]. Similarly, at the local scale, malaria risk is known to be associated with microepidemiological variation in risk factors, including greater odds of infection in those residing in proximity to mosquito breeding sites (e.g., ponds or forests) or living with other infected individuals [15–17]. The observed spatial heterogeneity in infected individuals also has implications for quantifying and understanding transmission intensity [18]. As described as part of the hotspot model, the high burden households within an endemic area may amplify transmission by acting as a constant parasite reservoir, or equally they could absorb infectious bites, attenuating observed transmission events [19, 20]. If these households or groups of households are driving transmission within foci, then hotspot-targeted interventions would be justified [8, 21].

Although biologically plausible, the evidence to support the concept of hotspots, here considered as a single household or group of high burden households within foci, fueling transmission has been mixed. For example, a recent trial targeting serologically defined hotspots of exposure

failed to observe any sustained reduction in transmission outside of the targeted area [22]. Transmission in the study area may have been too high for well-defined hotspots, hotspot boundaries may not have been effectively defined, or hotspots may not have contributed to maintaining transmission in this setting [23]. Despite the limited evidence to support the use of hotspot-targeted approaches, several malaria elimination programs have engaged in hotspot-inspired strategies [3, 21, 24].

In this study, we conducted a spatio-temporal analysis on a full population cohort distributed in six pairs of villages across The Gambia. The aim of this research was to establish if predicted risk of malaria transmission intensity exhibits a consistent pattern, meaning the risk of malaria moving from a high burden household or a group of households to neighboring households, over time. If the expected pattern exists, we aimed to identify at what transmission intensity this dynamic becomes apparent. In case of limited evidence to support the hotspot pattern, some potential drivers of any observed heterogeneity were explored.

Methods

Malaria transmission in The Gambia is highly seasonal and occurs during and soon after the rainy season, typically between August and December. Epidemiological data from the study cohort has been recently described [25]. Briefly, monthly blood samples were collected during the 2013 and 2014 malaria transmission seasons (June–December) from all people residing in every household in the study villages (Fig. 1). An additional blood sample was collected during the dry season, in April 2014. Village pairs were approximately 1–3 km apart and were considered as discrete spatial units. Populations ranged between 100 and 700 individuals per village, and all residents were included in the study. All households were geo-located. The number of households per village ranged from 13 to 69, and the distance between households within a village ranged from 0.4 to a maximum of 986.8 m (Table 1).

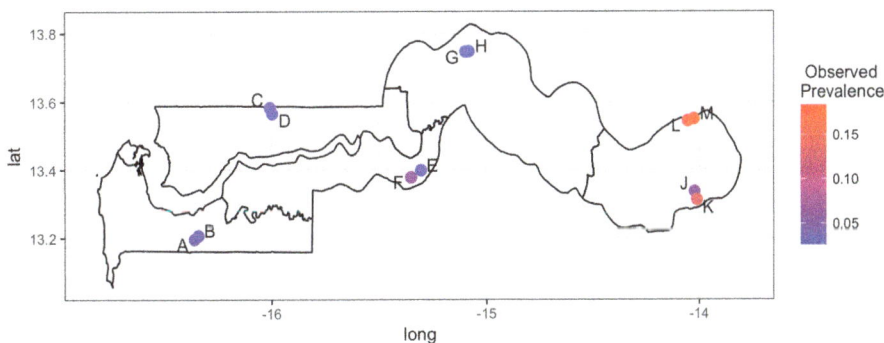

Fig. 1 Map of The Gambia showing the location of the 12 study villages. The study villages are represented as *circles* and labeled A–H and J–M. The circles are *colored* according to the overall observed malaria prevalence

Table 1 Key characteristics of study villages including demographics and the observed malaria burden

Region	Village	No. people	No. HH	Distance (meters) between HH (min-max)	Median age (IQR)	Median visits per person (IQR)	No. observed infections	Observed PCR prevalence
West Coast	A	670	68	16.6–986.8	13 (6–29)	10 (6–12)	240	0.039
	B	202	23	13.1–360.6	14 (7–32)	10 (6–12)	60	0.033
North Bank	C	273	19	4.7–191.2	12 (4–26)	13 (10–13)	107	0.036
	D	461	30	2.9–327.8	13 (5–27)	11 (5–12)	121	0.029
Lower River	E	112	10	22.7–179.3	13 (8–26)	12 (8–13)	34	0.031
	F	567	69	12.6–776.0	13 (5–27)	9 (4–11)	281	0.064
Central River	G	480	25	2.4–234.8	14 (5–30)	11 (7–12)	135	0.029
	H	204	13	0.4–196.8	13 (5–28)	10 (5–12)	45	0.026
Upper River South	J	418	28	8.1–216.0	14 (6–30)	9 (7–11)	224	0.062
	K	804	42	6.7–550.4	12 (5–27)	8 (6–10)	845	0.134
Upper River North	L	258	13	16.6–253.5	15 (6–26)	11 (9–12)	440	0.164
	M	217	20	8.1–242.8	16 (7–25)	10 (6–12)	345	0.183

HH household, *IQR* interquartile range

Furthermore, one round of mass drug administration (MDA) with dihydroartemisinin-piperaquine was carried out in June 2014.

Finger prick blood samples were collected on filter paper for identification of *Plasmodium falciparum* infections using polymerase chain reaction (PCR). All febrile individuals (auxiliary temperature ≥ 37.5 °C or history of fever in the last 24 h) were screened for malaria by rapid diagnostic test (RDT), and if positive they were treated with artemether-lumefantrine according to national guidelines. A study nurse was stationed within each village and recorded all malaria episodes between monthly visits, including administering an RDT and collecting a blood sample on filter paper.

Malaria parasites are transmitted to humans via the bite of an infected *Anopheles* mosquito and can be directly measured using the entomological inoculation rate (EIR) [26, 27]. The *P. falciparum* parasite rate (*Pf*PR) is a known correlate to EIR; it provides a measure of transmission intensity and is a more operationally feasible metric to generate [28]. Using PCR infection as the dependent variable as a proxy for transmission intensity, geostatistical analysis was conducted using the PrevMap package in R (v3.3.2) to determine the predicted malaria prevalence per household per month within each village accounting for spatial autocorrelation as well as temporal trends [29]. A Bayesian geostatistical probit model was used to predict the spatial variation in malaria parasite prevalence within each village. More details on the model specification are provided in Additional file 1. Because the cohort was a full population sample, no interpolation at unsampled locations was required. Predicted prevalence per household was estimated using the median of the posterior distribution, and maps of the combined and monthly predicted prevalence were generated.

Models were adjusted for sample date, distance to road, distance to river, and mean monthly rainfall. The distance to river and road variables were determined by extracting the relevant features from pan-sharpened Landsat 8 imagery and using the gDistance function in the rgeos package [30] to estimate the straight-line distance in kilometers. Monthly rainfall was obtained from weather stations located in each of the six study regions across the country.

The observed overdispersed distribution of infection counts has been used to support the notion of malaria hotspots [1]. However, it is possible that the skewed distribution is due to measurement bias in how infections are defined. For example, PCR-detected infections were not treated in this study (until becoming symptomatic and detectable by RDT) and could represent an infection from a single infectious bite or repeated inoculations within the same individual until treatment is sought. For example, by considering each time point where a PCR infection is detected as unique would lead to counting a single infection detected at 5 sequential time points as 5 unique infections instead of 1, thereby driving the observed overdispersion. To demonstrate the degree of potential measurement bias as an alternative explanation to the skewed patterns of case counts, two different approaches for counting were employed. The first was to consider each time point when a PCR positive result was recorded as a unique infection irrespective of whether there was a confirmed treatment in between sampling. The second approach considered any infections detected at sequential time points as the same infection unless the individual had been treated for malaria as part of the study. Any negative sample between two PCR positive samples in a non-treated individual was assumed to be a false negative and considered as a single infection. Any subsequent infection detected after a known treatment event (e.g., symptomatic and RDT positive, or participated in the MDA) was considered as a new infection.

Results

In total, 41,548 monthly observations were available from 360 households across 14 sampling time points. The size of households ranged from a single person to 78 individuals, and the residents had a similar age distribution between villages (Table 1). The aggregated infection prevalence across the study period ranged from 2.6 to 18.3% across the 12 villages (Fig. 1). During the 2-year study period, 2877 samples were positive for malaria infection, with substantial heterogeneity between villages. The lowest transmission village recorded 34 infections in 10 households, whereas the village with the highest transmission had 845 infections in 42 households (Table 1). Across all time points, 12.5% (45/360) households did not record a single infection, while the number of households without any infection varied from 0 in village L to 12 in village F. Household-level observed monthly incidence ranged from 0 to 0.50 infection per person (interquartile range (IQR) = 0.02–0.10) across the sampling months.

The overall number of observed infections per individual (Fig. 2a) and per household (Fig. 2b) exhibit the expected overdispersion pattern, illustrating the

considerable heterogeneity in malaria exposure experienced by this population. Results of the geostatistical model exhibited 100 m as the range of spatial autocorrelation, suggesting that village pairs were discrete transmission units. However, the geostatistical model failed to provide evidence of a pronounced spatial pattern within villages at either low or high transmission intensities (Fig. 3; see Additional file 1 for model output). Across all villages, only a single village (Fig. 3, village F) showed a pattern of high burden households grouping together. When the predicted household-level prevalence is plotted over time, there is no evidence that infection dynamics around high burden households exhibit a regular pattern around neighboring households at the monthly time step; the patterns appear stochastic (Additional file 2). Furthermore, as a group of high burden households was only evident in a single village with moderate transmission levels, the presence of hotspots within villages does not appear to be associated with transmission intensity. The spatial patterns were similar irrespective of whether an infection was symptomatic or asymptomatic (Additional file 3) [25].

As a consistent spatio-temporal dynamic of malaria around high burden households was not observed, the next step was to explore alternative explanations for the overdispersion pattern of malaria burden in the study population. The first explanation examined was

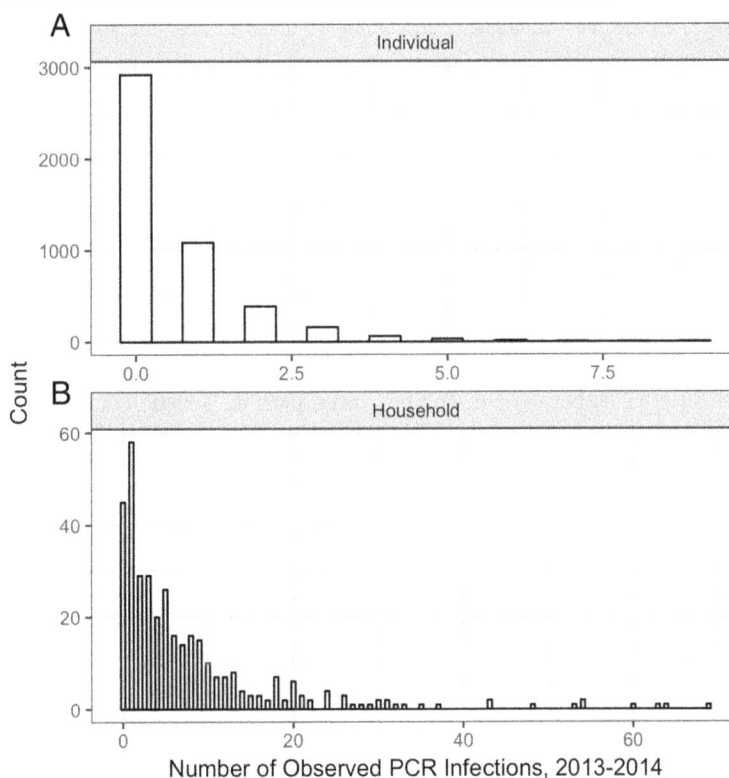

Fig. 2 Frequency distributions of malaria infections in the study population. Frequency of number of observed PCR positive infections **a** per individual and **b** per household

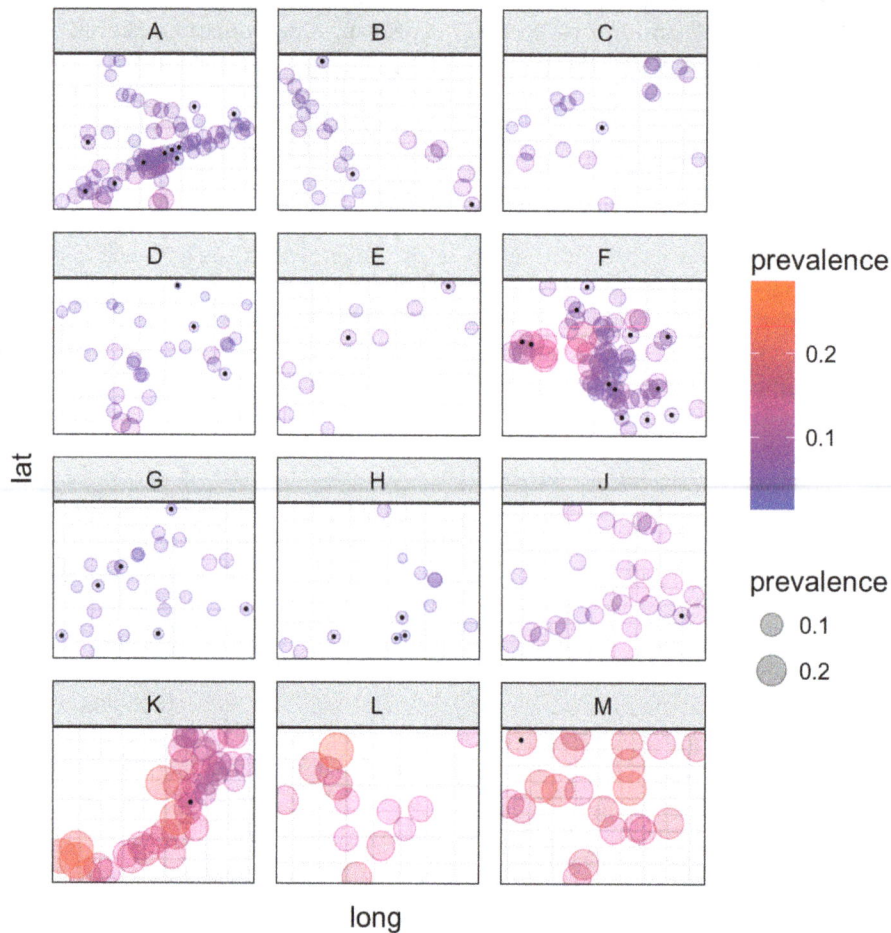

Fig. 3 Overall predicted PCR prevalence per household (*circles*), per village (panels **a-h**, **j-m**, corresponding to the village code) according to the spatio-temporal model. The *size* and *color* of the circles are scaled according to prevalence. The *black dots* identify those households with zero malaria infections recorded during the study

measurement bias in how infections were defined. If we consider the most conservative definition and assume only new infections as those after a recorded treatment event, the distribution becomes less skewed, with fewer households experiencing multiple malaria episodes (Fig. 4a). As expected, the differences between methods for counting infections are more pronounced in high transmission settings (Fig. 4b, village M) compared to low transmission settings (Fig. 4b, village A). Although neither method of counting infections is expected to fully capture the number of "true" infections experienced in the population, the heterogeneity in malaria burden was still present despite the most extreme definition of counting infections being applied.

The second explanation for the observed heterogeneity in malaria that we explored was to consider the household as the relevant spatial unit of transmission. Patterns of infections appearing within households suggested that three scenarios are evident: there are cases when several individuals are infected within the same month, there are cases

of infections appearing the month after another individual within the household becomes infected, and there are cases of stochastic introductions (Fig. 5). All patterns were observed in households in both the low (Fig. 5; village A) and high (Fig. 5; village M) transmission settings. However, parasite genetic data is required to confirm this hypothesis. See Additional file 4 for heat maps showing transmission dynamics within all study households.

Discussion

Heterogeneity in malaria burden is an inherent aspect of transmission, rooted in complex interactions between environmental, vector, and individual characteristics [9, 21, 31]. However, evidence on the importance of the observed heterogeneity within a village in maintaining or fueling transmission, consistent with the concept of hotspots, is required to support the use of such a strategy as part of control or elimination programs. In this study, we explored spatio-temporal trends of malaria transmission intensity to see if it shifted from high

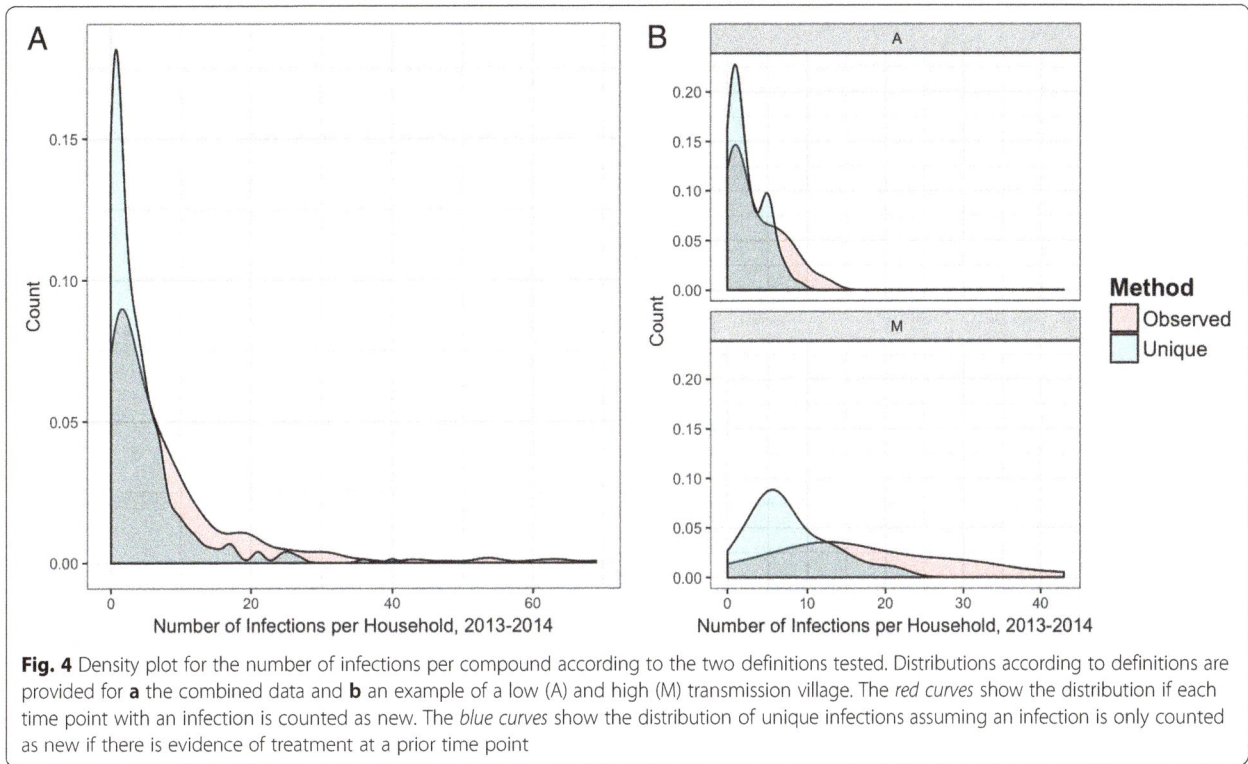

Fig. 4 Density plot for the number of infections per compound according to the two definitions tested. Distributions according to definitions are provided for **a** the combined data and **b** an example of a low (A) and high (M) transmission village. The *red curves* show the distribution if each time point with an infection is counted as new. The *blue curves* show the distribution of unique infections assuming an infection is only counted as new if there is evidence of treatment at a prior time point

burden households to the surrounding area. Though high burden households within villages exist, they were not consistently the same, and the risk of malaria was not observed to spread from high to low burden households at the monthly timescale. Together, these findings suggest that the relevant operational unit for targeting transmission in this setting is the household or the entire village, depending on the program goals and interventions being employed.

As heterogeneity in malaria infections was observed in the data, we next explored non-spatial factors that could be driving the pattern. In this study, participants were only treated if they had a symptomatic, RDT positive infection or participated in the MDA. Therefore, we hypothesized that each observed infection is unlikely to represent a unique infection event, and the overdispersion in burden may be partly driven by measurement bias. Assuming that new infections are only those identified after documented antimalarial treatment decreased but did not eliminate the observed heterogeneity. The "extreme" assumptions we used, namely that all detected infections are new ones or that new infections are only those occurring after treatment, are unlikely to represent the true number of infection events, as individuals may have cleared them spontaneously, received treatment outside of the study, or experienced superinfections [32–34]. Being able to account for superinfections and identify the role of these individuals in fueling onward transmission would help refine methods for counting

new or incident infections and determining which infections matter for maintaining transmission intensity [35]. The true incidence likely falls somewhere in between the two estimates used, but measurement bias is unlikely to contribute substantially to the levels of heterogeneity detected.

We next explored the extent to which transmission occurs within the household as a possible explanation for the observed overdispersion. Household-level risk has been identified in other settings whereby individuals residing within an infected house are more likely to also be or become infected [17, 25, 36, 37]. However, it is not known whether the increased burden is due to the aggregation of factors that increase risk of infection or because the household itself is the unit of transmission. In this setting, we observed sequential infections within households where new household members became infected in the month after the initial introduced infection. This pattern suggests that within-household transmission is plausible and supports the use of reactive case detection strategies, where households of any confirmed infection are visited and screened and/or treated for malaria to capture additional cases expected within households of index cases [17, 38]. Based on the limited spreading pattern observed, including neighboring households or those within a specific radius around index households would not be recommended in this setting. Also, a reactive approach for targeting residual infections within households is not likely to be

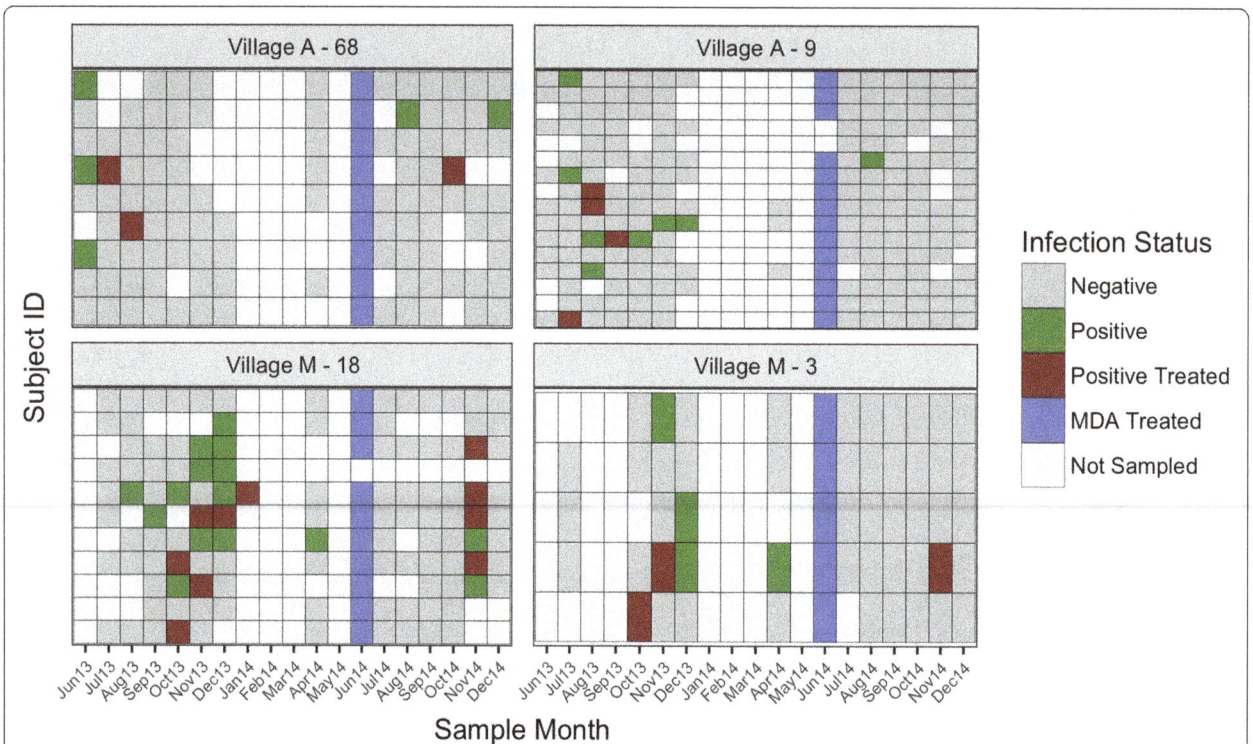

Fig. 5 Heat maps showing within-household transmission dynamics. Heat maps showing within-household transmission dynamics in a low transmission village (*village A*) and a high transmission village (*village M*). Each *grid* represents a household with each individual residing within the household shown in the *rows*. Each *column* within each grid represents a sampling month starting in June 2013 through December 2014. The *color* of each grid cell represents their infection and/or treatment status at that time point. Infection status is defined by those who are PCR positive with treatment being administered when there was a symptomatic infection confirmed by RDT in the field or the mass drug administration (MDA) administered between transmission seasons (June 2014)

appropriate in all settings. This is particularly true for those settings where transmission occurs outside of the household, for example, in forests, as is common in Southeast Asia [24, 39]. Furthermore, given the stochastic nature of infections across all villages, a reactive approach may not contribute to a reduction of transmission but may contribute to infections averted in household members, particularly if a drug with a longer prophylactic period is used. Given that all villages in this study are capable of supporting transmission and would therefore be considered as "active" according to the World Health Organization (WHO) definition of foci, one could argue that targeting the whole village population with interventions may be more appropriate as a way to accelerate malaria elimination [40].

It is possible that hotspots do exist and fuel transmission within foci, but it was not observed in this setting. It is unlikely that infections were missed, as routine sampling occurred every month during the transmission season with a study nurse capturing episodes between regular visits. Although the monthly time step was selected as it would account for the intrinsic and extrinsic incubation periods, it is possible that this temporal scale was not optimal or the monthly aggregated datasets too

small to detect the spreading of infections between households. The treatment of detectable infections as part of both the passive and active screenings may have altered or masked spatio-temporal patterns. However, the expected rate of treatments required to interrupt transmission is much higher than was administered as part of routine surveillance. Secondly, the spatio-temporal patterns observed pre- and post-MDA were similar, despite the magnitude of transmission intensity being lower in the second year. Therefore, the role of treatment likely had a minimal impact on the ability to observe any patterns. Alternative spatio-modeling approaches such as point pattern or dispersion models may have yielded different results. However, the number of points per village limited any point-based analysis, and understanding whether infections cluster would not directly address the question of interest. Incorporating the parasite genetic data into this analysis to track infections within and between households may help us understand the extent of within- and between-household transmission dynamics [41]. The detailed genetic data required for this analysis was not available. However, recent work supports the notion of microepidemiological clustering of parasite strains [33]. Next, the non-response bias experienced in this 2-year cohort may have masked any hotspot dynamics. It is possible that the individuals missed could have better illustrated any spreading between households. However, the participation rate across all villages was reasonably high and was consistent between villages, so although possible, we do not consider this as likely.

Conclusions

Approaches for more efficient targeting of malaria control and elimination activities have shifted to incorporating spatial dynamics of transmission and identifying lingering foci. Although hotspots fueling malaria transmission within a village or foci are biologically plausible, the limited evidence in field settings puts their role in sustaining transmission into question. The results presented here further support this shift in thinking [40, 42]. This population-level cohort in 12 villages across The Gambia showed that there is considerable heterogeneity in transmission both within and between study villages. Our results suggest that spatio-temporal patterns of malaria risk are stochastic at all endemicities and are inconsistent with the idea of hotspots fueling malaria transmission. Transmission was more likely to occur within households in this setting, supporting the use of reactive case detection strategies targeting the household only or to target the entire village as a focus, but not an approach targeting hotspots with the goal of interrupting transmission from high to low burden areas.

Additional files

Additional file 1: Description of the geostatistical model including outputs. (PDF 181 kb)

Additional file 2: Monthly predicted PCR prevalence per household (*circles*) for all study villages (*panels*) according to the spatio-temporal model. The *size* and *color* of the *circles* are scaled according to prevalence. Each household is identified by a black dot. Households with a predicted PCR prevalence between 0 and 1% are identified in greyscale. (MP4 285 kb)

Additional file 3: Results of analysis stratified by whether an infection was symptomatic or asymptomatic. Symptomatic infections were those individuals with fever and a confirmed infection by rapid diagnostic test (RDT), whereas asymptomatic infections were those who were febrile but RDT negative and positive by polymerase chain reaction (PCR) or were afebrile and positive for malaria by PCR. The distribution of prevalence of infection type per month per village as well as the predicted monthly prevalence of each infection type per village are shown. (DOCX 4478 kb)

Additional file 4: Heat maps for all villages, removing households with no infections and individuals with 5 or fewer time points sampled. Each *panel* represents a household, and each *row* within the panel represents an individual residing in that household. Individuals are ordered by increasing age with the youngest on top within each panel. Each *column* within each *grid* represents a sampling month starting in June 2013 through December 2014. (DOCX 4496 kb)

Abbreviations
IQR: Interquartile range; MDA: Mass drug administration; PCR: Polymerase chain reaction; RDT: Rapid diagnostic test

Acknowledgements
We would like to thank the teams involved in data collection as well as those in the laboratory who contributed to analyzing the generated samples. The authors would also like to acknowledge Dr. Nunu Sepulveda, who provided valuable input on the data and statistical analysis.

Funding
This study was funded by the UK Medical Research Council (MRC) and the UK Department for International Development (DFID) under the MRC/DFID Concordat agreement (MC_EX_MR/J002364/1) awarded to UD. The funders had no role in the study design, data collection and analysis, decision to publish, or preparation of the manuscript.

Authors' contributions
JM, JA, GLdT, JvG, and UD were responsible for the cohort study design. JM, AW, and MJ were involved in data collection and database management. Analysis and interpretation of the data was performed by GS, EG, JM, CD, TB, and UD. GS wrote the manuscript. All authors read and approved the final manuscript.

Competing interests
The authors declare that they have no competing interests.

Author details
[1]Department of Immunology and Infection, London School of Hygiene and Tropical Medicine, London, UK. [2]Medical Research Council Unit The Gambia at London School of Hygiene & Tropical Medicine, Fajara, The Gambia. [3]University of Antwerp, Antwerp, Belgium. [4]CHICAS, Lancaster Medical School, Lancaster University, Lancaster, UK. [5]Queen Mary University of London, London, UK. [6]Department of Medical Microbology, Radboud Medical University, Nijmegen, The Netherlands.

References
1. Woolhouse MEJ, Dye C, Etard J-F, Smith T, Charlwood JD, Garnett GP, Hagan P, Hii JLK, Ndhlovu PD, Quinnell RJ, et al. Heterogeneities in the transmission of infectious agents: implications for the design of control programs. Proc Natl Acad Sci U S A. 1997;94:338–42.
2. Bejon P, Williams TN, Nyundo C, Hay SI, Benz D, Gething PW, Otiende M, Peshu J, Bashraheil M, Greenhouse B, et al. A micro-epidemiological analysis of febrile malaria in coastal Kenya showing hotspots within hotspots. eLife. 2014;3:e02130.
3. Bjorkman A, Cook J, Sturrock H, Msellem M, Ali A, Xu W, Molteni F, Gosling R, Drakeley C, Martensson A. Spatial distribution of falciparum malaria infections in Zanzibar: implications for focal drug administration strategies targeting asymptomatic parasite carriers. Clin Infect Dis. 2017;64(9):1236–43.
4. Mogeni P, Omedo I, Nyundo C, Kamau A, Noor A, Bejon P, Hotspot Group A. Effect of transmission intensity on hotspots and micro-epidemiology of malaria in sub-Saharan Africa. BMC Med. 2017;15(1):121.
5. Gaudart J, Poudiougou B, Dicko A, Ranque S, Toure O, Sagara I, Diallo M, Diawara S, Ouattara A, Diakite M, et al. Space-time clustering of childhood malaria at the household level: a dynamic cohort in a Mali village. BMC Public Health. 2006;6:286.

6. Ernst KC, Adoka SO, Kowuor DO, Wilson ML, John CC. Malaria hotspot areas in a highland Kenya site are consistent in epidemic and non-epidemic years and are associated with ecological factors. Malar J. 2006;5:78.

7. Cook J, Kleinschmidt I, Schwabe C, Nseng G, Bousema T, Corran PH, Riley EM, Drakeley CJ. Serological markers suggest heterogeneity of effectiveness of malaria control interventions on Bioko Island, Equatorial Guinea. PLoS One. 2011;6(9):e25137.

8. Bousema T, Griffin JT, Sauerwein RW, Smith DL, Churcher TS, Takken W, Ghani A, Drakeley C, Gosling R. Hitting hotspots: spatial targeting of malaria for control and elimination. PLoS Med. 2012;9(1):e1001165.

9. Kangoye DT, Noor A, Midega J, Mwongeli J, Mkabili D, Mogeni P, Kerubo C, Akoo P, Mwangangi J, Drakeley C, et al. Malaria hotspots defined by clinical malaria, asymptomatic carriage, PCR and vector numbers in a low transmission area on the Kenyan coast. Malar J. 2016;15(1):213.

10. Paull SH, Song S, McClure KM, Sackett LC, Kilpatrick AM, Johnson PT. From superspreaders to disease hotspots: linking transmission across hosts and space. Front Ecol Environ. 2012;10(2):75–82.

11. Stresman GH. Beyond temperature and precipitation: ecological risk factors that modify malaria transmission. Acta Trop. 2010;116(3):167–72.

12. Gething PW, Patil AP, Smith DL, Guerra CA, Elyazar IR, Johnston GL, Tatem AJ, Hay SI. A new world malaria map: Plasmodium falciparum endemicity in 2010. Malar J. 2011;10:378.

13. Paajmans KP, Read AF, Thomas MB. Understanding the link between malaria risk and climate. Proc Natl Acad Sci U S A. 2009;106(33):13844–9.

14. Hay SI, Snow RW, Rogers DJ. Predicting malaria seasons in Kenya using multitemporal meteorological satellite sensor data. Trans R Soc Trop Med Hyg. 1998;92:12–20.

15. Bannister-Tyrrell M, Verdonck K, Hausmann-Muela S, Gryseels C, Muela Ribera J, Peeters Grietens K. Defining micro-epidemiology for malaria elimination: systematic review and meta-analysis. Malar J. 2017;16(1):164.

16. Tucker Lima JM, Vittor A, Rifai S, Valle D. Does deforestation promote or inhibit malaria transmission in the Amazon? A systematic literature review and critical appraisal of current evidence. Phil Trans R Soc London Ser B, Biol Sci. 2017;372(1722):20160125.

17. Sturrock HJ, Novotny JM, Kunene S, Dlamini S, Zulu Z, Cohen JM, Hsiang MS, Greenhouse B, Gosling RD. Reactive case detection for malaria elimination: real-life experience from an ongoing program in Swaziland. PLoS One. 2013;8(5):e63830.

18. Smith DL, Dushoff J, McKenzie FE. The risk of a mosquito-borne infection in a heterogeneous environment. PLoS Biol. 2004;2(11):e368.

19. Smith DL, McKenzie FE, Snow RW, Hay SI. Revisiting the basic reproductive number for malaria and its implications for malaria control. PLoS Biol. 2007;5(3):e42.

20. Smith DL, Perkins TA, Reiner RC Jr, Barker CM, Niu T, Chaves LF, Ellis AM, George DB, Le Menach A, Pulliam JR, et al. Recasting the theory of mosquito-borne pathogen transmission dynamics and control. Trans R Soc Trop Med Hyg. 2014;108(4):185–97.

21. Sturrock HJ, Hsiang MS, Cohen JM, Smith DL, Greenhouse B, Bousema T, Gosling RD. Targeting asymptomatic malaria infections: active surveillance in control and elimination. PLoS Med. 2013;10(6):e1001467.

22. Bousema T, Stresman G, Baidjoe AY, Bradley J, Knight P, Stone W, Osoti V, Makori E, Owaga C, Odongo W, et al. The impact of hotspot targeted interventions on malaria transmission in Rachuonyo South District in the western Kenyan highlands: a cluster-randomized controlled trial. PLoS Med. 2016;13(4):e1001993.

23. Stresman GH, Giorgi E, Baidjoe A, Knight P, Odongo W, Owaga C, Shagari S, Makori E, Stevenson J, Drakeley C, et al. Impact of metric and sample size on determining malaria hotspot boundaries. Sci Rep. 2017;7:45849.

24. van Eijk AM, Ramanathapuram L, Sutton PL, Kanagaraj D, Sri Lakshmi Priya G, Ravishankaran S, Asokan A, Tandel N, Patel A, Desai N, et al. What is the value of reactive case detection in malaria control? A case-study in India and a systematic review. Malar J. 2016;15(1):67.

25. Mwesigwa J, Achan J, Di Tanna GL, Affara M, Jawara M, Worwui A, Hamid-Adiamoh M, Kanuteh F, Ceesay S, Bousema T, et al. Residual malaria transmission dynamics varies across The Gambia despite high coverage of control interventions. PLoS One. 2017;12(11):e0187059.

26. Tusting LS, Bousema T, Smith DL, Drakeley C. Measuring changes in Plasmodium falciparum transmission: precision, accuracy and costs of metrics. Adv Parasitol. 2014;84:151–208.

27. Smith DL, Dushoff J, Snow RW, Hay SI. The entomological inoculation rate and Plasmodium falciparum infection in African children. Nature. 2005;438(7067):492–5.

28. Smith DL, Guerra CA, Snow RW, Hay SI. Standardizing estimates of the Plasmodium falciparum parasite rate. Malar J. 2007;6:131.

29. Giorgi E, Diggle P. PrevMap: an R package for prevalence mapping. J Stat Softw. 2017;78:1–29.

30. Bivand R, Rundel C, Pebesma E, Stuetz R, Hufthammer KO: Package 'rgeos'. The Comprehensive R Archive Network (CRAN) 2017(0.3–23).

31. Hardy A, Mageni Z, Dongus S, Killeen G, Macklin MG, Majambare S, Ali A, Msellem M, Al-Mafazy AW, Smith M, et al. Mapping hotspots of malaria transmission from pre-existing hydrology, geology and geomorphology data in the pre-elimination context of Zanzibar, United Republic of Tanzania. Parasites & vectors. 2015;8:41.

32. Chang HH, Childs LM, Buckee CO. Variation in infection length and superinfection enhance selection efficiency in the human malaria parasite. Sci Rep. 2016;6:26370.

33. Omedo I, Mogeni P, Bousema T, Rockett K, Amambua-Ngwa A, Oyier I, Stevenson JC, Baidjoe AY, de Villiers EP, Fegan G, et al. Micro-epidemiological structuring of Plasmodium falciparum parasite populations in regions with varying transmission intensities in Africa. Wellcome Open Research. 2017;2:10.

34. Karl S, White MT, Milne GJ, Gurarie D, Hay SI, Barry AE, Felger I, Mueller I. Spatial effects on the multiplicity of Plasmodium falciparum infections. PLoS One. 2016;11(10):e0164054.

35. Stone W, Goncalves BP, Bousema T, Drakeley C. Assessing the infectious reservoir of falciparum malaria: past and future. Trends Parasitol. 2015;31(7):287–96.

36. Stresman GH, Baidjoe AY, Stevenson J, Grignard L, Odongo W, Owaga C, Osoti V, Makori E, Shagari S, Marube E, et al. Focal screening to identify the subpatent parasite reservoir in an area of low and heterogeneous transmission in the Kenya highlands. J Infect Dis. 2015;212(11):1768–77.

37. Clark TD, Greenhouse B, Njama-Meya D, Nzarubara B, Maiteki-Sebuguzi C, Staedke SG, Seto E, Kamya MR, Rosenthal PJ, Dorsey G. Factors determining the heterogeneity of malaria incidence in children in Kampala, Uganda. J Infect Dis. 2008;198(3):393–400.

38. Stresman GH, Kamanga A, Moono P, Hamapumbu H, Mharakurwa S, Kobayashi T, Moss WJ, Shiff C. A method of active case detection to target reservoirs of asymptomatic malaria and gametocyte carriers in a rural area in Southern Province, Zambia. Malaria J. 2010;9:265.

39. Gerardin J, Bever CA, Bridenbecker D, Hamainza B, Silumbe K, Miller JM, Eisele TP, Eckhoff PA, Wenger EA. Effectiveness of reactive case detection for malaria elimination in three archetypical transmission settings: a modelling study. Malar J. 2017;16(1):248.

40. WHO. A framework for malaria elimination. Geneva: World Health Organization; 2017.

41. Reiner RC, Le Manach A, Kunene S, Ntshalintshali N, Hsiang MS, Perkins TA, Greenhouse B, Tatem AJ, Cohen JM, Smith DL. Mapping residual transmission for malaria elimination. eLife. 2015;4:e9520

42. Lessler J, McKay HS, Moore SM, Azman AS. What is a hotspot anyway? Am J Trop Med Hygiene. 2017;96(6):1270–3.

18

Frailty, nutrition-related parameters, and mortality across the adult age spectrum

Kulapong Jayanama[1,2], Olga Theou[2,3], Joanna M Blodgett[4], Leah Cahill[2,5] and Kenneth Rockwood[3,6*]

Abstract

Background: Nutritional status and individual nutrients have been associated with frailty in older adults. The extent to which these associations hold in younger people, by type of malnutrition or grades of frailty, is unclear. Our objectives were to (1) evaluate the relationship between individual nutrition-related parameters and frailty, (2) investigate the association between individual nutrition-related parameters and mortality across frailty levels, and (3) examine whether combining nutrition-related parameters in an index predicts mortality risk across frailty levels.

Methods: This observational study assembled 9030 participants aged ≥ 20 years from the 2003–2006 cohorts of the *National Health and Nutrition Examination Survey* who had complete frailty data. A 36-item frailty index (FI) was constructed excluding items related to nutritional status. We examined 62 nutrition-related parameters with established cut points: 34 nutrient intake items, 5 anthropometric measurements, and 23 relevant blood tests. The 41 nutrition-related parameters which were associated with frailty were combined into a nutrition index (NI). All-cause mortality data until 2011 were identified from death certificates.

Results: All 5 anthropometric measurements, 21/23 blood tests, and 19/34 nutrient intake items were significantly related to frailty. Although most nutrition-related parameters were directly related to frailty, high alcohol consumption and high levels of serum alpha-carotene, beta-carotene, beta-cryptoxanthin, total cholesterol, and LDL-c were associated with lower frailty scores. Only low vitamin D was associated with increased mortality risk across all frailty levels. Seventeen nutrition-related parameters were associated with mortality in the 0.1–0.2 FI group, 11 in the 0.2–0.3 group, and 16 in the > 0.3 group. Overall, 393 (5.8%) of the participants had an NI score less than 0.1 (abnormality in ≤ 4 of the 41 parameters examined). Higher levels of NI were associated with higher mortality risk after adjusting for frailty and other covariates (HR per 0.1: 1.19 [95%CI 1.133–1.257]).

Conclusions: Most nutrition-related parameters were correlated to frailty, but only low vitamin D was associated with higher risk for mortality across levels of frailty. As has been observed with other age-related phenomena, even though many nutrition-related parameters were not significantly associated with mortality individually, when combined in an index, they strongly predicted mortality risk.

Keywords: Nutrition, Dietary intake, Frailty, Frailty index, Mortality, NHANES

Background

Reflecting the increasing life expectancy of the global population [1], the number of adults aged 65 years or older is predicted to double by 2050 [2]. In parallel, the prevalence of age-related health deficits including cardiovascular, metabolic, cognitive, and musculoskeletal diseases is growing [3–6]. Frailty is a multiply determined, age-related state of vulnerability to adverse health outcomes compared with others of the same age [7, 8]. It is associated with a range of adverse outcomes, including morbidity, mortality, and increased healthcare costs [9, 10]. Frailty can be observed at all adult ages and is closely tied to ageing, suggesting that the prevalence of frailty is likely to increase as populations age [11]. Even so, two European cohorts have observed only very modest increases with age in the

* Correspondence: Kenneth.rockwood@nshealth.ca
[3]Centre for Health Care of the Elderly, QEII Health Sciences Centre, Nova Scotia Health Authority, Halifax, Nova Scotia, Canada
[6]Division of Geriatric Medicine, Department of Medicine, Dalhousie University, Camp Hill Veterans' Memorial Bldg., 5955 Veterans' Memorial Lane, Halifax, Nova Scotia B3H 2E1, Canada
Full list of author information is available at the end of the article

mean frailty, despite varying estimates in the extent of its lethality, especially in people with milder degrees of frailty [12, 13].

Against this background, two considerations motivate a more comprehensive understanding of the relationship between nutrition and frailty. First, the two are linked. The prevalence of malnourished individuals can be high in ageing populations, especially in rehabilitation, hospital, and nursing home settings [14, 15]. Malnutrition, which is affected by inadequate, excessive, or imbalance of energy or nutrient consumption, is associated with physical and cognitive impairment, poor quality of life, morbidity, and mortality in older individuals [16–20]. Malnutrition is also associated with higher levels of frailty [8, 21].

Second, optimal nutrition management can improve frailty [22, 23] and some nutrient intakes or supplements, for example, fish oil and antioxidants, are associated with reduced frailty levels [24–27]. Nutrition management therefore appears to make poor nutrition a modifiable risk factor in relation to frailty. Importantly too, nutrition management appears to work well, in both hospital and community settings, as part of multidimensional interventions that also include exercise, pharmacological treatment, and social support [28–31].

Despite these promising insights, the evidence about the relationship of nutrition-related parameters with frailty, and whether these associations hold in younger people and by type of malnutrition, is limited and inconsistent [32–35]. Further, the multiplicity of claims about which nutritional factors might be most important is a pragmatic obstacle to uptake [8, 36–38]. This obscures how the relationship might arise, and where new interventions might best be targeted. In other contexts in which the impact of age-related adverse outcomes varies by which items are studied, it has been useful to study deficits in the aggregate [39], something which has been variably applied in nutrition studies [40]. To help improve the understanding of the relationship between frailty and nutrition, this study aims (1) to evaluate the relationship between individual nutrition-related parameters and frailty, (2) to investigate the effect of these parameters on mortality risk across levels of frailty, and (3) to examine whether combining nutrition-related parameters in an index predicts mortality risk across frailty levels.

Methods

Study population and design

This observational study used data from 10,020 individuals aged 20 years or more from the 2003–2004 and 2005–2006 cohorts of the National Health and Nutrition Examination Survey (NHANES). NHANES is a series of publicly available, cross-sectional surveys focusing on the health and nutrition of non-institutionalized US residents [41, 42]. For the purpose of this study, 990 individuals with missing FI scores were excluded. The final sample included 9030 participants. Mortality status was identified from the death certificate records from the National Death Index in December 31, 2011, and survival time was counted from the date of the clinical examination to the death event.

Each participant signed written informed consent provided to participate. The NHANES protocol was approved by the institutional review board of the Centers for Disease Control and Prevention (CDC). As a matter of policy, our local Research Ethics Committee does not review secondary analyses of duly approved, publicly available data.

Nutrition-related data

Of 84 nutrition-related parameters included in NHANES, 62 items had established cut points. Among them, 34 energy and nutrient intake items were estimated from dietary information recalled during the 24-h period prior to the interview. Five anthropometric measurements and 23 blood tests related to nutrition were collected with standard techniques. The normal range of each parameter is shown in Table 5 in Appendix. These cut points were taken from a standard textbook, the Dietary Reference Intake (DRIs), published guidelines, and previous studies [11, 43–55].

Frailty index

The FI used in this study included 36 items and was modified from a previously validated FI in NHANES [11, 56] (Table 6 in Appendix). We excluded from the FI all items related to dietary intake or nutritional status (i.e. difficulty using fork and knife, difficulty preparing meals, glycohaemoglobin, triglyceride, creatinine, haemoglobin, mean corpuscular volume, total cholesterol, glucose, and sodium). The FI score, the number of deficits present divided by the total deficits considered, ranges between 0 and 1, and a higher score is associated with higher frailty. For stratification purposes, we grouped participants into 4 FI groups: FI ≤ 0.1 (fit), $0.1 < FI \leq 0.2$ (vulnerable), $0.2 < FI \leq 0.3$ (mildly frail), and FI > 0.3 (moderately/severely frail) [56].

Nutrition index

A nutrition index (NI) was constructed following the deficit accumulation approach [57] by combining the 41 nutrition-related parameters that were related with higher frailty: counting the number of nutritional deficits in an individual and dividing by the total deficits considered. Low-density lipoprotein cholesterol (LDL-

c) and subscapular skinfold were excluded from the NI due to high number of missing data: 53.9% for LDL-c and 23.8% for subscapular skinfold. Each nutritional parameter was scored "1" if the value fell outside the normal range and "0" otherwise. Abnormal values that were found to be protective for frailty (associated with lower levels of frailty) were also scored as 0 (Table 5 in Appendix). An NI score was only calculated for individuals with > 80% of the variables complete. The NI score ranges between 0 and 1; an NI score of 0 represents full nutritional health, while a score of 1 represents complete nutritional deficits. In the analysis, we used both the continuous NI score and a categorical variable: NI $\leq$ 0.2, 0.2 < NI $\leq$ 0.3, 0.3 < NI $\leq$ 0.4, 0.4 < NI $\leq$ 0.5, and NI > 0.5.

Statistical analysis

Demographic characteristics of the subjects are presented as mean ± standard deviation (SD) for continuous variables and as frequency (%) for binary or categorical variables. All percentages and mean values were weighted using the sampling weights provided by NHANES. Multiple linear regression analysis was used to assess the associations between each nutrition-related parameter, NI and FI scores and is presented by β-coefficient with 95% confidence interval (CI). The mortality risk from each parameter across the FI group was analysed using Cox regression models, and the odds of mortality risk was presented using the hazard ratios and the associated 95%CI. All regression models were adjusted for potential covariates including age, sex, race, energy intake, educational level, marital status, employment status, smoking, and study cohort. Models which included energy, energy per weight, dietary fiber per energy intakes, and NI as predictors were not adjusted for energy intake. Annual household income was not included as covariate due to missing data. Statistical significance was considered as a p value < 0.05, and all reported probability tests were two-sided. The statistical analysis was conducted using IBM SPSS Statistics for Windows, Version 24.0. Armonk, NY: IBM Corp.

Results

Of the 9030 included participants, 48% were male; their weighted mean age was 46.6 ± 16.9 years. When we stratified the sample by frailty, 5119 (56.7%), 2009 (22.2%), 1014 (11.2%), and 888 (9.8%) had an FI score < 0.1, 0.1–0.2, 0.2–0.3, and > 0.3, respectively. The weighted mortality rate was 6.5% (940/9030). The demographic characteristics of the sample by frailty categories are presented in Table 1. In the frailer groups, the mean age and number of people with female gender, lower education, non-full-time work, and

low income were significantly higher ($p < 0.001$) (Table 1).

Regarding objective 1 (to evaluate the relationship between individual nutrition-related parameters and frailty), many but not all nutrition-related parameters—especially those related to self-reported intake—varied in relation to the degree of frailty. The proportion of individuals who had abnormal dietary intakes differed significantly between FI groups in almost all variables, except high intake of saturated fat (%), vitamin A, iron, zinc, copper, selenium, and caffeine, and low intake of vitamin A and vitamin C (Table 2). Related to anthropometric measurement, only the percentage of individuals who were underweight and had low subscapular skinfold thickness did not significantly differ between FI groups (Table 3). Similarly, the proportion of individuals who had abnormal blood tests differed significantly between FI groups in almost all variables, except low MCV, low levels of folate in red blood cell and plasma glucose, and high levels of haemoglobin, serum beta-carotene, serum lutein/zeaxanthin, and serum iron (Table 4).

Linear regression models, adjusted for the potential covariates, revealed statistically significant associations between frailty and the inappropriate intake of many nutrients (Table 7 in Appendix), the abnormal range of many anthropometric measures (Table 8 in Appendix), and the abnormality of many nutrition-related blood tests (Table 9 in Appendix). To summarize, frailty was associated with 19 nutrient intakes (Fig. 1a). Low energy intake per weight showed the highest positive correlation with frailty (β-coefficient 0.018, 95%CI 0.014–0.021) followed by low protein per weight intake (0.016, 0.011–0.020), whereas high consumption of energy per weight, sodium, and alcohol were significantly associated with lower FI score. With regard to anthropometric measurements, only being overweight was significantly associated with lower frailty. Obesity, high waist circumference, triceps and subscapular skinfold thickness, and body weight change (loss and gain more than 10%) were significantly associated with higher FI score (Fig. 1b). Almost all blood tests (21/23) were significantly correlated with frailty. The highest association was found in low serum vitamin A (β-coefficient 0.085, 95%CI 0.030–0.139). High serum levels of alpha-carotene, beta-carotene, beta-cryptoxanthin, lutein/zeaxanthin, lycopene, total cholesterol, and LDL-c were inversely associated with FI score (Fig. 1c).

Results related to the relationship of the nutrition-related parameters with mortality risk (objective 2) are presented in Fig. 2 and Tables 10, 11, and 12 in Appendix. To summarize, only one abnormal blood test (low vitamin D which was associated with mortality risk at all grades of frailty) showed a relationship with mortality in people with

Table 1 Demographic characteristics of participants by frailty level

Characteristics	Frailty index score			
	≤ 0.1 N = 5119	> 0.1 to 0.2 N = 2009	> 0.2 to 0.3 N = 1014	> 0.3 N = 888
Age (year), mean ± SD	39.7 ± 13.2	54.8 ± 15.8	62.8 ± 14.5	65.3 ± 14.4
Sex, female, N (%)	2540 (48.3)	1114 (58.7)	529 (56.2)	504 (60.9)
Race, N (%)				
Non-Hispanic White	2478 (70.4)	1112 (75.6)	611 (79.9)	493 (73.1)
Non-Hispanic Black	1057 (10.6)	409 (10.8)	196 (10.7)	212 (15.1)
Hispanic	1356 (13.5)	416 (8.8)	179 (5.5)	144 (5.8)
Other	228 (5.5)	72 (4.7)	28 (4.0)	39 (5.9)
Education, N (%)				
Less than high school	1193 (14.3)	614 (19.5)	384 (27.6)	386 (33.1)
High school	1195 (24.4)	513 (27.4)	277 (30.3)	211 (29.3)
Some college/associated education	1560 (32.7)	528 (31.1)	226 (26.4)	204 (27.6)
College graduate or more	1167 (28.6)	352 (22.0)	127 (15.7)	80 (10.0)
Annual household Income (USD), N (%)				
0–19,999	802 (11.1)	478 (18.2)	335 (27.3)	385 (39.2)
20,000–44,999	1533 (27.0)	686 (33.0)	354 (38.3)	266 (34.6)
45,000–74,999	1149 (26.2)	391 (25.6)	143 (21.2)	120 (18.4)
≥ 75,000	1336 (35.7)	335 (23.3)	107 (13.2)	55 (7.8)
Marital status, N (%)				
Married	3376 (67.8)	1245 (65.4)	569 (59.9)	402 (50.0)
Widowed	129 (1.9)	280 (10.7)	225 (16.8)	260 (24.2)
Divorced or separated	500 (10.2)	294 (14.8)	154 (16.7)	164 (18.7)
Never married	1110 (20.2)	190 (9.1)	65 (6.6)	61 (7.2)
Full-time working, N (%)	3819 (80.7)	882 (53.4)	214 (28.1)	72 (11.7)
Smoking status, N (%)				
Never	2864 (53.5)	988 (47.4)	411 (40.1)	377 (41.2)
Former	1021 (20.5)	600 (29.7)	414 (38.1)	346 (37.7)
Current	1234 (26.0)	421 (22.9)	189 (21.8)	165 (21.1)

The percentages and mean values are weighted

USD United States Dollar

FI ≤ 0.1; four nutrient intakes, three anthropometric measurements, and ten blood tests in people with 0.1–0.2 FI; one nutrient intake, four anthropometric measurements, and six blood tests in people with 0.2–0.3 FI; and three nutrient intakes, three anthropometric measurements, and ten blood tests in people with FI > 0.3. Participants with FI > 0.1 who reported that they lost more than 10% of their weight in the past year had higher mortality risk. Being underweight and low serum creatinine levels were associated with higher mortality risk in individuals with FI > 0.2. Being overweight, having high waist circumference, and caffeine consumption were significantly associated with lower mortality risk in individuals with FI > 0.3.

Regarding objective 3 (to examine whether combining nutrition-related parameters in an index predicts mortality risk across frailty levels), we could not calculate the NI score for 500 individuals due to missing > 20% of the nutritional parameters included in the index (total included $n = 8530$). Overall, 393 (5.8%) of the participants had an NI score less than 0.1 (abnormality in ≤ 4 of the 41 parameters examined). This proportion decreased with higher frailty, from 7.4% among those with FI < 0.1 to 0.7% among those with FI > 0.3 (Fig. 3 and Table 13 in Appendix). The weighted mean NI score was 0.29 ± 0.13 (range 0.00–0.79) and was significantly higher for those people with higher frailty levels: 0.26 ± 0.12 for FI ≤ 1, 0.31 ± 0.13 for 0.1–0.2 FI, 0.35 ± 0.13 for 0.2–0.3 FI, and 0.40 ± 0.14 for FI > 0.3.

Table 2 Number of participants with abnormal range of daily nutrient intakes by frailty level

Nutrients, N (%)*		Frailty index score			
		≤ 0.1 N = 5119	> 0.1 to 0.2 N = 2009	> 0.2 to 0.3 N = 1014	> 0.3 N = 888
Energy (N = 8614)	Low	2218 (44.4)	1157 (55.3)	297 (63.8)	203 (71.7)
Energy per weight (N = 8510)	Low	1950 (39.8)	1051 (54.1)	605 (60.9)	566 (69.7)
	High	1479 (30.8)	307 (17.4)	108 (13.9)	64 (7.9)
Protein (N = 8614)	Low	821 (15.6)	450 (20.9)	297 (27.5)	303 (33.5)
Protein per weight (N = 8510)	Low	1524 (29.0)	955 (46.8)	563 (55.0)	524 (63.6)
Carbohydrate (N = 8614)	Low	1068 (22.8)	608 (31.1)	357 (35.5)	360 (41.2)
Simple sugar (N = 8614)	High	4633 (94.6)	1778 (92.9)	896 (93.1)	758 (91.7)
Dietary fiber per energy (N = 8613)	Low	4590 (94.6)	1713 (91.0)	870 (91.9)	755 (92.8)
Percentage of fat (N = 8614)	Low	119 (2.0)	83 (3.6)	41 (4.2)	46 (4.6)
	High	4413 (91.1)	1650 (88.1)	799 (85.0)	670 (82.7)
Percentage of saturated fat (N = 8613)	High	2827 (59.6)	1078 (59.0)	554 (57.4)	479 (60.8)
Cholesterol (N = 8614)	High	1924 (39.2)	652 (33.4)	312 (30.9)	255 (28.5)
Vitamin A, RAE (N = 8614)	Low	3725 (75.0)	1502 (76.8)	745 (76.1)	647 (76.7)
	High	31 (0.7)	5 (0.1)	11 (1.0)	4 (0.5)
Vitamin C (N = 8614)	Low	2903 (62.2)	1165 (61.8)	598 (63.2)	516 (65.1)
	High	0 (0.0)	0 (0.0)	0 (0.0)	1 (0.1)
Vitamin E (N = 8614)	Low	4548 (92.4)	1814 (93.2)	931 (94.9)	802 (95.9)
Vitamin K (N = 8614)	Low	3754 (74.4)	1503 (76.0)	776 (78.0)	679 (80.6)
Thiamin (N = 8614)	Low	1411 (27.3)	700 (34.3)	362 (35.2)	375 (42.6)
Riboflavin (N = 8614)	Low	831 (14.5)	359 (15.7)	189 (17.4)	212 (23.6)
Niacin (N = 8614)	Low	981 (18.0)	544 (25.3)	301 (26.2)	332 (37.1)
	High	1020 (23.0)	223 (13.1)	95 (13.0)	65 (8.7)
Pyridoxine (N = 8614)	Low	1596 (32.2)	898 (43.7)	507 (47.9)	470 (54.0)
Folate (N = 8614)	Low	2751 (54.8)	1236 (63.3)	658 (64.6)	606 (71.3)
	High	138 (3.2)	38 (2.1)	19 (2.7)	10 (1.3)
Cobalamin (N = 8614)	Low	1252 (24.5)	593 (28.5)	307 (30.5)	287 (32.8)
Calcium (N = 8614)	Low	3150 (63.7)	1457 (73.4)	787 (78.4)	698 (81.0)
	High	125 (2.8)	30 (1.8)	9 (1.2)	4 (0.8)
Phosphorous (N = 8614)	Low	551 (10.1)	322 (14.7)	187 (18.5)	217 (24.7)
	High	29 (0.5)	8 (0.5)	1 (0.3)	0 (0.0)
Magnesium (N = 8614)	Low	3656 (74.2)	1526 (76.9)	828 (82.7)	731 (87.1)
Iron (N = 8614)	Low	1750 (34.7)	579 (30.7)	223 (23.3)	228 (29.0)
	High	65 (1.4)	21 (1.1)	7 (1.0)	5 (0.7)
Zinc (N = 8614)	Low	1863 (36.3)	898 (42.8)	531 (49.7)	468 (52.5)
	High	56 (1.2)	14 (0.8)	8 (1.0)	3 (0.3)
Copper (N = 8614)	Low	1322 (25.5)	663 (31.9)	369 (34.8)	379 (44.4)
	High	10 (0.3)	1 (0.0)	2 (0.1)	1 (0.1)
Sodium (N = 8614)	Low	359 (6.7)	103 (8.0)	81 (7.5)	117 (12.4)
	High	3742 (79.2)	1219 (65.8)	599 (64.5)	435 (54.2)
Potassium (N = 8614)	Low	4484 (91.4)	1799 (92.4)	935 (95.6)	810 (96.7)
Selenium (N = 8614)	Low	571 (10.8)	344 (16.9)	203 (20.4)	228 (26.4)
	High	15 (0.3)	8 (0.5)	1 (0.1)	0 (0.0)

Table 2 Number of participants with abnormal range of daily nutrient intakes by frailty level *(Continued)*

Nutrients, N (%)*		Frailty index score			
		≤ 0.1 N = 5119	> 0.1 to 0.2 N = 2009	> 0.2 to 0.3 N = 1014	> 0.3 N = 888
Caffeine (N = 8614)	High	489 (14.2)	191 (13.5)	82 (12.3)	80 (11.4)
Alcohol (N = 8614)	High	885 (21.7)	270 (16.8)	111 (12.9)	59 (8.8)
Linoleic acid (N = 8614)	Low	2414 (47.9)	1030 (51.3)	562 (54.7)	531 (62.1)
α-Linolenic acid (N = 8614)	Low	2491 (49.8)	1100 (53.8)	603 (58.4)	552 (63.9)
Fish oil (N = 8614)	Low	4343 (88.7)	1700 (88.5)	872 (90.6)	764 (91.1)

RAE retinol activity equivalents
*The percentages are weighted

Higher NI score was significantly associated with higher frailty (β-coefficient 1.46, 95%CI 1.459–1.461) and higher mortality risk (HR per 0.1 NI score 1.30, 95%CI 1.23–1.36) after adjusting the models for potential covariates. After adjusting the survival analysis additionally for the FI, the HR per 0.1 NI score was 1.19 (95%CI 1.13–1.26). When analysis was stratified by frailty level, higher NI scores were significantly correlated with higher mortality in individual with FI > 0.1; HR per 0.1 NI score was 1.17 (1.06–1.30) for those with 0.1–0.2 FI, 1.20 (1.08–1.32) for those with 0.2–0.3 FI, and 1.27 (1.16–1.38) for those with FI > 0.3 (Fig. 4 and Table 14 in Appendix). When we examined the joint effect of nutrition and frailty status on mortality, we found a dose-response relationship (Fig. 5 and Table 15 in Appendix). People with FI > 0.3 had a higher mortality risk regardless of nutrition status, whereas having an FI ≤ 0.1 was not associated with frailty even for those with NI > 0.5. People with FI > 0.3 and NI > 0.5 had the highest mortality risk (HR 8.17, 95%CI 5.16–12.94).

Discussion

This observational study aimed to improve our understanding of the relationship between frailty and nutrition. As expected, we found that the two are related. When we looked at one nutritional parameter at a time (objective 1), the details are complicated: most but not all of the abnormal nutrition-related parameters included in NHANES were related to frailty (19/34 of nutrient intakes, all 5 anthropometric measurements and 21/23 of blood tests). Nevertheless, fewer than half were individually associated with higher mortality risk across frailty levels and their impact differed across levels of frailty (objective 2). A relationship with all-cause mortality was found with one parameter in the FI ≤ 0.1 group, 17 parameters in the 0.1–0.2 FI group, 11 parameters in the 0.2–0.3 FI group, and 16 parameters in the > 0.3 FI group. Only low serum vitamin D significantly increased the mortality risk across all levels of frailty. Even so, when we combined the nutrition-related parameters, including those not significantly associated with mortality, the resulting NI strongly predicted mortality risk, especially among those with higher FI scores (objective 3). In short, overall, the results show that frailty and nutrition are related, and for the most part, unless people are in good health, poor

Table 3 Number of participants with abnormal range of anthropometric measurement by frailty level

Anthropometric measurements, N (%)*		Frailty index score			
		≤ 0.1 N = 5119	> 0.1 to 0.2 N = 2009	> 0.2 to 0.3 N = 1014	> 0.3 N = 888
Body mass index (N = 8873)	Underweight	91 (1.9)	22 (1.3)	17 (1.8)	10 (1.2)
	Overweight	1816 (34.5)	702 (33.8)	341 (31.5)	244 (29.3)
	Obese	1519 (28.6)	735 (38.9)	408 (44.1)	359 (44.2)
Body weight change in past 1 year (N = 8852)	Loss > 10%	381 (6.8)	194 (9.7)	122 (10.9)	151 (15.6)
	Gain > 10%	872 (13.7)	252 (12.1)	115 (13.3)	104 (14.0)
Waist circumference (N = 8644)	High	3444 (67.2)	1603 (82.2)	815 (85.9)	643 (86.1)
Triceps skinfold (N = 7885)	Low	538 (11.3)	147 (8.1)	84 (8.6)	76 (10.3)
	High	415 (9.3)	184 (12.3)	108 (15.9)	93 (13.5)
Subscapular skinfold (N = 6884)	Low	428 (11.1)	143 (9.3)	66 (8.4)	62 (11.2)
	High	281 (7.2)	140 (9.0)	62 (10.0)	45 (6.8)

*The percentages and mean values are weighted

Table 4 Number of participants with abnormal range of blood levels by frailty level

Blood tests, N (%)*		Frailty index score			
		≤ 0.1 N = 5119	> 0.1 to 0.2 N = 2009	> 0.2 to 0.3 N = 1014	> 0.3 N = 888
Total lymphocyte count (N = 8965)	Low	862 (17.8)	451 (20.9)	272 (24.2)	304 (34.6)
Haemoglobin (N = 9017)	Low	304 (3.4)	224 (7.4)	175 (12.6)	216 (20.9)
	High	40 (1.0)	25 (1.4)	13 (2.1)	9 (0.8)
Mean corpuscular volume (N = 9017)	Low	170 (2.4)	130 (5.3)	30 (2.3)	43 (4.2)
	High	43 (0.9)	74 (3.7)	56 (5.8)	56 (6.6)
Albumin (N = 8916)	Low	308 (1.8)	84 (1.8)	28 (2.2)	68 (7.2)
Vitamin A (N = 8889)	Low	1 (0.0)	2 (0.1)	3 (0.1)	5 (0.6)
	High	168 (4.4)	148 (8.9)	128 (13.7)	159 (19.0)
Vitamin C (N = 8886)	Low	264 (6.6)	147 (7.4)	78 (8.3)	82 (8.0)
	High	77 (1.8)	66 (3.4)	44 (4.6)	36 (4.4)
Vitamin D (N = 8976)	Low	1906 (29.4)	740 (30.5)	422 (35.6)	438 (44.6)
	High	59 (1.5)	9 (0.6)	2 (0.2)	2 (0.3)
Pyridoxine (N = 8926)	Low	869 (15.0)	380 (16.5)	206 (19.4)	231 (25.6)
Folate, RBC (N = 8959)	Low	249 (4.1)	73 (2.7)	40 (3.1)	31 (3.5)
Cobalamin (N = 8865)	Low	112 (2.0)	50 (2.4)	43 (4.4)	39 (5.3)
α-carotene (N = 8885)	Low	1045 (21.4)	396 (20.4)	220 (22.5)	241 (30.3)
	High	562 (11.4)	223 (11.1)	72 (6.1)	54 (6.6)
β-carotene (N = 8501)	Low	908 (19.5)	345 (20.0)	197 (21.9)	189 (24.7)
	High	565 (11.9)	277 (13.4)	131 (11.8)	101 (11.0)
β-cryptoxanthin (N = 8865)	Low	619 (15.5)	368 (21.4)	247 (28.8)	257 (35.6)
	High	876 (12.3)	294 (12.1)	122 (8.7)	76 (7.0)
Lutein/Zeaxanthin (N = 8889)	Low	1131 (26.5)	531 (32.0)	307 (34.8)	346 (46.5)
	High	229 (3.8)	109 (4.8)	46 (4.5)	34 (3.5)
Lycopene (N = 8889)	Low	584 (10.7)	401 (16.3)	317 (29.2)	369 (40.3)
	High	666 (14.0)	163 (10.0)	55 (6.3)	34 (5.4)
Iron, serum (N = 8910)	Low	669 (11.6)	309 (13.8)	145 (15.3)	180 (20.8)
	High	84 (1.8)	22 (1.1)	10 (1.0)	7 (1.0)
Creatinine (N = 8916)	Low	337 (3.4)	103 (3.7)	40 (3.3)	30 (4.1)
	High	68 (1.2)	145 (6.0)	166 (13.9)	232 (24.7)
Total cholesterol (N = 8950)	High	2380 (46.1)	1053 (52.6)	445 (44.2)	367 (43.7)
Triglyceride (N = 8911)	High	1574 (29.1)	734 (39.2)	402 (42.2)	370 (44.1)
HDL-c (N = 8949)	Low	1453 (30.1)	576 (30.9)	290 (29.8)	312 (37.9)
LDL-c (N = 4161)	High	789 (32.7)	318 (32.5)	119 (24.0)	115 (29.0)
Glucose (N = 8916)	Low	141 (2.0)	25 (1.0)	16 (1.4)	20 (2.6)
	High	814 (15.3)	666 (31.5)	439 (39.7)	423 (46.5)
Homocysteine (N = 8979)	High	21 (0.5)	25 (1.1)	26 (2.1)	46 (5.0)

HDL-c high-density lipoprotein cholesterol, LDL-c low-density lipoprotein cholesterol, RBC red blood cell
*The percentages are weighted

nutritional status increases mortality in a dose-dependent fashion, independent of age, sex, marital status, and education.

Several features of these results require additional comment. Regarding the individual items, vitamin D plays an important role in both bone metabolism and non-bony tissue function including skeletal muscles which relate with function in elderly people [58]. Previous observational studies [59, 60] including one using the NHANES III data [61] showed that serum

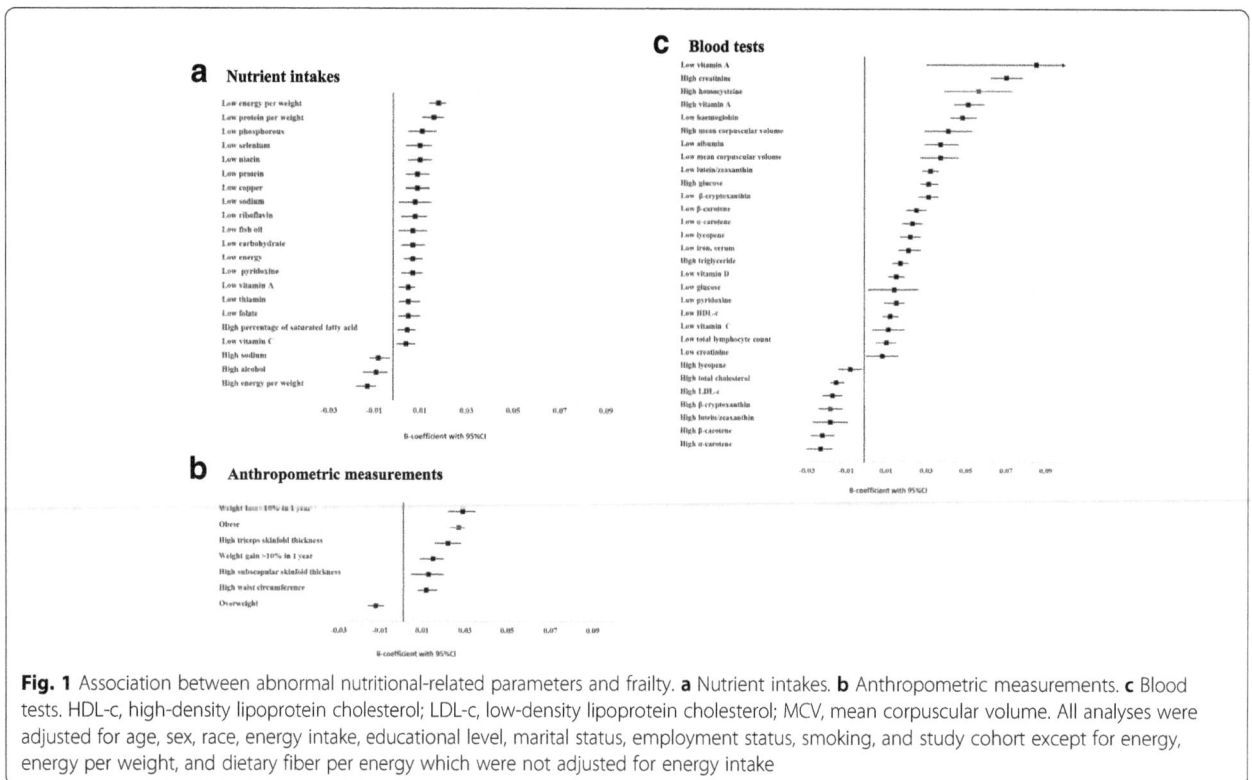

Fig. 1 Association between abnormal nutritional-related parameters and frailty. **a** Nutrient intakes. **b** Anthropometric measurements. **c** Blood tests. HDL-c, high-density lipoprotein cholesterol; LDL-c, low-density lipoprotein cholesterol; MCV, mean corpuscular volume. All analyses were adjusted for age, sex, race, energy intake, educational level, marital status, employment status, smoking, and study cohort except for energy, energy per weight, and dietary fiber per energy which were not adjusted for energy intake

vitamin D levels were correlated with frailty and all-cause mortality in older adults. Moreover, a meta-analysis of RCTs [62] reported the benefit of daily vitamin D supplementation on muscle strength and balance in older people. Concerning cognitive function, severe vitamin D deficiency was also correlated with visual memory decline [63]. The current study confirmed the association between low serum vitamin D levels and both frailty levels and mortality risk across levels of frailty, not only in older people but also in younger people.

According to World Health Organization (WHO), the normal range of weight in healthy adults is defined by body mass index (BMI) or Quetelet index between 18.5 and 24.9 kg/m^2 [64]. Even so, human physiology and mortality risk factors change with ageing. A previous meta-analysis [65] showed that a BMI < 23 kg/m^2 was associated with higher mortality risk in older people. BMI alone may not be a good indicator of adiposity in this population and this has been widely demonstrated based on the obesity paradox seen in the older people [66, 67]. The present study showed that obesity was associated with higher frailty but had no relationship with mortality. In contrast, being underweight increased mortality risk in individuals with FI > 0.2 and the mortality risk was lower in people with FI > 0.3 who were overweight. It is possible that body composition and weight change may be

better predictors in older people than BMI. This study revealed that excessive fat accumulation, high triceps and subscapular skinfold thickness, waist circumference, and change of body weight (loss and gain) more than 10% in the past year were correlated with higher frailty. Moreover, low triceps skinfold in people with 0.1–0.3 FI and weight loss more than 10% in the past year in people with FI > 0.1 were associated with higher mortality risk.

On the subject of phytochemicals, previous studies [68, 69] showed that low serum carotenoids levels were associated with higher frailty. This study also confirmed that low serum alpha-carotene, beta-carotene, beta-cryptoxanthin, lutein/zeaxanthin, and lycopene levels increased the risks of frailty and mortality; high serum levels of these carotenoids were associated with lower frailty levels. The relationship between the amount of dietary carotenoid intakes and their serum levels in older adults should be explored further. Recommending carotenoids-rich fruits and vegetables consumption could be the focus of dietary interventions to improve frailty status.

This study illustrates the virtue of considering deficit accumulation as a means of providing context in age-related disorders. As put pithily in a 2014 Nature commentary, "the problems of old age come as a package" [70]. Deficit accumulation indices can quantify those packages of age-associated problems [71] and

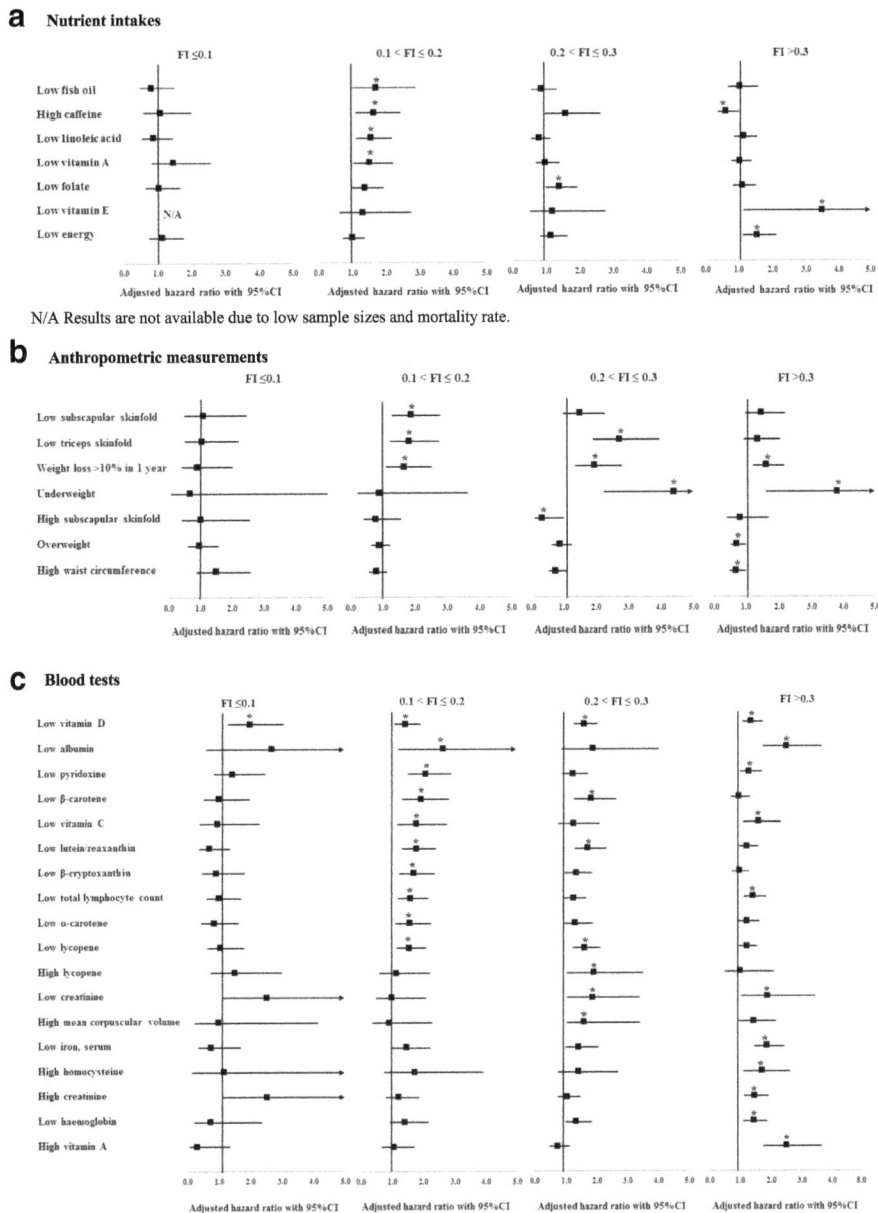

Fig. 2 Association between abnormal nutritional-related parameters and mortality across levels of frailty. **a** Nutrient intakes. N/A, results are not available due to low sample sizes and mortality rate. **b** Anthropometric measurements. **c** Blood tests. FI, frailty index. All analyses were adjusted for age, sex, race, energy intake, educational level, marital status, employment status, smoking, and study cohort except for energy and energy per weight which were not adjusted for energy intake. *p value < 0.05

have been used by our group and others in a variety of contexts to quantify the cumulative impact of brain MRI changes [72], social vulnerability measures [73], laboratory measures [74], and ageing biomarkers [75]. An NI, constructed using the deficit accumulation approach, was a stronger prediction of frailty and mortality risk than were single nutritional parameters. This study, similarly to previous studies [76, 77], highlights that the accumulation of small deficits, even

those that may not result in clinically detectable problems, corresponds to the ability of the organism to respond and recover from stressors [78]. A recent report noted the benefit to considering 11 nutrition-related parameters in mortality prediction, but did not evaluate frailty [40]. The findings from that work do not contradict our key clinical message: patient management should reflect not just nutritional parameters that cross an illness threshold, but the overall nutritional status.

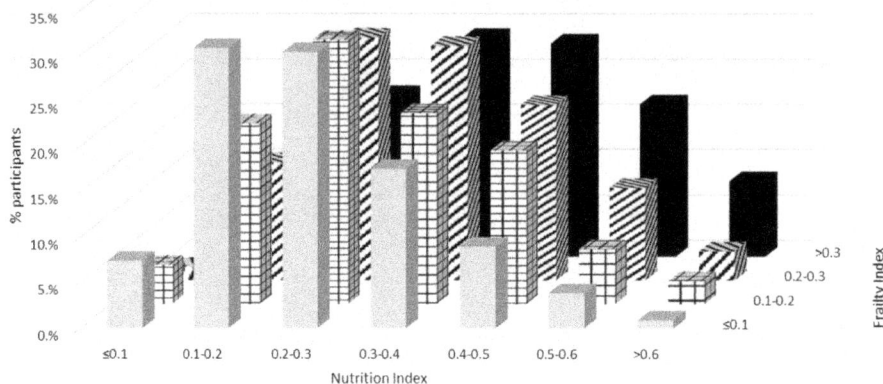

Fig. 3 Percentage of participants in each level of nutritional index score by frailty level. The percentages are weighted

In addition, there appears to be some merit in broader modeling of the nutrition risk as part of age-related deficit accumulation [79]. For example, the doubling time of biomarker deficits appears to be longer than laboratory ones, which in turn are longer than clinical deficits [74, 75, 80], something which appears to reflect their relative connectivity as nodes in a network. How the various types of nutritional deficits fit in this spectrum is of interest, with an initial hypothesis that their variable relationships with mortality might reflect their connectivity (or other network properties). Recent work suggests that information theory might help better analyse factors that influence the health trajectories of individuals [79], offering pragmatic new approaches to studying age-related disease [81].

Here, participants with low energy consumption for their body weight were more likely to be frail. Lower than recommended calorie intake can cause malnutrition; high levels of frailty are common among malnourished people [8]. We also showed a strong association between frailty and body weight changes of more than 10%, both losing and gaining weight in 1 year. Weight loss is a major sign of malnutrition, is included in most of the nutritional screening tools, and is one of the five criteria used in defining the "frailty phenotype" [82]. Weight loss can be caused not only by loss of fat but also by loss of muscle and bony mass [83]. On the other hand, weight gain leads to more fat mass than muscle mass in sedentary young individuals. The fat accumulation itself is associated with many health deficits, especially the metabolic syndrome and metabolic-related diseases. Even so, how the metabolic syndrome and frailty interact in relation to mortality appears to change across the life course [84].

The causes of frailty may be different at each age group. For example, younger people may accumulate deficits due to a chronic condition whereas older people may accumulate deficits even when few comorbidities are present [85]. Similarly, nutritional problems are altered across the lifespan. For example, older people may require more protein and calcium

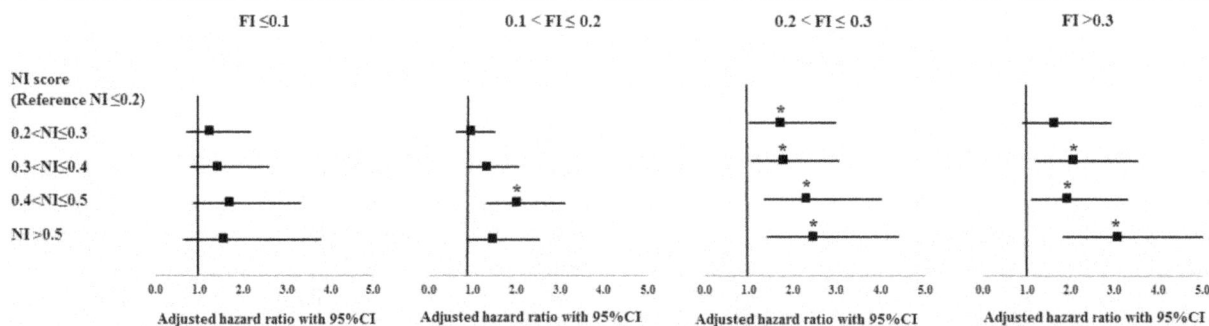

Fig. 4 Association between nutritional index and mortality across levels of frailty. FI, frailty index; NI, nutritional index. All analyses were adjusted for age, sex, race, educational level, marital status, employment status, smoking, and study cohort except for energy and energy per weight which were not adjusted for energy intake. *p value < 0.05

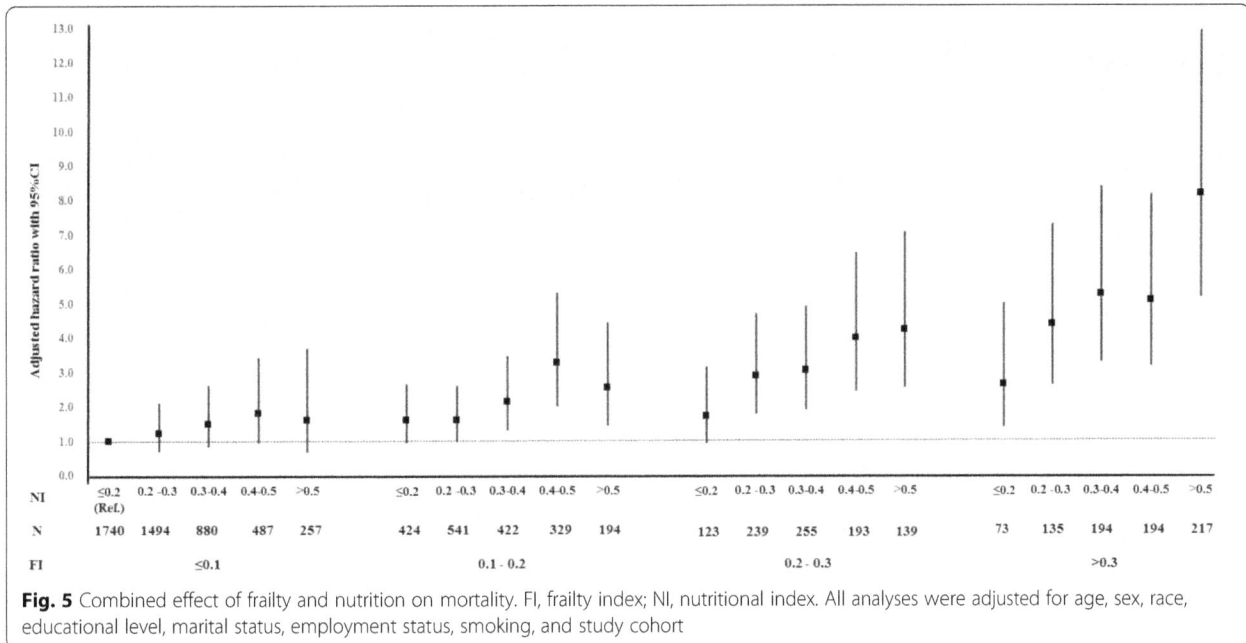

Fig. 5 Combined effect of frailty and nutrition on mortality. FI, frailty index; NI, nutritional index. All analyses were adjusted for age, sex, race, educational level, marital status, employment status, smoking, and study cohort

intake than do younger people [45, 86] whereas the requirement for iron typically declines after the menopause [52]. Here, we recognized this by using cutoff points of normal intake according to the recommendation for each age and gender group. Even so, the effect of abnormal nutrition on frailty can be different in each age group and future interventional studies need to investigate this.

We used publicly available data from NHANES, a large population-based study with a well-controlled and rigorous protocol. We analysed a huge number of nutrition-related parameters. Mortality was extracted from death certificate data and was examined 5–8 years after testing. However, our data must be interpreted with caution: (a) Due to the cross-sectional design, the causal relationship between frailty and nutrition cannot be examined and the duration of exposure to each parameter cannot be explored. For example, here, daily alcohol consumption of more than 2 standard drinks (28 g) in men and 1 standard drink in women (14 g) was associated with lower frailty but was not related with mortality risk. Nevertheless, alcohol consumption more than 3 standard drinks (42 g) per day was not associated with frailty (data not shown). (b) Since dietary data (including alcohol use) were recorded by 24-h recall, day-to-day variation could not be counted, and food intake could be altered along the study period. (c) People who have chronic abnormal serum levels of some nutrients may have experienced temporally normal levels during testing.

The absence of longitudinal data also makes it difficult to discern age from period and cohort effects. Our data do however demonstrate that both frailty and nutritional deficiencies can be detected at all adult ages. Nutritional deficiencies, at least in the aggregate, can also be seen more commonly at higher ages and with frailty, and increase the lethality of frailty. Here, for similar levels of deficit accumulation, at all ages, impaired nutrition reduced survival in people whose FI score were higher than 0.1.

Conclusions

This study revealed that most nutritional parameters were related with frailty, but the impact of individual parameters on mortality differed across levels of frailty. Only low vitamin D was associated with higher levels of frailty and higher risk for mortality across all levels of frailty. Weight loss more than 10% in the past year also increased mortality risk, except in very fit people. Nevertheless, mortality risk was decreased by being overweight, having high waist circumference and subscapular skinfold and consuming more than 400 mg of caffeine daily in people FI > 0.3. Even though many nutrition-related parameters were not significantly associated with mortality, we found that in people with FI > 0.1, they strongly predicted mortality risk when combined in an index. The combined effect of frailty and nutrition deficits had the most impact on mortality risk. Balanced nutritional interventions appear to be reasonable approaches to remediating frailty. Further studies are needed to examine the impact of nutritional interventional studies on frailty levels and to evaluate whether the number of nutritional deficits relates to other health outcomes such as hospitalization, institutionalization, and quality of life.

Appendix

Table 5 Normal range of parameter

Parameter	Normal range	Score in nutritional index	
		0	1
Nutrient intakes			
Energy (kcal/day)	M ≥ 2400, F ≥ 1800	Normal range	M < 2400, F < 1800
Energy per weight (kcal/kg/day)	25–35	≥ 25	< 25
Protein (g/day)	M ≥ 56, F ≥ 46	Normal range	M < 56, F < 46
Protein per weight (g/kg/day)	< 65 years, ≥ 0.8 ≥65 years, ≥ 1	Normal range	< 65 years, < 0.8 ≥ 65 years, < 1
Carbohydrate (g/day)	≥ 180	Normal range	< 180
Simple sugar (mg/day)	M < 36, F < 25	–	–
Dietary fiber (g/1000 kcal/day)	> 14	–	–
Percentage of fat (%)	20–35	–	–
Percentage of saturated fat (%)	< 10	–	–
Cholesterol (mg/day)	< 300	–	–
Vitamin A, RAE (mcg/day)	M 900–3000, F 700–3000	–	–
Vitamin C (mg/day)	M 90–2000, F 75–2000	–	–
Vitamin E (mg/day)	15–1000	–	–
Vitamin K (mcg/day)	M ≥ 120, F ≥ 90	Normal range	M < 120, F < 90
Thiamin (mg/day)	M ≥ 1.2, F ≥ 1.1	Normal range	M < 1.2, F < 1.1
Riboflavin (mg/day)	M ≥ 1.3, F ≥ 1.1	Normal range	M < 1.3, F < 1.1
Niacin (mg/day)	M 16–35, F 14–35	–	–
Pyridoxine (mg/day)	≤ 50 years, 1.3–100 > 50 years, M 1.7–100 > 50 years, F 1.5–100	Normal range	≤50 years, < 1.3 or > 100 > 50 years, M < 1.7 or > 100 > 50 years, F < 1.5 or > 100
Folate (mcg/day)	400–1000	Normal range	< 400 or > 1000
Cobalamin (mcg/day)	≥ 2.4	Normal range	< 2.4
Calcium (mg/day)	M ≤ 70 years, 1000–2500 M > 70 years, 1200–2500 F ≤ 50 years, 1000–2500 F > 50 years, 1200–2500	Normal range	M ≤ 70 years, < 1000 or > 2500 M > 70 years, < 1200 or > 2500 F ≤ 50 years, < 1000 or > 2500 F > 50 years, < 1200 or > 2500
Phosphorous (mg/day)	700–4000	Normal range	< 700 or > 4000
Magnesium (mg/day)	M ≥ 420, F ≥ 320	Normal range	M < 420, F < 320
Iron (mg/day)	M 8–45 F ≤ 50 years, 18–45 F > 50 years, 8–45	–	–
Zinc (mg/day)	M 11–40, F 8–40	Normal range	M < 11 or > 40, F < 8 or > 40
Copper (mg/day)	0.9–10	Normal range	< 0.9 or > 10
Sodium (mg/day)	≤ 50 years, 1500–2300 > 50–70 years, 1300–2300 > 70 years, 1200–2300	–	–
Potassium (mg/day)	≥ 4700	–	–
Selenium (mcg/day)	55–400	Normal range	< 55 or > 400
Caffeine (mg/day)	≤ 400	–	–
Alcohol (g/day)	M ≤ 28, F ≤ 14	M > 28, F > 14	M ≤ 28, F ≤ 14
Linoleic acid (g/day)	≤ 50 years, M ≥ 17, F ≥ 12 > 50 years, M ≥ 14, F ≥ 11	Normal range	≤ 50 years, M < 17, F < 12, > 50 years, M < 14, F < 11
α-Linolenic acid (g/day)	M ≥ 1.6, F ≥ 1.1	Normal range	M < 1.6, F < 1.1
Fish oil (g/day)*	≥ 0.25	–	–

Table 5 Normal range of parameter *(Continued)*

Parameter	Normal range	Score in nutritional index	
		0	1
Anthropometric measurements			
Body mass index (kg/m^2)	18.5–24.9**	18.5–29.9	< 18.5 or ≥ 30
Body weight change in past 1 year (%)	≤ 10	–	–
Waist circumference (cm)	M < 94, F < 80	Normal range	M > 94, F > 80
Triceps skinfold (mm)	M 7.5–24.3, F 14–33.7	–	–
Subscapular skinfold (mm)	M10.3–30.5, F10.3–33.9	–	–
Blood tests			
Total lymphocyte count (cells/mm^3)	> 1500	Normal range	≤ 1500
Haemoglobin (g/dL)	M 13.5–18, F 12–16	Normal range	M < 13.5 or > 18, F < 12 or > 16
MCV (fL)	80–100	–	–
Albumin (g/L)	35–55	–	–
Vitamin A (mcmol/L)	0.35–3.00	Normal range	< 0.35 or > 3.00
Vitamin C (mg/dL)	0.2–2.0	Normal range	< 0.2 or > 2.0
Vitamin D (ng/mL)	20–50	–	–
Pyridoxine (nmol/L)	> 20	–	–
Folate, RBC (ng/mL)	≥ 140	–	–
Cobalamin (pg/L)	> 200	Normal range	≤ 200
α-carotene (mcg/dL)	1.3–9.2	–	–
β-carotene (mcg/dL)	6.4–35.1	–	–
β-cryptoxanthin (mcg/dL)	4.0–16.4	≥ 4.0	< 4.0
Lutein/Zeaxanthin (mcg/dL)	11.1–33.0	–	–
Lycopene (mcg/dL)	11.9–36.1	≥ 11.9	< 11.9
Iron, serum (mcg/dL)	50–180	–	–
Creatinine (mg/dL)	M 0.80–1.40, F 0.56–1.00	Normal range	M < 0.80 or > 1.40, F < 0.56 or > 1.00
Total cholesterol (mg/dL)	< 200	–	–
Triglyceride (mg/dL)	< 150	Normal range	≥ 150
HDL-c (mg/dL)	M > 40, F > 50	–	–
LDL-c (mg/dL)	< 130	–	–
Glucose (mg/dL)	70–100	Normal range	< 70 or > 100
Homocysteine (mcmol/L)	≤ 21.6	Normal range	> 21.6

F female, *HDL-c* high-density lipoprotein cholesterol, *LDL-c* low-density lipoprotein cholesterol, *M* male, *MCV* mean corpuscular volume, *RAE* retinol activity equivalents, *RBC* red blood cell. These variables were excluded from the nutrition index due to high missing data or no relationship with high frailty. *Dietary fish oil is the combination between docosahexaenoic acid (DHA) and eicosapentaenoic acid (EPA) in dietary intake. ** < 18.5 kg/m^2 (underweight), 25–29.9 kg/m^2 (overweight), ≥ 30 kg/m^2 (obese)

Table 6 36-item frailty index

Self-reported items

1. Angina/angina pectoris	14. Difficulty lifting or carrying
2. Heart attack	15. Difficulty walking between rooms on same floor
3. Coronary heart disease	16. Difficulty standing up from armless chair
4. Stroke	17. Difficulty getting in and out of bed
5. Thyroid condition	18. Difficulty dressing yourself difficulty
6. Cancer	19. Difficulty grasping/holding small objects
7. Arthritis	20. Difficulty attending social event
8. High blood pressure	21. Self-reported health
9. Diabetes mellitus	22. Frequency of healthcare use
10. Weak/failing kidneys	23. Health compared to 1 year ago
11. Confusion or inability to remember things	24. Overnight hospital stays
12. Difficulty managing money	25. Medications
13. Difficulty stooping, crouching, kneeling	

Laboratory items

26. Pulse rate (60–99 bpm)	32. Red cell distribution width (≤ 14.6%)
27. Systolic blood pressure (90–140 mmHg)	33. Lactate dehydrogenase (≤ 190 U/L)
28. Pulse pressure (30–60 mmHg)	34. Alkaline phosphatase (≤ 115 U/L)
29. Platelet count SI (150–450 unit 1000 cells/uL)	35. Uric acid (M: 240–510, F: 160–430 umol/L)
30. Blood urea nitrogen (3–20 mg/dL)	36. Total calcium (2.0–2.5 mmol/L)
31. Bicarbonate (≤ 28 mmol/L)	

F female, *M* male

Table 7 Association between abnormal nutrient intakes and frailty

Nutrients		Linear regression analysis	
		β-coefficient (95%CI)	p value
Energy	Low	0.007 (0.003, 0.011)	0.001*
Energy per weight	Low	0.018 (0.014, 0.021)	< 0.001*
	High	− 0.013 (− 0.018,− 0.009)	< 0.001*
Protein	Low	0.009 (0.004, 0.014)	0.001*
Protein per weight	Low	0.016 (0.011, 0.020)	< 0.001*
Carbohydrate	Low	0.007 (0.002, 0.012)	0.004*
Simple sugar	High	− 0.004 (− 0.012, 0.003)	0.267
Dietary fiber per energy	Low	0.005 (− 0.002, 0.012)	0.170
Percentage of fat	Low	0.003 (− 0.008, 0.014)	0.597
	High	− 0.001 (− 0.007, 0.005)	0.737
Percentage of saturated fat	High	0.005 (0.001, 0.008)	0.018*
Cholesterol	High	0.003 (− 0.002, 0.007)	0.213
Vitamin A, RAE	Low	0.005 (0.001, 0.010)	0.027*
	High	− 0.018 (− 0.043, 0.006)	0.148
Vitamin C	Low	0.004 (0.001, 0.008)	0.027*
	High	–	
Vitamin E	Low	− 0.004 (− 0.013, 0.004)	0.297
Vitamin K	Low	0.002 (− 0.002, 0.007)	0.328
Thiamin	Low	0.005 (0.001, 0.010)	0.027*
Riboflavin	Low	0.008 (0.002, 0.013)	0.006*
Niacin	Low	0.010 (0.005, 0.015)	< 0.001*
	High	0.000 (− 0.006, 0.006)	0.956
Pyridoxine	Low	0.007 (0.002, 0.011)	0.003*
Folate	Low	0.005 (0.001, 0.010)	0.023*
	High	0.006 (− 0.006, 0.019)	0.339
Cobalamin	Low	0.002 (− 0.002, 0.007)	0.354
Calcium	Low	− 0.003 (− 0.008, 0.002)	0.189
	High	0.011 (− 0.003, 0.025)	0.134
Phosphorous	Low	0.011 (0.005, 0.017)	< 0.001*
	High	0.019 (− 0.010, 0.048)	0.201
Magnesium	Low	0.004 (− 0.002, 0.009)	0.187
Iron	Low	0.001 (− 0.004, 0.006)	0.826
	High	0.012 (− 0.006, 0.030)	0.183
Zinc	Low	0.002 (− 0.003, 0.006)	0.499
	High	0.010 (− 0.010, 0.030)	0.323
Copper	Low	0.009 (0.004, 0.014)	< 0.001*
	High	− 0.014 (− 0.061, 0.032)	0.547
Sodium	Low	0.008 (0.001, 0.015)	0.022*
	High	− 0.008 (− 0.012, − 0.003)	0.002*
Potassium	Low	0.000 (− 0.008, 0.009)	0.971
Selenium	Low	0.010 (0.004, 0.015)	0.001*
	High	0.004 (− 0.032, 0.041)	0.809

Table 7 Association between abnormal nutrient intakes and frailty *(Continued)*

Nutrients		Linear regression analysis	
		β-coefficient (95%CI)	p value
Caffeine	High	0.000 (− 0.007, 0.006)	0.911
Alcohol	High	− 0.009 (− 0.015, − 0.004)	0.001*
Linoleic acid	Low	0.004 (0.000, 0.009)	0.060
α-Linolenic acid	Low	0.004 (− 0.001, 0.008)	0.107
Fish oil	Low	0.007 (0.001, 0.013)	0.025*

RAE retinol activity equivalents

All analyses were adjusted for age, sex, race, energy intake, educational level, marital status, employment status, smoking and study cohort except for energy, energy per weight and dietary fiber per energy which were not adjusted for energy intake

− Results are not available due to low sample sizes and mortality rate, *p value < 0.05

Table 8 Association between abnormal anthropometric measurements and frailty

Anthropometric measurements		Linear regression analysis	
		β-coefficient (95%CI)	p value
Body mass index	Underweight	− 0.008 (− 0.023, 0.007)	0.323
	Overweight	− 0.012 (− 0.016, − 0.008)	< 0.001*
	Obese	0.027 (0.023, 0.030)	< 0.001*
Body weight change in past 1 year	Loss > 10%	0.029 (0.022, 0.035)	< 0.001*
	Gain > 10%	0.015 (0.009, 0.020)	< 0.001*
Waist circumference	High	0.012 (0.008, 0.017)	< 0.001*
Triceps skinfold	Low	0.000 (− 0.006, 0.006)	0.989
	High	0.022 (0.016, 0.028)	< 0.001*
Subscapular skinfold	Low	− 0.004 (− 0.011, 0.003)	0.224
	High	0.013 (0.005, 0.020)	0.001*

All analyses were adjusted for age, sex, race, energy intake, educational level, marital status, employment status, smoking and study cohort, *p value < 0.05

Table 9 Association between abnormal blood tests and frailty

Blood tests		Linear regression analysis	
		β-coefficient (95%CI)	p value
Total lymphocyte count	Low	0.010 (0.005, 0.015)	< 0.001*
Haemoglobin	Low	0.048 (0.042, 0.055)	< 0.001*
	High	− 0.003 (− 0.022, 0.017)	0.798
Mean corpuscular volume	Low	0.037 (0.027, 0.046)	< 0.001*
	High	0.041 (0.029, 0.053)	< 0.001*
Albumin	Low	0.037 (0.029, 0.046)	< 0.001*
Vitamin A	Low	0.085 (0.030, 0.139)	0.002*
	High	0.051 (0.044, 0.059)	< 0.001*
Vitamin C	Low	0.011 (0.003, 0.019)	0.005*
	High	− 0.001 (− 0.013, 0.011)	0.845
Vitamin D	Low	0.015 (0.011, 0.019)	< 0.001*
	High	− 0.150 (− 0.036, 0.006)	0.160
Pyridoxine	Low	0.015 (0.010, 0.020)	< 0.001*
Folate, RBC	Low	− 0.008 (− 0.017, 0.001)	0.093
Cobalamin	Low	0.006 (− 0.005, 0.018)	0.287
α-carotene	Low	0.023 (0.018, 0.028)	< 0.001*
	High	− 0.023 (− 0.030, − 0.017)	< 0.001*
β-carotene	Low	0.025 (0.020, 0.030)	< 0.001*
	High	− 0.022 (− 0.028, − 0.016)	< 0.001*
β-cryptoxanthin	Low	0.031 (0.026, 0.036)	< 0.001*
	High	− 0.017 (− 0.022, − 0.012)	< 0.001*
Lutein/Zeaxanthin	Low	0.032 (0.028, 0.036)	< 0.001*
	High	− 0.018 (− 0.027, − 0.009)	< 0.001*
Lycopene	Low	0.022 (0.017, 0.027)	< 0.001*
	High	− 0.008 (− 0.014, − 0.002)	0.014*
Iron, serum	Low	0.021 (0.016, 0.027)	< 0.001*
	High	0.001 (− 0.015, 0.016)	0.947
Creatinine	Low	0.008 (0.000, 0.016)	0.048*
	High	0.070 (0.062, 0.078)	< 0.001*
Total cholesterol	High	− 0.015 (− 0.019, − 0.011)	< 0.001*
Triglyceride	High	0.017 (0.013, 0.021)	< 0.001*
HDL-c	Low	0.012 (0.008, 0.016)	< 0.001*
LDL-c	High	− 0.018 (− 0.024, − 0.012)	< 0.001*
Glucose	Low	0.014 (0.001, 0.026)	0.029*
	High	0.031 (0.027, 0.036)	< 0.001*
Homocysteine	High	0.056 (0.039, 0.073)	< 0.001*

All analyses were adjusted for age, sex, race, energy intake, educational level, marital status, employment status, smoking and study cohort
HDL-c high-density lipoprotein cholesterol, *LDL-c* low-density lipoprotein cholesterol, *RBC* red blood cell, *p value < 0.05

Table 10 Associations between abnormal nutrient intakes and mortality across levels of frailty

Nutrients		Frailty index score							
		≤0.1 HR (95%CI)	p value	> 0.1 to 0.2 HR (95%CI)	p value	> 0.2 to 0.3 HR (95%CI)	p value	> 0.3 HR (95%CI)	p value
Energy	Low	1.14 (0.74, 1.77)	0.554	1.00 (0.73, 1.35)	0.976	1.16 (0.83, 1.61)	0.384	1.55 (1.14, 2.10)	0.005*
Energy per weight	Low	1.16 (0.72, 1.86)	0.547	0.87 (0.64, 1.18)	0.373	0.93 (0.69, 1.25)	0.632	1.36 (1.00, 1.86)	0.052
	High	0.77 (0.40, 1.47)	0.427	1.11 (0.73, 1.68)	0.620	1.04 (0.63, 1.73)	0.868	1.38 (0.85, 2.25)	0.195
Protein	Low	1.09 (0.64, 1.84)	0.758	0.93 (0.65, 1.32)	0.675	0.84 (0.61, 1.15)	0.266	0.93 (0.71, 1.22)	0.607
Protein per weight	Low	0.90 (0.56, 1.45)	0.670	1.05 (0.76, 1.45)	0.765	0.80 (0.59, 1.09)	0.161	0.84 (0.62, 1.12)	0.238
Carbohydrate	Low	1.25 (0.75, 2.11)	0.394	1.30 (0.92, 1.83)	0.134	1.25 (0.90, 1.74)	0.178	0.88 (0.66, 1.71)	0.367
Simple sugar	High	1.02 (0.46, 2.26)	0.964	0.73 (0.45, 1.17)	0.189	0.92 (0.57, 1.48)	0.720	1.15 (0.77, 1.81)	0.505
Dietary fiber per energy	Low	0.57 (0.32, 1.03)	0.064	1.42 (0.98, 2.26)	0.140	0.99 (0.66, 1.48)	0.941	0.89 (0.62, 1.27)	0.510
Percentage of fat	Low	1.16 (0.31, 4.36)	0.822	0.62 (0.27, 1.43)	0.265	1.42 (0.91, 2.21)	0.335	0.56 (0.31, 1.02)	0.990
	High	1.29 (0.61, 2.73)	0.509	0.68 (0.44, 1.04)	0.072	0.96 (0.76, 122)	0.121	1.049 (0.75, 1.48)	0.784
Percentage of saturated fat	High	0.87 (0.58, 1.32)	0.523	1.27 (0.96, 1.67)	0.092	1.11 (0.85, 1.44)	0.450	0.97 (0.78, 1.21)	0.800
Cholesterol	High	1.17 (0.74, 1.84)	0.502	1.03 (0.76, 1.39)	0.857	1.21 (0.89, 1.66)	0.225	1.08 (0.84, 1.40)	0.552
Vitamin A, RAE	Low	1.47 (0.83, 2.59)	0.184	1.51 (1.03, 2.21)	0.033*	0.99 (0.71, 1.38)	0.935	1.03 (0.78, 1.37)	0.818
	High	1.22 (0.16, 9.41)	0.849	–		2.01 (0.72, 5.63)	0.182	–	
Vitamin C	Low	0.95 (0.62, 1.45)	0.814	1.26 (0.94, 1.67)	0.121	1.19 (0.90, 1.57)	0.223	1.23 (0.97, 1.56)	0.091
	High	–		–		–		–	
Vitamin E	Low	–		1.31 (0.62, 2.73)	0.478	1.20 (0.53, 2.74)	0.658	3.49 (1.15, 11.00)	0.033*
Vitamin K	Low	1.13 (0.65, 1.97)	0.657	1.35 (0.92, 1.98)	0.121	1.06 (0.74, 1.51)	0.755	0.97 (0.72, 1.31)	0.842
Thiamin	Low	1.61 (0.99, 2.60)	0.055	1.31 (0.95, 1.80)	0.095	1.17 (0.86, 1.58)	0.310	1.15 (0.89, 1.48)	0.288
Riboflavin	Low	0.83 (0.45, 1.53)	0.548	0.93 (0.62, 1.40)	0.733	1.17 (0.83, 1.65)	0.361	1.00 (0.75, 1.32)	0.992
Niacin	Low	1.15 (0.70, 1.91)	0.581	1.16 (0.83, 1.61)	0.388	1.05 (0.77, 1.43)	0.754	0.99 (0.76, 1.29)	0.945
	High	0.81 (0.39, 1.70)	0.580	1.10 (0.68, 1.77)	0.699	0.58 (0.32, 1.05)	0.074	1.37 (0.89, 2.11)	0.148
Pyridoxine	Low	0.87 (0.55, 1.39)	0.566	0.96 (0.71, 1.31)	0.815	1.26 (0.95, 1.67)	0.106	1.03 (0.80, 1.32)	0.818
Folate	Low	1.04 (0.64, 1.66)	0.885	1.37 (0.98, 1.91)	0.068	1.39 (1.01, 1.91)	0.042*	1.13 (0.84, 1.51)	0.413
	High	1.97 (0.59, 6.57)	0.269	1.35 (0.53, 3.45)	0.526	1.00 (0.31, 3.21)	0.996	0.77 (0.19, 3.16)	0.714
Cobalamin	Low	1.10 (0.68, 1.77)	0.695	1.09 (0.79, 1.49)	0.605	1.15 (0.86, 1.54)	0.351	0.94 (0.73, 1.21)	0.635
Calcium	Low	1.20 (0.67, 2.14)	0.548	1.09 (0.73, 1.62)	0.679	1.06 (0.74, 1.53)	0.747	1.05 (0.74, 1.50)	0.773
	High	0.74 (0.10, 5.69)	0.769	1.42 (0.34, 5.99)	0.629	–		–	
Phosphorous	Low	0.67 (0.34, 1.33)	0.251	0.85 (0.56, 1.29)	0.446	1.03 (0.71, 1.49)	0.888	1.14 (0.85, 1.53)	0.380
	High	–		–		–		–	
Magnesium	Low	0.74 (0.41, 1.32)	0.307	1.49 (0.94, 2.36)	0.089	1.40 (0.86, 2.28)	0.179	1.11 (0.73, 1.69)	0.634
Iron	Low	1.32 (0.75, 2.31)	0.338	1.09 (0.75, 1.60)	0.650	1.17 (0.81, 1.67)	0.402	1.06 (0.79, 1.42)	0.703
	High	–		1.34 (0.42, 4.30)	0.620	–		–	
Zinc	Low	1.04 (0.65, 1.67)	0.855	1.21 (0.89, 1.66)	0.228	0.90 (0.66, 1.23)	0.509	0.96 (0.74, 1.25)	0.761
	High	–		2.47 (0.59, 10.41)	0.217	–		–	
Copper	Low	1.24 (0.74, 2.06)	0.410	1.20 (0.87, 1.68)	0.270	1.25 (0.92, 1.71)	0.154	0.79 (0.60, 1.04)	0.098
	High	6.35 (0.86, 46.98)	0.070	–		–		–	
Sodium	Low	0.79 (0.37, 1.71)	0.550	1.04 (0.62, 1.72)	0.893	0.82 (0.47, 1.42)	0.475	0.96 (0.67, 1.38)	0.845
	High	0.64 (0.38, 1.09)	0.099	0.84 (0.60, 1.17)	0.303	1.08 (0.79, 1.48)	0.609	1.13 (0.85, 1.48)	0.403
Potassium	Low	0.83 (0.33, 2.08)	0.695	0.86 (0.45, 1.64)	0.646	1.18 (0.50, 2.80)	0.700	1.00 (0.43, 2.32)	0.996
Selenium	Low	1.61 (0.93, 2.77)	0.088	1.03 (0.70, 1.52	0.885	1.05 (0.76, 1.47)	0.757	1.06 (0.80, 1.39)	0.700
	High	–		–		–		–	

Table 10 Associations between abnormal nutrient intakes and mortality across levels of frailty *(Continued)*

Nutrients		≤ 0.1 HR (95%CI)	p value	> 0.1 to 0.2 HR (95%CI)	p value	> 0.2 to 0.3 HR (95%CI)	p value	> 0.3 HR (95%CI)	p value
		Frailty index score							
Caffeine	High	1.07 (0.58, 1.98)	0.834	1.63 (1.09, 2.43)	0.016*	1.59 (0.97, 2.60)	0.064	0.61 (0.37, 0.99)	0.047*
Alcohol	High	0.92 (0.49, 1.74)	0.805	1.17 (0.81, 1.74)	0.386	1.18 (0.76, 1.83)	0.465	0.72 (0.43, 1.22)	0.223
Linoleic acid	Low	0.88 (0.54, 1.43)	0.599	1.55 (1.12, 2.16)	0.009*	0.81 (0.57, 1.13)	0.216	1.16 (0.87, 1.54)	0.312
α-Linolenic acid	Low	1.12 (0.69, 1.83)	0.652	1.18 (0.86, 1.63)	0.311	0.84 (0.60, 1.16)	0.279	1.21 (0.91, 1.61)	0.193
Fish oil	Low	0.82 (0.45, 1.50)	0.522	1.70 (1.00, 2.88)	0.048*	0.86 (0.57, 1.30)	0.466	1.04 (0.69, 1.57)	0.850

RAE Retinol activity equivalents
All analyses were adjusted for age, sex, race, energy intake, educational level, marital status, employment status, smoking and study cohort except for energy, energy per weight and dietary fiber per energy which were not adjusted for energy intake
– Results are not available due to low sample sizes and mortality rate, *p value < 0.05

Table 11 Associations between abnormal anthropometric measurements and mortality across levels of frailty

Anthropometric measurements		≤ 0.1 HR (95%CI)	p value	> 0.1 to 0.2 HR (95%CI)	p value	> 0.2 to 0.3 HR (95%CI)	p value	> 0.3 HR (95%CI)	p value
		Frailty index score							
Body mass index	Underweight	0.69 (0.09, 5.21)	0.723	0.88 (0.22, 3.61)	0.861	4.41 (2.23, 8.74)	< 0.001*	3.80 (1.60, 9.03)	0.002*
	Overweight	0.97 (0.61, 1.57)	0.915	0.88 (0.64, 1.21)	0.421	0.90 (0.65, 1.23)	0.499	0.72 (0.54, 0.98)	0.036*
	Obese	0.91 (0.52, 1.60)	0.742	0.82 (0.56, 1.19)	0.293	0.77 (0.54, 1.11)	0.161	0.89 (0.66, 1.19)	0.424
Body weight change in past 1 year	Loss > 10%	0.91 (0.41, 2.01)	0.812	1.66 (1.10, 2.50)	0.016*	1.95 (1.36, 2.79)	< 0.001*	1.61 (1.21, 2.13)	0.001*
	Gain > 10%	1.41 (0.66, 3.00)	0.380	1.66 (0.97, 2.85)	0.063	1.56 (0.98, 2.47)	0.061	1.35 (0.91, 2.01)	0.139
Waist circumference	High	1.50 (0.88, 2.56)	0.135	0.80 (0.57, 1.11)	0.185	0.77 (0.55, 1.09)	0.146	0.70 (0.50, 0.98)	0.037*
Triceps skinfold	Low	1.07 (0.53, 2.18)	0.842	1.83 (1.22, 2.74)	0.003*	2.73 (1.90, 3.94)	< 0.001*	1.36 (0.93, 2.00)	0.113
	High	1.16 (0.50, 2.71)	0.731	1.41 (0.85, 2.35)	0.184	0.74 (0.44, 1.25)	0.259	0.98 (0.64, 1.51)	0.924
Subscapular skinfold	Low	1.10 (0.50, 2.45)	0.807	1.89 (1.29, 2.77)	0.001*	1.49 (0.98, 2.26)	0.060	1.46 (0.99, 2.15)	0.058
	High	1.02 (0.41, 2.54)	0.970	0.78 (0.39, 1.54)	0.470	0.36 (0.13, 0.98)	0.046*	0.83 (0.41, 1.66)	0.589

All analyses were adjusted for age, sex, race, energy intake, educational level, marital status, employment status, smoking, and study cohort, *p value < 0.05

Table 12 Associations between abnormal blood tests and mortality across levels of frailty

Blood tests		Frailty index score							
		≤ 0.1 HR (95%CI)	p value	> 0.1 to 0.2 HR (95%CI)	p value	> 0.2 to 0.3 HR (95%CI)	p value	> 0.3 HR (95%CI)	p value
Total lymphocyte count	Low	1.03 (0.63, 1.70)	0.908	1.61 (1.21, 2.15)	0.001*	1.26 (0.96, 1.65)	0.102	1.43 (1.14, 1.81)	0.002*
Haemoglobin	Low	0.74 (0.23, 2.36)	0.609	1.41 (0.93, 2.15)	0.110	1.33 (0.98, 1.81)	0.064	1.45 (1.13, 1.86)	0.003*
	High	0.70 (0.10, 5.09)	0.724	0.94 (0.23, 3.84)	0.934	3.04 (0.72, 12.76)	0.129	–	
Mean corpuscular volume	Low	1.60 (0.38, 6.64)	0.519	0.92 (0.37, 2.28)	0.863	1.72 (0.74, 3.97)	0.208	1.07 (0.56, 2.04)	0.842
	High	1.00 (0.24, 4.14)	0.999	1.19 (0.69, 2.03)	0.533	1.58 (1.02, 2.47)	0.043*	1.45 (0.99, 2.14)	0.059
Albumin	Low	2.70 (0.63, 11.62)	0.183	2.66 (1.23, 5.74)	0.013*	1.88 (0.88, 4.02)	0.105	2.51 (1.74, 3.64)	< 0.001*
Vitamin A	Low	–		–		–		–	
	High	0.33 (0.08, 1.34)	0.121	1.06 (0.66, 1.71)	0.795	0.74 (0.49, 1.10)	0.131	1.34 (1.02, 1.75)	0.035*
Vitamin C	Low	0.98 (0.42, 2.29)	0.958	1.80 (1.19, 2.75)	0.006*	1.25 (0.76, 2.07)	0.376	1.61 (1.13, 2.30)	0.009*
	High	0.69 (0.17, 2.83)	0.605	0.81 (3.94, 1.65)	0.554	1.02 (0.57, 1.85)	0.936	1.18 (0.72, 1.93)	0.520
Vitamin D	Low	2.01 (1.32, 3.06)	0.001*	1.45 (1.10, 1.92)	0.009*	1.62 (1.23, 2.12)	< 0.001*	1.38 (1.10, 1.73)	0.006*
	High	–		–		–		–	
Pyridoxine	Low	1.47 (0.87, 2.48)	0.151	2.11 (1.54, 2.89)	< 0.001*	1.24 (0.90, 1.71)	0.192	1.31 (1.01, 1.70)	0.04*
Folate, RBC	Low	0.92 (0.33, 2.55)	0.877	0.93 (0.43, 2.03)	0.863	1.27 (0.67, 2.41)	0.462	0.83 (0.39, 1.77)	0.630
Cobalamin	Low	1.34 (0.49, 3.68)	0.572	1.14 (0.54, 2.43)	0.728	0.68 (0.34, 1.39)	0.294	0.97 (0.57, 1.64)	0.900
α-carotene	Low	0.87 (0.46, 1.63)	0.657	1.58 (1.12, 2.23)	0.009*	1.31 (0.92, 1.85)	0.131	1.23 (0.95, 1.61)	0.121
	High	0.78 (0.40, 1.53)	0.469	0.80 (0.48, 1.32)	0.382	0.80 (0.48, 1.33)	0.383	1.00 (0.62, 1.62)	0.997
β-carotene	Low	1.04 (0.55, 1.99)	0.902	1.94 (1.33, 2.82)	0.001*	1.82 (1.26, 2.61)	0.001*	0.97 (0.71, 1.32)	0.854
	High	0.92 (0.51, 1.67)	0.784	0.91 (0.60, 1.36)	0.636	0.91 (0.63, 1.31)	0.623	0.97 (0.69, 1.36)	0.846
β-cryptoxanthin	Low	0.95 (0.49, 1.81)	0.867	1.71 (1.24, 2.36)	0.001*	1.34 (0.97, 1.84)	0.074	0.99 (0.76, 1.29)	0.951
	High	1.05 (0.62, 1.80)	0.849	0.73 (0.45, 1.17)	0.194	0.98 (0.66, 1.46)	0.916	0.94 (0.62, 1.42)	0.768
Lutein/Zeaxanthin	Low	0.73 (0.39, 1.36)	0.322	1.79 (1.33, 2.41)	< 0.001*	1.72 (1.30, 2.29)	< 0.001*	1.25 (0.99, 1.58)	0.055
	High	1.09 (0.50, 2.40)	0.822	0.96 (0.51, 1.78)	0.891	1.20 (0.63, 2.30)	0.576	1.08 (0.62, 1.88)	0.772
Lycopene	Low	1.08 (0.65, 1.79)	0.774	1.56 (1.16, 2.08)	0.003*	1.60 (1.22, 2.09)	0.001*	1.24 (0.98, 1.56)	0.075
	High	1.52 (0.77, 3.00)	0.227	1.16 (0.60, 2.22)	0.661	1.91 (1.04, 3.52)	0.037*	1.02 (0.50, 2.08)	0.965
Iron, serum	Low	0.78 (0.36, 1.69)	0.524	1.48 (0.98, 2.22)	0.061	1.41 (0.98, 2.03)	0.066	1.87 (1.46, 2.41)	< 0.001*
	High	–		0.27 (0.04, 1.90)	0.187	–		–	
Creatinine	Low	2.54 (1.15, 5.62)	0.021	1.01 (0.49, 2.09)	0.974	1.87 (1.02, 3.41)	0.042*	1.89 (1.05, 3.42)	0.034*
	High	2.46 (1.04, 5.78)	0.039	1.22 (0.80, 1.86)	0.363	1.04 (0.75, 1.45)	0.798	1.48 (1.15, 1.90)	0.002*
Total cholesterol	High	1.05 (0.69, 1.59)	0.824	0.95 (0.72, 1.26)	0.740	0.84 (0.64, 1.10)	0.200	0.92 (0.73, 1.16)	0.458
Triglyceride	High	1.33 (0.88, 2.02)	0.178	0.78 (0.58, 1.06)	0.116	0.95 (0.72, 1.26)	0.728	0.95 (0.75, 1.20)	0.676
HDL-c	Low	1.50 (0.67, 2.32)	0.071	1.08 (0.79, 1.46)	0.639	0.93 (0.68, 1.28)	0.673	1.18 (0.94, 1.49)	0.158
LDL-c	High	0.97 (0.51, 1.87)	0.936	0.93 (0.61, 1.41)	0.729	0.60 (0.36, 0.10)	0.050	1.20 (0.81, 1.77)	0.364
Glucose	Low	1.99 (0.27, 14.73)	0.499	1.20 (0.38, 3.78)	0.758	0.44 (0.11, 1.81)	0.256	1.49 (0.77, 2.87)	0.236
	High	1.34 (0.86, 2.09)	0.195	1.17 (0.89, 1.55)	0.263	1.09 (0.83, 1.42)	0.537	1.06 (0.85, 1.34)	0.593
Homocysteine	High	1.19 (0.16, 8.69)	0.865	1.73 (0.76, 3.90)	0.190	1.41 (0.74, 2.69)	0.298	1.71 (1.13, 2.60)	0.011*

HDL-c high-density lipoprotein cholesterol, LDL-c low-density lipoprotein cholesterol, RBC red blood cell
All analyses were adjusted for age, sex, race, energy intake, educational level, marital status, employment status, smoking and study cohort
– Results are not available due to low sample sizes and mortality rate, *p value < 0.05

Table 13 Number of participants in each level of nutritional index score by frailty level

	Frailty index			
	≤ 0.1 N = 4858	> 0.1 to 0.2 N = 1910	> 0.2 to 0.3 N = 949	> 0.3 N = 813
Nutritional index, N (%) (N = 8530)				
≤ 0.1 (N = 393)	305 (7.4)	70 (4.3)	13 (1.5)	5 (0.7)
> 0.1 to 0.2 (N = 1967)	1435 (30.9)	354 (19.9)	110 (13.0)	68 (8.5)
> 0.2 to 0.3 (N = 2409)	1494 (30.5)	541 (29.2)	239 (26.8)	135 (17.8)
> 0.3 to 0.4 (N = 1751)	880 (17.6)	422 (21.0)	255 (25.9)	194 (24.2)
> 0.4 to 0.5 (N = 1203)	487 (9.0)	329 (16.9)	193 (19.3)	194 (23.5)
> 0.5 to 0.6 (N = 602)	209 (3.8)	139 (6.0)	104 (10.2)	150 (16.8)
> 0.6 (N = 205)	48 (0.9)	55 (2.6)	35 (3.2)	67 (8.4)

The percentages are weighted

Table 14 Association between nutritional index and mortality across levels of frailty

Nutritional index	Frailty index score							
	≤ 0.1 HR (95%CI)	p value	> 0.1 to 0.2 HR (95%CI)	p value	> 0.2 to 0.3 HR (95%CI)	p value	> 0.3 HR (95%CI)	p value
Nutritional index score (per 0.1 score)	1.15 (0.98, 1.35)	0.082	1.17 (1.06, 1.30)	0.002*	1.20 (1.08, 1.32)	< 0.001*	1.27 (1.16, 1.38)	< 0.001*
Nutritional index score in group								
≤ 0.2	1.00		1.00		1.00		1.00	
> 0.2 to 0.3	1.26 (0.72, 2.18)	0.420	0.99 (0.64, 1.53)	0.958	1.73 (1.01, 2.97)	0.046*	1.63 (0.91, 2.91)	0.100
> 0.3 to 0.4	1.44 (0.80, 2.59)	0.219	1.35 (0.88, 2.06)	0.164	1.80(1.06, 3.05)	0.029*	2.05 (1.20, 3.52)	0.009*
> 0.4 to 0.5	1.70 (0.88, 3.31)	0.117	2.04 (1.34, 3.11)	0.001*	2.34 (1.36, 4.01)	0.002*	1.92 (1.12, 3.31)	0.019*
> 0.5	1.58 (0.66, 3.76)	0.302	1.49 (0.89, 2.51)	0.130	2.49 (1.42, 4.38)	0.001*	3.09 (1.81, 5.27)	< 0.001*
P for trend across nutritional index group		0.097		0.001*		0.001*		< 0.001*

All analyses were adjusted for age, sex, race, educational level, marital status, employment status, smoking, and study cohort, *p value < 0.05

Table 15 Combined effect of frailty and nutrition on mortality

Frailty index score	Nutrition index score	N (%)	Cox regression analysis	
			Hazard ratio (95%CI)	p value
≤ 0.1	≤ 0.2	1740 (24.5)	1.00 (reference)	
	> 0.2 to 0.3	1494 (19.5)	1.23 (0.71, 2.12)	0.468
	> 0.3 to 0.4	880 (11.2)	1.48 (0.84, 2.64)	0.178
	> 0.4 to 0.5	487 (5.7)	1.80 (0.95, 3.42)	0.073
	> 0.5	257 (3.0)	1.59 (0.68, 3.69)	0.281
> 0.1 to 0.2	≤ 0.2	424 (5.0)	1.59 (0.95, 2.65)	0.079
	> 0.2 to 0.3	541 (6.0)	1.59 (0.95, 2.65)	0.069
	> 0.3 to 0.4	422 (4.3)	2.13 (1.31, 3.46)	0.002*
	> 0.4 to 0.5	329 (3.5)	3.26 (2.01, 5.29)	< 0.001*
	> 0.5	194 (1.8)	2.53 (1.44, 4.45)	0.001*
> 0.2 to 0.3	≤ 0.2	123 (1.3)	1.70 (0.92, 3.15)	0.092
	> 0.2 to 0.3	239 (2.4)	2.88 (1.77, 4.68)	< 0.001*
	> 0.3 to 0.4	255 (2.3)	3.04 (1.88, 4.91)	< 0.001*
	> 0.4 to 0.5	193 (1.7)	3.97 (2.44, 6.46)	< 0.001*
	> 0.5	139 (1.2)	4.23 (2.53, 7.08)	< 0.001*
> 0.3	≤ 0.2	73 (0.6)	2.64 (1.39, 5.01)	< 0.001*
	> 0.2 to 0.3	135 (1.2)	4.38 (2.62, 7.31)	< 0.001*
	> 0.3 to 0.4	194 (1.6)	5.26 (3.29, 8.39)	< 0.001*
	> 0.4 to 0.5	194 (1.6)	5.09 (3.16, 8.18)	< 0.001*
	> 0.5	217 (1.7)	8.17 (5.16, 12.94)	< 0.001*

The percentages are weighted
All analyses were adjusted for age, sex, race, educational level, marital status, employment status, smoking, and study cohort, *p value < 0.05

Abbreviations
BMI: Body mass index; CI: Confidential interval; FI: Frailty index; LDL-c: Low-density lipoprotein cholesterol; NHANES: National Health and Nutrition Examination Survey; NI: Nutrition index

Acknowledgements
We are grateful to the Faculty of Medicine Ramathibodi Hospital, Mahidol University, for supporting KJ with a research fellowship to conduct this research; our colleagues in Geriatric Medicine Research, at Dalhousie University & Nova Scotia Health Authority for their support; all NHANES participants; and the NHANES researchers for making this data publicly available.

Funding
This study was not funded entirely or partially by an outside source.

Authors' contributions
KJ, OT, and KR conceived and designed the study, interpreted the data, and co drafted the manuscript. JB assisted with data analysis and revised the manuscript. LC designed the study and revised the manuscript. All authors reviewed and approved the final manuscript before submission.

Competing interests
All authors declare that they have no competing interests.

Author details
[1]Chakri Naruebodindra Medical Institute, Faculty of Medicine Ramathibodi Hospital, Mahidol University, Bangkok, Thailand. [2]Department of Medicine, Dalhousie University, Halifax, Nova Scotia, Canada. [3]Centre for Health Care of the Elderly, QEII Health Sciences Centre, Nova Scotia Health Authority, Halifax, Nova Scotia, Canada. [4]MRC Unit for Lifelong Health and Ageing, UCL, London, UK. [5]Department of Nutrition, Harvard T.H. Chan School of Public Health, Boston, MA, USA. [6]Division of Geriatric Medicine, Department of Medicine, Dalhousie University, Camp Hill Veterans' Memorial Bldg., 5955 Veterans' Memorial Lane, Halifax, Nova Scotia B3H 2E1, Canada.

References
1. Lutz W, Sanderson W, Scherbov S. The coming acceleration of global population ageing. Nature. 2008;451(7179):716–9.
2. Ferrucci L, Giallauria F, Guralnik JM. Epidemiology of aging. Radiol Clin N Am. 2008;46(4):643–52 v.
3. Yazdanyar A, Newman AB. The burden of cardiovascular disease in the elderly: morbidity, mortality, and costs. Clin Geriatr Med. 2009;25(4):563–77 vii.
4. Saad MA, Cardoso GP, Martins Wde A, Velarde LG, Cruz Filho RA. Prevalence of metabolic syndrome in elderly and agreement among four diagnostic criteria. Arq Bras Cardiol. 2014;102(3):263–9.
5. Plassman BL, Langa KM, Fisher GG, Heeringa SG, Weir DR, Ofstedal MB, et al. Prevalence of dementia in the United States: the aging, demographics, and memory study. Neuroepidemiology. 2007;29(1–2):125–32.
6. Gheno R, Cepparo JM, Rosca CE, Cotten A. Musculoskeletal disorders in the elderly. J Clin Imaging Sci. 2012;2:39.
7. Hubbard RE, Theou O. Frailty: enhancing the known knowns. Age Ageing. 2012;41(5):574–5.
8. Lorenzo-Lopez L, Maseda A, de Labra C, Regueiro-Folgueira L, Rodriguez-Villamil JL, Millan-Calenti JC. Nutritional determinants of frailty in older adults: a systematic review. BMC Geriatr. 2017;17(1):108.
9. Muscedere J, Waters B, Varambally A, Bagshaw SM, Boyd JG, Maslove D, et al. The impact of frailty on intensive care unit outcomes: a systematic review and meta-analysis. Intensive Care Med. 2017;43(8):1105–22.
10. Walters K, Frost R, Kharicha K, Avgerinou C, Gardner B, Ricciardi F, et al. Home-based health promotion for older people with mild frailty: the HomeHealth intervention development and feasibility RCT. Health Technol Assess. 2017;21(73):1–128.
11. Blodgett JM, Theou O, Howlett SE, Rockwood K. A frailty index from common clinical and laboratory tests predicts increased risk of death across the life course. GeroScience. 2017. https://doi.org/10.1007/s11357-017-9993-7.
12. Backman K, Joas E, Falk H, Mitnitski A, Rockwood K, Skoog I. Changes in the lethality of frailty over 30 years: evidence from two cohorts of 70-year-olds in Gothenburg Sweden. J Gerontol A Biol Sci Med Sci. 2017;72(7):945–50.
13. Mousa A, Savva GM, Mitnitski A, Rockwood K, Jagger C, Brayne C, et al. Is frailty a stable predictor of mortality across time? Evidence from the Cognitive Function and Ageing Studies. Age Ageing. 2018;47(5):721-7.
14. Constans T, Bacq Y, Brechot JF, Guilmot JL, Choutet P, Lamisse F. Protein-energy malnutrition in elderly medical patients. J Am Geriatr Soc. 1992;40(3):263–8.
15. Kaiser MJ, Bauer JM, Ramsch C, Uter W, Guigoz Y, Cederholm T, et al. Frequency of malnutrition in older adults: a multinational perspective using the mini nutritional assessment. J Am Geriatr Soc. 2010;58(9):1734–8.
16. Kiesswetter E, Pohlhausen S, Uhlig K, Diekmann R, Lesser S, Heseker H, et al. Malnutrition is related to functional impairment in older adults receiving home care. J Nutr Health Aging. 2013;17(4):345–50.
17. Rasheed S, Woods RT. Malnutrition and quality of life in older people: a systematic review and meta-analysis. Ageing Res Rev. 2013;12(2):561–6.
18. Correia MI, Waitzberg DL. The impact of malnutrition on morbidity, mortality, length of hospital stay and costs evaluated through a multivariate model analysis. Clin Nutr. 2003;22(3):235–9.
19. Ruengurairoek T, Vathesatogkit P, Boonhat H, Warodomwichit D, Thongmuang N, Matchariyakul D, et al. The association between processed meat intake and the prevalence of type 2 diabetes in Thais: a cross-sectional study from the Electricity Generating Authority of Thailand. Ramathibodi Med J. 2017;40(3):1–10.

20. Ribeiro RV, Hirani V, Senior AM, Gosby AK, Cumming RG, Blyth FM, et al. Diet quality and its implications on the cardio-metabolic, physical and general health of older men: the Concord Health and Ageing in Men Project (CHAMP). Br J Nutr. 2017;118(2):130–43.

21. Sao Romao Preto L, Dias Conceicao MDC, Figueiredo TM, Pereira Mata MA, Barreira Preto PM, Mateo Aguilar E. Frailty, body composition and nutritional status in non-institutionalised elderly. Enferm Clin. 2017;27(6):339–45.

22. Shlisky J, Bloom DE, Beaudreault AR, Tucker KL, Keller HH, Freund-Levi Y, et al. Nutritional considerations for healthy aging and reduction in age-related chronic disease. Adv Nutr. 2017;8(1):17–26.

23. Theou O, Chapman I, Wijeyaratne L, Piantadosi C, Lange K, Naganathan V, et al. Can an intervention with testosterone and nutritional supplement improve the frailty level of under-nourished older people? J Frailty Aging. 2016;5(4):247–52.

24. Strike SC, Carlisle A, Gibson EL, Dyall SC. A high omega-3 fatty acid multinutrient supplement benefits cognition and mobility in older women: a randomized, double-blind, placebo-controlled pilot study. J Gerontol A Biol Sci Med Sci. 2016;71(2):236–42.

25. Hutchins-Wiese HL, Kleppinger A, Annis K, Liva E, Lammi-Keefe CJ, Durham HA, et al. The impact of supplemental n-3 long chain polyunsaturated fatty acids and dietary antioxidants on physical performance in postmenopausal women. J Nutr Health Aging. 2013;17(1):76–80.

26. van Dijk M, Dijk FJ, Hartog A, van Norren K, Verlaan S, van Helvoort A, et al. Reduced dietary intake of micronutrients with antioxidant properties negatively impacts muscle health in aged mice. J Cachexia Sarcopenia Muscle. 2018;9(1):146–59.

27. Bonnefoy M, Berrut G, Lesourd B, Ferry M, Gilbert T, Guerin O, et al. Frailty and nutrition: searching for evidence. J Nutr Health Aging. 2015; 19(3):250–7.

28. Cesari M, Theou O. Frailty: The Broad View. In: Fillit HM, Rockwood K, Young JB. editor. Brocklehurst's Textbook of Geriatric Medicine and Gerontology. 8th ed. Philadelphia: Elsevier, Inc.; 2017. p. 84–7.

29. Aguirre LE, Villareal DT. Physical exercise as therapy for frailty, Nestle Nutrition Institute workshop series, vol. 83; 2015. p. 83–92.

30. Kelaiditi E, van Kan GA, Cesari M. Frailty: role of nutrition and exercise. Curr Opin Clin Nutr Metab Care. 2014;17(1):32–9.

31. Theou O, Stathokostas L, Roland KP, Jakobi JM, Patterson C, Vandervoort AA, et al. The effectiveness of exercise interventions for the management of frailty: a systematic review. J Aging Res. 2011;2011:569194.

32. Soysal P, Isik AT, Carvalho AF, Fernandes BS, Solmi M, Schofield P, et al. Oxidative stress and frailty: a systematic review and synthesis of the best evidence. Maturitas. 2017;99:66–72.

33. Ble A, Cherubini A, Volpato S, Bartali B, Walston JD, Windham BG, et al. Lower plasma vitamin E levels are associated with the frailty syndrome: the InCHIANTI study. J Gerontol A Biol Sci Med Sci. 2006;61(3):278–83.

34. Bollwein J, Volkert D, Diekmann R, Kaiser MJ, Uter W, Vidal K, et al. Nutritional status according to the mini nutritional assessment (MNA(R)) and frailty in community dwelling older persons: a close relationship. J Nutr Health Aging. 2013;17(4):351–6.

35. Shikany JM, Barrett-Connor E, Ensrud KE, Cawthon PM, Lewis CE, Dam TT, et al. Macronutrients, diet quality, and frailty in older men. J Gerontol A Biol Sci Med Sci. 2014;69(6):695–701.

36. Beasley JM, LaCroix AZ, Neuhouser ML, Huang Y, Tinker L, Woods N, et al. Protein intake and incident frailty in the Women's Health Initiative observational study. J Am Geriatr Soc. 2010;58(6):1063–71.

37. Rahi B, Colombet Z, Gonzalez-Colaço Harmand M, Dartigues J-F, Boirie Y, Letenneur L, et al. Higher protein but not energy intake is associated with a lower prevalence of frailty among community-dwelling older adults in the French three-city cohort. J Am Med Dir Assoc. 2016;17(7):672.e7–11.

38. Cruz-Jentoft AJ, Kiesswetter E, Drey M, Sieber CC. Nutrition, frailty, and sarcopenia. Aging Clin Exp Res. 2017;29(1):43–8.

39. Theou O, Rockwood K. China's oldest-old-prospects for good health in late life. Lancet. 2017;389(10079):1584–6.

40. Huang YC, Wahlqvist ML, Lo YC, Lin C, Chang HY, Lee MS. A non-invasive modifiable Healthy Ageing Nutrition Index (HANI) predicts longevity in free-living older Taiwanese. Sci Rep. 2018;8(1):7113.

41. National Center for Health Statistics (NCHS) of the Centers for Disease Control and Prevention (CDC). https://www.cdc.gov/nchs/nhanes/. Cited 28 Dec 2017.

42. Zipf G, Chiappa M, Porter KS, Ostchega Y, Lewis BG, Dostal J. National health and nutrition examination survey: plan and operations, 1999-2010. Vital and health statistics Ser 1, Programs and collection procedures. 2013(56):1–37.

43. Aparicio-Ugarriza R, Palacios G, Alder M, Gonzalez-Gross M. A review of the cut-off points for the diagnosis of vitamin B12 deficiency in the general population. Clin Chem Lab Med. 2015;53(8):1149–59.

44. Ross C, Caballero B, Tucker KL, Cousins RJ. Modern nutrition in health and disease. 11th ed. Baltimore: Lippincott Williams & Wilkins; 2014.

45. Institute of Medicine. Dietary Reference Intakes for Calcium, Phosphorus, Magnesium, Vitamin D, and Fluoride. Washington, DC: The National Academies Press; 1997. https://doi.org/10.17226/5776.

46. Institute of Medicine. Dietary Reference Intakes for Thiamin, Riboflavin, Niacin, Vitamin B6, Folate, Vitamin B12, Pantothenic Acid, Biotin, and Choline. Washington, DC: The National Academies Press; 1998. https://doi.org/10.17226/6015.

47. Kromhout D, Giltay EJ, Geleijnse JM, Alpha Omega Trial G. n-3 fatty acids and cardiovascular events after myocardial infarction. N Engl J Med. 2010; 363(21):2015–26.

48. Genuth S, Alberti KG, Bennett P, Buse J, Defronzo R, Kahn R, et al. Follow-up report on the diagnosis of diabetes mellitus. Diabetes Care. 2003;26(11):3160–7.

49. National Cholesterol Education Program Expert Panel on Detection E, Treatment of High Blood Cholesterol in A. Third Report of the National Cholesterol Education Program (NCEP) Expert Panel on Detection, Evaluation, and Treatment of High Blood Cholesterol in Adults (Adult Treatment Panel III) final report. Circulation. 2002;106(25):3143–421.

50. Fryar CD, Gu Q, Ogden CL, Flegal KM. Anthropometric Reference Data for Children and Adults: United States, 2011–2014, Vital and health statistics series 3, Analytical Studies, no. 39; 2016. p. 1–46.

51. Alberti KG, Zimmet P, Shaw J, Group IDFETFC. The metabolic syndrome--a new worldwide definition. Lancet. 2005;366(9491):1059–62.

52. Trumbo P, Yates AA, Schlicker S, Poos M. Dietary reference intakes: vitamin A, vitamin K, arsenic, boron, chromium, copper, iodine, iron, manganese, molybdenum, nickel, silicon, vanadium, and zinc. J Am Diet Assoc. 2001; 101(3):294–301.

53. U.S. Department of Health and Human Services, U.S. Department of Agriculture. 2015 – 2020 Dietary guidelines for Americans. 8th ed; 2015.

54. Prevention and management of osteoporosis. World Health Organ Tech Rep Ser. 2003;921:1-164, back cover.

55. Hosten AO. BUN and Creatinine. In: Walker HK, Hall WD, Hurst JW, editors. Clinical Methods: The History, Physical, and Laboratory Examinations. Boston: Butterworths; 1990. p. 874–8.

56. Theou O, Blodgett JM, Godin J, Rockwood K. Association between sedentary time and mortality across levels of frailty. CMAJ. 2017;189(33):E1056–E64.

57. Mitnitski AB, Mogilner AJ, Rockwood K. Accumulation of deficits as a proxy measure of aging. TheScientificWorldJOURNAL. 2001;1:323–36.

58. Halfon M, Phan O, Teta D. Vitamin D: a review on its effects on muscle strength, the risk of fall, and frailty. Biomed Res Int. 2015;2015:953241.

59. Vogt S, Decke S, de Las Heras Gala T, Linkohr B, Koenig W, Ladwig KH, et al. Prospective association of vitamin D with frailty status and all-cause mortality in older adults: results from the KORA-Age Study. Prev Med. 2015; 73:40–6.

60. Vaes AMM, Brouwer-Brolsma EM, Toussaint N, de Regt M, Tieland M, van Loon LJC, et al. The association between 25-hydroxyvitamin D concentration, physical performance and frailty status in older adults. Eur J Nutr. 2018.

61. Wilhelm-Leen ER, Hall YN, Deboer IH, Chertow GM. Vitamin D deficiency and frailty in older Americans. J Intern Med. 2010;268(2):171–80.

62. Muir SW, Montero-Odasso M. Effect of vitamin D supplementation on muscle strength, gait and balance in older adults: a systematic review and meta-analysis. J Am Geriatr Soc. 2011;59(12):2291–300.

63. Kuzma E, Soni M, Littlejohns TJ, Ranson JM, van Schoor NM, Deeg DJ, et al. Vitamin D and memory decline: two population-based prospective studies. J Alzheimers Dis. 2016;50(4):1099–108.

64. World Health Organization: Body mass index – BMI. http://www.euro.who.int/en/health-topics/disease-prevention/nutrition/a-healthy-lifestyle/body-mass-index-bmi. Cited 27 Apr 2018.

65. Winter JE, MacInnis RJ, Wattanapenpaiboon N, Nowson CA. BMI and all-cause mortality in older adults: a meta-analysis. Am J Clin Nutr. 2014;99(4):875–90.

66. Chapman IM. Obesity paradox during aging. Interdiscip Top Gerontol. 2010; 37:20–36.

67. Chang SH, Beason TS, Hunleth JM, Colditz GA. A systematic review of body fat distribution and mortality in older people. Maturitas. 2012;72(3):175–91.

68. Rietman ML, Spijkerman AMW, Wong A, van Steeg H, Burkle A, Moreno-Villanueva M, et al. Antioxidants linked with physical, cognitive and psychological frailty: analysis of candidate biomarkers and markers derived from the MARK-AGE study. Mech Ageing Dev. 2018.

69. Semba RD, Bartali B, Zhou J, Blaum C, Ko CW, Fried LP. Low serum micronutrient concentrations predict frailty among older women living in the community. J Gerontol A Biol Sci Med Sci. 2006;61(6):594–9.
70. Fontana L, Kennedy BK, Longo VD, Seals D, Melov S. Medical research: treat ageing. Nature. 2014;511(7510):405–7.
71. Howlett SE, Rockwood K. Ageing: develop models of frailty. Nature. 2014; 512(7514):253.
72. Guo H, Siu W, D'Arcy RC, Black SE, Grajauskas LA, Singh S, et al. MRI assessment of whole-brain structural changes in aging. Clin Interv Aging. 2017;12:1251–70.
73. Armstrong JJ, Andrew MK, Mitnitski A, Launer LJ, White LR, Rockwood K. Social vulnerability and survival across levels of frailty in the Honolulu-Asia Aging Study. Age Ageing. 2015;44(4):709–12.
74. Howlett SE, Rockwood MR, Mitnitski A, Rockwood K. Standard laboratory tests to identify older adults at increased risk of death. BMC Med. 2014;12:171.
75. Mitnitski A, Collerton J, Martin-Ruiz C, Jagger C, von Zglinicki T, Rockwood K, et al. Age-related frailty and its association with biological markers of ageing. BMC Med. 2015;13:161.
76. Wallace LM, Theou O, Kirkland SA, Rockwood MR, Davidson KW, Shimbo D, et al. Accumulation of non-traditional risk factors for coronary heart disease is associated with incident coronary heart disease hospitalization and death. PLoS One. 2014;9(3):e90475.
77. Brothers TD, Kirkland S, Theou O, Zona S, Malagoli A, Wallace LMK, et al. Predictors of transitions in frailty severity and mortality among people aging with HIV. PLoS One. 2017;12(10):e0185352.
78. Howlett SE, Rockwood K. New horizons in frailty: ageing and the deficit-scaling problem. Age Ageing. 2013;42(4):416–23.
79. Rutenberg AD, Mitnitski AB, Farrell SG, Rockwood K. Unifying aging and frailty through complex dynamical networks. Exp Gerontol. 2018;107:126–9.
80. Mitnitski A, Rockwood K. The rate of aging: the rate of deficit accumulation does not change over the adult life span. Biogerontology. 2016;17(1):199–204.
81. Pincus Z. Ageing: A stretch in time. Nature. 2016;530(7588):37–8.
82. Fried LP, Tangen CM, Walston J, Newman AB, Hirsch C, Gottdiener J, et al. Frailty in older adults: evidence for a phenotype. J Gerontol A Biol Sci Med Sci. 2001;56(3):M146–56.
83. Huo YR, Suriyaarachchi P, Gomez F, Curcio CL, Boersma D, Gunawardene P, et al. Comprehensive nutritional status in sarco-osteoporotic older fallers. J Nutr Health Aging. 2015;19(4):474–80.
84. Kane AE, Gregson E, Theou O, Rockwood K, Howlett SE. The association between frailty, the metabolic syndrome, and mortality over the lifespan. Geroscience. 2017;39(2):221–9.
85. Theou O, Rockwood MR, Mitnitski A, Rockwood K. Disability and co-morbidity in relation to frailty: how much do they overlap? Arch Gerontol Geriatr. 2012;55(2):e1–8.
86. Deutz NE, Bauer JM, Barazzoni R, Biolo G, Boirie Y, Bosy-Westphal A, et al. Protein intake and exercise for optimal muscle function with aging: recommendations from the ESPEN Expert Group. Clin Nutr. 2014;33(6):929–36.

19

Racial differences in comorbidity profile among patients with chronic obstructive pulmonary disease

Hyun Lee[1], Sun Hye Shin[2], Seonhye Gu[3], Di Zhao[5], Danbee Kang[3,4], Yeong Rae Joi[3], Gee Young Suh[2], Roberto Pastor-Barriuso[6], Eliseo Guallar[4,5], Juhee Cho[3,4,5†] and Hye Yun Park[2*†]

Abstract

Background: Chronic obstructive pulmonary disease (COPD) is often accompanied by multiple comorbidities, which are associated with an increased risk of exacerbation, a poor health-related quality of life, and high mortality. However, differences in comorbidity profile by race and ethnicity in COPD patients have not been fully elucidated.

Methods: Participants aged 40 to 79 years with spirometry-defined COPD from the U.S. National Health and Nutrition Examination Survey (NHANES) (2007–2012) and from the Korea NHANES (2007–2015) were analyzed to compare the prevalence of comorbidities by race and ethnicity group. Comorbidities were defined using questionnaire data, physical exams, and laboratory tests.

Results: Non-Hispanic Whites had the highest prevalence of dyslipidemia (65.5%), myocardial infarction (6.2%), osteoarthritis (40.1%), and osteoporosis (13.6%), while non-Hispanic Blacks had the highest prevalence of asthma (24.0%), hypertension (70.2%), stroke (7.3%), diabetes mellitus (DM) (23.3%), anemia (16.4%), and rheumatoid arthritis (11.9%). Compared to non-Hispanic Whites, non-Hispanic Blacks had a significantly higher prevalence of hypertension, stroke, DM, anemia, and rheumatoid arthritis after adjusting for age, sex, body mass index, and smoking status, while Hispanics had a significantly higher prevalence of DM and anemia, and Koreans had significantly lower prevalences of all comorbidities except stroke, DM, and anemia.

Conclusions: COPD-related comorbidities varied significantly by race and ethnicity, and different strategies may be required for the optimal management of COPD and its comorbidities in different race and ethnicity groups.

Keywords: COPD, Comorbidity, Race, Ethnicity

Background

Chronic obstructive pulmonary disease (COPD) is a common respiratory disease characterized by persistent respiratory symptoms and airflow limitations [1]. Due to the ongoing epidemic of smoking and to prolonged life expectancy, COPD is projected to increase in prevalence and to contribute over 4.5 million annual deaths worldwide by 2030 [2, 3].

Since aging and smoking are independent risk factors not only for COPD, but also for multiple chronic diseases, COPD is often accompanied by comorbidities, including cardiovascular disease (CVD), osteoporosis, metabolic syndrome, depression, and several types of cancer [4]. Furthermore, in COPD patients, these comorbidities are associated with an increased risk of exacerbation [5], a poor health-related quality of life [6], increased utilization of health services [7], and high mortality [8]. As a consequence, recent COPD guidelines give special emphasis to the management of comorbid conditions in COPD [1].

COPD guidelines, however, have been developed using data primarily from populations of European descent. COPD and associated comorbidities have multiple genetic, behavioral, environmental, and socioeconomic risk factors, which may vary substantially across racial

---

* Correspondence: hyeyunpark@skku.edu
†Juhee Cho and Hye Yun Park contributed equally to this work.
2Division of Pulmonary and Critical Care Medicine, Department of Medicine, Samsung Medical Center, Sungkyunkwan University School of Medicine, Seoul, South Korea
Full list of author information is available at the end of the article

groups, like other diseases [9–11], but differences in co-morbidity profile by race and ethnicity in COPD patients have not been fully elucidated. This study aimed to evaluate differences in comorbidity profile by race and ethnicity in subjects with COPD participating in nationally representative surveys from the United States and South Korea.

Methods

Participants

We used data from the 2007–2012 cycles of the U.S. National Health and Nutrition Examination Survey (NHANES) and from the 2007–2015 cycles of the Korea NHANES (KNHANES). Both surveys provide nationally representative data of the non-institutionalized population using a multi-stage cluster sampling design. We restricted our analysis to men and women 40 to 79 years old with spirometry-defined COPD [pre-bronchodilator forced expiratory volume in 1 s (FEV_1) / forced vital capacity (FVC) < 70%] [12]. Among U.S. NHANES participants, we further restricted the analysis to those who self-identified as Non-Hispanic White (n = 944), Non-Hispanic Black (n = 324), or Hispanic (n = 227). KNHANES provided a representation of Asians (n = 3808), as the number of Asian participants with COPD in U.S. NHANES was too small for comparisons (Fig. 1).

Spirometric measurement

In both surveys, spirometry was performed according to the recommendations of the American Thoracic Society and European Respiratory Society [13]. Absolute values of FEV_1 and FVC were obtained, and the percentage of predicted values for FEV_1 and FVC were calculated using the reference equation obtained from an analysis of the general U.S. population for U.S. NHANES [14] and a representative Korean sample for KNHANES [15].

Definitions

COPD was defined based on pre-bronchodilator FEV_1 / FVC < 0.7, and COPD severity was classified as mild ($FEV_1 \geq 80\%$ predicted), moderate ($50\% \leq FEV_1 < 80\%$ predicted), or severe-to-very severe ($FEV_1 < 50\%$ predicted) [1]. Height and weight were measured and body mass index (BMI) was calculated as weight in kilograms divided by height in meters squared. Obesity was defined as $BMI \geq 30.0$ kg/m^2 and overweight was defined as BMI = 25.0–29.9 kg/m^2 in Non-Hispanic Whites, Non-Hispanic Blacks, and Hispanics, and as $BMI \geq 25$ kg/m^2 for obesity and as BMI = 23.0–24.9 for overweight in Koreans according to World Health Organization guidelines [16].

Comorbidities were defined as a self-reported physician diagnosis. In addition, hypertension was defined as the use of antihypertensive medication, a systolic

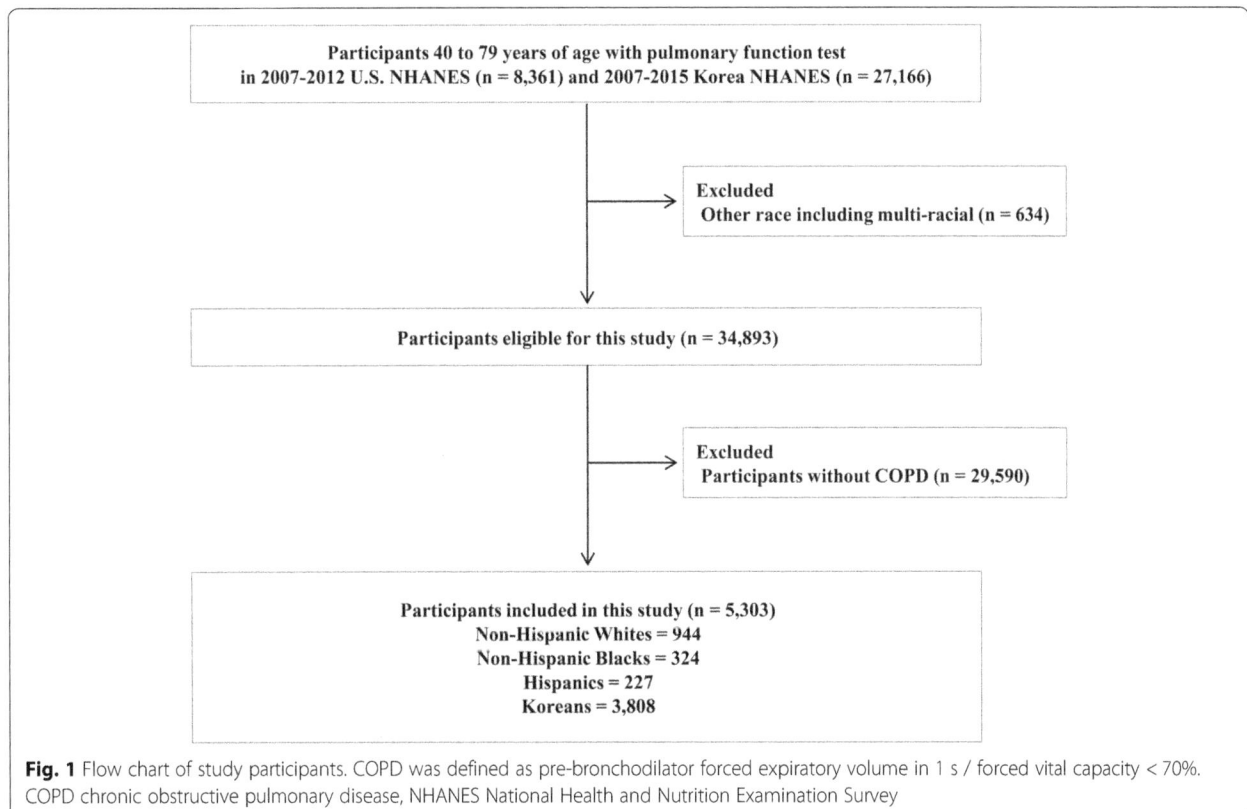

Fig. 1 Flow chart of study participants. COPD was defined as pre-bronchodilator forced expiratory volume in 1 s / forced vital capacity < 70%. COPD chronic obstructive pulmonary disease, NHANES National Health and Nutrition Examination Survey

blood pressure ≥ 140 mmHg, or a diastolic blood pressure ≥ 90 mmHg. Dyslipidemia was defined as the use of lipid-lowering medications or a low-density lipoprotein cholesterol level greater than 130 mg/dL or high-density lipoprotein cholesterol level less than 40 mg/dL [17]. Diabetes mellitus (DM) was defined as the use of glucose-lowering medications or a fasting plasma glucose level ≥ 126 mg/dL. Anemia was defined as hemoglobin level < 13 g/dL in men and < 12 g/dL in women [18].

Outcomes

We compared the comorbidity profile by race and ethnicity in subjects with COPD participating in U.S. and Korea NHANES. As comorbidities, we included asthma, hypertension, dyslipidemia, stroke, myocardial infarction, DM, and osteoporosis, which were recommended for screening and management in the Global Initiative for COPD guideline [1], plus anemia, osteoarthritis, and rheumatoid arthritis (RA), three common conditions having a substantial impact on the quality of life.

Statistical analysis

Statistical analysis used the *svy* commands in Stata (release 13.1; StataCorp LP, College Station, TX, USA) to account for survey weights and for the complex sampling design. For each comorbidity, we calculated its prevalence and 95% confidence interval (CI) by race and ethnicity group and used log binomial regression to estimate adjusted prevalence ratios (aPRs) and 95% CIs comparing each race and ethnicity group to Non-Hispanic Whites, adjusting for age, sex, BMI, and smoking status.

Table 1 Characteristics of participants with COPD aged 40–79 by race and ethnicity, U.S. NHANES 2007–2012 and Korea NHANES 2007–2015[a]

	U.S. NHANES			Korea NHANES	
	Non-Hispanic White (n = 944)	Non-Hispanic Black (n = 324)	Hispanic[b] (n = 227)	Korean (n = 3808)	p value
Age, years	59.8(0.4)	59.6 (0.7)	59.6 (0.8)	63.6 (0.2)	< 0.001
Age group, years					< 0.001
40–49	18.7 (1.7)	20.7 (2.9)	19.7 (3.1)	11.3 (0.7)	
50–59	31.2 (2.2)	30.9 (2.6)	29.9 (3.9)	23.2 (0.9)	
60–69	30.3 (2.4)	24.1 (1.8)	32.0 (3.0)	31.2 (0.9)	
70–79	19.8 (1.3)	24.2 (2.5)	18.3 (2.7)	34.3 (1.0)	
Men, %	59.1 (2.4)	60.2 (2.3)	69.2 (4.2)	73.8 (0.9)	< 0.001
BMI, kg/m^2	27.7 (0.2)	27.8 (0.4)	28. 6 (0.4)	23.7 (0.1)	< 0.001
BMI group					0.023
Underweight	1.9 (0.5)	3.1 (1.2)	0	2.7 (0.4)	
Normal	32.3 (1.6)	35.1 (2.8)	27.4 (3.4)	38.9 (1.1)	
Overweight	37.8 (1.5)	33.4 (2.3)	41.9 (3.7)	27.6 (0.9)	
Obese	27.9 (1.4)	28.4 (2.6)	30.7 (3.8)	30.7 (1.0)	
Smoking					< 0.001
Current	33.5 (2.4)	42.4 (3.4)	26.4 (2.8)	41.6 (1.0)	
Former	39.9 (2.1)	26.4 (2.2)	35.5 (2.9)	27.9 (0.9)	
Never	26.6 (2.1)	31.3 (2.8)	38.1 (3.3)	30.5 (1.0)	
Spirometry					
FVC, % predicted	96.5 (0.7)	96.7 (1.1)	97.9 (1.4)	90.5 (0.3)	< 0.001
FEV$_1$, % predicted	80.3 (0.7)	77.5 (1.1)	82.6 (1.3)	77.8 (0.3)	< 0.001
COPD severity[c]					0.106
Mild	52.3 (2.3)	46.5 (3.1)	60.4 (4.1)	46.4 (1.0)	
Moderate	41.3 (2.2)	44.4 (3.1)	36.0 (4.3)	48.7 (1.1)	
Severe-to-very severe	6.4 (0.8)	9.2 (2.3)	3.6 (1.1)	4.9 (0.4)	

[a]Values are presented as weighted means (standard error of the mean) or weighted percentage (standard error of the percentage)
[b]Hispanic was defined as Mexican American or other Hispanic
[c]Participants were categorized as having mild (FEV$_1$ / FVC < 0.7 and FEV$_1$ ≥ 80% predicted), moderate (FEV$_1$ / FVC < 0.7 and 50% ≤ FEV$_1$ < 80% predicted), or severe-to-very severe (FEV$_1$ / FVC < 0.7 and FEV$_1$ < 50% predicted) disease based on the Global Initiative for Chronic Obstructive Lung Disease guideline
COPD chronic obstructive pulmonary disease, *NHANES* National Health and Nutrition Examination Survey (NHANES), *BMI* body mass index, *FEV$_1$* forced expiratory volume in 1 s, *FVC* forced expiratory vital capacity

Results

The average age of non-Hispanic Whites, non-Hispanic Blacks, and Hispanics was similar (59.8, 59.6, and 59.6 years, respectively), but Koreans were older on average (63.6 years, $p < 0.001$; Table 1). By sex, the proportions of men among non-Hispanic Whites and non-Hispanic Blacks were similar (59.1 and 60.2%, respectively), and lower than among Hispanic (69.2%) and Korean (73.8%) participants. Hispanic participants were the most likely to be overweight or obese (72.6%), while Non-Hispanic Blacks and Koreans were the most likely to be current smokers (42.4 and 41.6%, respectively). By severity, non-Hispanic Blacks had the highest proportion of severe-to-very-severe COPD (9.2%), while Hispanics had the lowest (3.6%).

Non-Hispanic White participants had the highest prevalence of dyslipidemia (65.5%), myocardial infarction (6.2%), osteoarthritis (40.1%), and osteoporosis (13.6%), while non-Hispanic Blacks had the highest prevalence of asthma (24.0%), hypertension (70.2%), stroke (7.3%), DM (23.3%), anemia (16.4%), and RA (11.9%) (Table 2 and Fig. 2). Hispanics had very high prevalences of all comorbidities except for stroke, ranking second in the prevalence of asthma, hypertension, myocardial infarction, DM, anemia, RA, and osteoporosis compared to other race and ethnicity groups. Koreans had the lowest prevalence of all comorbidities except for stroke, DM, and anemia.

Compared to non-Hispanic Whites, non-Hispanic Black participants had a significantly higher prevalence of hypertension (aPR 1.36, 95% CI 1.23 to 1.51), stroke (aPR 2.01, 95% CI 1.16 to 3.47), DM (aPR 1.76, 95% CI 1.34 to 2.31), anemia (aPR 3.82, 95% CI 2.42 to 6.04),

and RA (aPR 1.83, 95% CI, 1.16 to 2.89) after adjusting for age, sex, BMI, and smoking status, while Hispanics had a higher prevalence of DM (aPR 1.64, 95% CI 1.18 to 2.29) and anemia (aPR 2.18, 95% CI 1.23 to 3.86). Koreans had significantly lower prevalences of all comorbidities except stroke, DM, and anemia (Table 3).

Discussion

We found major differences in the comorbidity profile among race and ethnicity groups in subjects with COPD. Non-Hispanic Whites had a comorbidity pattern characterized by dyslipidemia, myocardial infarction, osteoarthritis, and osteoporosis. Non-Hispanic Blacks had a high prevalence of current smokers as well as a high prevalence of multiple comorbidities, especially asthma, hypertension, stroke, DM, anemia, and RA. Hispanics had the highest average BMI levels, as well as high prevalences of asthma and DM. Finally, Koreans had the highest prevalence of current smokers, but lower prevalences of other comorbidities except for stroke, DM, and anemia. Given that coexisting comorbidities have an adverse impact on COPD prognosis, early recognition and management of prevalent disease based on racial differences could reduce the clinical burden of disease in COPD patients.

CVD is a key comorbidity in COPD patients and a major determinant of mortality and functional status [19]. In our study, non-Hispanic Whites had a pattern of CVD comorbidities characterized by a high prevalence of dyslipidemia and coronary disease, while non-Hispanic Blacks had a pattern driven by hypertension, DM, and stroke. These were like the results of a previous study that compared COPD

Table 2 Prevalence of comorbidities (95% confidence intervals) among participants with COPD aged 40–79 by race and ethnicity, U.S. NHANES 2007–2012 and Korea NHANES 2007–2015

	U.S. NHANES			Korea NHANES	
	Non-Hispanic White ($n = 944$)	Non-Hispanic Black ($n = 324$)	Hispanic[a] ($n = 227$)	Korean ($n = 3808$)	P value
Asthma	19.9 (16.5 to 23.7)	24.0 (19.4 to 29.3)	20.7 (14.3 to 29.0)	9.1 (8.0 to 10.4)	< 0.001
Cardiovascular disease					
Hypertension	51.5 (47.4 to 55.7)	70.2 (64.0 to 75.6)	54.1 (46.4 to 61.5)	48.8 (46.8 to 50.8)	< 0.001
Dyslipidemia	65.5 (61.2 to 69.7)	53.9 (47.3 to 60.3)	57.2 (48.5 to 65.4)	44.8 (42.7 to 47.0)	< 0.001
Stroke	3.6 (2.6 to 4.8)	7.3 (4.6 to 11.3)	1.6 (0.5 to 5.3)	2.5 (2.0 to 3.1)	0.003
Myocardial infarction	6.2 (4.7 to 8.1)	4.2 (2.6 to 6.6)	5.4 (3.3 to 8.8)	1.7 (1.2 to 2.3)	< 0.001
Diabetes mellitus	13.3 (10.8 to 16.4)	23.3 (18.6 to 28.8)	23.1 (17.5 to 29.7)	18.4 (16.8 to 20.1)	< 0.001
Anemia	4.4 (3.0 to 6.3)	16.4 (12.3 to 21.6)	9.2 (5.8 to 14.3)	6.6 (5.7 to 7.6)	< 0.001
Musculoskeletal disease					
Osteoarthritis	40.1 (36.4 to 44.0)	38.0 (33.0 to 43.2)	31.2 (24.5 to 38.8)	14.9 (13.5 to 16.5)	< 0.001
Rheumatoid arthritis	6.3 (4.3 to 9.1)	11.9 (8.4 to 16.4)	7.9 (5.2 to 12.0)	2.2 (1.6 to 2.8)	< 0.001
Osteoporosis	13.6 (10.9 to 16.9)	9.1 (6.5 to 12.7)	9.9 (6.1 to 15.4)	3.3 (2.7 to 4.1)	< 0.001

[a]Hispanic was defined as Mexican American or other Hispanic
COPD chronic obstructive pulmonary disease, *NHANES* National Health and Nutrition Examination Survey

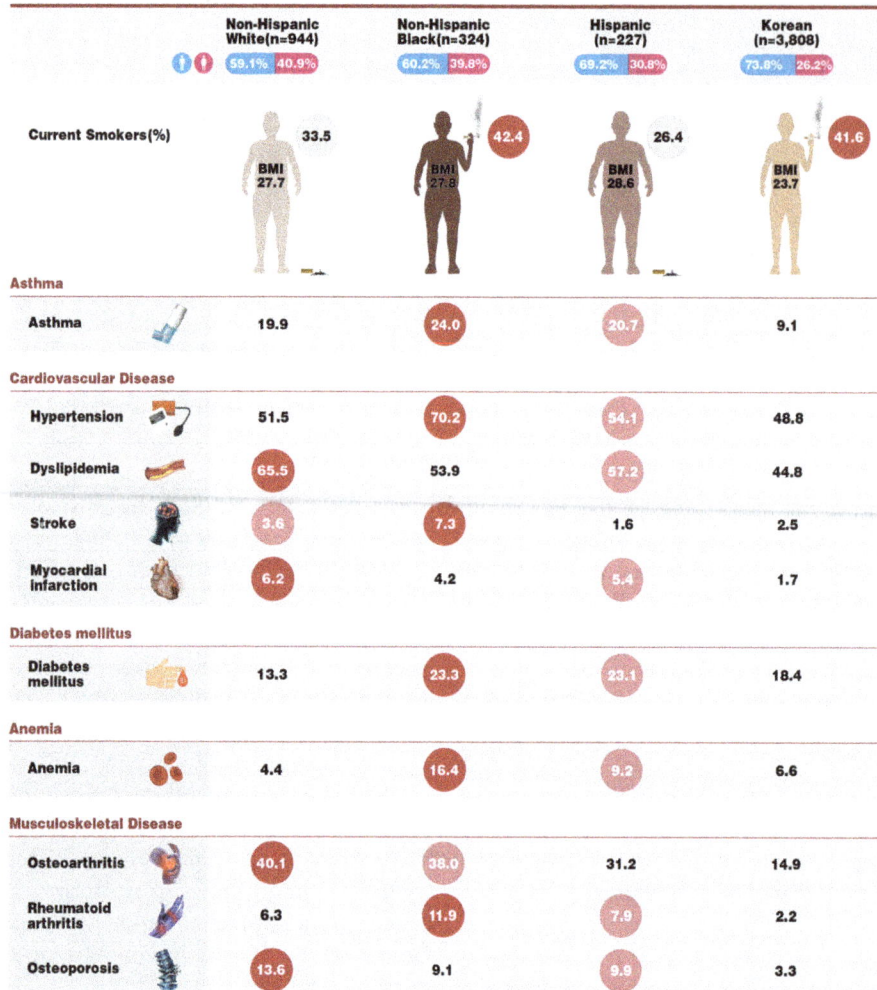

Fig. 2 Prevalence of comorbidities among participants with COPD aged 40–79 by race and ethnicity, U.S. NHANES 2007–2012 and Korea NHANES 2007–2015. COPD chronic obstructive pulmonary disease, NHANES National Health and Nutrition Examination Survey

comorbidities between non-Hispanic Whites and non-Hispanic Blacks [20]. In comparison, Hispanics had a pattern driven by obesity and DM. In addition to CVD, asthma is a major comorbidity as well as a risk factor in COPD, complicating treatment and further impairing functional status. Asthma prevalence was particularly high among non-Hispanic Blacks, although non-Hispanics Whites and Hispanics also had a relatively high prevalence. Considering their high prevalence and disease burden, clinicians should consider active screening and management of CVD and asthma in COPD patients.

Anemia has recently been recognized as an independent prognostic predictor of increased hospitalization and mortality in COPD [21–24]. It is also an important comorbidity linked to nutritional deficiency and poor exercise performance among COPD patients [23]. Previous studies have suggested the possibility of improving

functional outcomes by correcting anemia [25, 26], and active screening and management of anemia among COPD patients may be beneficial for clinical outcomes, especially among non-Hispanic Blacks and Hispanics.

Non-Hispanic Blacks had very high prevalences of COPD risk factors and comorbidities. Multiple sources of health disparities and inequalities, including socioeconomic factors, environmental hazards, behavioral factors, and access to health care and preventive services, contribute to the excess burden of disease and mortality among non-Hispanic Blacks in the U.S. [27]. The presence of multiple comorbidities may further complicate management and prognosis in these patients [28, 29]. It may be necessary, however, to develop integrated approaches to prevention and management to reduce the burden of chronic disease-related morbidity and mortality, particularly among non-Hispanic Black subjects with COPD.

Table 3 Adjusted prevalence ratios and 95% confidence intervals for comorbidities in participants with COPD aged 40–79, U.S. NHANES 2007–2012 and Korea NHANES 2007–2015[a]

	U.S. NHANES			Korea NHANES
	Non-Hispanic White (n = 944)	Non-Hispanic Black (n = 324)	Hispanic[b] (n = 227)	Korean (n = 3808)
Asthma	Reference	1.23 (0.92 to 1.65)	1.05 (0.72 to 1.53)	0.56 (0.43 to 0.72)
Cardiovascular disease				
Hypertension	Reference	1.36 (1.23 to 1.51)	1.03 (0.89 to 1.20)	0.88 (0.81 to 0.95)
Dyslipidemia	Reference	0.83 (0.72 to 0.96)	0.86 (0.73 to 1.00)	0.68 (0.63 to 0.73)
Stroke	Reference	2.01 (1.16 to 3.47)	0.47 (0.14 to 1.61)	0.69 (0.45 to 1.06)
Myocardial infarction	Reference	0.66 (0.39 to 1.12)	0.86 (0.49 to 1.53)	0.21 (0.14 to 0.33)
Diabetes mellitus	Reference	1.76 (1.34 to 2.31)	1.64 (1.18 to 2.29)	1.11 (0.90 to 1.38)
Anemia	Reference	3.82 (2.42 to 6.04)	2.18 (1.23 to 3.86)	1.31 (0.90 to 1.91)
Musculoskeletal disease				
Osteoarthritis	Reference	0.95 (0.82 to 1.10)	0.81 (0.65 to 1.01)	0.35 (0.30 to 0.40)
Rheumatoid arthritis	Reference	1.83 (1.16 to 2.89)	1.40 (0.85 to 2.31)	0.31 (0.20 to 0.50)
Osteoporosis	Reference	0.68 (0.45 to 1.03)	0.74 (0.46 to 1.20)	0.22 (0.16 to 0.32)

[a]Adjusted for age, sex, BMI group (underweight, normal, overweight, or obese using World Health Organization criteria for the U.S. population and Asian criteria for the Korean population), and smoking status (current, former, or never)
[b]Hispanic was defined as Mexican American or other Hispanic
COPD chronic obstructive pulmonary disease, NHANES National Health and Nutrition Examination Survey

Hispanic subjects with COPD had a very high burden of overweight and obesity and DM, although the prevalence of myocardial infarction was lower than in non-Hispanic Whites. The lower prevalence of CVD, despite relatively high levels of metabolic risk factors among Hispanics, has been termed the Hispanic paradox [30], but the reasons for this paradox are controversial. Irrespective of the implications of elevated BMI in Hispanic patients, the high prevalence of overweight and obesity in this group should prompt proper management, as morbid obesity is a risk for poor management and functional decline in COPD [31, 32].

Finally, although Korean COPD patients were older, more likely to be smokers, and more likely to be male than other race or ethnicity groups, they had the lowest prevalences of most comorbidities. A similar pattern has been observed in other Asian countries [33]. In particular, the low prevalence of myocardial infarction in Koreans may reflect lower background rates of the disease due to environmental or genetic factors. Since smoking is a predominant risk factor for COPD among Asians and considering the increasing number of Asians in the U.S., more active surveillance regarding COPD and its comorbidities may be warranted.

Several limitations need to be considered when interpreting our findings. First, we used a cross-sectional study and we do not have information on the timing of the development of each comorbidity. We were, thus, unable to establish causal inferences. Our objective, however, was to compare the comorbidity patterns across race and ethnicity groups, not to identify causal pathways of comorbidities. The different comorbidity patterns may be due to different prevalences of risk factors such as smoking, obesity, socioeconomic status, or environmental exposures, but race and ethnicity may affect the development of comorbidities. Second, we could not evaluate the prevalence of some important COPD-related comorbidities or conditions, such as obstructive sleep apnea or use of long-term oxygen therapy, due to lack of data in either U.S. NHANES or KNHANES. Third, we did not have data that would allow us to evaluate the outcomes of the different comorbidities. This information is important for understanding the impact of the differences in comorbidity profile by race and ethnicity. Given the racial differences in outcomes such as emergency room visits and duration of hospital stays [7], further studies should evaluate the management and outcomes of COPD, including exacerbations and mortality, by comorbidity profile. Fourth, we used data for Koreans as we did not have data for other Asian groups. However, Korean COPD patients had similar overall characteristics as other Asian COPD patients, including Taiwanese, Japanese, or Chinese patients, although the degree of exposure to biomass fuels differed across Asian groups [33].

Conclusions

In our study, COPD-related comorbidities occurred disproportionally according to race and ethnicity, and different strategies may be required for the optimal management of COPD and its comorbidities for different race and ethnicity groups. Furthermore, the generation of local maps of COPD-related comorbidities may help in planning different strategies for the diagnosis, treatment, and prevention of COPD and its associated comorbidities.

Abbreviations

aPR: adjusted prevalence ratio; BMI: body mass index; CI: confidence interval; COPD: chronic obstructive lung disease; CVD: cardiovascular disease; DM: diabetes mellitus; FEV_1: forced expiratory volume in 1 s; FVC: forced vital capacity; KNHANES: Korea National Health and Nutrition Examination Survey; NHANES: National Health and Nutrition Examination Survey; RA: rheumatoid arthritis

Funding

Not applicable.

Acknowledgements

Not applicable.

Authors' contributions

HL, JC, and HYP were responsible for the conception and design of the study. HL, SS, SG, JC, and HYP conducted the experiments and data acquisition. HL, SS, SG, DZ, DK, YRJ, GYS, RP, EG, JC, and HYP undertook the analysis and interpretation of the data. HL, SG, EG, JC, and HYP drafted the manuscript. HL, SS, SG, DZ, DK, YRJ, GYS, RP, EG, JC, and HYP made a critical revision of the manuscript. All authors read and approved the final manuscript.

Competing interests

HYP has received lecture fees from AstraZeneca, Novartis, and Boehringer-Ingelheim. HL, SHS, SG, DZ, DK, YRJ, GYS, RP, EG, and JC have no competing interests to declare.

Author details

[1]Division of Pulmonary Medicine and Allergy, Department of Internal Medicine, Hanyang University College of Medicine, Seoul, South Korea. [2]Division of Pulmonary and Critical Care Medicine, Department of Medicine, Samsung Medical Center, Sungkyunkwan University School of Medicine, Seoul, South Korea. [3]Center for Clinical Epidemiology, Samsung Medical Center, Seoul, South Korea. [4]Department of Clinical Research Design and Evaluation, SAIHST, Sungkyunkwan University, Seoul, South Korea. [5]Department of Epidemiology and Welch Center for Prevention, Epidemiology, and Clinical Research, Johns Hopkins University Bloomberg School of Public Health, Baltimore, MD, USA. [6]National Center for Epidemiology, Instituto de Salud Carlos III, and Consortium for Biomedical Research in Epidemiology and Public Health (CIBERESP), Madrid, Spain.

References

1. GOLD. Global strategy for the diagnosis, management and prevention of chronic obstructive pulmonary disease. (2018 Report) Available from www.goldcopd.org. Assessed 1 June 2018.
2. Lopez AD, Shibuya K, Rao C, Mathers CD, Hansell AL, Held LS, et al. Chronic obstructive pulmonary disease: current burden and future projections. Eur Respir J. 2006;27:397–412.
3. World Health Organization. Projecitons of mortaity and causes of death, 2015 and 2030. Available at: http://www.who.int/healthinfo/global_burden_disease/projections/en/. Assessed 1 June 2018.
4. Vanfleteren LE, Spruit MA, Groenen M, Gaffron S, van Empel VP, Bruijnzeel PL, et al. Clusters of comorbidities based on validated objective measurements and systemic inflammation in patients with chronic obstructive pulmonary disease. Am J Respir Crit Care Med. 2013;187:728–35.
5. Westerik JA, Metting EI, van Boven JF, Tiersma W, Kocks JW, Schermer TR. Associations between chronic comorbidity and exacerbation risk in primary care patients with COPD. Respir Res. 2017;18:31.
6. Huber MB, Wacker ME, Vogelmeier CF, Leidl R. Comorbid influences on generic health-related quality of life in COPD: a systematic review. PLoS One. 2015;10:e0132670.
7. Westney G, Foreman MG, Xu J, Henriques King M, Flenaugh E, Rust G. Impact of comorbidities among Medicaid enrollees with chronic obstructive pulmonary disease, United States, 2009. Prev Chronic Dis. 2017;14:E31.
8. Sin DD, Anthonisen NR, Soriano JB, Agusti AG. Mortality in COPD: role of comorbidities. Eur Respir J. 2006;28:1245–57.
9. Haiman CA, Stram DO, Wilkens LR, Pike MC, Kolonel LN, Henderson BE, et al. Ethnic and racial differences in the smoking-related risk of lung cancer. N Engl J Med. 2006;354:333–42.
10. Bahrami H, Kronmal R, Bluemke DA, Olson J, Shea S, Liu K, et al. Differences in the incidence of congestive heart failure by ethnicity: the multi-ethnic study of atherosclerosis. Arch Intern Med. 2008;168:2138–45.
11. Gutierrez J, Williams OA. A decade of racial and ethnic stroke disparities in the United States. Neurology. 2014;82:1080–2.
12. Lange P, Celli B, Agusti A, Boje Jensen G, Divo M, Faner R, et al. Lung-function trajectories leading to chronic obstructive pulmonary disease. N Engl J Med. 2015;373:111–22.
13. Miller MR, Hankinson J, Brusasco V, Burgos F, Casaburi R, Coates A, et al. Standardisation of spirometry. Eur Respir J. 2005;26:319–38.
14. Hankinson JL, Odencrantz JR, Fedan KB. Spirometric reference values from a sample of the general U.S. population. Am J Respir Crit Care Med. 1999;159:179–87.
15. Choi JK, Paek D, Lee JO. Normal predictive values of spirometry in Korean population. Tuberc Respir Dis. 2005;58:230–42.
16. WHO. Physical Status: The use and interpretation of anthropometry: report of a World Health Organization (WHO) expert committee. Geneva: World Health Organization; 1995.
17. Force USPST, Bibbins-Domingo K, Grossman DC, Curry SJ, Davidson KW, Epling JW Jr, et al. Statin use for the primary prevention of cardiovascular disease in adults: US preventive services task force recommendation statement. JAMA. 2016;316:1997–2007.
18. World Health Organization. Haemoglobin concentrations for the diagnosis of Anaemia and assessment of severity. Vitamin and mineral nutrition information system. Geneva: World Health Organization; 2011. Available from: http://www.who.int/vmnis/indicators/haemoglobin.pdf. Accessed 1 July 2018
19. Sin DD, Man SF. Chronic obstructive pulmonary disease as a risk factor for cardiovascular morbidity and mortality. Proc Am Thorac Soc. 2005;2:8–11.
20. Putcha N, Han MK, Martinez CH, Foreman MG, Anzueto AR, Casaburi R, et al. Comorbidities of COPD have a major impact on clinical outcomes, particularly in African Americans. Chronic Obstr Pulm Dis. 2014;1:105–14.
21. Chambellan A, Chailleux E, Similowski T. Prognostic value of the hematocrit in patients with severe COPD receiving long-term oxygen therapy. Chest. 2005;128:1201–8.
22. Martinez-Rivera C, Portillo K, Munoz-Ferrer A, Martinez-Ortiz ML, Molins E, Serra P, et al. Anemia is a mortality predictor in hospitalized patients for COPD exacerbation. COPD. 2012;9:243–50.
23. Oh YM, Park JH, Kim EK, Hwang SC, Kim HJ, Kang DR, et al. Anemia as a clinical marker of stable chronic obstructive pulmonary disease in the Korean obstructive lung disease cohort. J Thorac Dis. 2017;9:5008–16.
24. Park SC, Kim YS, Kang YA, Park EC, Shin CS, Kim DW, et al. Hemoglobin and mortality in patients with COPD: a nationwide population-based cohort study. Int J Chron Obstruct Pulmon Dis. 2018;13:1599–605.
25. Schonhofer B, Wenzel M, Geibel M, Kohler D. Blood transfusion and lung function in chronically anemic patients with severe chronic obstructive pulmonary disease. Crit Care Med. 1998;26:1824–8.
26. Silverberg DS, Mor R, Weu MT, Schwartz D, Schwartz IF, Chernin G. Anemia and iron deficiency in COPD patients: prevalence and the effects of correction of the anemia with erythropoiesis stimulating agents and intravenous iron. BMC Pulm Med. 2014;14:24.
27. Centers for Disease Control and Prevention. CDC Health Disparities and Inequalities Report — United States, 2013. https://www.cdc.gov/mmwr/pdf/other/su6203.pdf. Accessed 1 June 2018.

28. Decramer M, Janssens W. Chronic obstructive pulmonary disease and comorbidities. Lancet Respir Med. 2013;1:73–83.

29. Hillas G, Perlikos F, Tsiligianni I, Tzanakis N. Managing comorbidities in COPD. Int J Chron Obstruct Pulmon Dis. 2015;10:95–109.

30. Rodriguez CJ, Allison M, Daviglus ML, Isasi CR, Keller C, Leira EC, et al. Status of cardiovascular disease and stroke in Hispanics/Latinos in the United States: a science advisory from the American Heart Association. Circulation. 2014;130:593–625.

31. O'Donnell DE, Ciavaglia CE, Neder JA. When obesity and chronic obstructive pulmonary disease collide. Physiological and clinical consequences. Ann Am Thorac Soc. 2014;11:635–44.

32. Katz P, Iribarren C, Sanchez G, Blanc PD. Obesity and functioning among individuals with chronic obstructive pulmonary disease (COPD). COPD. 2016; 13:352–9.

33. Oh YM, Bhome AB, Boonsawat W, Gunasekera KD, Madegedara D, Idolor L, et al. Characteristics of stable chronic obstructive pulmonary disease patients in the pulmonology clinics of seven Asian cities. Int J Chron Obstruct Pulmon Dis. 2013;8:31–9.

20

External validation of the Scandinavian guidelines for management of minimal, mild and moderate head injuries in children

Johan Undén[16,17], Stuart R. Dalziel[11,12], Meredith L. Borland[4,5], Natalie Phillips[6], Amit Kochar[7], Mark D. Lyttle[2,13,14], Silvia Bressan[2,15], John A. Cheek[1,2,9], Jocelyn Neutze[10], Susan Donath[2,3], Stephen Hearps[2], Ed Oakley[1,2,3], Sarah Dalton[8], Yuri Gilhotra[6], Franz E. Babl[1,2,3]* and on behalf of the Paediatric Research in Emergency Departments International Collaborative (PREDICT)

Abstract

Background: Clinical decision rules (CDRs) aid in the management of children with traumatic brain injury (TBI). Recently, the Scandinavian Neurotrauma Committee (SNC) has published practical, evidence-based guidelines for children with Glasgow Coma Scale (GCS) scores of 9–15. This study aims to validate these guidelines and to compare them with other CDRs.

Methods: A large prospective cohort of children (< 18 years) with TBI of all severities, from ten Australian and New Zealand hospitals, was used to assess the SNC guidelines. Firstly, a validation study was performed according to the inclusion and exclusion criteria of the SNC guideline. Secondly, we compared the accuracy of SNC, CATCH, CHALICE and PECARN CDRs in patients with GCS 13–15 only. Diagnostic accuracy was calculated for outcome measures of need for neurosurgery, clinically important TBI (ciTBI) and brain injury on CT.

Results: The SNC guideline could be applied to 19,007/20,137 of patients (94.4%) in the validation process. The frequency of ciTBI decreased significantly with stratification by decreasing risk according to the SNC guideline. Sensitivities for the detection of neurosurgery, ciTBI and brain injury on CT were 100.0% (95% CI 89.1–100.0; 32/32), 97.8% (94.5–99.4; 179/183) and 95% (95% CI 91.6–97.2; 262/276), respectively, with a CT/admission rate of 42% (mandatory CT rate of 5%, 18% CT or admission and 19% only admission). Four patients with ciTBI were missed; none needed specific intervention. In the homogenous comparison cohort of 18,913 children, the SNC guideline performed similar to the PECARN CDR, when compared with the other CDRs.

Conclusion: The SNC guideline showed a high accuracy in a large external validation cohort and compares well with published CDRs for the management of paediatric TBI.

Keywords: Head trauma, Head injury, Guideline, Clinical decision rule, Infant, Child, Computed tomography, Scandinavia

Background

Traumatic brain injury (TBI) is a major global health problem [1] with a general incidence of 262 per 100,000 per year [2], which does not seem to be declining despite increased knowledge and prevention strategies [3]. TBI is common in both developed and also in low- and middle-income countries and is associated with considerable mortality and morbidity [3, 4]. The incidence of TBI is higher in children than in adults [5], children are often more difficult to assess and neuroradiological management is associated with concerning health risks [6, 7].

Initial management is focused on the detection or exclusion of significant brain injury, in particular injuries that would need neurosurgical procedures. The gold-standard investigation is computed tomography (CT), which reliably detects and excludes intracranial complications following

* Correspondence: franz.babl@rch.org.au
[1]Department of Emergency Medicine, Royal Children's Hospital, 50 Flemington Rd, Parkville, Victoria 3052, Australia
[2]Murdoch Children's Research Institute, Melbourne, 50 Flemington Rd, Parkville, Victoria 3052, Australia
Full list of author information is available at the end of the article

head injury. However, the concerns of economic, logistic and radiation burden of increasing CT use limits its use for all children with head injury [8–11]. An alternative option is admission to hospital of intermediate risk groups for clinical observation with deferred CT imaging if signs and symptoms worsen or do not improve, a practice which has been demonstrated to be safe but may be associated with higher health care costs [12, 13].

Clinical decision rules (CDRs) have been developed to stratify patients according to the risk of important outcomes and hence indication for CT, with the goal of optimising resource use while assuring detection of important intracranial injuries. Several CDRs for children have been developed including the Pediatric Emergency Care Applied Research Network (PECARN) rule, the Canadian Assessment of Tomography for Childhood Head Injury (CATCH) rule and the Children's Head Injury Algorithm for the Prediction of Important Clinical Events (CHALICE) rule [14–16]. These were derived using high-quality methods and have recently been externally validated in a large prospective cohort [17]. Although the PECARN rule seems to display the best accuracy [17], in particular a very high sensitivity for relevant outcomes, the actual impact of such a rule will depend on the target population and baseline management routines. Although not borne out by recent data [18, 19], there is an ongoing concern that these rules may increase CT use in some settings [20].

Recently, the Scandinavian Neurotrauma Committee (SNC), a non-profit organisation of neurosurgeons, anaesthesiologists, intensivists, neurologists and other specialties from Sweden, Norway, Denmark, Finland and Iceland, with an interest in TBI, developed and published evidence-based guidelines for management of minimal, mild and moderate head injuries in adults [21] and children [20]. These guidelines offer a comprehensive guide to TBI management, including selection of patients for CT scan and/or hospital observation, in the context of the Scandinavian health care system, see Fig. 1. As these guidelines were not based on a derivation cohort, validation, in particular external validation, is required before widespread clinical implementation.

Recently, Babl et al. published an appropriately powered multicentre validation and comparison study, the Australian Paediatric Head Injury Rules Study (APHIRST), comparing the accuracy of the PECARN, CHALICE and CATCH CDRs [17, 22]. This study included sufficient predictor variables to externally validate the SNC guidelines. In addition to an external validation as the primary aim, we set out to compare the SNC guidelines to the PECARN, CHALICE and CATCH CDRs.

Methods
Design and setting
The APHIRST study was a prospective multicentre observational study, which enrolled 20,137 children (age < 18 years) with head injury of all severities at ten Australian and New Zealand centres of the Paediatric Research in Emergency Departments International Collaborative (PREDICT) network [23]. Predictor variables from the PECARN, CATCH and CHALICE were collected, and the performance accuracy of these rules was externally validated. Detailed information on this study can be found in the primary publication [16] and the protocol publication [22].

The SNC guideline is intended for all children (< 18 years) with head injury and a GCS of 9–15, presenting within 24 h of injury [20]. Being a tool for selecting children for imaging, those children who have already had imaging are excluded.

Procedure
In most cases, the clinical predictors elicited in the APHIRST study were identical to the ones used in the SNC guideline. In the few instances where variables were different, assumptions were made a priori to analysis, see Table 1. SNC guideline parameters were applied to the APHIRST dataset, and suggested management was noted.

As with the APHIRST parent publication [17], the SNC guideline was assessed in two ways. Firstly, the cohort was inputted into the SNC guideline according to the guideline inclusion criteria and with the intended SNC primary outcomes, neurosurgical intervention and intracranial injury [20]. Secondly, the same comparison cohort used in the parent publication [17], i.e. children with a GCS of 13–15 who presented within 24 h of injury, was used in order to compare the SNC guideline with PECARN, CHALICE and CATCH CDRs. The common outcome variable used to compare the accuracy of the SNC guideline and the three CDRs was the presence of clinically important TBI (ciTBI) [14].

Definitions
Neurosurgery was defined as any neurosurgical procedure for TBI.

ciTBI was defined according to the PECARN definition; death from TBI, neurosurgical intervention for TBI, intubation of more than 24 h from TBI or hospital admission of two nights or more for TBI, associated with TBI on CT [14].

TBI on CT was defined as any acute intracranial finding revealed on CT that was attributable to acute injury, including closed depressed skull fractures and pneumocephalus, but excluding non-depressed skull fractures and basilar skull fractures [14].

As the SNC guideline recommends both CT and/or hospital admission with observation, depending on the

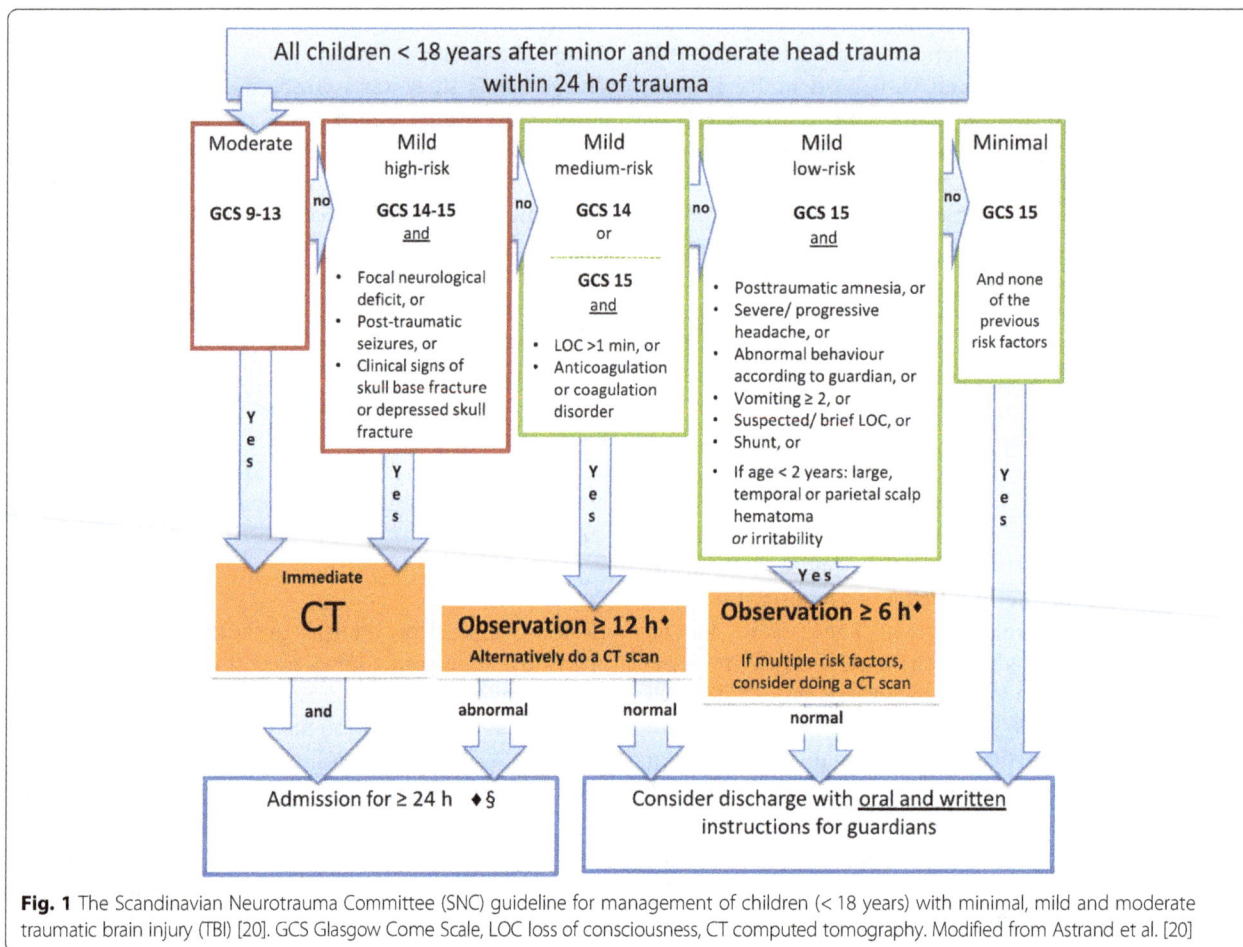

Fig. 1 The Scandinavian Neurotrauma Committee (SNC) guideline for management of children (< 18 years) with minimal, mild and moderate traumatic brain injury (TBI) [20]. GCS Glasgow Come Scale, LOC loss of consciousness, CT computed tomography. Modified from Astrand et al. [20]

risk group, a binary variable was assumed where CT and/or observation was compared to discharge. This is similar to the method used for the external validation of the PECARN rule [17].

Analysis

We did not undertake a separate sample size calculation beyond the sample size calculation undertaken for the APHIRST parent study [22].

Sensitivity, specificity and predictive values were calculated with corresponding 95% confidence intervals. Differences between risk groups were assessed by Fisher's exact test.

Results

From the original sample of 20,137 children, we applied SNC guideline eligibility criteria and excluded 1013 children who presented > 24 h after injury and 117 with GCS < 9. Therefore, a total of 19,007 children (94% of the total cohort) were applicable to the SNC guideline. Selected patient characteristics are shown in Table 2.

Validation of SNC guideline

Thirty-two (0.17%) children needed neurosurgery, 183 (1.0%) had ciTBI, 276 (1.5%) had a TBI on CT and one patient died (TBI was not the cause of death in this patient). The distribution of children in the different SNC risk categories, with corresponding neurosurgery, ciTBI and brain injury on CT outcomes, is shown in Fig. 2. There were significant differences between the risk groups in terms of ciTBI frequency. When combining groups to represent the recommendations of 'immediate CT', 'observation or CT', 'observation' and 'discharge', there were also highly significant differences, see Fig. 2. In the primary analysis of the SNC guideline, point sensitivities for the detection of neurosurgery, ciTBI and TBI on CT were 100, 98 and 95%, respectively, and point specificities were 58, 59 and 59%, respectively (Table 3).

SNC guideline comparison with CDRs

Of 18,913 children included in the comparison cohort, we further omitted patients with a GCS of 9–12. Twenty-four (0.13%) children needed neurosurgery, 160 (0.85%) had ciTBI, 251 (1.3%) had TBI on CT and one patient died. Point sensitivities and specificities for the

Table 1 Comparison of inclusion criteria, exclusion criteria and clinical predictors between the Australasian Paediatric Head Injury Rules Study (APHIRST) cohort and the Scandinavian Neurotrauma Committee (SNC) guidelines

APHIRST	SNC
Inclusion criteria	
All children < 18 years, all GCS	All children < 18 years with head injury within 24 h of trauma, GCS 9–15
Exclusion criteria	
Trivial facial injury only	Prior imaging
Referral from ER to external provider	
Neuroimaging before transfer to site	
Did not wait to be seen	
Predictor variables	
GCS 9–13	GCS 9–13
GCS 14	GCS 14
Positive focal neurology	Focal neurological deficit
Seizure in patient with no history of epilepsy	Post-traumatic seizures
(Clinical signs of basal skull fracture) OR (suspicion of penetrating or depressed skull injury)	Clinical signs of skull base fracture or depressed skull fracture
LOC > 5 s	LOC > 1 min
Any bleeding disorder or anticoagulation therapy	Anticoagulation or coagulation disorder
Amnesia (antegrade or retrograde; > 5 min)	Post-traumatic amnesia
(Severe headache) OR (history of worsening headache)	Severe/progressive headache
Not acting normally per parent report	Abnormal behaviour according to guardian
Vomiting ≥ 2 episodes	Vomiting ≥ 2 episodes
Any or suspected LOC	Suspected/brief LOC
Shunt	Shunt
(Age < 2 and irritability on examination) OR (age < 2 and temporal or parietal hematoma) OR (age < 2 and large, boggy scalp hematoma)	If age < 2 years, large, temporal or parietal scalp hematoma OR irritability
Combination of at least two risk factors from the SNC predictors	Multiple risk factors

GCS Glasgow Come Scale, *ER* emergency room, *LOC* loss of consciousness

detection of neurosurgery, ciTBI and TBI on CT were similar to the validation cohort (Table 4). Four patients with ciTBI and 14 with TBI on CT were missed by the SNC guideline (Table 5). All the missed ciTBIs were classified as such due to admission to hospital > 2 days for TBI, with none needing any specific intervention.

CT and observation rate

Applying the SNC guideline would have resulted in a CT/in-hospital observation rate of 42% in both the validation sample and in the comparison cohort. When strictly applied, the mandatory CT rate for the SNC guideline (Fig. 1) would have been only 5% in both the validation and comparison cohorts, with an 18% rate of observation *or* CT and a 19% rate for only observation (no CT). If children with multiple risk factors and medium-risk factors (observation or CT according to the guideline) were all to receive a CT, the rate would be 23%.

Discussion

In this study, we were able to apply a multinational clinical head injury guideline from Scandinavia to a large, previously collected data set of head injured children and externally assess the accuracy of the guideline. This study appears to adequately validate the accuracy of the SNC guidelines for the management of minimal, mild and moderate head injury in children. In the validation cohort, the guideline displayed a high sensitivity for important outcomes, missing four patients with ciTBI, 14 patients with TBI on CT scan, but no patients requiring neurosurgery out of over 19,000 patients. The SNC guideline was designed to be a pragmatic and universal aid [20]; as demonstrated by the large number of patients, the guideline could be applied to the current APHIRST cohort. Only patients with severe head injury, those who already had neuroimaging and those seeking medical care after 24 h are excluded by the guideline.

When comparing the applicability of the SNC guideline with well-known CDRs, when used as designed [24],

Table 2 Patient characteristics in the entire Australasian Paediatric Head Injury Rules Study (APHIRST) cohort, the APHIRST comparison cohort and the patients eligible for the Scandinavian Neurotrauma Committee (SNC) guideline

	APHIRST validation n = 20,137	APHIRST comparison n = 18,913	SNC n = 19,007
DEMOGRAPHICS			
Mean age	5.7 (sd 4.7)	5.7 (sd 4.6)	5.7 (sd 4.6)
< 2 years	5374 (26.7%)	5046 (26.7%)	5067 (26.7%)
≥ 2 years	14,763 (73.3%)	13,867 (73.3%)	13,940 (73.3%)
Boys	12,828 (63.7%)	12,073 (63.8%)	12,136 (63.9%)
Girls	7309 (36.3%)	6840 (36.2%)	6871 (36.1%)
Injury mechanism			
Fall	14,119 (70.1%)	13,337 (70.5%)	13,401 (70.5%)
Motor vehicle incident	849 (4.2%)	745 (3.9%)	759 (4.0%)
High-impact projetile or object	1320 (6.6%)	1228 (6.5%)	1232 (6.5%)
Suspected non-accidental injury	112 (0.6%)	81 (0.4%)	85 (0.4%)
High-energy/velocity trauma	1669 (8.3%)	1523 (8.1%)	1543 (8.1%)
Predictor examples			
GCS3–8	121 (0.6%)	–	–
GCS 9–13	231 (1.2%)	132 (0.7%)	226 (1.2%)
GCS 14	578 (2.9%)	567 (3.0%)	567 (3.0%)
GCS 15	19,207 (95.4%)	18,214 (96.3%)	18,214 (95.8%)
LOC	2707 (13.5%)	2468 (13.0%)	2506 (13.2%)
Vomiting	3452 (17.1%)	3094 (16.4%)	3138 (16.5%)
Headache	4127 (20.5%)	3785 (20.0%)	3810 (20.0%)
Multiple risk factors	2597 (12.9%)	2324 (12.3%)	2359 (12.4%)
Outcomes			
Cranial CT	2106 (10.5%)	1691 (8.9%)	1760 (9.3%)
Admission	4544 (22.6%)	4164 (22.0%)	4229 (22.2%)
ER discharge	15,594 (77.4%)	14,749 (78.0%)	14,778 (77.8%)
Neurosurgery	83 (0.4%)	24 (0.1%)	32 (0.2%)
Death	15 (0.1%)	1 (< 0.01%)	1 (< 0.01%)
Clinically important TBI (PECARN)	280 (1.4%)	160 (0.8%)	183 (1.0%)
Clinically significant intracranial injury (CHALICE)	403 (2.0%)	251 (1.3%)	276 (1.5%)

GCS Glasgow Come Scale, ER emergency room, LOC loss of consciousness, CT computed tomography, TBI traumatic brain injury, PECARN Paediatric Emergency Care Applied Research Network, CHALICE Children's Head Injury Algorithm for the Prediction of Important Clinical Events, NS neurosurgery, ciTBI clinically important traumatic brain injury, sd standard deviation

the SNC guideline was applicable to a high percentage of the patient cohort (94%); similar to the CHALICE rule (99.5%), a rule including all severities of head injury, and more inclusive than the CATCH (24.6%) and PECARN rules (75.3%) [17]. Adherence to clinical guidelines and CDRs may be problematic [25, 26], especially when dealing with specific and multiple inclusion criteria for guideline applicability [24]. A pragmatic guideline with near-universal inclusion is therefore desirable to ensure clinical use as intended.

Comparing guidelines is difficult due to the differing inclusion criteria, clinical predictors and outcome variables used. Using the APHIRST dataset, a comparison cohort (identical to the SNC inclusion criteria with the exception of patients with GCS 9–12) could be used to directly compare the accuracy of the different rules. The performance of the SNC guideline was similar to the PECARN CDR (high sensitivity, lower specificity) rather than the CATCH and CHALICE CDRs (lower sensitivities but higher specificities). However, the confidence intervals overlap, meaning a statistical difference cannot formally be established. Nonetheless, for the outcome of neurosurgery (the primary outcome variable of the SNC guideline and arguably the most important outcome variable in TBI [17, 20]), the SNC guideline was 100% sensitive, with a relatively high lower 95% confidence

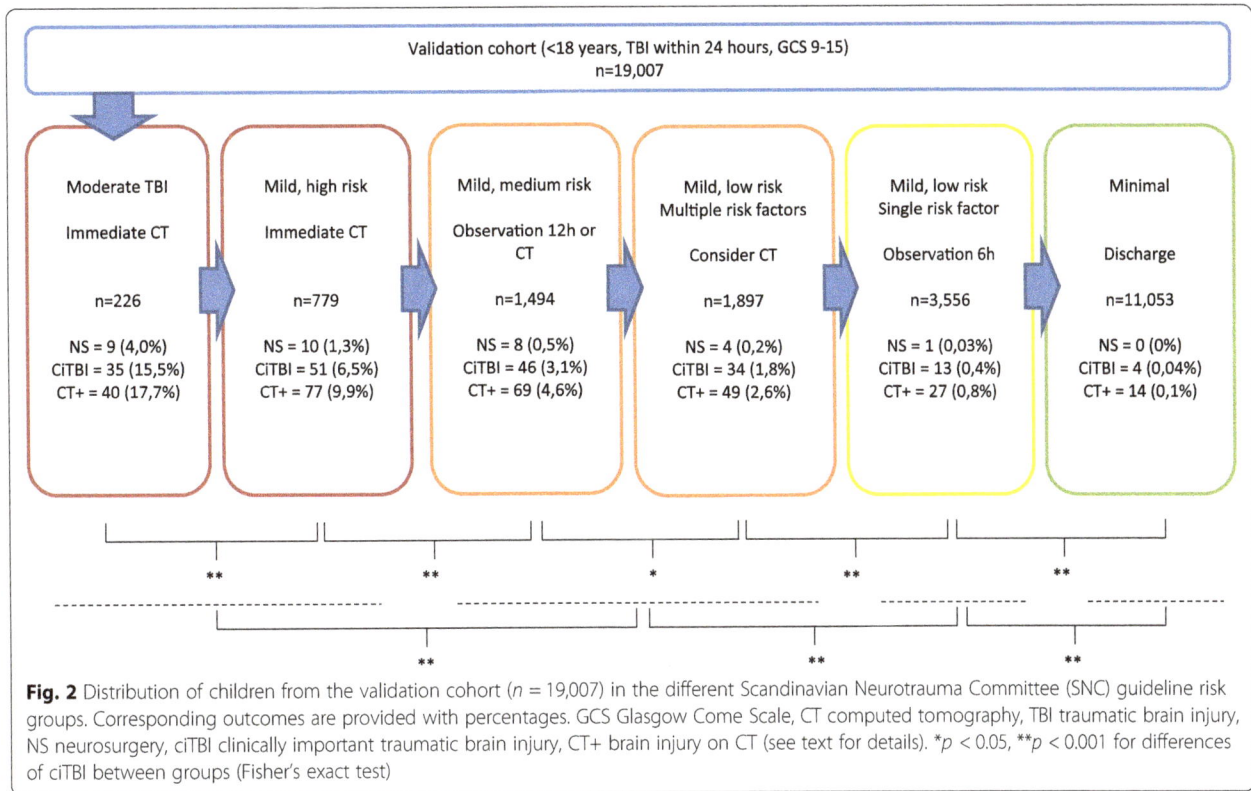

Fig. 2 Distribution of children from the validation cohort (*n* = 19,007) in the different Scandinavian Neurotrauma Committee (SNC) guideline risk groups. Corresponding outcomes are provided with percentages. GCS Glasgow Come Scale, CT computed tomography, TBI traumatic brain injury, NS neurosurgery, ciTBI clinically important traumatic brain injury, CT+ brain injury on CT (see text for details). *p < 0.05, **p < 0.001 for differences of ciTBI between groups (Fisher's exact test)

interval (85.8%) and a higher overall specificity than PECARN. As an evidence-based guideline, the largest individual evidence contributor for the synthesis of the SNC guideline was derived from the PECARN study, which likely explains the similarities in performance.

The projected CT or admission rate for SNC of 42%, in both the validation and comparison sample, is difficult to compare with the CATCH or CHALICE CDRs. Both dichotomise patients into CT/no CT, without consideration of observation, with projected CT rates for CATCH of 30% (using all predictors) and for the CHALICE rule of 22%, for the comparison cohorts. However, as with the PECARN CDR [14], the SNC guideline has both a CT and in-hospital observation management

option, depending on the risk group. The rate for mandatory CT (moderate or high-risk mild TBI according to the guidelines) was only 5%, which increases to 23% if children with medium-risk mild TBI or multiple risk factors (observation or CT according to the guideline) were all to receive a CT.

No patients requiring neurosurgery would be discharged according to the SNC guideline. One patient needing neurosurgery was assigned to the 6-h in-hospital observation group and another 12 patients needing neurosurgery to the in-hospital observation or CT groups. The present study did not include necessary details to examine if the SNC observation routines, mandating a CT scan when a fall in GCS or new/progressive

Table 3 Performance of the Scandinavian Neurotrauma Committee (SNC) guidelines in the validation cohort (*n* = 19,007)

Outcome	Neurosurgery[a]	ciTBI[a]	Brain injury on CT[a]
SNC CT or observation, with outcome	32	179	262
SNC CT or observation, without outcome	7921	7775	7692
SNC discharge, with outcome	0	4	14
SNC discharge, without outcome	11,052	11,049	11,039
Sensitivity (95% CI)	100% (89.1–100)	97.8% (94.5–99.4)	94.9% (91.6–97.2)
Specificity (95% CI)	58.3% (57.5–59.0)	58.7% (58.0–59.4)	58.9% (58.2–59.6)
PPV (95% CI)	0.4% (0.3–0.6)	2.3% (1.9–2.6)	3.3% (2.9–3.7)
NPV (95% CI)	100% (100–100)	100% (99.9–100)	99.9% (99.8–99.9)

CT computed tomography, *PPV* positive predictive value, *NPV* negative predictive value, *ciTBI* clinically important traumatic brain injury
[a]See text for detailed definitions

Table 4 Performance of the PECARN, CATCH, CHALICE and SNC guidelines in the comparison cohort with all children presenting within 24 h of injury and GCS 13–15 (n = 18,913)

	PECARN				CATCH		CHALICE		SNC	
	< 2 years		2 years							
	n = 5046		n = 13,867							
Primary outcome										
	Positive	Negative	Positive	Negative	Positive	Negative	Positive	Negative	Positive	Negative
Clinically important traumatic brain injury *	Yes 42	0	Yes 117	1	Yes 147	13	Yes 148	12	Yes 156	4
	No 2047	2957	No 6606	7143	No 5560	13,193	No 4018	14,735	No 7704	11,049
Sens (95% CI)	42/42		117/118		147/160		148/160		156/160	
	100·0% (91·6–100·0)		99·2% (95·4–100·0)		91·9% (86·5–95·6)		92·5% (87·3–96·1)		97·5% (93·7–99·3)	
Spec (95% CI)	2957/5004		7143/13749		13,193/18753		14,735/18753		11,049/18753	
	59·1% (57·7–60·5)		52·0% (51·1–52·8)		70·4% (69·7–71·0)		78·6% (78·0–79·2)		58·9% (58·2–59·6)	
PPV (95% CI)	42/2089		117/6723		147/5707		148/4166		156/7860	
	2·0% (1·5–2·7)		1·7% (1·4–2·1)		2·6% (2·2–3·0)		3·6% (3·0–4·2)		2·0% (1·7–2·3)	
NPV (95% CI)	2957/2957		7143/7144		13,193/13206		14,735/14747		11,049/11053	
	100·0% (99·9–100·0)		100·0% (99·9–100·0)		99·9% (99·8–99·9)		99·9% (99·9–100·0)		100% (99·9–100·0)	
Secondary outcomes										
	Positive	Negative	Positive	Negative	Positive	Negative	Positive	Negative	Positive	Negative
Traumatic brain injury on CT*	Yes 70	0	Yes 180	1	Yes 220	31	Yes 227	24	Yes 237	14
	No 2019	2957	No 6543	7143	No 5487	13,175	No 3939	14,723	No 7623	11,039
Sens (95% CI)	70/70		180/181		220/251		227/251		237/251	
	100·0% (94·9–100·0)		99·4% (97·0–100·0)		87·6% (82·9–91·5)		90·4% (86·1–93·8)		94·4% (90·8–96·9)	
Spec (95% CI)	2957/4976		7143/13686		13,175/18662		14,723/18662		11,039/18662	
	59·4% (58·0–60·8)		52·2% (51·4–53·0)		70·6% (69·9–71·3)		78·9% (78·3–79·5)		59·2% (58·4–59·9)	
PPV (95% CI)	70/2089		180/6723		220/5707		227/4166		237/7860	
	3·4% (2·6–4·2)		2·7% (2·3–3·1)		3·9% (3·4–4·4)		5·4% (4·8–6·2)		3·0% (2·6–3·4)	
NPV (95% CI)	2957/2957		7143/7144		13,175/13206		14,723/14747		11,039/11053	
	100·0% (99·9–100·0)		100·0% (99·9–100·0)		99·8% (99·7–99·8)		99·8% (99·8–99·9)		99·9% (99·8–99·9)	
	Positive	Negative	Positive	Negative	Positive	Negative	Positive	Negative	Positive	Negative
Neurosurgery*	Yes 6	0	Yes 18 0		Yes 23	1	Yes 22	2	Yes 24	0
	No 2083	2957	No 6705	7144	No 5684	13, 205	No 4144	14,745	No 7835	11,052
Sens (95% CI)	6/6		18/18		23/24		22/24		24/24	
	100·0% (54·1–100·0)		100·0% (81·5–100·0)		95·8% (78·9–99·9)		91·7% (73·0–99·0)		100·0% (85·8–100·0)	
Spec (95% CI)	2957/5040		7144/13849		13,205/18889		14,745/18889		11,052/18889	
	58·7% (57·3–60·0)		51·6% (50·7–52·4)		69·9% (69·2–70·6)		78·1% (77·5–78·6)		58·5% (57·8–59·2)	
PPV (95% CI)	6/2089		18/6723		23/5707		22/4166		24/7859	
	0·3% (0·1–0·6)		0·3% (0·2–0·4)		0·4% (0·3–0·6)		0·5% (0·3–0·8)		0·3% (0·2–0·5)	
NPV (95% CI)	2957/2957		7144/7144		13,205/13206		14,745/14747		11,052/11052	
	100·0 (99·9–100·0)		100·0% (99·9–100·0)		100·0% (100·0–100·0)		100·0% (100·0–100·0)		100·0% (100·0–100·0)	

PECARN Paediatric Emergency Care Applied Research Network, *CATCH* Canadian Assessment of Tomography for Childhood Head Injury, *CHALICE* Children's Head Injury Algorithm for the Prediction of Important Clinical Events, *Sens* sensitivity, *Spec* specificity, *PPV* positive predictive value, *NPV* negative predictive value
[a]See text for detailed definitions

neurological symptoms are observed, would have led to a prompt CT scan for these patients. Children are not to be discharged from hospital until their symptoms (i.e. clinical predictors) have resolved [20]. Overall, this approach may be more expensive than a CT option [13], but removes the logistics and potential radiation risks associated with CT scans.

The corresponding numbers for mandatory CT for the PECARN CDR are not known, though the CT rate

Table 5 Characteristics of patients with Glasgow Come Score (GCS) 13–15 presenting within 24 h after injury in the comparison cohort with clinically important traumatic brain injury (CiTBI) not identified by Scandinavian Neurotrauma Committee (SNC) guideline

Age	Gender	GCS	Mechanism of injury	Injury recorded on CT	Neurosurgery	Clinically important traumatic brain injury
6 years	F	15	Fall 1.5 m–3 m	Intracranial haemorrhage/contusion—extra-axial Pneumocephalus Skull fracture—non depressed	No	Yes Admitted > 2 days
10 years	F	15	Fall from motorised vehicle	Intracranial haemorrhage/contusion—extra-axial and parenchymal Pneumocephalus Basilar skull fracture	No	Yes Admitted > 2 days
15 years	M	15	Unclear	Intracranial haemorrhage/contusion—parenchymal	No	Yes Admitted > 2 days
2 years	M	15	Kicked by animal	Intracranial contusion—parenchymal Depressed skull fracture	No	Yes Admitted > 2 days

CT computed tomography

would probably be higher due to presence of GCS 14 and altered mental status as predictors for mandatory CT. The presence of these risk factors was a major issue when the SNC workgroup were deciding on the adaptation of an external guideline (PECARN) or synthesising a new, evidence-based guideline. We chose to use the latter strategy, as the group found GCS 14 to be too unreliable as a risk factor to recommend a mandatory CT [27–29] and altered mental status too complicated to use effectively, with potential to lead to unacceptable increases in CT rates in Scandinavia. For this reason, allowing an element of physician judgement in the medium-risk group was chosen.

Unlike other guidelines, the SNC stratifies patients into multiple risk groups for important outcomes. This allows physicians to further understand the potential impact of management in patients. Our analysis confirms the stratification, with higher risk groups showing significantly higher rates of important outcome, such as ciTBI, with gradual reduction of these rates with decreasing risk Fig. 2.

High-energy trauma mechanism is not a strict risk factor in the SNC guidelines. These patients are relatively uncommon in Scandinavia and are managed according to separate clinical trauma protocols. Most receive CT scanning and all of these children are admitted. This risk factor was also judged as complicated to use, having a specific definition and often including assessment of fall height, vehicle speed and number of stairs. In the validation cohort, 1543 patients were involved in high-energy trauma, 65 had brain injury on CT, 50 had ciTBI and 9 needed neurosurgery. All patients needing neurosurgery were identified by other predictors included in the SNC guideline. This suggests that omitting this risk factor is safe in the presence of other risk factors included in the guideline.

Children with suspicion of non-accidental injury (NAI) are always admitted to hospital in Scandinavia and generally receive diagnostic imaging. However, this is not a defined risk factor in the actual guideline, although it is clearly stated that these children should be admitted independent of TBI predictors [20].

In adult TBI management, biomarkers, specifically S100B, have been recommended in clinical guidelines as they could reduce CT rates and overall costs [30] and studies in children have shown promise [31]. Such a biomarker would be most valuable in the intermediate risk groups, such as the medium- and low-risk groups from the SNC guidelines (i.e. the groups presently managed with in-hospital observation), especially considering that today's clinical predictors seem to have reached their full potential for decision making. Indeed, the actual CT rate from the APHIRST study was only 8.9% in the comparison cohort [17], indicating that clinical guidelines may have limited effect in situations with high-baseline clinician accuracy and low CT rates [32]. However, the evidence base for S100B is too weak for a clinical recommendation in children. Other potential biomarkers have shown promise in adults [33], but studies in children are lacking.

Ultimately, the choice of a guideline will be dependent on the baseline situation and intended effect in the health care setting. Before the SNC guideline, most Swedish hospitals did not have official management pathways for paediatric head injury [34] and many used the SNC guideline from 2000 [13], intended for adults. Although the PECARN rules are based upon a rigorously powered cohort and are externally validated, Scandinavian experts were reluctant to recommend these rules for clinical practice, instead opting for a pragmatic, universal and comprehensive evidence-based option [20]. The results of this study support this approach.

The main strength of this study is the large dataset which was robustly powered and prospectively collected. Also, the dataset was adopted into the guideline by an author (SH) unconnected with the SNC group. However, a limitation is that the dataset was not designed with the

SNC guidelines in mind (published first after the study was commenced), but to assess the accuracy of PECARN, CHALICE and CATCH. Clinical predictors were, however, identical in most cases. The few cases where clinical predictors were approximated would likely not have affected the overall performance of the guideline. Additionally, the clinical setting was that of Australian and New Zealand emergency predominately tertiary departments, which may differ from care in the Scandinavian countries for which the SNC guideline was developed.

Conclusion

In this study, we were able to apply the clinical SNC head injury guideline to a large, previously collected data set of head injured children. The evidence-based SNC head injury guideline was externally assessed in terms of its accuracy and found to have a high sensitivity, missing very few patients with ciTBI and none needing neurosurgery. The present validation study supports the clinical use of the guideline, although national validation in Scandinavian countries may also be warranted.

Abbreviations
CATCH: Canadian Assessment of Tomography for Childhood Head Injury; CDR: Clinical Decision Rule; CHALICE: Children's Head Injury Algorithm for the Prediction of Important Clinical Events; ciTBI: Clinically important TBI; CT: Computed tomography; PECARN: Pediatric Emergency Care Applied Research Network; PREDICT: Paediatric Research in Emergency Departments International Collaborative; SNC: Scandinavian Neurotrauma Committee; TBI: Traumatic brain injury

Acknowledgements
We would like to thank all the participating centres for the collection of data.

Funding
This present study was funded by non-commercial Swedish state sources Region Skåne and Region Halland, Sweden.
The APHIRST parent study was funded by grants from the National Health and Medical Research Council (project grant GNT1046727, Centre of Research Excellence for Paediatric Emergency Medicine GNT1058560), Canberra, Australia; the Murdoch Children's Research Institute, Melbourne, Australia; the Emergency Medicine Foundation (EMPJ-11162), Brisbane, Australia; Perpetual Philanthropic Services (2012/1140), Australia; Auckland Medical Research Foundation (No. 3112011) and the A + Trust (Auckland District Health Board), Auckland, New Zealand; WA Health Targeted Research Funds 2013, Perth, Australia; the Townsville Hospital and Health Service Private Practice Research and Education Trust Fund, Townsville, Australia; and supported by the Victorian Government's Infrastructure Support Program, Melbourne, Australia. FEB's time was part funded by a grant from the Royal Children's Hospital Foundation, Melbourne, Australia, an NHMRC Practitioner Fellowship GNT1124466 and a Melbourne Children's Clinician Scientist Fellowship. SRD's time was part funded by the Health Research Council of New Zealand (HRC13/556).

Authors' contributions
SH did the data calculations, and the results were overviewed by JU. JU drafted the manuscript with input from all authors. All other authors collected the data. All authors have approved the final manuscript.

Competing interests
The authors declare that they have no competing interests.

Author details
[1]Department of Emergency Medicine, Royal Children's Hospital, 50 Flemington Rd, Parkville, Victoria 3052, Australia. [2]Murdoch Children's Research Institute, Melbourne, 50 Flemington Rd, Parkville, Victoria 3052, Australia. [3]Department of Paediatrics, Faculty of Medicine, Dentistry and Health Sciences, University of Melbourne, Melbourne, Grattan St, Parkville, Victoria 3010, Australia. [4]Emergency Department, Princess Margaret Hospital for Children, Roberts Rd, Subiaco, Perth, Western Australia 6008, Australia. [5]Divisions of Paediatrics and Emergency Medicine, School of Medicine, University of Western Australia, 35 Stirling Hwy, Crawley, Western Australia 6009, Australia. [6]Emergency Department, Lady Cilento Children's Hospital, Brisbane and Child Health Research Centre, School of Medicine, The University of Queensland, 501 Stanley St, South Brisbane, Queensland 4101, Australia. [7]Emergency Department, Women's & Children's Hospital, Adelaide, 72 King William St, North Adelaide, South Australia 5006, Australia. [8]Emergency Department, The Children's Hospital at Westmead, 212 Hawkesbury Rd, Westmead, New South Wales 2145, Australia. [9]Emergency Department, Monash Medical Centre, 246 Clayton Rd, Clayton, Victoria 3186, Australia. [10]Emergency Department, Kidzfirst Middlemore Hospital, 100 Hospital Rd, Auckland 2025, New Zealand. [11]Emergency Department, Starship Children's Health, 2 Park Rd, Grafton, Auckland 1023, New Zealand. [12]Liggins Institute, University of Auckland, 85 Park Ave, Grafton, Auckland 1023, New Zealand. [13]Emergency Department, Bristol Children's Hospital, Paul O'Gorman Building, Upper Maudlin St, Bristol BS2 8BJ, UK. [14]Academic Department of Emergency Care, University of the West of England, Blackberry Hill, Bristol BS16 1XS, UK. [15]Department of Women's and Children's Health, University of Padova, Via Giustiniani3, 2, 35128 Padova, Padova, Italy. [16]Department of Operation and Intensive Care, Hallands Hospital, Halmstad, Sweden. [17]Lund University, Lund, Sweden.

References
1. Maas AI, Stocchetti N, Bullock R. Moderate and severe traumatic brain injury in adults. Lancet Neurol. 2008;7(8):728–41.
2. Peeters W, van den Brande R, Polinder S, Brazinova A, Steyerberg EW, Lingsma HF, et al. Epidemiology of traumatic brain injury in Europe. Acta Neurochir. 2015;157(10):1683–96.
3. Maas AIR, Menon DK, Adelson PD, Andelic N, Bell MJ, Belli A, InTBIR Participants and Investigators, et al. Traumatic brain injury: integrated approaches to improve prevention, clinical care, and research. Lancet Neurol. 2017;16(12):987–1048.
4. Hyder AA, Wunderlich CA, Puvanachandra P, Gururaj G, Kobusingye OC. The impact of traumatic brain injuries: a global perspective. NeuroRehabilitation. 2007;22(5):341–53.
5. McKinlay A, Grace RC, Horwood LJ, Fergusson DM, Ridder EM, MacFarlane MR. Prevalence of traumatic brain injury among children, adolescents and young adults: prospective evidence from a birth cohort. Brain Inj. 2008;22(2): 175–81.
6. Brenner DJ, Hall EJ. Computed tomography—an increasing source of radiation exposure. N Engl J Med. 2007;357(22):2277–84.
7. Mathews JD, Forsythe AV, Brady Z, Butler MW, Goergen SK, Byrnes GB, et al. Cancer risk in 680,000 people exposed to computed tomography scans in childhood or adolescence: data linkage study of 11 million Australians. BMJ. 2013;346:f2360.
8. Larson DB, Johnson LW, Schnell BM, Goske MJ, Salisbury SR, Forman HP. Rising use of CT in child visits to the emergency department in the United States, 1995–2008. Radiology. 2011;259(3):793–801.
9. Sodickson A, Baeyens PF, Andriole KP, Prevedello LM, Nawfel RD, Hanson R, et al. Recurrent CT, cumulative radiation exposure, and associated radiation-induced cancer risks from CT of adults. Radiology. 2009;251(1):175–84.
10. Pearce MS, Salotti JA, Little MP, McHugh K, Lee C, Kim KP, et al. Radiation exposure from CT scans in childhood and subsequent risk of leukaemia and brain tumours: a retrospective cohort study. Lancet. 2012;380(9840):499–505.
11. Miglioretti DL, Johnson E, Williams A, Greenlee RT, Weinmann S, Solberg LI, et al. The use of computed tomography in pediatrics and the associated radiation exposure and estimated cancer risk. JAMA Pediatr. 2013;167(8): 700–7.

12. af Geijerstam JL, Oredsson S, Britton M, Study Investigators OCTOPUS. Medical outcome after immediate computed tomography or admission for observation in patients with mild head injury: randomised controlled trial. BMJ. 2006;333(7566):465.

13. Ingebrigtsen T, Romner B, Kock-Jensen C. Scandinavian guidelines for initial management of minimal, mild, and moderate head injuries. Scand Neurotrauma Comm J Trauma. 2000;48(4):760–6.

14. Kuppermann N, Holmes JF, Dayan PS, Hoyle JD Jr, Atabaki SM, Holubkov R, et al. Identification of children at very low risk of clinically-important brain injuries after head trauma: a prospective cohort study. Lancet. 2009; 374(9696):1160–70.

15. Osmond MH, Klassen TP, Wells GA, Correll R, Jarvis A, Joubert G, et al. CATCH: a clinical decision rule for the use of computed tomography in children with minor head injury. CMAJ. 2010;182(4):341–8.

16. Dunning J, Daly JP, Lomas JP, Lecky F, Batchelor J, Mackway-Jones K, et al. Derivation of the children's head injury algorithm for the prediction of important clinical events decision rule for head injury in children. Arch Dis Child. 2006;91(11):885–91.

17. Babl FE, Borland ML, Phillips N, Kochar A, Dalton S, McCaskill M, et al. Accuracy of PECARN, CATCH, and CHALICE head injury decision rules in children: a prospective cohort study. Lancet. 2017;389(10087):2393–402.

18. Bressan S, Romanato S, Mion T, Zanconato S, Da Dalt L. Implementation of adapted PECARN decision rule for children with minor head injury in the pediatric emergency department. Acad Emerg Med. 2012;19(7):801–7.

19. Nigrovic LE, Stack AM, Mannix RC, Lyons TW, Samnaliev M, Bachur RG, et al. Quality improvement effort to reduce cranial CTs for children with minor blunt head trauma. Pediatrics. 2015;136(1):e227–33.

20. Astrand R, Rosenlund C, Unden J, Scandinavian Neurotrauma Committee (SNC). Scandinavian guidelines for initial management of minor and moderate head trauma in children. BMC Med 2016;14:33–016-0574.

21. Unden J, Ingebrigtsen T, Romner B, Scandinavian Neurotrauma Committee (SNC). Scandinavian guidelines for initial management of minimal, mild and moderate head injuries in adults: an evidence and consensus-based update. BMC Med 2013;11:50–7015-11-50.

22. Babl FE, Lyttle MD, Bressan S, Borland M, Phillips N, Kochar A, et al. A prospective observational study to assess the diagnostic accuracy of clinical decision rules for children presenting to emergency departments after head injuries (protocol): the Australasian Paediatric Head Injury Rules Study (APHIRST). BMC Pediatr. 2014;14:148. https://doi.org/10.1186/1471-2431-14-148.

23. Babl F, Borland M, Ngo P, Acworth J, Krieser D, Pandit S, et al. Paediatric Research in Emergency Departments International Collaborative (PREDICT): first steps towards the development of an Australian and New Zealand research network. Emerg Med Australas. 2006;18(2):143–7.

24. Lyttle MD, Cheek JA, Blackburn C, Oakley E, Ward B, Fry A, et al. Applicability of the CATCH, CHALICE and PECARN paediatric head injury clinical decision rules: pilot data from a single Australian centre. Emerg Med J. 2013;30(10):790–4.

25. Gupta A, Ip IK, Raja AS, Andruchow JE, Sodickson A, Khorasani R. Effect of clinical decision support on documented guideline adherence for head CT in emergency department patients with mild traumatic brain injury. J Am Med Inform Assoc. 2014;21(e2):e347–51.

26. Stiell IG, Bennett C. Implementation of clinical decision rules in the emergency department. Acad Emerg Med. 2007;14(11):955–9.

27. Gill M, Martens K, Lynch EL, Salih A, Green SM. Interrater reliability of 3 simplified neurologic scales applied to adults presenting to the emergency department with altered levels of consciousness. Ann Emerg Med. 2007; 49(4):403–7, 407.e1.

28. Gill MR, Reiley DG, Green SM. Interrater reliability of Glasgow Coma Scale scores in the emergency department. Ann Emerg Med. 2004;43(2):215–23.

29. Bledsoe BE, Casey MJ, Feldman J, Johnson L, Diel S, Forred W, et al. Glasgow Coma Scale scoring is often inaccurate. Prehosp Disaster Med. 2015;30(1):46–53.

30. Calcagnile O, Anell A, Unden J. The addition of S100B to guidelines for management of mild head injury is potentially cost saving. BMC Neurol. 2016;16(1):200.

31. Bouvier D, Fournier M, Dauphin JB, Amat F, Ughetto S, Labbé A, Sapin V. Serum S100B determination in the management of pediatric mild traumatic brain injury. Clin Chem. 2012;58(7):1116–22.

32. Babl FE, Oakley E, Dalziel SR, Borland ML, Phillips N, Kochar A, Dalton S, Cheek JA, Gilhotra Y, Furyk J, Neutze J, Donath S, Hearps S, Molesworth C, Crowe L, Bressan S, Lyttle MD. Accuracy of clinician practice compared with three head injury decision rules in children: a prospective cohort study. Ann Emerg Med. 2018;71(6):703-10.

33. Bazarian JJ, Biberthaler P, Welch RD, Lewis LM, Barzo P, Bogner-Flatz V, Gunnar Brolinson P, Büki A, Chen JY, Christenson RH, Hack D, Huff JS, Johar S, Jordan JD, Leidel BA, Lindner T, Ludington E, Okonkwo DO, Ornato J, Peacock WF, Schmidt K, Tyndall JA, Vossough A, Jagoda AS. Serum GFAP and UCH1-L1 in prediction of absence of intracranial injuries on head CT (ALERT-TBI): a multicenter observational study. Lancet Neurol. 2018;17(9):782-9.

34. Astrand R, Unden J, Bellner J, Romner B. Survey of the management of children with minor head injuries in Sweden. Acta Neurol Scand. 2006; 113(4):262–6.

21

The hidden burden of measles in Ethiopia: how distance to hospital shapes the disease mortality rate

Piero Poletti[1*], Stefano Parlamento[1], Tafarraa Fayyisaa[2], Rattaa Feyyiss[2], Marta Lusiani[3], Ademe Tsegaye[3], Giulia Segafredo[4], Giovanni Putoto[4], Fabio Manenti[4] and Stefano Merler[1]

Abstract

Background: A sequence of annual measles epidemics has been observed from January 2013 to April 2017 in the South West Shoa Zone of the Oromia Region, Ethiopia. We aimed at estimating the burden of disease in the affected area, taking into account inequalities in access to health care due to travel distances from the nearest hospital.

Methods: We developed a dynamic transmission model calibrated on the time series of hospitalized measles cases. The model provided estimates of disease transmissibility and incidence at a population level. Model estimates were combined with a spatial analysis to quantify the hidden burden of disease and to identify spatial heterogeneities characterizing the effectiveness of the public health system in detecting severe measles infections and preventing deaths.

Results: A total of 1819 case patients and 36 deaths were recorded at the hospital. The mean age was 6.0 years (range, 0–65). The estimated reproduction number was 16.5 (95% credible interval (CI) 14.5–18.3) with a cumulative disease incidence of 2.34% (95% CI 2.06–2.66). Three thousand eight hundred twenty-one (95% CI 1969–5671) severe cases, including 2337 (95% CI 716–4009) measles-related deaths, were estimated in the Woliso hospital's catchment area (521,771 inhabitants). The case fatality rate was found to remarkably increase with travel distance from the nearest hospital: ranging from 0.6% to more than 19% at 20 km. Accordingly, hospital treatment prevented 1049 (95% CI 757–1342) deaths in the area.

Conclusions: Spatial heterogeneity in the access to health care can dramatically affect the burden of measles disease in low-income settings. In sub-Saharan Africa, passive surveillance based on hospital admitted cases might miss up to 60% of severe cases and 98% of related deaths.

Keywords: Mathematical model, Sub-Saharan Africa, Access to health care, Case fatality rate, Measles epidemic, Infectious diseases

Background

Measles is one of the most contagious vaccine-preventable viral diseases and represents an important cause of child mortality in sub-Saharan Africa [1, 2]. Despite considerable progress has been made during the last decade in measles mortality reduction [3], the persistent circulation of measles in the WHO African Region [1, 4–6] reflects the challenge of achieving sufficiently high herd immunity levels in areas with limited financial resources.

In low-income countries, a strong heterogeneity both in the measles case fatality rate [47] and in the access to health care infrastructures has been widely documented [8–10], although rarely quantified and little understood [8–12].

In particular, some recent epidemiological studies, focusing on a variety of illness conditions, have shown that larger travel distances to large health care facilities are associated with lower hospital admission rates [8–10] and higher mortality [8, 9, 12]. However, these studies

* Correspondence: poletti@fbk.eu
[1]Center for Information Technology, Fondazione Bruno Kessler, via Sommarive, 18, I-38123 Trento, Italy
Full list of author information is available at the end of the article

do not always differentiate between causes of hospitalization and death [11] and few recent works have documented measles mortality in sub-Saharan Africa [13]. As a matter of fact, the burden of disease is still often estimated on the basis of admitted hospital cases, representing a biased sample that does not reflect the severity of measles within the community [7].

In recent years, recurrent measles outbreaks, primarily affecting children below 5 years of age [1], have been reported in several areas of Ethiopia [1, 14], including the Oromia Region [4]. In Ethiopia, the national Expanded Programme on Immunization was established in 1980 and consists of the first dose of measles-containing vaccine (MCV1) administered at 9 months of age. Routine immunization of infants is supplemented by planned campaigns at 2- and 5-year intervals [3], aimed at increasing vaccination coverage and providing the opportunity for a second dose of vaccine to children who did not respond to the first one [3].

Here we analyze a sequence of annual measles epidemics, with 1819 hospitalized cases and 36 deaths, occurring from January 2013 to April 2017 in the South West Shoa Zone of the Oromia Region. Specifically, we describe the epidemiological characteristics of the observed epidemic, providing estimates of the disease transmissibility, incidence, and mortality at population level. In addition, we investigate the spatial heterogeneity characterizing both the detection and treatment of measles infections as a consequence of travel distance to the nearest hospital. The performed analysis highlights the potential hidden burden of disease caused by the heterogeneous access to primary health care in the region.

Methods
Study population and measles case patients
This study was conducted in the South West Shoa Zone of the Oromia Region in Ethiopia (Fig. 1a), with an estimated population of 1,341,702 inhabitants in 2014, of whom 50.3% were men and 49.7% were women. The main hospital is located in Woliso town, 114 km southwest of the capital Addis Ababa, representing the nearest hospital for 521,771 individuals living within an area of 30 km radius from Woliso town (53,065 inhabitants). The hospital has 200 beds with an annual average bed-occupation rate of 84%; single-patient air-borne infection isolation rooms are not available in the hospital.

Data on age, sex, residence at woreda (i.e., district) and kebele (i.e., neighborhood) level, date of hospital admission, and death/discharge of measles case patients from 2013 to 2017 were obtained from the registers of Woliso hospital. Incidence of hospitalizations by woreda and kebele were calculated by assuming population projections for the 2014, based on the 2007 census conducted by the Central Statistical Agency of Ethiopia (Table 1) [15]. Travel distances to the Woliso hospital for different kebeles and woredas were obtained from administrative hospital records on distances of all health posts and largest villages distributed in the main hospital's catchment area (see Table 1). The case fatality rate (CFR) for hospital admitted cases was calculated as the percentage of fatal cases among measles patients recorded. Routine vaccination coverage for this area was derived from administrative records: on average, 88% of children are routinely vaccinated against measles at 9 months of age. Two immunization campaigns were conducted in the area from May 29 to June 5, 2013, and from March 13 to March 20, 2017, targeting children 9–59 months of age [16]; the achieved vaccination coverage is unknown. In 2016, the vaccination status of case patients was assessed for 295 children in the age group 9 months to 5 years.

Patients' records related to different illness conditions recorded at the Woliso hospital between 2014 and 2016 were considered to estimate hospitalization incidence over time and to assess differences in the access to health care and related outcomes with respect to travel distances from the hospital.

Collected data consisted of routine health data and medical records, were encrypted and anonymous, and did not contain any information that might be used to identify individual patients; therefore, the study did not require informed consent.

Synchrony of local epidemics
Synchrony in the timing of epidemics across different woredas was assessed by calculating the cross-correlation of time series at different time lags. The aim of this analysis is twofold: (i) to evaluate whether the observed seasonal pattern is an artifact of averaging asynchronous local epidemics and (ii) to support the hypothesis that observed measles cases were the result of a unique synchronous epidemic with similar epidemiological characteristics across different woredas.

The modeling approach
The baseline analysis combines results of a dynamic transmission model, calibrated on the time series of hospitalized measles cases occurring between 2013 and 2017, with a spatial regression analysis, providing estimates of the measles hospitalization rate at different distances from the Woliso hospital. We restricted the analysis to measles cases from Woliso, Wonchi, Ameya, and Goro woredas, which represent the main hospital catchment area, consisting of 521,771 inhabitants and accounting for 83.1% of recorded case patients. Under the assumption of homogeneous mixing transmission, the baseline model provided estimates

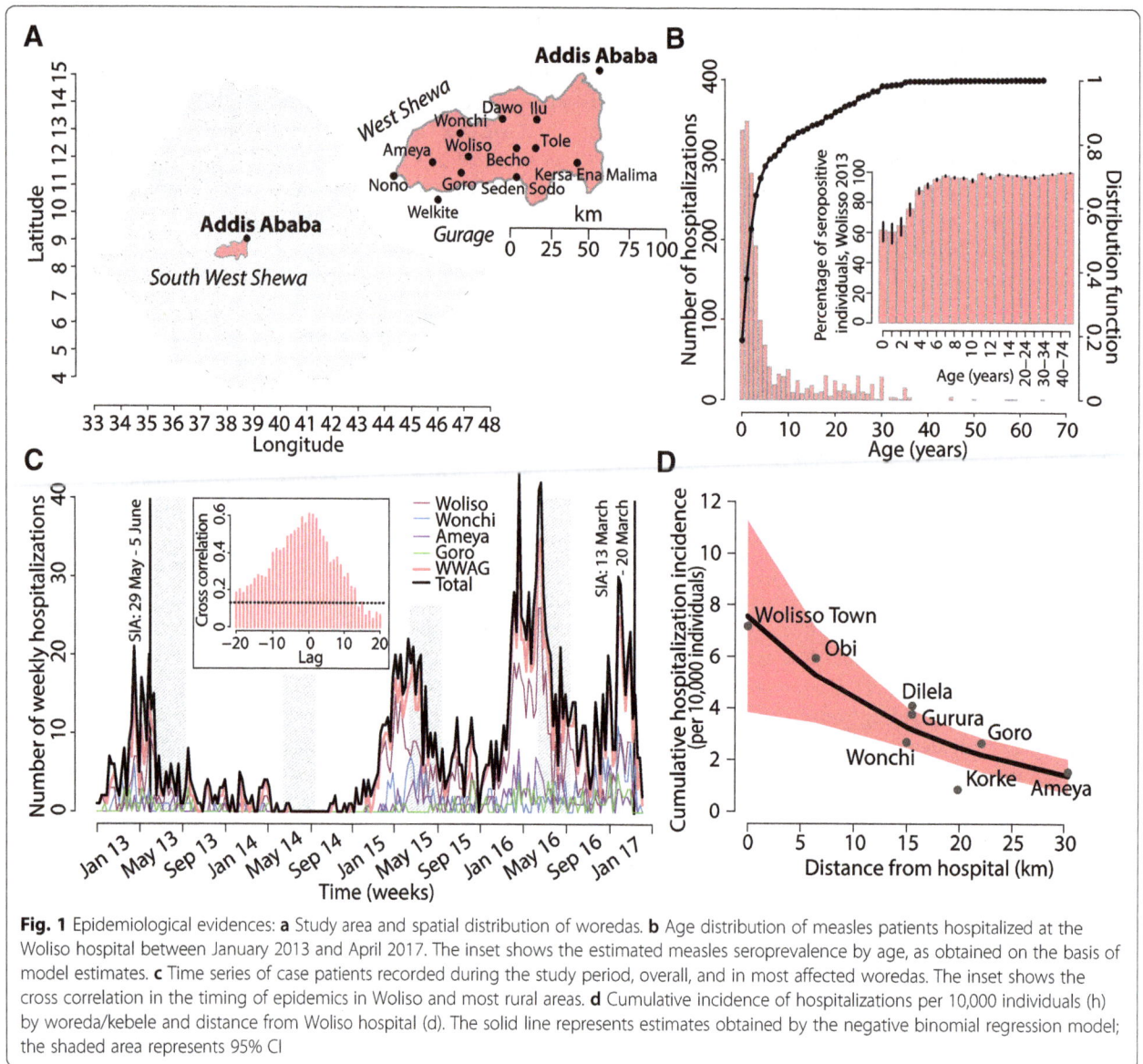

Fig. 1 Epidemiological evidences: **a** Study area and spatial distribution of woredas. **b** Age distribution of measles patients hospitalized at the Woliso hospital between January 2013 and April 2017. The inset shows the estimated measles seroprevalence by age, as obtained on the basis of model estimates. **c** Time series of case patients recorded during the study period, overall, and in most affected woredas. The inset shows the cross correlation in the timing of epidemics in Woliso and most rural areas. **d** Cumulative incidence of hospitalizations per 10,000 individuals (h) by woreda/kebele and distance from Woliso hospital (d). The solid line represents estimates obtained by the negative binomial regression model; the shaded area represents 95% CI

of the basic reproductive number (R_0), the age-specific immunity profile, and the average measles incidence in the considered area. The estimated total number of infection cases in the population was disaggregated into smaller spatial units (woredas and kebeles), by assuming the same incidence rate across all spatial units and proportionally to the population size of each spatial unit. A regression model was applied to counts of observed hospitalized cases in each spatial unit to estimate the corresponding hospitalization rate; distance from the hospital was used as the independent variable and the estimated total number of cases in each spatial unit as offset. Obtained results were used to quantify the hidden burden of measles disease.

In the rest of this section, we detail the dynamic transmission model, the performed spatial analysis, how we calculated the hidden burden of disease, and the performed sensitivity analyses.

The dynamic transmission model

Measles transmission dynamics between 2013 and 2017 is simulated through a deterministic, non-stationary, age-structured transmission model. In the model, the population is stratified in 86 1-year age classes, according to available data on the age distribution of the Ethiopian population in 2013 [17]. The crude birth rate of the population is 0.0325 years^{-1}; individuals die according to age-specific mortality rates as reported between

Table 1 Measles cases patients. Epidemiological characteristics of measles cases admitted to Woliso hospital (South West Shewa Zone, Oromia Region, Ethiopia) from January 1, 2013, to April 9, 2017

Mean age (years)	6.1 (SD 8.9; range 0–65)				
Deaths	36/1819 (2.0%)				
Females	855/1819 (47.0%)				
Vaccinated measles patients (2016)	120/295 (40.6%)				
Hospital main catchment area					
Woreda	Kebele	Patients	Deaths	Population	Distance (km)
Woliso	All kebeles	843	19	209,321	0–19.9
Woliso	Woliso town	379	8	52,849	0
Woliso	Obi	91	5	15.341	6.4
Woliso	Dilela	182	3	48,353	15.5
Woliso	Gurura	141	0	34,477	15.5
Woliso	Korke	50	3	58,301	19.9
Wonchi	All kebeles	296	1	110,275	15.0
Goro	All kebeles	147	3	55,640	22.1
Ameya	All kebeles	226	5	146,535	30.4
Woredas outside the hospital main catchment area					
Becho		41	3	91,116	33.7
Welkite (Gurage Zone)		31	1	55,097	40.1
Seden Sodo		19	1	82,969	45.0
Dawo		23	0	101,133	49.5
Ilu		19	0	75,326	55.9
Tole		48	0	75,438	73.6
Nono (West Shoa Zone)		45	1	108,356	82.7
Kersa Ena Malima		1	1	97,761	137.0
Other		80	1	Unknown	Unknown

2013 and 2015 and reflecting a crude mortality rate of 0.0083 days^{-1} [17]. The population of any age a is divided into five epidemiological classes: individuals protected by maternal antibodies (M_a), susceptible individuals (S_a), exposed individuals (E_a), infectious individuals (I_a), and individuals who acquired immunity against measles through either vaccination or natural infection (R_a).

We assume that newborn individuals are protected against measles infection for 6 months on average by the passive transfer of maternal immunity [1], after which they become susceptible to the infection.

Susceptible individuals can acquire infection after contact with an infectious individual under the assumption of homogeneous mixing and become exposed without symptoms; at the end of the latent period, lasting 7.5 days on average, infectious individuals can transmit the infection for 6.5 days on average; the resulting generation time is 14 days [18]. After recovery, individuals are assumed to gain lifelong immunity. Newly infected individuals are hospitalized with a certain, age-independent, probability p_h,

representing the average hospitalization rate in the main hospital catchment area.

Seasonal variations in the transmission rate are considered: during school holidays, overlapping with the rainy season [14], the transmission rate is decreased by a factor r.

Routine vaccination of children is simulated at 9 months of age [3] with homogenous coverage across woredas at 88%. The latter estimate was obtained by administrative records on infant immunization occurring between 2013 and 2016 in the main hospital catchment area. Vaccine efficacy at the first dose of routine administration is assumed at 85% [19].

The follow-up campaigns conducted in 2013 (from May 29 to June 5) and in 2017 (from March 13 to March 20), targeting children 9–59 months of age [16], are also considered. The coverage of the 2013 supplementary immunization activities (SIAs), c_S, was estimated among free model parameters. Vaccine efficacy during SIAs is assumed to be 95% [19].

Epidemiological transitions are described by the following system of ordinary differential equations:

$$
\begin{cases}
M_a{}'(t) &= bN(t) - \mu M_a(t) - (\varepsilon_R c_R(t,a) + \varepsilon_S c_S(t,a))M_a(t) - d(t,a)M_a(t) \\
S_a{}'(t) &= \mu M_a(t) - (\varepsilon_R c_R(t,a) + \varepsilon_S c_S(t,a))S_a(t) - \beta(t)S_a(t)I(t)/N(t) - d(t,a)S_a(t) \\
E_a{}'(t) &= \beta(t)S_a(t)I(t)/N(t) - \omega E_a(t) - d(t,a)E_a(t) \\
I_a{}'(t) &= \omega E_a(t) - \gamma I_a(t) - d(t,a)I_a(t) \\
R_a{}'(t) &= \gamma I_a(t) + (\varepsilon_R c_R(t,a) + \varepsilon_S c_S(t,a))(S_a(t) + M_a(t)) - d(t,a)R_a(t) \\
H_a{}'(t) &= p_h \omega E_a(t) \\
I(t) &= \sum_{a=0}^{85} I_a(t) \\
H(t) &= \sum_{a=0}^{85} H_a(t) \\
N(t) &= \sum_{a=0}^{85} [M_a(t) + S_a(t) + E_a(t) + I_a(t) + R_a(t)]
\end{cases}
$$

where t represents time and a the individuals' chronological age; $b(t)$ and $d(t,a)$ are the crude birth and the age-specific mortality rates at time t; $1/\mu$ is the average duration of protection provided by maternal antibodies; $1/\omega$ and $1/\gamma$ are the average duration of the latent and the infectivity periods; $c_R(t,a)$ and $c_S(t,a)$ are the coverage associated with the first-dose routine vaccination and SIAs for individuals of age a, at time t; ε_R and ε_S represent the vaccine efficacy associated with routine vaccination of infants and SIAs. Specifically, c_S denotes the vaccinated fraction of individuals who were not yet immunized by natural infection or routine programs. $N(t)$ and $H(t)$ represent the total population of the hospital main catchment area and the cumulative number of hospitalized measles cases at time t; p_h is the fraction of measles infections that are hospitalized, and $\beta(t)$ is the measles transmission rate defined as follows:

$$
\beta(t) = \begin{cases} r\,\beta, & \text{1st Jun} < t < \text{12th Sep} \\ \beta, & \text{otherwise} \end{cases}
$$

At the end of the year, the chronological age of individuals is incremented by 1. The number of hospitalized measles cases in a time interval $[t_1, t_2]$ is computed as $H(t_2) - H(t_1)$.

Model estimates were obtained by simulating measles transmission between January 1, 2013, and March 20, 2017. Simulations are initialized on January 1, 2013. As the result of past natural infection and immunization campaigns, only a fraction s_0 of the population is assumed to be susceptible to the infection. The age distribution of susceptibles at the beginning of 2013 was assumed to mirror the age distribution of hospitalized cases between January 2013 and March 2017. Specifically, the initial fraction of susceptible and immune individuals in each age group are $S_a(0) = N_a s_0 Z_a / \sum_{a=0}^{85} Z_a$ and $R_a(0) = N_a - S_a(0)$, respectively, where N_a is the number of individuals of age a at the beginning of 2013 in Woliso, Ameya, Goro, and Wonchi [17] and Z_a is the observed total number of hospitalized measles cases of age a.

Free model parameters (s_0, β, r_β, p_h, c_S) were calibrated using a Markov Chain Monte Carlo (MCMC) approach based on the negative binomial likelihood of observing the weekly number of hospitalized case patients reported between January 1, 2013, and the beginning of the 2017 SIA. The scale parameter defining the negative binomial distribution was jointly estimated with other free parameters within the MCMC procedure. Details are provided in the Additional file 1.

Reproduction number and disease elimination

The fundamental quantity regulating disease dynamics is the basic reproduction number (defined as $R_0 = \langle \beta \rangle / \gamma$, where $\langle \beta \rangle$ is the average of $\beta(t)$ over the year), which represents the average number of secondary infections in a fully susceptible population generated by a typical index case during the entire period of infectiousness. The larger the R_0, the higher the disease transmissibility. If $R_0 > 1$, the infection will be able to spread in a population. Otherwise, the infection will die out. For endemic diseases like measles, R_0 provides insights into the proportion p of population to be successfully vaccinated to achieve disease elimination; the equation $p = 1 - 1/R_0$ is widely accepted (e.g., [5, 18, 20]). For instance, if $R_0 = 10$, at least 90% of children have to be routinely immunized to eliminate the disease.

Spatial analysis

A negative binomial regression was used to study the relationship between incidence of hospitalization by kebeles/woredas and distance from Woliso hospital. Specifically, the observed number of hospitalized cases from each spatial unit is the response variable, the distance from the hospital is the independent variable, and the estimated total number of measles cases in each spatial unit (as estimated by the transmission model) is used as the offset.

Detailed origin of patients at the kebele level was used to better identify the travel distances for patients living within the Woliso woreda, where the hospital is located (Table 1).

In the negative binomial regression, we assume that counts of hospitalized cases h_i (the response variable) associated with a given location i are distributed as a negative binomial of mean μ_i determined by the number of infection in the location c_i (the offset) and the distance of location from the hospital d_i (the regressor) as follows:

$$\mu_i = \exp(\ln(c_i) + b_1 + b_2 d_i)$$

where b_1, b_2 are unknown parameters that are estimated from the observed hospitalized cases h_i.

In order to take into account the uncertainty on incidence estimates obtained with the dynamic model, 10,000 draws from the posterior distribution of incidence estimates associated with 10,000 samples of the posterior distribution of free model parameters were considered to generate a distribution of regression model fits. Obtained results therefore account for the combined uncertainty due to the regression model and the dynamic transmission model.

We investigate the spatial variation in the incidence of hospitalized patients in the population as a consequence of different illness conditions. The aim is to characterize the relationship between hospitalization and distance from the hospital. The relative risk of being hospitalized at different distances from the hospital was computed by considering the incidence of hospitalization in each kebele/woreda divided by the incidence of hospitalized cases from Woliso town. The relative risk was fitted by an exponential function using distance as the independent variable (i.e., by fitting a linear model to the logarithm of the relative risk without intercept). Finally, a proportional test was used to assess possible statistical differences in the case fatality rate at hospital between cases coming from different sites.

The hidden burden of disease

Persons living in Woliso town do not have distance barriers to access to the Woliso hospital. The probability of severe disease after measles infection was therefore computed as the fraction of measles patients from Woliso town that have been hospitalized for two nights or more among all measles infections estimated by the transmission model for this spatial unit. For severe cases, we indicate here those cases that from a clinical point of view are physiologically unstable and require supportive care (fluid resuscitation, oxygen, etc.) that can be provided only inside a well-resourced hospital. The resulting probability of developing severe measles illness p^s was used in combination with the estimated number of measles infections at different kebeles and woredas c_i to estimate the potential number of severe cases occurring at different distances from the hospital as $p^s c_i$. For each considered spatial unit i, missed severe cases were computed as the difference between the estimated number of severe cases and the number of patients recorded at the hospital, namely $m_i^s = p^s c_i - h_i$. Missed severe cases were considered untreated and counted as additional deaths. The overall number of deaths caused by measles was estimated as the sum of missed deaths and measles deaths observed among hospital admitted patients. Averted deaths due to hospital treatment were estimated by considering all severe cases $p^s c_i$ as counterfactual deaths that would have occurred in the absence of adequate treatment.

Sensitivity analyses

A variety of sensitivity analyses were conducted to evaluate to what extent some crucial assumptions made in the above described analysis may affect the obtained results.

We evaluated whether the assumption of decreased transmissibility during school holidays (or rainy season) is necessary to explain the observed pattern, by fitting a model with constant transmission rate against the time series of measles hospitalized cases.

Since the fraction of immunized individuals during the SIA in 2013 is unknown, we also considered two alternative models with $c_S = 0$ (SIA not conducted in 2013 in the considered area) and $c_S = 0.92$ (the highest coverage reported for past campaigns, namely 92% [3]).

We explored whether the assumption of homogeneous mixing, consisting in applying the same transmission rate to all age groups, can affect the model ability in reproducing the observed epidemiological patterns. To do this, we fitted the time series of cases with a transmission model encoding age-specific contacts as recently estimated for Ethiopia by Prem et al. [21]. In this case, increased mixing in schools corresponds to higher transmission rate among school-age children.

Models' performances were assessed through the Deviance Information Criterion (DIC).

A sensitivity analysis was also conducted by fitting a transmission model to the time series of measles cases observed in Woliso, Wonchi, Ameya, and Goro separately. Specifically, a single epidemic was simulated in the four woredas simultaneously, by assuming the same initial conditions and by assuming that populations from different locations mix homogeneously. All epidemiological parameters were assumed to be equal across different woredas, but a different hospitalization rate was considered for each woreda.

An additional sensitivity analysis was performed to test whether estimates on the spatial variation of the hospitalization rates change when patients recorded from all woredas of the South West Shoa Zone are considered or when patients' sex is considered.

Finally, estimates on the overall number of measles deaths and on the overall case fatality rate were estimated by relaxing the assumption that all missed/untreated severe measles cases die.

Details are provided in Additional file 1.

Results

Measles case patients

A total of 1819 case patients were recorded in Woliso hospital from January 1, 2013, to April 9, 2017 (Table 1). Of these, 855 (47.0%) were female and 964 (53.0%) were male; 1512 patients (83.1%) were resident in the main hospital's catchment area, consisting of Woliso, Wonchi, Goro, and Ameya woredas. The mean age was 6.0 years (range, 0–65); 1259 case patients (69.2%) were aged ≤ 4 years and 1486 (81.7%) were aged ≤ 10 years (Fig. 1b). Records obtained during 2016 show that vaccinated admitted cases between 9 months and 5 years of age were 40.6%. In sub-Saharan Africa, different immunization rates may correspond to rural and urban areas [22, 23]. However, by looking at the vaccination status of hospitalized measles cases, though only recorded for a small fraction of cases, we found that the fraction of vaccinated individuals among measles cases was not significantly different across woredas (proportional test p value, 0.663) and consistent with administrative records of routine coverage in the area (see Additional file 1). This simple analysis partially supports the assumption of homogeneous coverage in the main catchment area.

The CFR based on hospital admitted cases was 1.98% (36/1819, 95% credible interval (CI) 1.43–2.72). The mean age of fatal cases was 3.3 years (range, 0–30). The time series of case patients is shown in Fig. 1c. Epidemic peaks were observed in June of 2013, 2015, and 2016, with marked incidence decrease after closure of schools for holidays and at the beginning of rainy seasons. A much lower number of case patients was recorded in 2014. In 2017, the epidemic peak was observed in late winter with marked incidence decrease after the conducted SIA (13–20 March).

Measles transmissibility and seasonal patterns in measles circulation

Simpler transmission models with $r = 1$, $c_S = 0$, or $c_S = 0.92$ and the one based on heterogeneous mixing by age were all ruled out by the DIC analysis. Best model performances were obtained with the baseline transmission model. Remarkably, even if based on the assumption of homogeneous mixing, the baseline transmission model well reproduced the number of measles cases observed over time, among different age groups: 0–6 years, 7–14 years, and > 15 years (details in Additional file 1). Interestingly, we found that considering different transmission rate by age groups, as a consequence of heterogeneous mixing by age, does not improve the model ability in reproducing the observed time series of measles cases. The average reproduction number estimated with the baseline transmission model was $R_0 = 16.5$ (95% CI 14.5–18.3).

A strong seasonal pattern of transmission was consistently observed across the different woredas. Significant synchrony in the timing of epidemics in Woliso and most rural areas was observed (inset of Fig. 1c and Additional file 1), so that the observed seasonal pattern was not an artifact of averaging asynchronous local epidemics. Model estimates suggest an average decrease in the force of infection of 27.8% (95% CI 21.6–33.2) between June and September, corresponding to school holidays and the rainy season.

The estimated average hospitalization rate in the main hospital's catchment area was 12.4% (95% CI 10.9–14.1), similar to results found in [24]. Accordingly, 12,194 infections (95% CI 10,723–13,872), corresponding to a disease incidence of 234 per 10,000 individuals (95% CI 206–266), may have occurred in the area from January 1, 2013, to March 13, 2017.

The coverage of the 2013 SIA among residual susceptible individuals was estimated to be 18.7% (95% CI 11.9–24.3). The percentage of susceptible individuals at the beginning of 2013 was estimated to be 6.5% (95% CI 6.0–7.3). By assuming that the age distribution of observed measles cases mirrored the distribution of susceptible individuals across different age segments, we estimated the corresponding age-specific immunity profile of the population. This analysis showed that about 40% of children aged ≤ 2 years were not immunized against measles, while less than 10% of individuals aged > 5 years were susceptible to measles (inset of Fig. 1b).

Spatial analysis

Differences in the case fatality rate among hospital admitted patients from different sites were not found statistically significant (see Fig. 2b). Significantly different cumulative incidences of hospitalizations by woreda and kebele were observed, with the largest values at 71 per 10,000 inhabitants in Woliso town (Fig. 1d). Cumulative incidence of hospitalizations by kebele/woreda was significantly correlated to travel distance from Woliso (Pearson $\rho = - 0.90$, $p = 0.003$) (Fig. 1d).

Estimated measles hospitalization rate dramatically decreases with travel distance from the hospital: from 31.0% (95% CI 15.9–45.0) in Woliso town to 5.7% (95% CI 3.0, 8.1) at 30 km from the hospital (Fig. 2a). Remarkably, similar estimates were obtained by fitting the transmission model to cases observed in Woliso (Woliso town and Obi, Dilela, Gurura, and Korke kebeles), Wonchi, Ameya, and Goro separately (see Additional file 1). In this case, estimates of woredas' specific hospitalization rates range between 6.1% (95% CI

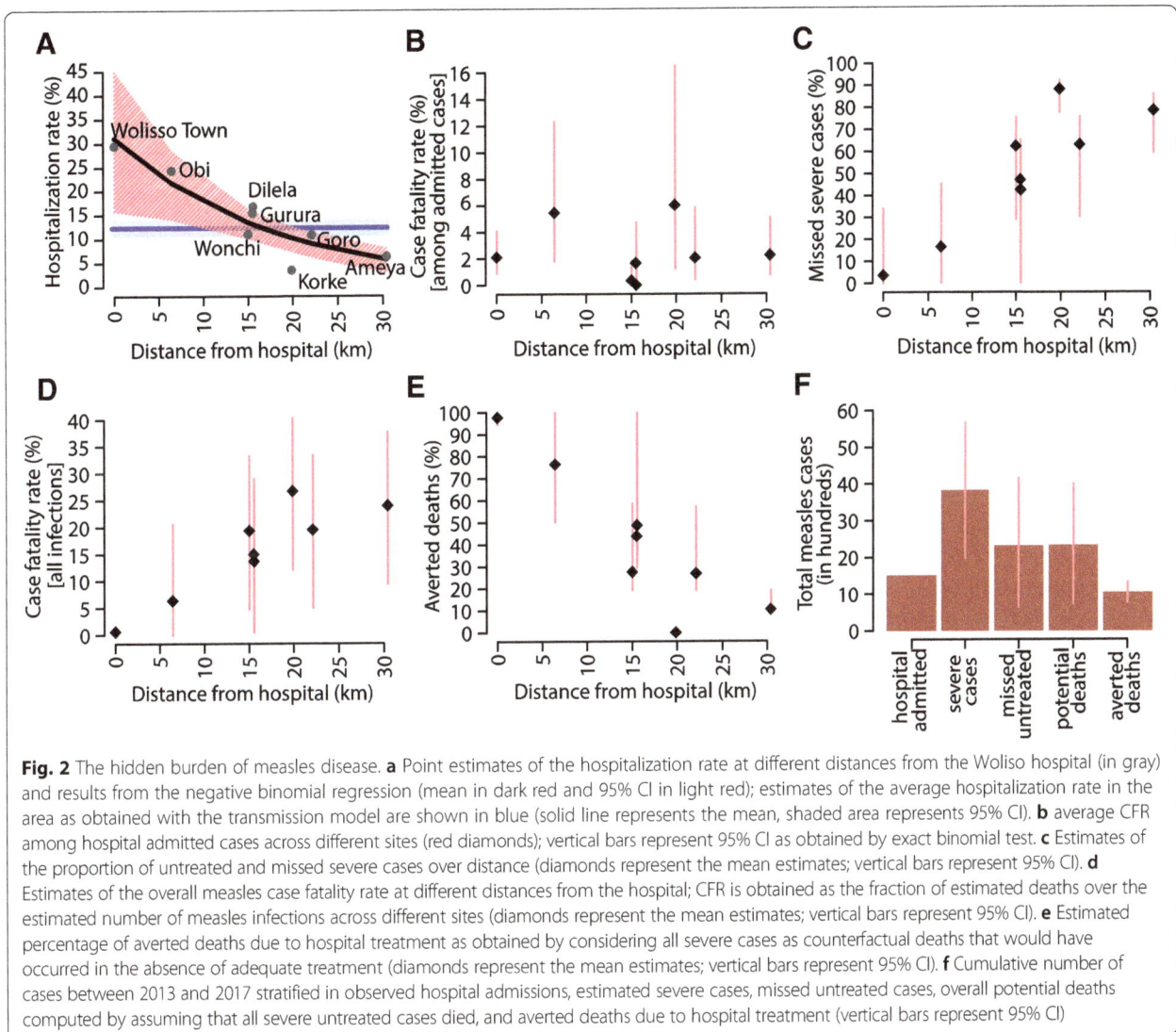

Fig. 2 The hidden burden of measles disease. **a** Point estimates of the hospitalization rate at different distances from the Woliso hospital (in gray) and results from the negative binomial regression (mean in dark red and 95% CI in light red); estimates of the average hospitalization rate in the area as obtained with the transmission model are shown in blue (solid line represents the mean, shaded area represents 95% CI). **b** average CFR among hospital admitted cases across different sites (red diamonds); vertical bars represent 95% CI as obtained by exact binomial test. **c** Estimates of the proportion of untreated and missed severe cases over distance (diamonds represent the mean estimates; vertical bars represent 95% CI). **d** Estimates of the overall measles case fatality rate at different distances from the hospital; CFR is obtained as the fraction of estimated deaths over the estimated number of measles infections across different sites (diamonds represent the mean estimates; vertical bars represent 95% CI). **e** Estimated percentage of averted deaths due to hospital treatment as obtained by considering all severe cases as counterfactual deaths that would have occurred in the absence of adequate treatment (diamonds represent the mean estimates; vertical bars represent 95% CI). **f** Cumulative number of cases between 2013 and 2017 stratified in observed hospital admissions, estimated severe cases, missed untreated cases, overall potential deaths computed by assuming that all severe untreated cases died, and averted deaths due to hospital treatment (vertical bars represent 95% CI)

5.7–6.5) in Ameya and 15.9% (95% CI 15.0–17.0) in Woliso, with an average hospitalization rate in the hospital catchment area of 12.7% (95% CI 11.1–14.1) that is consistent with estimates obtained with the baseline model (see Additional file 1).

Similar results were also obtained when all woredas of the South West Shoa Zone were considered, although it is likely that measles cases occurring beyond 30 km from Woliso town have been partially detected, recovered, and treated in other health care facilities. A sensitivity analysis suggested that males had a higher access to health facilities with respect to females. However, the impact of distance on individuals' access to care was found to not depend on the individual sex.

Interestingly, we found that the relative risk of hospitalization at the Woliso hospital associated with different illness conditions and health care treatments decreases with distance as well (see Additional file 1).

These results suggest that the estimated decrease in measles hospitalization with the distance from the hospital is ascribable to inequalities in access to health care due to travel distances from the nearest hospital. These results, combined with those coming from the cross-correlation analysis of time series of cases from distinct woredas, suggest that observed measles cases were the result of a unique synchronous epidemic with similar epidemiological characteristics across different woredas. More details are provided in Additional file 1.

The hidden burden of disease

The probability of severe illness once infected, based on measles inpatients from Woliso town, resulted in 0.30 (95% CI 0.16–0.43). The total number of severe measles cases in the Woliso hospital catchment area was consequently estimated to be 3821 (95% CI 1969–5671), only 1512 of which have been recorded among hospital admissions (Fig. 2c, f). By assuming that all untreated severe measles cases died, a total number of 2337 deaths (95% CI 716–4009) were estimated, 28 of which were detected at the hospital. Accordingly, 98% of deaths remained unobserved.

By estimating for each site the overall number of infected cases, the number of severe cases, and deaths, we found that the overall case fatality rate in the whole area (defined as the number of deaths per measles infection) might have been as high as 18.4% (95% CI 5.9–30.2).

Averted deaths due to hospitalization in the main hospital's catchment area resulted to be 1049 (95% 757–1342). However, our results suggest that hospital effectiveness in preventing deaths dramatically reduces with travel distance from the hospital, becoming negligible beyond 20–30 km from the hospital (Fig. 2e). Our estimates suggest that the case fatality rate increases from 0.62% (95% CI 0.60–0.65) in Woliso town to more than 20%, on average, for sites that are more than 20 km far from the hospital (Fig. 2d).

The estimated number of deaths and the resulting CFR in the main catchment area decrease with the fatality rate assumed among severe cases that were not hospitalized (see Fig. 3). However, if only half of the severe cases that were not hospitalized are assumed to die, the estimated average number of measles deaths exceeds 1100, only 3% of which were recorded at the hospital; the estimated CFR among all infections results larger than 9% (see Fig. 3).

Discussion

The epidemic in South West Shoa Zone highlights that measles still represents a major public health issue in Ethiopia. The synchrony of local epidemics and the consistent negative relationship between hospitalization incidence for different illness conditions and the distance from the referral hospital support the hypothesis of a large epidemic, spreading in the entire zone with similar transmission characteristics, but characterized by a significant heterogeneity in access to health care infrastructures.

The estimated average reproduction number of the observed epidemic was $R_0 = 16.5$ (95% CI 14.5–18.3), slightly larger than values recently found for Niger (4.7–15.7) [20] and Zambia (12.6) [5]. Accordingly, the herd immune level required in the area to progress towards measles elimination is around 94%, far beyond possible achievements with routine administration of a single dose at 85% of vaccine efficacy [19, 25] and coverage at 88%. In particular, the estimated age-specific serological profile is consistent with estimates recently provided for Ethiopia [26], showing that, in 2015, 60% of susceptible individuals in Ethiopia were less than 5 years of age. These results suggest critically low immunization rates in recent birth cohorts.

Our analysis highlighted a significant reduction of measles transmission between June and September.

Such a reduction may reflect changes in contact rates induced by either school closure or rainfalls. Indeed, in the Oromia Region, school holidays occur during the rainy season [14]. Changes in measles transmission during this period was already observed in Ethiopia [14], and the decrease in measles circulation caused by rainfalls was suggested for other African countries [6], possibly due to relatively low connectivity or an increase in urban density during the dry season as a consequence of migration from agricultural areas. As already observed in Niger [6], the strong seasonality in measles

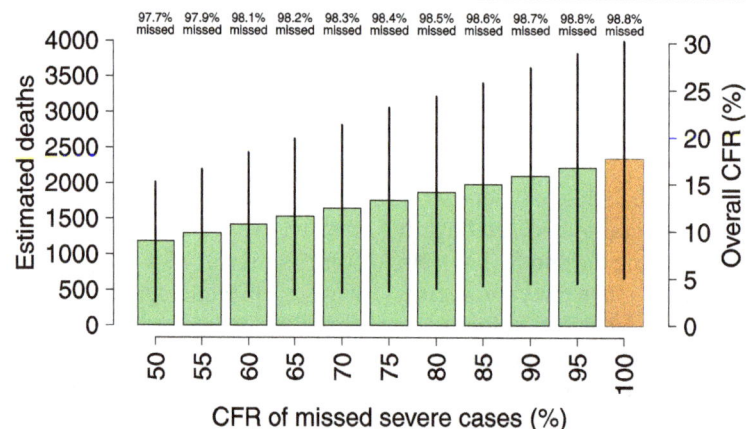

Fig. 3 Sensitivity analysis. Total number of measles deaths (scaled on the left) and overall measles case fatality rate (scaled on the right) in the main hospital catchment area as estimated for different values of the fatality rate among severe cases that were not hospitalized. Estimates obtained with the baseline assumption are shown in orange. Vertical bars represent 95% of credible intervals. Percentages shown on top of the figure represent the estimated average proportions of deaths that were not reported at the hospital obtained with different values of the fatality rate among missed/untreated severe cases

transmission, combined with variations in vaccine uptake and in fertility rates may lead to erratic epidemiological patterns [27], characterized by frequent stochastic fadeouts, and irregular large epidemics. Occasional large outbreaks may be followed by years of very few cases, with inter-epidemic periods of unpredictable length and frequency, during which the high fertility characterizing the country can produce a fast, possibly unnoticed, recruitment of susceptible individuals [6, 26–28]. These considerations apply also to the South West Shoa Zone.

We found that the 2013 SIA might have reached less than 20% of residual susceptible individuals, which is much lower than the observed 75% reduction in the susceptible proportion produced by the first regional SIA conducted in southern Ethiopia in 1999 [29] and than the coverage levels estimated for SIAs conducted in other sub-Saharan countries (66–77%) [30]. The low impact of 2013 vaccination campaign with respect to past SIAs might have been influenced by problems in cold chain operations or vaccine maintenance [25] and the short duration of this campaign. However, the low impact of 2013 SIA may also reflect difficulties in immunizing individuals who escaped routine programs and past immunization efforts, especially through vaccination activities performed as a response strategy to ongoing epidemics [31].

Remarkably, we found that hospitalization rates and the effectiveness of passive surveillance based on hospital admissions, in both detecting measles and preventing measles-related deaths, dramatically decrease with travel distances from the hospital, becoming negligible beyond 20–30 km from the hospital. In particular, our estimates suggest that measles hospitalization rate decreases by about 80% within a 30-km travel distance from the hospital. These results are consistent with what observed in Kenya where all-cause admission rates were found to decrease by 11–20% with every 5-km increase in distance from the hospital [10]. A decrease of hospital admissions with increasing distance from the hospital was also found when estimating the global and regional burden of severe acute lower respiratory infections [32].

The overall estimated cumulative incidence was 2.34% (95% CI 2.06–2.66) of the population in less than 5 years. CFR among hospitalized cases was 1.98% (95% CI 1.43–2.72). However, while only 36 deaths were recorded at the hospital, the spatial epidemiological analysis performed highlighted that the observed epidemics may have caused about 2300 additional deaths, consisting of severe cases that did not received any hospital treatment. These results suggest that the overall case fatality rate among all measles infections might have been between 5 and 30%, significantly higher than published estimates for epidemics occurred in 2005–2006 in Niger, Chad,

and Nigeria, namely 4.2–8.1% [13]. Obtained estimates for the measles CFR are consistent with those obtained for low-income countries during outbreaks occurring in isolated populations (above 15%) [7]. The assumed CFR among untreated measles cases essentially reflects our estimate of the percentage of most severe cases (around 30%), and it is in line with estimates of measles CFR in Ethiopia dating back to more than 30 years ago (around 27%) [7]. Estimates obtained on the total number of deaths and on the overall case fatality rate strongly depend on the assumption that all unobserved severe measles cases died. On the one hand, this represents a worst-case scenario. On the other hand, it is worth considering that cases here defined as severe are those with critical complications requiring to occupy, for two or more consecutive nights, one out of the 200 beds of a hospital in Ethiopia serving a potential catchment area of roughly 1.3 Million people and representing the closest well-resourced heath facility that can provide adequate treatments and supportive care for 521,771 inhabitants.

Obtained results are supported by spatial trends we identified in the relative risk of being hospitalized as a consequence of other illness conditions (see Additional file 1) and are consistent with what observed in previous studies on a variety of illness conditions [10, 22]. The role of distance as a barrier to health care access and affecting individuals' mortality has been well documented by recent population-based studies [8, 9], although most of them do not differentiate between causes of death [11] and between levels of care available in facilities [11], and none of these are focused on measles. In particular, a cross-sectional survey recently conducted in Ethiopia highlighted that children who lived more than 30 km from the health center had a two- to threefold greater risk of death than children who lived near to the health center [8]. Similar results were found when considering either traveling distances or travel times [8]. In rural Tanzania, direct obstetric mortality was found to be four times higher at 35 km from hospital [11]. Finally, geographical clusters of acute abdominal conditions in India were found to have a nine times higher mortality rate and significantly greater distance to a well-resourced hospital [12].

All these epidemiological evidences suggest that what was observed for measles in the South West Shoa zone may likely affect other diseases and characterize other low-income settings of sub-Saharan Africa. Obtained results highlight that epidemiological estimates, based on hospitalization records only, may dramatically underestimate the burden of measles and should be carefully considered to design adequate and effective surveillance activities. More, in general, as already suggested in [10, 11], disease burden estimates based on hospital data may be strongly affected by distance from the hospital, although the amount of underestimation of disease burden may differ by disease [10, 11] and region considered.

The analysis has several limitations that should be considered in interpreting the results. The most important ones relate to the short observational period, the limited area considered, and the difficult task of quantifying unobserved severe measles cases. In particular, we assume that severe cases occurring within the main hospital's catchment area that have not been reported at the Woliso hospital were not treated at all for measles disease. Although past studies have not found any association between child mortality and distance to small health facilities (e.g., health posts) [8], most severe infections might have seek treatment at hospitals that are more distant than the Woliso one. In addition, factors other than distance such as individual sex, age, family's income, and geographical heterogeneity in incidence levels of comorbidities and social support provided to families might have strongly affected the access to health care and the disease outcome of patients coming from different locations [9]. Finally, misclassification of measles patients may always occur [7]. These limitations make it particularly difficult to reliably quantify untreated cases and estimate their fatality rate and the number of measles deaths, especially in absolute terms [7]. Other limitations of the proposed approach are determined by the lack of suitable data to model heterogeneous vaccination coverage within the hospital main catchment area, possible changes in the measles hospitalization rates over time, variations in the individual transmission rate of hospitalized cases, and seasonal variations of the population density as a consequence of migration flows between rural and urban areas.

Conclusions

The carried out analysis represents a first attempt to investigate the impact of spatial heterogeneity in hospital accessibility on measles epidemiology, to quantify the hidden burden of measles in low-income settings, and to assess the effect of hospitalization in preventing death from severe measles disease. Epidemiological patterns identified through the performed analysis should be tested in other settings and may strongly depend on both levels of care available in health facilities [11] and infection rates in the considered community. If similar results will be confirmed, geographical heterogeneity in the hospitalization rates should be taken into account when estimating the burden of diseases and the effectiveness of the public healthcare system [7].

Abbreviations

CFR: Case fatality rate; CI: Credible interval; DIC: Deviance Information Criterion; MCMC: Markov Chain Monte Carlo; MCV1: First dose of measles-containing vaccine; R_0: Basic reproductive number; SIA: Supplementary immunization activity; WHO: World Health Organization

Acknowledgements

The authors would like to thank the three reviewers of this manuscript for their constructive feedback on the manuscript.

Funding

This work was supported by the Italian Ministry of Foreign Affairs and International Cooperation within the project entitled "Rafforzamento del sistema di sorveglianza e controllo delle malattie infettive in Etiopia"—AID 011330. The funders had no role in the study design, data collection and analysis, interpretation, or preparation of the manuscript. The corresponding author had full access to all the data in the study and had the final responsibility for the decision to submit for publication.

Authors' contributions

PP, SP, GP, FM, and SM conceived of the study. TF, RF, ML, AT, GS, GP, and FM collected the data. PP, SP, GP, FM, and SM analyzed the data. PP and SM performed the experiments. PP drafted the first version of the manuscript. All authors contributed to the interpretation of the results and edited and approved the final manuscript.

Competing interests

The authors declare that they have no competing interests.

Author details

[1]Center for Information Technology, Fondazione Bruno Kessler, via Sommarive, 18, I-38123 Trento, Italy. [2]South West Shoa Zone Health Office, P.O. Box 253, Woliso, Oromia, Ethiopia. [3]Doctors with Africa CUAMM, Woliso Hospital, P.O. Box 250, Woliso, Oromia, Ethiopia. [4]Doctors with Africa CUAMM, via S. Francesco, 126, I-35121, Padova, Italy.

References

1. Goodson JL, Masresha BG, Wannemuehler K, Uzicanin A, Cochi S. Changing epidemiology of measles in Africa. J Infect Dis. 2011;204(suppl 1):S205–14.
2. Otten M, Kezaala R, Fall A, Masresha B, Martin R, Cairns L, et al. Public-health impact of accelerated measles control in the WHO African Region 2000–03. Lancet. 2005;366:9488.

3. Mitiku K, Bedada T, Masresha BG, Kegne W, Nafo-Traoré F, Tesfaye N, Yigzaw A. Progress in measles mortality reduction in Ethiopia, 2002–2009. J Infect Dis. 2011;204(suppl 1):S232–8.

4. Beyene BB, Tegegne AA, Wayessa DJ, Enqueselassie F. National measles surveillance data analysis, 2005 to 2009, Ethiopia. J Public Health Epidemiol. 2016;8:3.

5. Lessler J, Moss WJ, Lowther SA, Cummings DAT. Maintaining high rates of measles immunization in Africa. Epidemiol Infect. 2011;139(07):1039–49.

6. Ferrari MJ, Grais RF, Bharti N, Conlan AJ, Bjørnstad ON, Wolfson LJ, et al. The dynamics of measles in sub-Saharan Africa. Nature. 2008;451(7179):679–84.

7. Wolfson LJ, Grais RF, Luquero FJ, Birmingham ME, Strebel PM. Estimates of measles case fatality ratios: a comprehensive review of community-based studies. Int J Epidemiol. 2009;38(1):192–205.

8. Okwaraji YB, Cousens S, Berhane Y, Mulholland K, Edmond K. Effect of geographical access to health facilities on child mortality in rural Ethiopia: a community based cross sectional study. Plos One. 2012;7:3.

9. Rutherford ME, Mulholland K, Hill PC. How access to health care relates to under-five mortality in sub-Saharan Africa: systematic review. Tropical Med Int Health. 2010;15(5):508–19.

10. Etyang AO, Munge K, Bunyasi EW, Matata L, Ndila C, Kapesa S, et al. Burden of disease in adults admitted to hospital in a rural region of coastal Kenya: an analysis of data from linked clinical and demographic surveillance systems. Lancet Glob Health. 2014;2(4):e216–24.

11. Hanson C, Cox J, Mbaruku G, Manzi F, Gabrysch S, Schellenberg D, et al. Maternal mortality and distance to facility-based obstetric care in rural southern Tanzania: a secondary analysis of cross-sectional census data in 226000 households. Lancet Glob Health. 2015;3:7.

12. Dare AJ, Ng-Kamstra JS, Patra J, Fu SH, Rodriguez PS, Hsiao M, et al. Deaths from acute abdominal conditions and geographical access to surgical care in India: a nationally representative spatial analysis. Lancet Glob Health. 2015;3:10.

13. Grais RF, Dubray C, Gerstl S, Guthmann JP, Djibo A, Nargaye KD, et al. Unacceptably high mortality related to measles epidemics in Niger, Nigeria, and Chad. PLoS Med. 2007;4(1):e16.

14. Getahun M, Beyene B, Ademe A, Teshome B, Tefera M, Asha A, et al. Epidemiology of laboratory confirmed measles virus cases in Amhara Regional State of Ethiopia, 2004–2014. BMC Infect Dis. 2016;16:1.

15. Central Statistical Agency of Ethiopia. Population Projection of Ethiopia for All Regions At Wereda Level from 2014–2017. National report 2013; http://www.csa.gov.et. Accessed Mar 2018.

16. Federal Ministry of Health of Ethiopia. Ethiopia National Expanded Programme on Immunization. National report 2015; http://www.nationalplanningcycles.org. Accessed Mar 2018.

17. Population Division of the Department of Economic and Social Affairs of the United Nations Secretariat. Revision of World Population Prospects 2015; https://esa.un.org. Accessed Mar 2018.

18. Anderson RM, May RM, Anderson B. Infectious diseases of humans: dynamics and control (Vol. 28). Oxford: Oxford university press; 1992.

19. Uzicanin A, Zimmerman L. Field effectiveness of live attenuated measles-containing vaccines: a review of published literature. J Infect Dis. 2011;204(Suppl 1):S133–49.

20. Grais RF, Ferrari MJ, Dubray C, Bjørnstad ON, Grenfell BT, Djibo A, et al. Estimating transmission intensity for a measles epidemic in Niamey, Niger: lessons for intervention. Trans R Soc Trop Med Hyg. 2006;100(9):867–73.

21. Prem K, Cook AR, Jit M. Projecting social contact matrices in 152 countries using contact surveys and demographic data. PLoS Comput Biol. 2017;13(9):e1005697.

22. Utazi CE, Thorley J, Alegana VA, Ferrari MJ, Takahashi S, Metcalf CJ, et al. High resolution age-structured mapping of childhood vaccination coverage in low and middle income countries. Vaccine. 2018;36(12):1583–91.

23. Takahashi S, Metcalf CJ, Ferrari MJ, Tatem AJ, Lessler J. The geography of measles vaccination in the African Great Lakes region. Nat Commun. 2017;8:15585.

24. Odega CC, Fatiregun AA, Osaghemi GK. Completeness of suspected measles reporting in a southern district of Nigeria. Public Health. 2010;124(1):24–7.

25. Allam MF. Measles vaccination. J Prev Med Hyg. 2009;50:201–205.

26. Trentini F, Poletti P, Merler S, Melegaro A. Measles immunity gaps and the progress towards elimination: a multi-country modeling analysis. Lancet Infect Dis. 2017;17:10.

27. Earn DJ, Rohani P, Bolker BM, Grenfell BT. A simple model for complex dynamical transitions in epidemics. Science. 2000;287:5453.

28. Merler S, Ajelli M. Deciphering the relative weights of demographic transition and vaccination in the decrease of measles incidence in Italy. Proc R Soc B. 2014;281(1777):20132676.

29. Nigatu W, Samuel D, Cohen B, Cumberland P, Lemma E, Brown DW, et al. Evaluation of a measles vaccine campaign in Ethiopia using oral-fluid antibody surveys. Vaccine. 2008;26(37):4769–74.

30. Lessler J, Metcalf CJE, Grais RF, Luquero FJ, Cummings DA, Grenfell BT. Measuring the performance of vaccination programs using cross-sectional surveys: a likelihood framework and retrospective analysis. PLoS Med. 2011;8(10):e1001110.

31. Lessler J, Metcalf CJE, Cutts FT, Grenfell BT. Impact on epidemic measles of vaccination campaigns triggered by disease outbreaks or serosurveys: a modeling study. PLoS Med. 2016;13(10):e1002144.

32. Nair H, Simões EA, Rudan I, Gessner BD, Azziz-Baumgartner E, Zhang JSF, et al. Global and regional burden of hospital admissions for severe acute lower respiratory infections in young children in 2010: a systematic analysis. Lancet. 2013;381:9875.

Permissions

All chapters in this book were first published in MEDICINE, by BioMed Central; hereby published with permission under the Creative Commons Attribution License or equivalent. Every chapter published in this book has been scrutinized by our experts. Their significance has been extensively debated. The topics covered herein carry significant findings which will fuel the growth of the discipline. They may even be implemented as practical applications or may be referred to as a beginning point for another development.

The contributors of this book come from diverse backgrounds, making this book a truly international effort. This book will bring forth new frontiers with its revolutionizing research information and detailed analysis of the nascent developments around the world.

We would like to thank all the contributing authors for lending their expertise to make the book truly unique. They have played a crucial role in the development of this book. Without their invaluable contributions this book wouldn't have been possible. They have made vital efforts to compile up to date information on the varied aspects of this subject to make this book a valuable addition to the collection of many professionals and students.

This book was conceptualized with the vision of imparting up-to-date information and advanced data in this field. To ensure the same, a matchless editorial board was set up. Every individual on the board went through rigorous rounds of assessment to prove their worth. After which they invested a large part of their time researching and compiling the most relevant data for our readers.

The editorial board has been involved in producing this book since its inception. They have spent rigorous hours researching and exploring the diverse topics which have resulted in the successful publishing of this book. They have passed on their knowledge of decades through this book. To expedite this challenging task, the publisher supported the team at every step. A small team of assistant editors was also appointed to further simplify the editing procedure and attain best results for the readers.

Apart from the editorial board, the designing team has also invested a significant amount of their time in understanding the subject and creating the most relevant covers. They scrutinized every image to scout for the most suitable representation of the subject and create an appropriate cover for the book.

The publishing team has been an ardent support to the editorial, designing and production team. Their endless efforts to recruit the best for this project, has resulted in the accomplishment of this book. They are a veteran in the field of academics and their pool of knowledge is as vast as their experience in printing. Their expertise and guidance has proved useful at every step. Their uncompromising quality standards have made this book an exceptional effort. Their encouragement from time to time has been an inspiration for everyone.

The publisher and the editorial board hope that this book will prove to be a valuable piece of knowledge for researchers, students, practitioners and scholars across the globe.

List of Contributors

Anna Meyer-Weitz, Kwaku Oppong Asante and Bukenge J. Lukobeka
Discipline of Psychology, University of KwaZulu-Natal, Durban, South Africa

Kwaku Oppong Asante
Department of Psychology, University of Ghana, Legon, Accra, Ghana

Ankur Pandya
Department of Health Policy and Management, Harvard T.H. Chan School of Public Health, 718 Huntington Ave, 2nd Floor, Boston, MA 02115, USA

Tim Doran
Department of Health Sciences, University of York, Heslington, York, UK

Ankur Pandya and Jinyi Zhu
Center for Health Decision Science, Harvard T.H. Chan School of Public Health, Boston, MA, USA

Simon Walker
Centre for Health Economics, University of York, Heslington, York, UK

Emily Arntson and Andrew M. Ryan
Department of Health Management and Policy, University of Michigan School of Public Health, Ann Arbor, MI, USA

Susanna C. Larsson
Unit of Nutritional Epidemiology, Institute of Environmental Medicine, Karolinska Institutet, 171 77 Stockholm, Sweden

Stephen Burgess
MRC Biostatistics Unit, University of Cambridge, Cambridge, UK

Stephen Burgess
Department of Public Health and Primary Care, University of Cambridge, Cambridge, UK

Karl Michaëlsson
Department of Surgical Sciences, Uppsala University, Uppsala, Sweden

Yirong Chen and Alex R. Cook
Saw Swee Hock School of Public Health, National University of Singapore and National University Health System, 12 Science Drive 2, Singapore 117549,Singapore

Janet Hui Yi Ong, Jayanthi Rajarethinam, Grace Yap and Lee Ching Ng
Environmental Health Institute, 11 Biopolis Way, Singapore 138667, Singapore

Nathaniel J. Pollock and Shree Mulay
Division of Community Health and Humanities, Faculty of Medicine, Memorial University, Prince Philip Drive, St. John's, Newfoundland and Labrador A1B 3V6, Canada

Nathaniel J. Pollock
Labrador Institute of Memorial University, Stn. B, 219 Hamilton River Road, Happy Valley-Goose Bay, ,Newfoundland and Labrador A0P 1E0, Canada

Kiyuri Naicker, Alex Loro and Ian Colman
School of Epidemiology and Public Health, Faculty of Medicine, University of Ottawa, 600 Peter Morand Cr, Room 308C, Ottawa, ON K1G 5Z3, Canada

Cristina Mussini
Clinic of Infectious Diseases, University Hospital, University of Modena and Reggio Emilia, Via del Pozzo, 71, 41124 Modena, Italy

Patrizia Lorenzini and Andrea Antinori
National Institute for Infectious Diseases L. Spallanzani, Rome, Italy

Alessandro Cozzi-Lepri
Department of Infection and Population Health Division of Population Health, University College London, Hampstead Campus, London, UK

Giulia Marchetti, Stefano Rusconi, Andrea Gori and Antonella d'Arminio Monforte
Clinic of Infectious Diseases, Department of Health Sciences San Paolo Hospital, DIBIC Luigi Sacco, University of Milan,Milan, Italy

Silvia Nozza
Clinic of Infectious Diseases, San Raffaele Hospital, University Vita e Salute, Milan, Italy

Miriam Lichtner
Department of Public Health and Infectious Diseases, Sapienza University of Rome, Polo Pontino, Italy

Andrea Cossarizza
Pathology and Immunology, University of Modena and Reggio Emilia, Modena, Italy

Gregg S. Gonsalves, J. Tyler Copple and Tyler Johnson
Department of Epidemiology of Microbial Diseases, Yale School of Public Health, 60 College Street, New Haven, CT, USA

J. Tyler Copple
Independent Consultant, Yale School of Public Health, 60 College Street, New Haven, CT, USA

A. David Paltiel
Department of Health Policy and Management, Yale School of Public Health, 60 College Street, New Haven, CT, USA

Joshua L. Warren
Department of Biostatistics, Yale School of Public Health, 60 College Street, New Haven, CT, USA

Department of Biostatistics, Yale University, New Haven, CT 06510, USA

Louis Grandjean
Paediatric Infectious Diseases, Section of Paediatrics, Department of Medicine, Imperial College, London W2 1NY, UK

Louis Grandjean, David A. J. Moore, Jorge Coronel and Patricia Sheen
Laboratorio de Investigacion y Desarrollo, Universidad Peruana Cayetano Heredia, San Martin de Porres, Lima, Peru

David A. J. Moore and Anna Lithgow
TB Centre and Department of Clinical Research, London School of Hygiene and Tropical Medicine, London, UK

Jonathan L. Zelner
Department of Epidemiology, University of Michigan, Ann Arbor, MI 48109, USA

Jason R. Andrews
Department of Medicine, Stanford University, Stanford, CA 94305, USA

Ted Cohen
Department of Epidemiology of Microbial Diseases, Yale University, New Haven, CT 06510, USA

Minah Park, Mark Jit and Joseph T. Wu
WHO Collaborating Centre for Infectious Disease Epidemiology and Control, School of Public Health, Li Ka Shing Faculty of Medicine, The University of Hong Kong, G/F, Patrick Manson Building (North Wing), 7 Sassoon Road, Hong Kong SAR, People's Republic of China

Mark Jit
Department of Infectious Disease Epidemiology, London School of Hygiene and Tropical Medicine, Keppel Street, London WC1E 7HT, UK

Modelling and Economics Unit, Public Health England, 61 Colindale Avenue, London NW9 5EQ, UK

Cecilia Galbete, Janine Kröger, Franziska Jannasch and Matthias B. Schulze
Department of Molecular Epidemiology, German Institute of Human Nutrition Potsdam-Rehbruecke (DIfE), Nuthetal, Germany

Khalid Iqbal, Lukas Schwingshackl, Carolina Schwedhelm and Heiner Boeing
Department of Epidemiology, German Institute of Human Nutrition Potsdam-Rehbruecke, Nuthetal, Germany

Cornelia Weikert
Department of Food Safety, Federal Institute for Risk Assessment, Berlin, Germany

Matthias B. Schulze
University of Potsdam, Institute of Nutritional Sciences, Nuthetal, Germany
German Center for Diabetes Research (DZD), München-Neuherberg, Germany
DZHK (German Centre for Cardiovascular Research), partner site Berlin, Berlin, Germany

Cecilia Galbete, Khalid Iqbal, Lukas Schwingshackl, Carolina Schwedhelm, Cornelia Weikert, Heiner Boeing and Matthias B. Schulze
NutriAct – Competence Cluster Nutrition Research Berlin-Potsdam, Nuthetal, Germany

Samia A. Hurst
Institute for Ethics, History, and the Humanities, Geneva University Medical School, 1211 Genève, Switzerland

Ueli Zellweger and Matthias Bopp
Epidemiology, Biostatistics and Prevention Institute, University of Zurich, Hirschengraben 84, CH-8001 Zürich, Switzerland

Georg Bosshard
Clinic for Geriatric Medicine, Zurich University Hospital, and Center on Aging and Mobility, University of Zurich and City Hospital Waid, Rämistrasse 100, 8091 Zürich, Switzerland

Hawkar Ibrahim, Verena Ertl, Claudia Catani and Frank Neuner
Department of Psychology, Clinical Psychology and Psychotherapy, Bielefeld University, Bielefeld, Germany

Hawkar Ibrahim and Azad Ali Ismail
Department of Clinical Psychology, Koya University, Koya, Kurdistan Region, Iraq

Hawkar Ibrahim, Verena Ertl, Claudia Catani and Frank Neuner
vivo International, Konstanz, Germany

Myriam Alexander, Jolyon Fairburn-Beech, Peter Egger, Stuart Kendrick and Dawn M. Waterworth
GlaxoSmithKline, London, UK

A. Katrina Loomis
Worldwide Research and Development, Pfizer, Connecticut, USA

Johan van der Lei, Peter Rijnbeek and Mees Mosseveld
Erasmus Universitair Medisch Centrum, Rotterdam, The Netherlands

Talita Duarte-Salles
Fundació Institut Universitari per a la Recerca a l'Atenció Primària de Salut Jordi Gol i Gurina, Barcelona, Spain

Daniel Prieto-Alhambra
Centre for Statistics in Medicine, NDORMS, University of Oxford, Oxford, UK

David Ansell
Quintile IMS, London, UK.

Alessandro Pasqua and Francesco Lapi
Health Search, Italian College of General Practitioners and Primary Care, Florence, Italy

Paul Avillach
Harvard Medical School, Harvard, Boston, MA, USA

Naveed Sattar
University of Glasgow, BHF Glasgow Cardiovascular Research Centre, Glasgow, UK

William Alazawi
Barts Liver Centre, Blizard Institute, Queen Mary, University of London, London, UK

Julia Moreira Pescarini and Eliseu Alves Waldman
Faculdade de Saúde Pública, Universidade de São Paulo, São Paulo, Brazil

Vera Simonsen, Lucilaine Ferrazoli and Rosangela S. Oliveira
Instituto Adolfo Lutz, São Paulo, Brazil

Julia Moreira Pescarini and Laura C. Rodrigues
Department of Infectious Disease Epidemiology, Faculty of Epidemiology and Public Health, London School of Hygiene and Tropical Medicine, London, UK

Rein Houben
TB Modelling Group, TB Centre, London School of Hygiene and Tropical Medicine, London, UK

Gwenan M. Knight, Céire Costelloe, Luke S. P. Moore, Susan Hopkins, Alan P. Johnson, Julie V. Robotham and Alison H. Holmes
National Institute of Health Research Health Protection Research Unit in Healthcare Associated Infections and Antimicrobial Resistance, Department of Infectious Diseases, Imperial College London, London W12 0NN, UK

Sarah R. Deeny
Data Analytics, The Health Foundation, London, UK

Luke S. P. Moore and Alison H. Holmes
Imperial College Healthcare NHS Trust, London, UK

Susan Hopkins and Julie V. Robotham
Antimicrobial Resistance Programme, Public Health England, London, UK

Susan Hopkins
Royal Free London NHS Foundation Trust Healthcare, London, UK

Susan Hopkins and Alan P. Johnson
Division of Healthcare-Associated Infection & Antimicrobial Resistance, National Infection Service, Public Health England, London, UK

Julie V. Robotham
Modelling and Economics Unit, National Infection Service, Public Health England and Health Protection Research Unit in Modelling Methodology, London, UK

Po-Wen Ku
Graduate Institute of Sports and Health, National Changhua University of Education, Changhua City, Taiwan

Andrew Steptoe
Department of Behavioural Science and Health, University College London, London, UK

Yung Liao
Department of Health Promotion and Health Education, National Taiwan Normal University, Taipei, Taiwan

Ming-Chun Hsueh
Department of Physical Education, National Taiwan Normal University, NO.162, He-ping East Road, Section 1, Taipei 106, Taiwan

Li-Jung Chen
Department of Exercise Health Science, National Taiwan University of Sport, No. 16, Section 1, Shuang-Shih Rd., Taichung 404, Taiwan

Gillian H. Stresman, Chris Drakeley and Umberto D'Alessandro
Department of Immunology and Infection, London School of Hygiene and Tropical Medicine, London, UK

Julia Mwesigwa, Jane Achan, Archibald Worwui, Musa Jawara and Umberto D'Alessandro
Medical Research Council Unit The Gambia at London School of Hygiene & Tropical Medicine, Fajara, The Gambia

Julia Mwesigwa, Jane Achan, Archibald Worwui, Musa Jawara, Jean-Pierre Van Geertruyden and Umberto D'Alessandro
University of Antwerp, Antwerp, Belgium

Emanuele Giorgi
CHICAS, Lancaster Medical School, Lancaster University, Lancaster, UK

Gian Luca Di Tanna
Queen Mary University of London, London, UK

Teun Bousema
Department of Medical Microbology, Radboud Medical University, Nijmegen, The Netherlands

Kulapong Jayanama, Olga Theou, Leah Cahill and Kenneth Rockwood
Chakri Naruebodindra Medical Institute, Faculty of Medicine Ramathibodi Hospital, Mahidol University, Bangkok, Thailand

Kulapong Jayanama, Olga Theou and Leah Cahill
Department of Medicine, Dalhousie University, Halifax, Nova Scotia, Canada

Olga Theou and Kenneth Rockwood
Centre for Health Care of the Elderly, QEII Health Sciences Centre, Nova Scotia Health Authority, Halifax, Nova Scotia, Canada

Joanna M Blodgett
MRC Unit for Lifelong Health and Ageing, UCL, London, UK

Leah Cahill
Department of Nutrition, Harvard T.H. Chan School of Public Health, Boston, MA, USA

Kenneth Rockwood
Division of Geriatric Medicine, Department of Medicine, Dalhousie University, Camp Hill Veterans' Memorial Bldg., 5955 Veterans' Memorial Lane, Halifax, Nova Scotia B3H 2E1, Canada

Hyun Lee
Division of Pulmonary Medicine and Allergy, Department of Internal Medicine, Hanyang University College of Medicine, Seoul, South Korea

Sun Hye Shin, Gee Young Suh and Hye Yun Park
Division of Pulmonary and Critical Care Medicine, Department of Medicine, Samsung Medical Center, Sungkyunkwan University School of Medicine,Seoul, South Korea

Seonhye Gu, Danbee Kang, Yeong Rae Joi and Juhee Cho
Center for Clinical Epidemiology, Samsung Medical Center, Seoul, South Korea

Danbee Kang, Eliseo Guallar and Juhee Cho
Department of Clinical Research Design and Evaluation, SAIHST, Sungkyunkwan University, Seoul, South Korea

Di Zhao, Eliseo Guallar and Juhee Cho
Department of Epidemiology and Welch Center for Prevention, Epidemiology, and Clinical Research, Johns Hopkins University Bloomberg School of Public Health, Baltimore, MD, USA

Roberto Pastor-Barriuso
National Center for Epidemiology, Instituto de Salud Carlos III, and Consortium for Biomedical Research in Epidemiology and Public Health (CIBERESP), Madrid, Spain

Johan Undén
Department of Operation and Intensive Care, Hallands Hospital, Halmstad, Sweden
Lund University, Lund, Sweden

Stuart R. Dalziel
Emergency Department, Starship Children's Health, 2 Park Rd, Grafton, Auckland 1023, New Zealand
Liggins Institute, University of Auckland, 85 Park Ave, Grafton, Auckland 1023, New Zealand

Meredith L. Borland
Emergency Department, Princess Margaret Hospital for Children, Roberts Rd, Subiaco, Perth, Western Australia 6008, Australia
Divisions of Paediatrics and Emergency Medicine, School of Medicine, University of Western Australia

Sarah Dalton
Emergency Department, The Children's Hospital at Westmead, 212 Hawkesbury Rd, Westmead, New South Wales 2145, Australia

Yuri Gilhotra
Emergency Department, Lady Cilento Children's Hospital, Brisbane and Child Health Research Centre, School of Medicine, The University of Queensland, 501 Stanley St, South Brisbane, Queensland 4101, Australia

Piero Poletti, Stefano Parlamento and Stefano Merler
Center for Information Technology, Fondazione Bruno Kessler, via Sommarive, 18, I-38123 Trento, Italy

Tafarraa Fayyisaa and Rattaa Feyyiss
South West Shoa Zone Health Office, Woliso, Oromia, Ethiopia

Marta Lusiani and Ademe Tsegaye
Doctors with Africa CUAMM, Woliso Hospital, Woliso, Oromia, Ethiopia

Giulia Segafredo, Giovanni Putoto and Fabio Manenti
Doctors with Africa CUAMM, via S. Francesco, 126, I-35121, Padova, Italy

Index